S. Sakuma T. Ishigaki T. Takeuchi

Diagnostic Imaging of the Liver Biliary Tract and Pancreas

Data Analysis and Diagnostic Procedures

With 312 Figures in 932 Separate Illustrations

Springer-Verlag Berlin Heidelberg New York
London Paris Tokyo

Sadayuki Sakuma, M.D.
Professor and Chairman
Department of Radiology
Nagoya University
School of Medicine
65 Tsurumai-Cho, Showa-Ku
Nagoya, Japan

Takeo Ishigaki, M.D.
Associate Professor
Department of Radiology
Nagoya University
School of Medicine
65 Tsurumai-Cho, Showa-Ku
Nagoya, Japan

Toshihiko Takeuchi, M.D.
Professor and Chairman
Department of 1st Internal Medicine
Nagoya City University
Medical School
1 Kawasumi-cho, Showa-Ku
Nagoya, Japan

First published in Japan by Shujunsha Co., Ltd.

ISBN-13: 978-3-642-71309-5 e-ISBN-13: 978-3-642-71307-1
DOI: 10.1007/978-3-642-71307-1

Library of Congress Cataloging in Publication Data

Diagonstic imaging of the liver, biliary tract, and pancreas. Translated from the Japanese orginal. Includes index. 1. Diagnostic imaging. 2. Liver–Diseases–Diagnosis. 3. Biliary tract–Diseases–Diagnosis. 4. Pancreas–Diseases–Diagnosis. I. Sakuma, Sadayuki. II. Ishigaki, Takeo, 1942- . III. Takeuchi, Toshihiko, 1931- . [DNLM: 1. Biliary Tract Diseases–diagnosis. 2. Liver Diseases–diagnosis. 3. Pancreatic Diseases–diagnosis. WI 700 D5346]
RC847.D467 1987 616.3'60757 86-31609

ISBN 0-387-16667-X (U. S.)

Softcover reprint of the hardcover 1st edition 1987

2121/3145-543210

Preface

The development and the widespread clinical application of various diagnostic imaging modalities, such as diagnostic ultrasonography, X-ray computed tomography, single photon emission computed tomography, and magnetic resonance imaging, have been beyond all expectation. In particular, ultrasonography and X-ray computed tomography have become major diagnostic tools for diseases of the liver, the biliary tract, and the pancreas. They often have virtually replaced other conventional imaging modalities including invasive angiography and percutaneous transhepatic cholangiography. One modality may complement or conflict with another or other modalities. Each modality should be carefully selected with due regard for its diagnostic efficacy.

In this book, the first section contains nine chapters dealing with current techniques of each diagnostic modality applicable to the liver, the biliary tract, and the pancreas. The second section deals with diseases of the liver, the biliary tract, and the pancreas and takes the form of case presentation with discussion of the significance of diagnostic imagings and diagnostic procedure.

Preparation of the manuscript was made possible by the help of Dr. S. Fujita, who prepared the photographs, and Mrs. Sobajima, who typed the original manuscript. Dr. S. Miura and Miss Y. Shimizu undertook the labor of translating our manuscript from Japanese into English.

I would like to express my deep appreciation to all these persons, as well as to the contributors to this book, and also to the publishers, Shujunsha, Japan and Springer-Verlag.

Nagoya, January 1987 Sadayuki Sakuma

Table of Contents

Part I General Considerations

A Main Imaging Modalities

1 *Plain Abdominal Radiography* 3
1.1 Positioning and Roentgenographic Conditions 5
1.2 Roentgenographic Findings in the Normal Liver 5
1.3 Abnormal Roentgenographic Findings in the Liver 6
1.4 Abnormal Roentgenographic Findings in the Biliary Tract . . 8
1.5 Abnormal Roentgenographic Findings in the Pancreas . . . 11

2 *Ultrasonography* 13
2.1 Instrumentation 13
2.2 Examination Procedures 14
2.3 Liver 17
2.4 Gallbladder and Bile Duct 25
2.5 Pancreas 33

3 *Nuclear Examination* 42
3.1 Colloid Liver Scintigraphy 42
3.2 Radioisotope Angiography of the Liver 46
3.3 Hepatobiliary Scintigraphy 48

4 *X-ray Computed Tomography* 54
4.1 Equipment 54
4.2 Premedication 54
4.3 Examination Procedures 55
4.4 Contrast Medium Administration 56
4.5 Viewing of the Images 58
4.6 CT Images of the Normal Liver, Biliary Tract, and Pancreas . 58
4.7 CT Images of the Diseased Liver 67
4.8 CT Images of Gallbladder and Biliary Tract Diseases 75
4.9 CT Images of Diseases of the Pancreas 79

5 *Angiography* 87
5.1 Examination Procedures 87
5.2 Hepatic Vasculature and Its Findings 88
5.3 Angiographic Findings in Diseases of the Liver 94
5.4 Vessels of the Biliary Tract and Gallbladder
and Their Angiograms 109
5.5 Angiographic Findings in the Pancreas 115

B Other Imaging Modalities

6 Hypotonic Duodenography 127
6.1 Application 127
6.2 Roentgenographic Anatomy of the Duodenal Loop 128
6.3 Hypotonic Duodenography in Diseases of the Biliary Tract and Pancreas 130

7 Excretory Cholecystocholangiography 134
7.1 Oral Cholecystography 134
7.2 Intravenous Cholangiography 135
7.3 Examination Procedures 137
7.4 Side Effects 137
7.5 Roentgenographic Findings 138

8 Endoscopic Retrograde Cholangiopancreatography (ERCP) . 143
8.1 Examination Procedures 143
8.2 Findings from Opacification of the Pancreas 144
8.3 Findings from Opacification of the Bile Duct 147

9 Percutaneous Transhepatic Cholangiography (PTC) 149
9.1 Opacification Procedure 149
9.2 Roentgenographic Anatomy of the Biliary Tract 149
9.3 PTC Images of Diseases of the Pancreas and Biliary Tract . . 151

Part II Clinical Presentation

Introductory Remarks 156

A Diagnostic Imaging in Diseases of the Liver

1 Procedure 157

2 Cases 161
2.1 Liver Cyst 161
2.2 Parenchymal Hamartoma 165
2.3 Chronic Active Hepatitis (Lupoid Hepatitis) 169
2.4 Liver Cirrhosis 173
2.5 Liver Cirrhosis 177
2.6 Fatty Liver 183
2.7 Hemochromatosis 189
2.8 Liver Abscess 193
2.9 Hemangioma of the Liver 199
2.10 Hepatoblastoma 203
2.11 Hepatocellular Carcinoma 209
2.12 Hepatocellular Carcinoma 215
2.13 Cholangiocarcinoma 221
2.14 Liver Metastasis (Carcinoma of the Rectum) 227
2.15 Hepatic Injury 233

B Diagnostic Imaging of Diseases of the Biliary Tract

1 *Procedure* . . . 239

2 *Cases* . . . 245
2.1 Hepatolithiasis and Choledocholithiasis . . . 245
2.2 Congenital Dilatation of the Bile Duct . . . 251
2.3 Primary Sclerosing Cholangitis . . . 259
2.4 Carcinoma of the Gallbladder . . . 267
2.5 Carcinoma of the Common Bile Duct . . . 273
2.6 Carcinoma of the Common Hepatic Duct . . . 279

C Diagnostic Imaging of Diseases of the Pancreas

1 *Procedure* . . . 287

2 *Cases* . . . 289
2.1 Acute Pancreatitis . . . 289
2.2 Chronic Pancreatitis . . . 293
2.3 Chronic Pancreatitis (Pancreatolithiasis, Pseudocyst of the Pancreas . . . 299
2.4 Cyst of the Pancreas (Pseudocyst) . . . 303
2.5 Carcinoma of the Pancreas (Body and Tail) . . . 309
2.6 Carcinoma of the Pancreas (Head) . . . 315
2.7 Cystadenocarcinoma of the Pancreas . . . 321
2.8 Insulinoma of the Pancreas . . . 325
2.9 Nonfunctioning Islet Cell Tumor . . . 329

Appendix, Methods of Measurement and Normal Values for Laboratory Data . . . 337

Subject Index . . . 339

Contributors

Ishigaki, Takeo, M.D., Associate Professor
Department of Radiology
Nagoya University, School of Medicine

Ishiguchi, Tsuneo, M.D.,
Department of Radiology
Nagoya University, School of Medicine

Ito, Makoto, M.D., Associate Professor
Department of 1st Internal Medicine
Nagoya City University

Matsuyama, Koji, M.D., Chief
Department of 3rd Pediatrics
1st Nagoya Red Cross Hospital

Miyaji, Makoto, M.D., Associate Professor
Division of Medical Information
Nagoya City University Hospital

Sakuma, Sadayuki, M.D., Professor, Chairman
Department of Radiology
Nagoya University, School of Medicine

Takeuchi, Toshihiko, M.D., Professor, Chairman
Department of 1st Internal Medicine
Nagoya City University

Part I
General Considerations

A: Main Imaging Modalities

1 Plain Abdominal Radiography

Presumptive diagnosis of diseases of the liver, gallbladder, biliary tract, and pancreas can often be made from plain abdominal radiograms alone. The outline of the liver can be estimated even in normal cases from the surrounding fat pad which forms its contour, the gas in the intestine, and the relationship with the diaphragm.

The gallbladder and pancreas, however, cannot normally be observed on the plain abdominal radiogram. They may be visible on plain abdominal radiograms if abnormal images of calcification and gas are visualized due to disease.

In general, fine radiograms cannot be obtained because a great deal of X-ray absorption and scatter occur in the upper abdomen including the liver due to its thickness. For this reason, diagnosis by plain abdominal radiography is often not treated seriously.

Figure 1.1 shows the distribution of abdominal thickness among different age groups of Japanese, and Fig. 1.2 indicates the relationship between the distance from the center of the X-ray beam and the doses at the depth of 10 cm from the phantom surface, using tube voltage as a parameter. The field size is 30 × 30 cm. This figure shows the curves for disturbances due to scattering of X-rays in plain X-ray diagnosis of the abdominal organs. Image quality, however, could be improved to some degree by highly effective radiography [10] and computed radiography with an imaging plate [17] (Fig. 1.3).

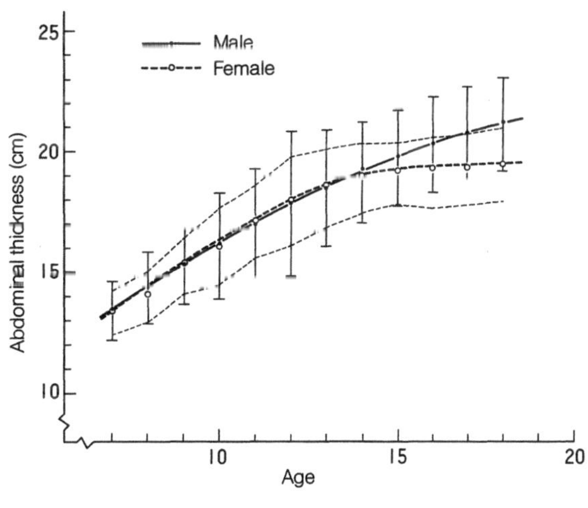

Fig. 1.1. Relationship between abdominal thickness and age

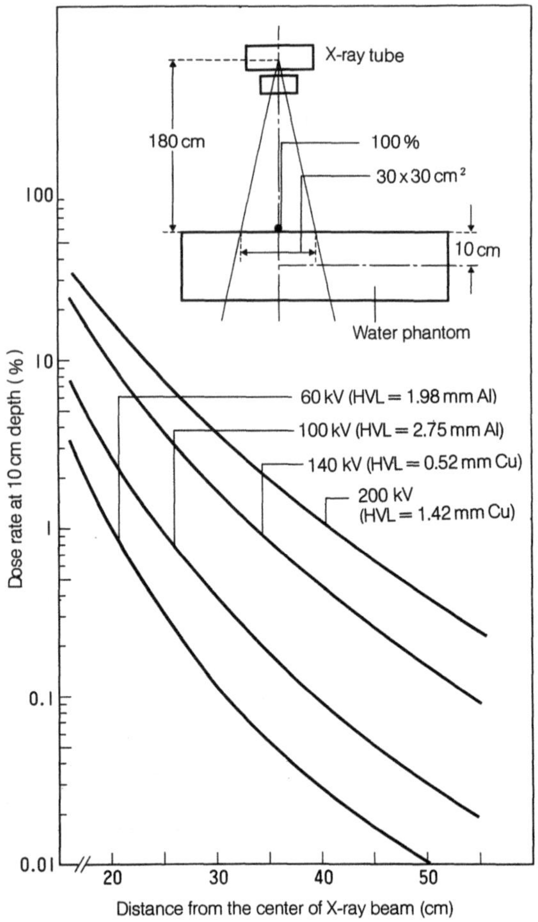

Fig. 1.2. Changes in X-ray dose distribution at 10 cm depth due to differences in X-ray tube voltage in a radiation field of 30 × 30 cm

Fig. 1.3 A, B. Cholecystolithiasis with a calcified stone in the right upper abdomen. Exposure obtained with computed radiography using an imaging plate.
A Contrast enhancement and spatial frequency enhancement are similar to conventional radiography.
B Spatial enhancement peaks in the vicinity of 0.38 lp/mm frequency

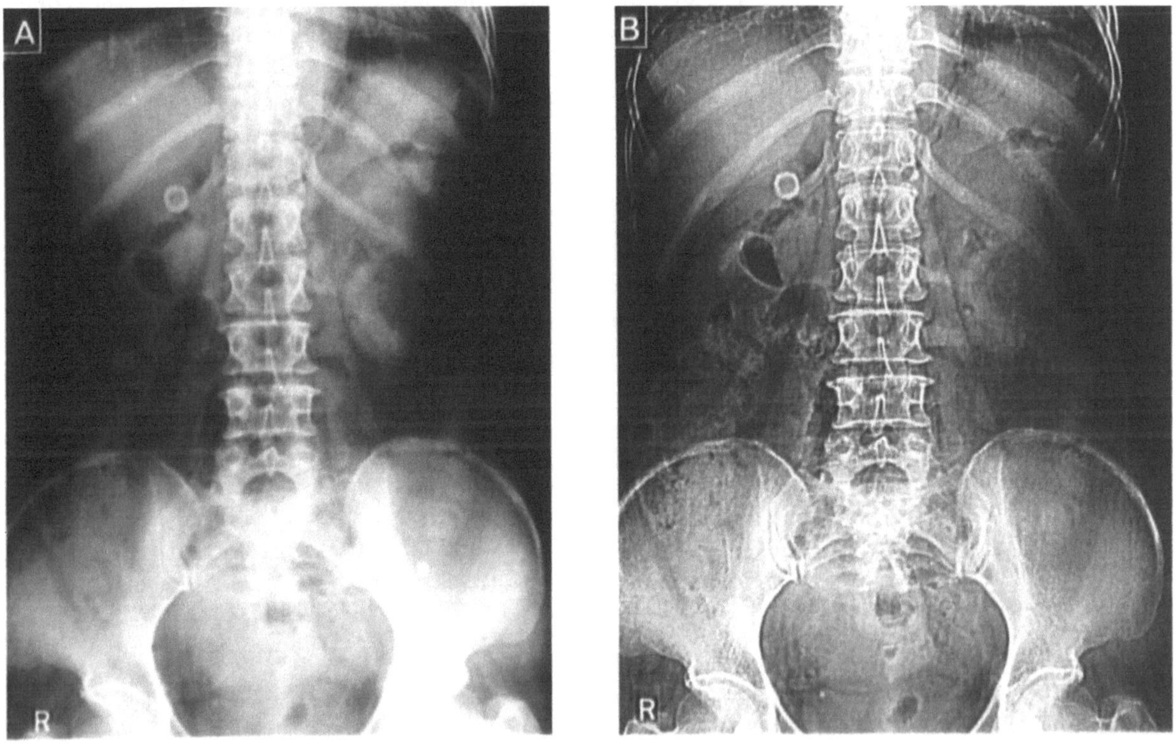

1.1 Positioning and Roentgenographic Conditions

Generally, the anteroposterior projection is radiographed in the supine position. The lower edge of the liver, however, is demonstrated more clearly in the posteroanterior projection in the prone position. For observation of intestinal gas or air-fluid levels, frontal views in upright or recumbent positions may be needed.

To perceive the spatial relationships in abnormal findings such as calcification or gas in organs, lateral views are required. A right anteroposterior projection image is necessary to obtain the liver volume from a plain abdominal radiogram [22]. On a 35.4×43.0 cm film, the radiogram should cover an area framed by the domes of the diaphragm, the pubic symphysis, and the flank.

1.2 Roentgenographic Findings in the Normal Liver

A normal liver on the plain abdominal radiogram appears as an image of homogeneous soft tissue density from the right upper abdomen to the medial region. The lower edge is distinctly visualized with the aid of a fat pad; thus, it is particularly clearly observed in obese patients (Fig. 1.4). This radiographic image of the lower edge of the liver does not necessarily represent the anatomical lower edge of the liver [24, 25]. It may depend on the shape of the liver, body type, and the angle of the X-ray beam. Nevertheless, the radiographic image of the lower border of the liver is straight or slightly concave. The lower edge may become convex if a large space-occupying lesion is present in the liver.

The presence of gas in the hepatic flexure of the colon or the transverse colon makes the lower edge of the liver more clearly visible. In normal cases, the lower edge of the left hepatic lobe is usually indistinct.

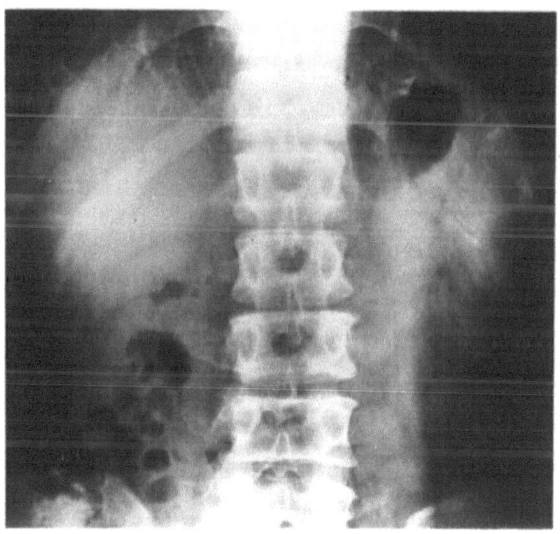

Fig. 1.4. Plain radiogram of normal upper abdomen (prone position)

1.3 Abnormal Roentgenographic Findings in the Liver

1.3.1 Size and Density. In the case of a massive hepatomegaly the liver itself displays a high soft tissue density. Even if no major change is seen in the film density the enlargement of the liver can be inferred. In other words, an enlargement of the right lobe results in an elevation of the right dome of the diaphragm and restricts respiratory movement. A downward displacement of the hepatic flexure, displacement of the stomach to the left, and inferior displacement of the right kidney are also observed (Fig. 1.5).

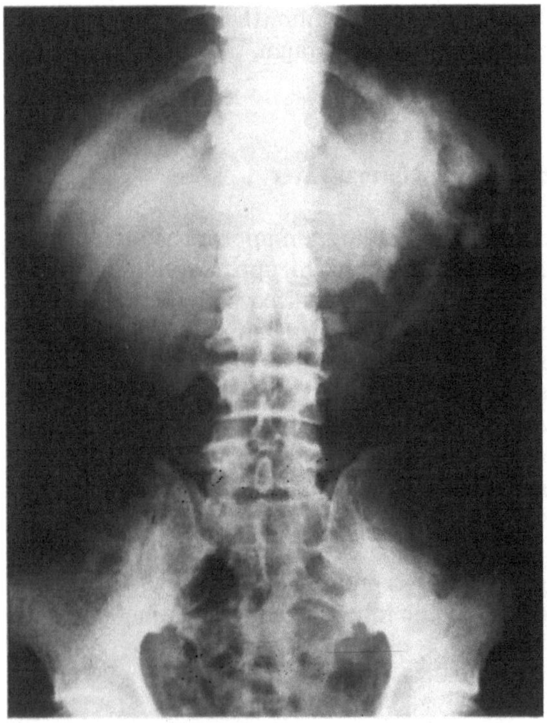

Fig. 1.5. Hepatocellular carcinoma (downward displacement of the hepatic flexure due to right lobe swelling)

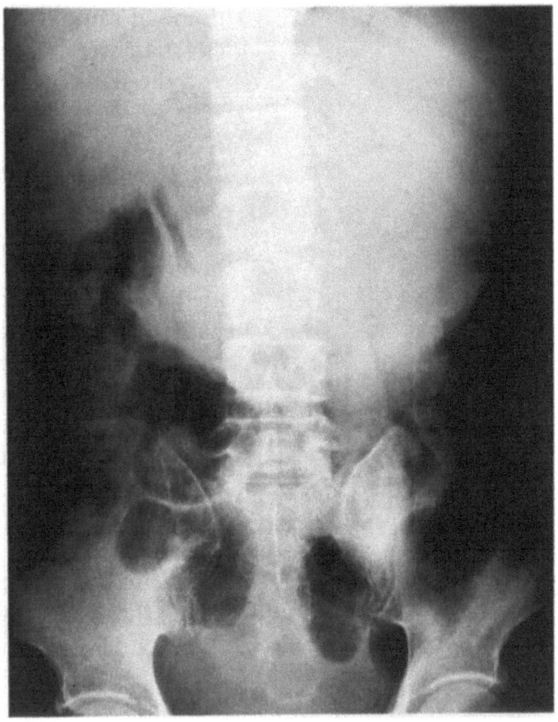

Fig. 1.6. Hepatocellular carcinoma (downward displacement of bowel gas due to massive tumor in the left lobe)

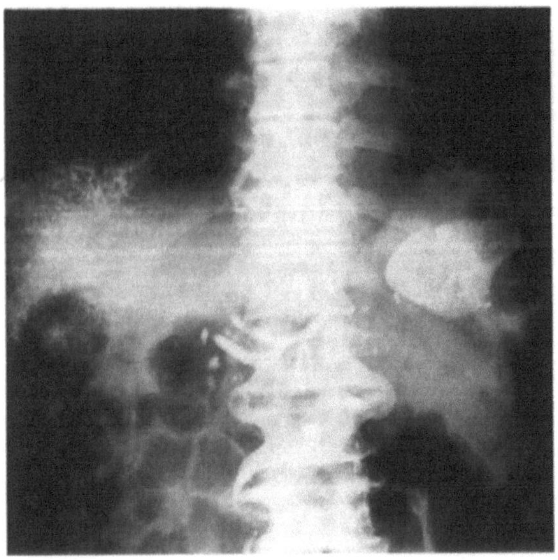

Fig. 1.7. Thorotrast deposits in the liver, spleen, and lymph nodes

Enlargement of the left lobe causes elevation of the left dome of the diaphragm and downward displacement of the splenic flexure of the colon (Fig. 1.6).

Occasionally, the gastric fundus and the diaphragm are observed separately. Besides enlargement of the liver, high density of the liver on the plain film may occasionally also be seen. Thorotrast deposits in the liver are an example (Fig. 1.7).

Sometimes, there may be a decrease in density of the liver on the plain film. Fatty liver and liver abscesses are examples of this [6, 19, 27].

If image quality is improved, using highly effective radiography (see p. 193, "liver abscess") or computed radiography (Fig. 1.3), decreased density of the liver is observed more clearly.

1.3.2 Calcification. In addition to calcification in the parenchyma, calcifications in the gallbladder, biliary tract, portal vein, hepatic artery, subphrenic area, the base of the right lung, right adrenal gland, lymph nodes in the porta hepatis, and abdominal wall are easily observed in a frontal view of plain film [8, 11].

Generally, calcification in the liver indicates existence of some lesions. Hydatid disease of the liver is a typical example of this [21] (Fig. 1.8). With *Echinococcus granulosis*, curvilinear calcification often appears along the wall of the hydatid cyst, and often the entire cyst may be calcified. Occasionally, daughter cysts within the mother cyst calcify the wall and show eggshell calcification smaller than 1.5 cm. Ring calcifications gathering at 2–4 mm radius with a radiolucent may be observed with *Echinococcus multilocularis*.

As for the nonparasitic cyst, the walls calcify occasionally and may be observed in a liver abscess, histoplasmosis, brucellosis, and gumma [1, 21].

Tuberculosis can be suspected from calcification in both the liver and the psoas muscle. However, calcification in liver tumors is very rare. Vascular calcification may be seen in the liver.

In the case of arterial sclerosis, aneurysm, and arterial thrombosis, clacification in the hepatic artery will be observed presenting various patterns such as parallel curvilinear lines, round, or oval. Calcification of portal vein thrombus is sometimes observed. Most of the calcification of the lymph nodes in the porta hepatis is usually caused by tuberculosis.

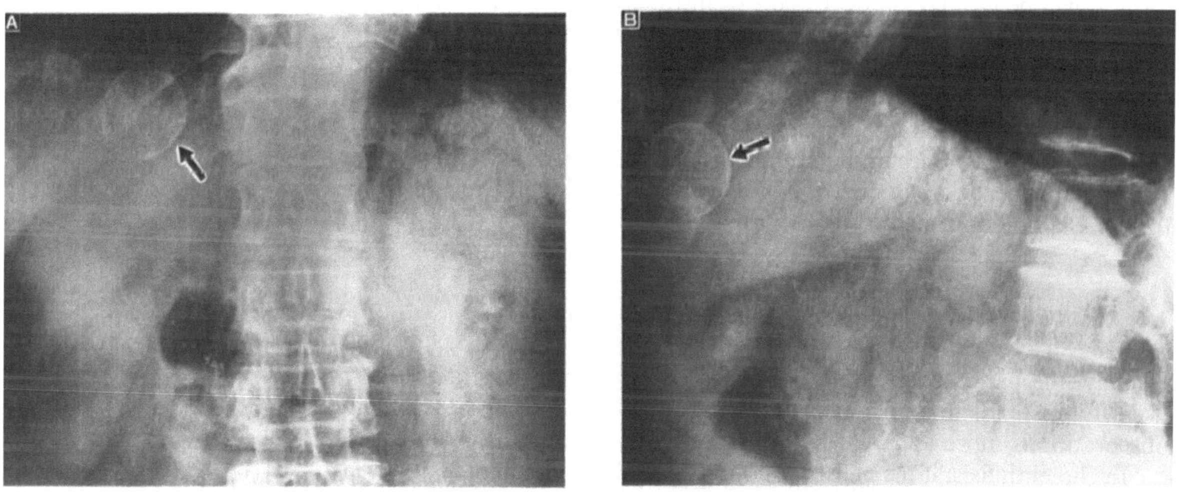

Fig. 1.8 A, B. Hydatid disease. Spherical calcification in the superior anterior segment of the right lobe (→). **A** frontal view; **B** lateral view. Same case as shown in Fig. 5.16

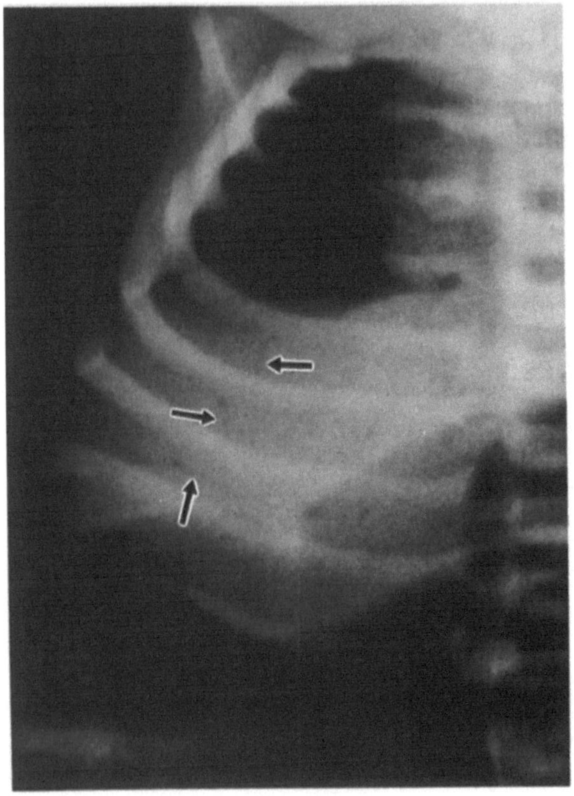

Fig. 1.9. Gas in the portal vein (necrotizing enteritis); branch-formed gas image (→)

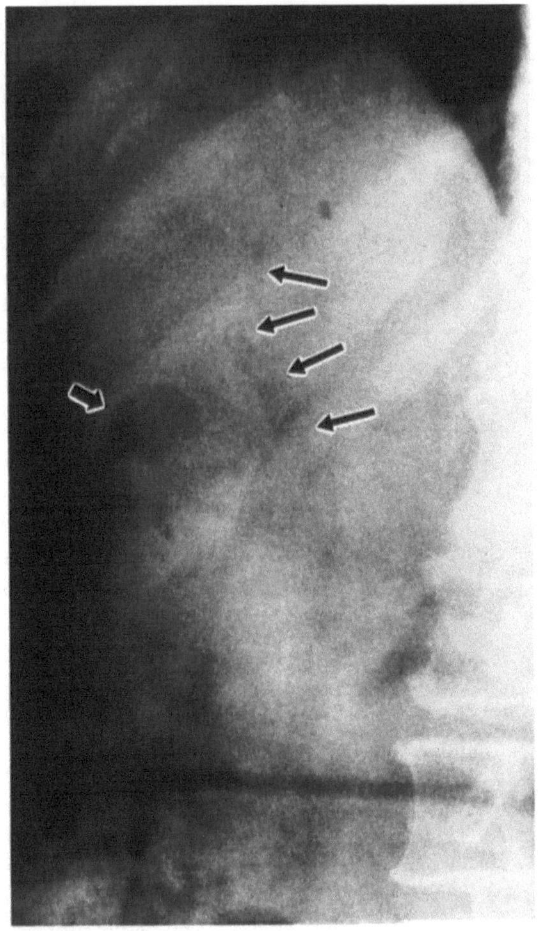

Fig. 1.10. Gas in the biliary tract: →, in the intra- and extrahepatic bile ducts; →, in the gallbladder

1.3.3 Gas in the Liver. Gas in the liver parenchyma is observed in penetrating injuries, liver abscess, and gas gangrene of the liver. An air-fluid level may be shown in liver abscesses. If gas in the liver is observed in a branch form, it will be gas in the portal veins or intrahepatic bile duct. Gas in the portal vein is seen in the case of necrotizing enteritis [5, 26] (Fig. 1.9).

Gas in the intrahepatic bile duct is seen in the case of incompetence of Oddi's sphincter, internal fistula between the gastroinestinal tract and the bile duct, and biliary tract infections (Fig. 1.10).

The major difference in the findings of the gas image in the portal vein and the intrahepatic bile duct is observed at the peripheral region in the former example but more proximal area in the latter case.

1.4 Abnormal Roentgenographic Findings in the Biliary Tract

Usually, the gallbladder cannot be observed on plain radiograms. However, if it distends to a certain extent, a part of its outline can be seen, and observation is more apparent by radiography in the upright position.

In cholelithiasis, if the gallstone contains calcium bilirubinate, it is visible on a plain abdominal radiogram (Figs. 1.11 and 1.3), although it only occurs in about 15% of all patients with cholelithiasis. In about 90% of

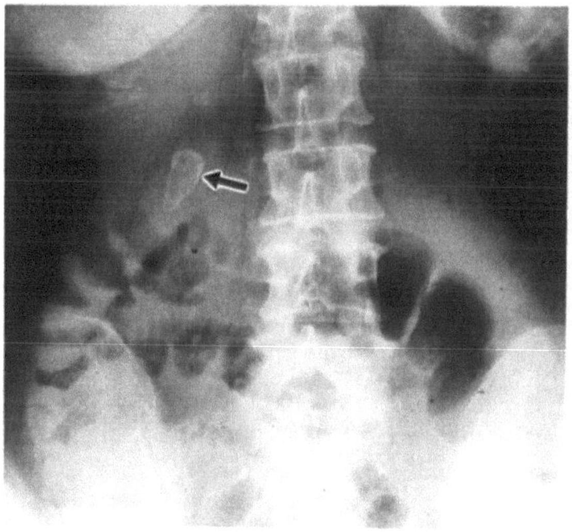

Fig. 1.11. Cholecystolithiasis with a calcified stone in the right upper abdomen (→)

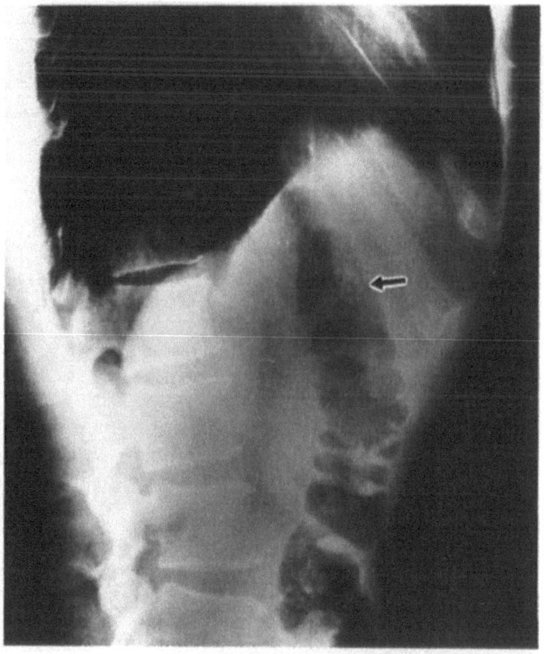

Fig. 1.12. Hepatolithiasis (→)

these cases, stones exist in the gallbladder, but a calcified stone is rarely observed in the common bile duct or intrahepatic bile duct (Fig. 1.12). Two-directional views are necessary to differentiate gallstones from a right kigney stone.

On plain abdominal radiograms, a calcification which conforms to the shape of a gallbladder is observed occasionally in the cases of large calcified gallstones, limy bile (milk of calcium bile), and porcelain gallbladder (calcified gallbladder) [2]. Limy bile is an accumulation of the bile-dense calcium carbonate in the gallbladder caused by the obstruction of the cystic duct by a gallstone. Thus, its form presents in the same way as a normally opacified gallbladder following oral cholecystography. In this case, however, the shape of the gallbladder changes according to the patient's position, so differentiation from cholelithiasis is possible (Figs. 1.13 and 1.14).

Calcification of the wall of the gallbladder is called porcelain gallbladder or calcified gallbladder [13], and it is supposed to occur secondary to cholecystitis (Fig. 1.15). However, some authors believe that it occurs due to intramural hemorrhage or an imbalance of calcium metabolism. Such calcification occurs widely in the muscular layer or in multiple punctate form in the glandular spaces of the mucosa. It occurs frequently in females patients; the male-to-female ratio is 1:5. It combines gallstones, obstructing the cystic duct, and the gallbladder becomes hydropic. In this case, carcinoma of the gallbladder occurs at a high rate. Calcification in the gallbladder is rarely seen in carcinoma of the gallbladder. Calcification sometimes occurs in the common bile duct such as calcified calculi, limy bile, and calcified carcinoma of the bile duct. Calcification of the bile duct is observed as a linear shadow, and it is similar to the calcified vascular wall. Gas in the gallbladder can be observed on plain abdominal radiograms (Fig. 1.10). It is caused by imcompetence of Oddi's sphincter, an internal fistula between the gastrointestinal tract and the intrahepatic bile duct, and infection by gas-producing organisms. In emphysematous cholecystitis, gas sometimes occurs in the wall of the gallbladder.

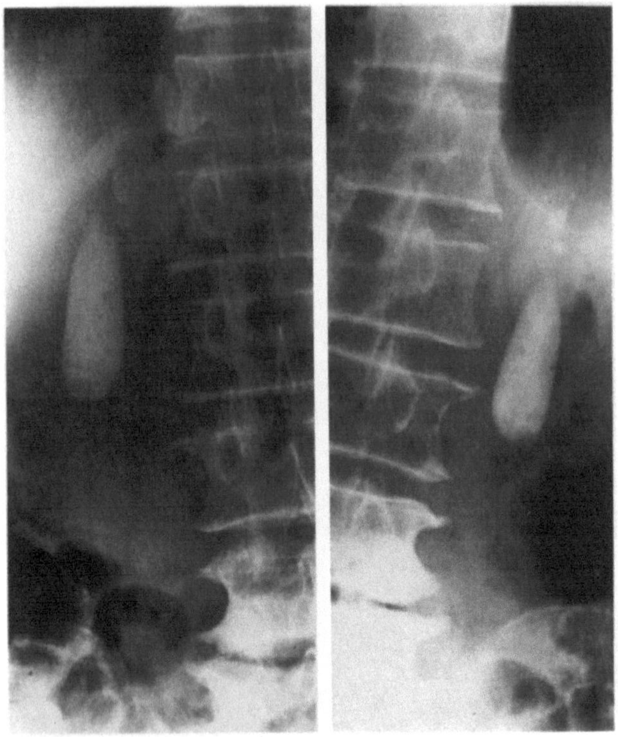

Fig. 1.13. Limy bile. Highly dense gallbladder with multiple tiny stones can be seen without contrast medium

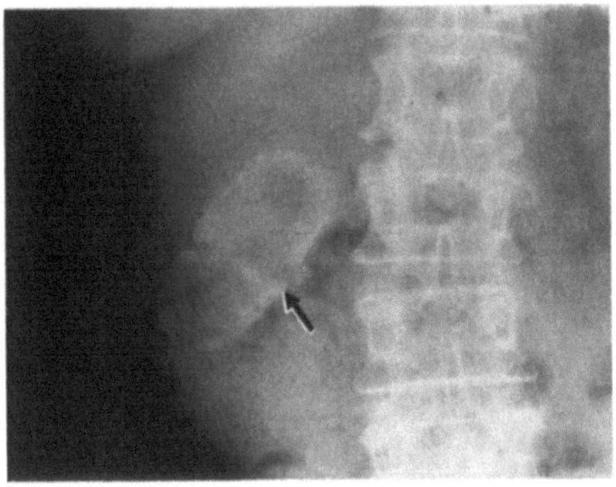

Fig. 1.15. Calcified gallbladder (→)

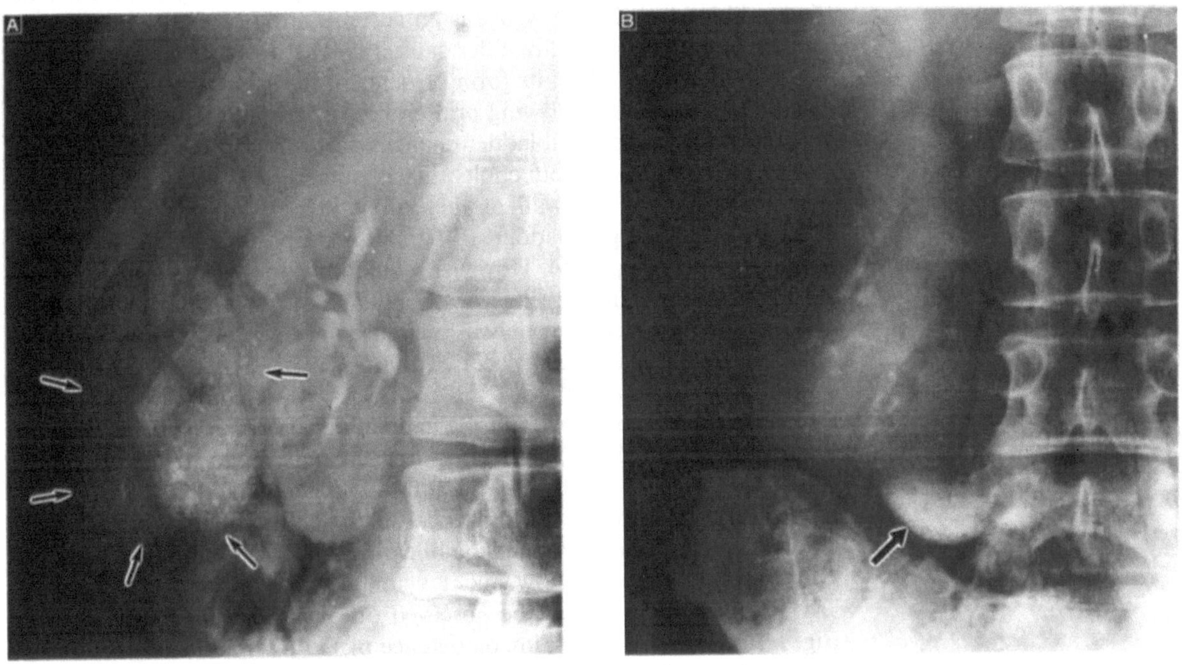

Fig. 1.14 A, B. Limy bile (diagnosed accidentally during pyelography). A Left anterior oblique supine position showing multiple tiny stones in the low-density opacified gallbladder without contrast medium (→). B Erect position with fluid level formation. Same case as in Figs. 2.27 and 4.32

1.5 Abnormal Roentgenographic Findings in the Pancreas

Usually, the pancreas cannot be observed on plain abdominal radiograms. However, if there is a swelling in the pancreas, the swollen tail of the pancreas is sometimes observed lying over the stomach bubble in the erect position.

In acute pancreatitis, the intestine causes localized paralytic ileus due to extension of the inflammatory process [12], and the gas-filled dilated intestine can be observed. This is called the sentinel-loop sign [4,18]. This finding is not peculiar to acute pancreatitis and also occurs in acute cholecystitis [7, 23].

Some authors mention the "colon cut-off" sign [15, 16, 20], which is peculiar to acute pancreatitis, rather than the sentinel-loop sign [3]. Some believe that by the extension of the transverse colon with gas from the ascending colon, gas suddenly disappears in the splenic flexure of the colon or midtransverse colon.

Abscess formation is observed in 3%–4% of all pancreatitis cases. In such cases, multiple small gas bubbles are observed in the pancreas. However, in these cases, differentiation from emphysematous gastritis, subphrenic abscesses, and pneumatosis cystoides intestinalis is required.

Calcification of the pancreas is observed on plain abdominal films. It is usually observed in chronic pancreatitis, and sometimes multiple small calcifications may be seen on the whole pancreas.

Calcification of pancreatic parenchyma is often observed when there is an intrapancreatic hemorrhage due to trauma and infarction. Calcification is observed in 12%–20% of pseudocysts of the pancreas; calcification surrounding the pseudocysts is sometimes observed. Pancreatic carcinoma is supposed to occur at a high rate in those who have calcification in the pancreas. Calcification is observed in 10% of cystadenoma or cystadenocarcinoma [14]. Calcification is not observed in adenocarcinoma [9].

References

Plain Radiography

1. Alergant CD (1956) Gumma of the liver with calcification. Arch Intern Med 98:340–343
2. Berk RN, Clemett AR (1977) Radiology of the galbladder and bile ducts. Saunders, Philadelphia
3. Braacho DJ, Reynolds TN, Zanca P (1962) The radiographic "Colon cut-off sign" in acute pancreatitis. Radiology 79:763–768
4. Eaton SB Jr, Ferrucci JT Jr (1973) Radiology of the pancreas and duodenum. Saunders, Philadelphia
5. Gold RP, Seaman WB (1977) Splenic flexure carcinoma as a source of hepatic portal venous gas. Radiology 122:329–330
6. Griscom NT, Capitanio MA, Wagoner ML, Culham G, Morris L (1975) The visibly fatty liver. Radiology 117:385–389
7. Grollman AI, Goodman S, Fine A (1950) Localized paralytic ileus. An early roentgen sign in acute pancreatitis. Surg Gynecol Obstet 91:65–70
8. Haddow RA, Kemp-Harper, RA (1967) Calcification in the liver and portal system. Clin Radiol 18:225–236
9. Imhof H, Frank P (1977) Pancreatic calcifications in malignant islet cell tumors. Radiology 122:333–337

10. Ishikawa T, Ishigaki T, Araki K, Sakuma S, Kato H, Takano M, Shinomiya K (1981) High effective radiography and its computer-processed image (in Japanese). J Med Imagings 1:70–74
11. McAfee, JG, Donner MW (1962) Differential diagnosis of calcifications encountered in abdominal radiographs. Am J Med Sci 243:609–650
12. Meyers MA, Evans JA (1973) Effects of pancreatitis on the small bowel and colon: spread along mesenteric planes. Am J Roentgenol 119:151–165
13. Ochsner, SF, Carrera GM (1963) Calcification of the gallbladder (porcelain gallbladder). Am J Roentgenol 89:847–853
14. Piper CE, ReMine WH, Priestley JR (1962) Pancreatic cystadenomata: report of 20 cases. JAMA 180:648–652
15. Price CWR (1956) The colon cut-off sign of pancreatitis. Med J Aust 1:313–314
16. Rosch J (1967) Roentgenologic diagnosis of pancreatic disease. Am J Roentgenol 100:664–672
17. Sonoda M, Takano M, Miyahara J, Kato H (1983) Computed radiography utilizing scanning laser simulated luminescence. Radiology 148:833–838
18. Stein GN, Kalser MH, Sarian NN, Finkelstein A (1959) an evaluation of the roentgen changes in acute pancreatitis: correlation with clinical findings. Gastroenterology 36:354–361
19. Steinbach HL, Crane JT, Bruyn HB (1954) The roentgen demonstration of cirrhosis of the liver with fatty metamorphosis. Radiology 62:858–861
20. Stuart C (1956) Acute pancreatitis: new radiodiagnostic sign. J Fac Radiol 8:50–58
21. Thompson WM, Chisholm D P, Tank R (1972) Plain film roentgenographic findings in alveolar hydatid disease. Am J Roentgenol 116:345–358
22. Walk L (1961) Roentgenologic determination of the liver volume. Acta Radiol 55:49–56
23. Weens HS, Walker LA (1964) The radiologic diagnosis of acute cholecystitis and pancreatitis. Radiol Clin North Am 2:89–106
24. Whalen JP, Berne AS, Riemenschneider, PA (1969) The extraperitoneal perivisceral fat pad. I. Its role in roentgenologic visualization of abdominal organs. Radiology 92:466–472
25. Whalen JP, Berne AS (1969) The extraperitoneal pervisceral fat pad. II. Roentgen interpretation of pathological alterations. Radiology 92:473–480
26. Wolfe, JN, Evans WA (1955) Gas in the portal veins of the liver in infants. A roentgenographic demonstration with postmortem anatomical correlation. Am J Roentgenol 74:486–489
27. Yousefzadeh DK, Lupetin AR, Jackson, JH (1979) The radiographic signs of fatty liver. Radiology 131:351–355

2 Ultrasonography

Ultrasonography has been deemed to be of high diagnostic value for morphological diagnosis of the liver, biliary tract, and pancreas. Continued technical developments and diversification of its uses have both markedly contributed to this rise in its status.

This presumably is due to the following points:

1. It is noninvasive and painless for patients.
2. No special preparation is needed, and the examination is easy even for outpatients.
3. No hazards, such as from radiation, are observed in the low-power levels used for diagnostic ultrasonography.
4. Image quality has been vastly improved by new developments in equipment.

Highly professional medical understanding is necessary to operate the ultrasonic apparatus because ultrasonic images adequate for diagnosis are a consequence of well-trained and skillful handling.

2.1 Instrumentation

The B-mode, in which an image is obtained according to the strength of the echo, is the one mostly used in the ultrasonic diagnosis of conditions affecting the upper abdominal organs. There are two methods of creating an ultrasonic image, contact scanning and real-time scanning. In contact scanning, the transducer is moved by hand across the patient's skin according to a given plane. In real-time scanning, the ultrasonic beam is moved automatically by mechanical or electronic methods so that the image is both continuous and dynamic. Formerly, a real-time scanning image was inferior to that of contact scanning. It has been greatly improved, and the same quality of the image as in contact scanning can be obtained today. However, in real-time scanning the observable range is limited, and it is preferable to use both methods together in diagnosis.

In the upper abdomen, because a view of the deep organs is required, it is impossible to use a high frequency of great attenuation. Usually, 2.25–5 MHz is used for examination of the upper abdomen.

Ultrasound waves make higher resolutions as the frequency becomes higher. On the other hand, attenuation becomes greater as the frequency becomes higher. Thus, it is necessary to consider all these points when the frequency is decided. In choosing a transducer, care must be taken with the various levels of focus length (Fig. 2.1).

The Doppler effect is used to measure the blood flow. Recently, a pulsed Doppler unit in which it is possible to measure a certain deep blood flow selctively has been developed.

We have recently employed a combination of an electronic sector scanning probe and a pulse Doppler probe. Blood flow measurement by the pulse Doppler method can be performed precisely by guidance from the sector scanning image. With this method it has become possible to determine blood flow and velocity at an arbitrary point of a blood vessel. Furthermore, blood flow throughout or in segmental portions of the liver can be measured noninvasively. Figure 2.2 shows the principles of our method and blood velocity distribution in the portal vein.

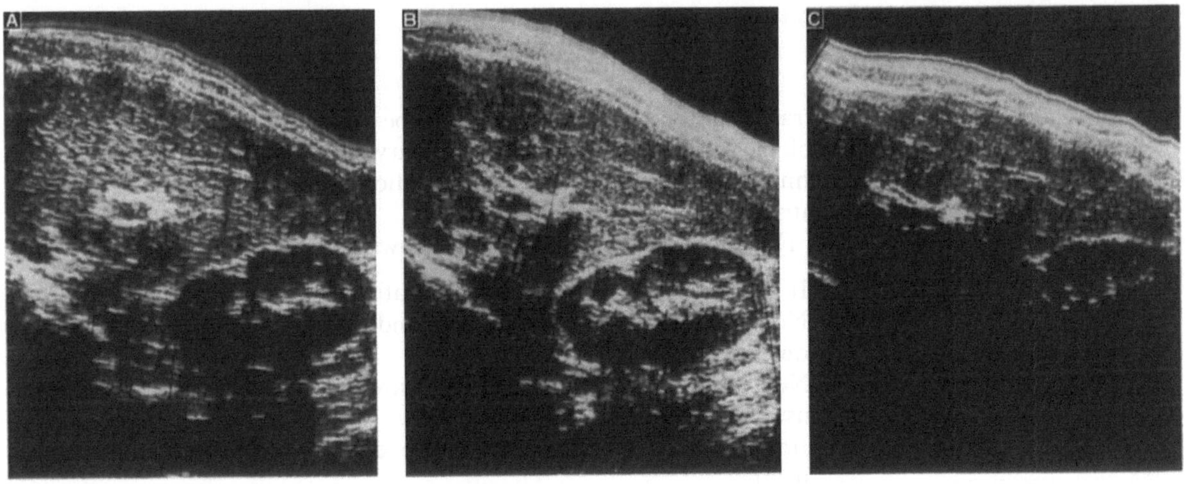

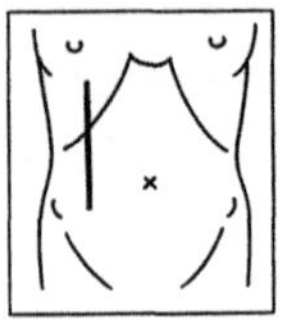

Fig. 2.1 A–C. Relationship of image quality to ultrasonic frequency. The quality of the ultrasonic image improves as ultrasonic frequency increases, although detail in deeper portions becomes less clear. **A** 2.25 MHz; **B** 3.5 MHz; **C** 5 MHz

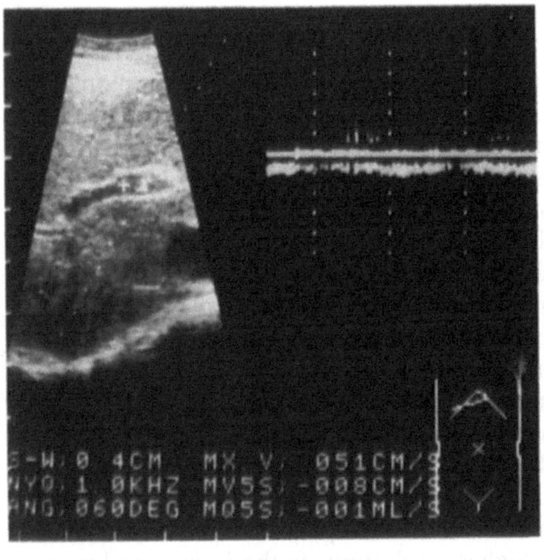

Fig. 2.2. Blood velocity pattern in the portal vein of the liver

2.2 Examination Procedures

In the ultrasonic examination of the gallbladder and pancreas, if gas exists in the intestinal tract, acoustic velocity is relatively low in air, so that these images are not observable. The patient must fast for a minimum of 8 h prior to the examination. An absorbent and carminative must be taken 2 or 3 days before the examination.

During the examination, the patient is usually in the supine position. Using the real-time ultrasonic scanner, the probe is flexible in its location and is moved according to need. However, the contact compound scanner has some limitations as an arbitrary cross-sectional image. Therefore, the patient's position is altered to some degree according to the examination.

While scanning the upper portion of the right hepatic lobe, it may be necessary to project the ultrasonic beam from the right intercostal space.

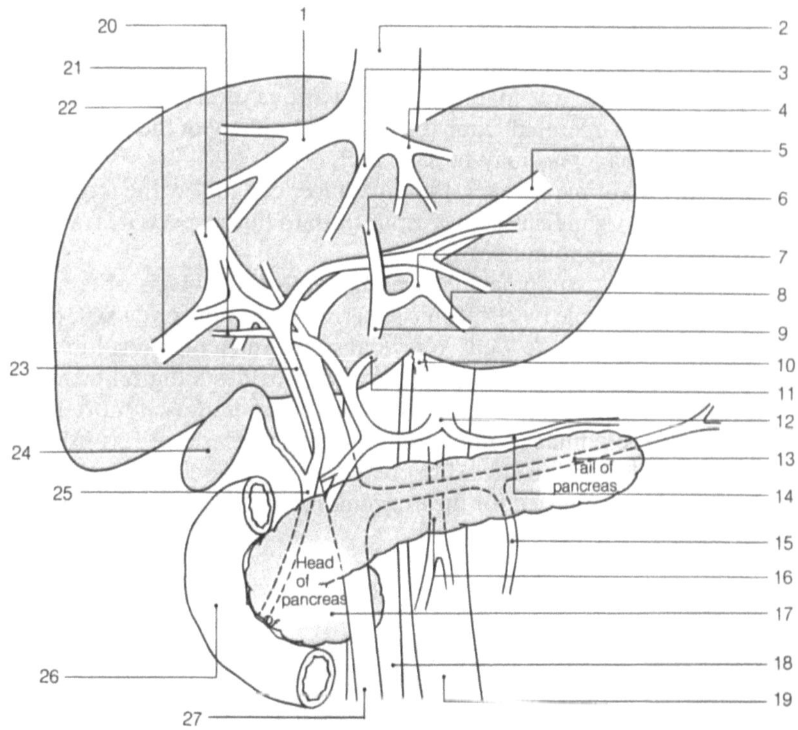

Fig. 2.3. Schema for ultrasonic diagnosis of the liver, biliary tract, and pancreas. 1) Right hepatic vein 2) Inferior vena cava 3) Middle hepatic vein 4) Left Hepatic vein 5) Superior branch of left portal vein to the lateral segment of the left lobe 6) Superior branch of left portal vein to the medial segment of the left lobe 7) Umbilical portion 8) Inferior branch of left portal vein to the lateral segment of the left lobe 9) Inferior branch of left portal vein to the medial segment of the left lobe 10) Ligamentum teres 11) Left hepatic artery 12) Celiac artery 13) Splenic vein 14) Splenic artery 15) Inferior mesenteric vein 16) Superior mesenteric artery 17) Uncinate process of the pancreas 18) Inferior vena cava 19) Aorta 20) Right hepatic artery 21) Posterior branch of right portal vein 22) Anterior branch of right portal vein 23) Common hepatic duct 24) Gallbladder 25) Common bile duct 26) Duodenum 27) Superior mesenteric vein

The left lateral decubitus position is suitable for this projection.

To examine the common bile duct, elevation of the right side, which is the right anterior oblique position, is suitable [5]. In this situation, an image of the common bile duct and portal vein may be visualized simultaneously.

Obtaining the ultrasonic image of the pancreas requires much skill. To obtain the entire image of the pancreas in the supine position, obstruction by gas in the stomach and intestinal tract must be nonexistent, although usually obstruction by gas exists. The tail of the pancreas is especially apt to be obscured by intestinal gas. In such a case, the gas must be moved by putting the patient in the sitting position or in the right or left lateral decubitus position. Having the patient drink an adequate quantity of degassed water and projecting the ultrasonic beam from above the stomach, forming an acoustic window, is also a good solution.

By changing the patient's position, the water in the stomach is made to shift, and consequently any part of the pancreas can be clearly shown. While contact scanning, be careful to have the patient stop respiration at the inspiratory phase, to stop the movement of the abdominal organs caused by respiration.

On real-time scanning, it is not always necessary to stop respiration. The entire image of the pancreas can be obtained quite easily by pressing the ultrasonic probe firmly against the abdominal wall in order to move the bowel gas. However, the tail of the pancreas may not be clearly observable even if the transducer is manipulated in various directions. In this case, if the transducer is operated from above the left kidney in the prone position, the tail of the pancreas may be seen [30].

With the real-time scanner, the transducer can follow the movements of the abdominal organs caused by respiration. In this respect, it is far superior to the contact compound scanner.

Recently, new equipment has been developed, which obtains a long focal beam as a whole by electronic superimpositioning and exchanging the ultrasonic beam with the focus in several steps, and a high resolution power has been obtained. Also, equipment which provides a digital memory and then freezes the ultrasonic image voluntarily is being used more frequently, and thus the contact compound scanner is becoming less used today. Figure 2.3 shows the relationships between the blood vessels and organs, which must be recognized for the examination of the liver, biliary tract, and pancreas.

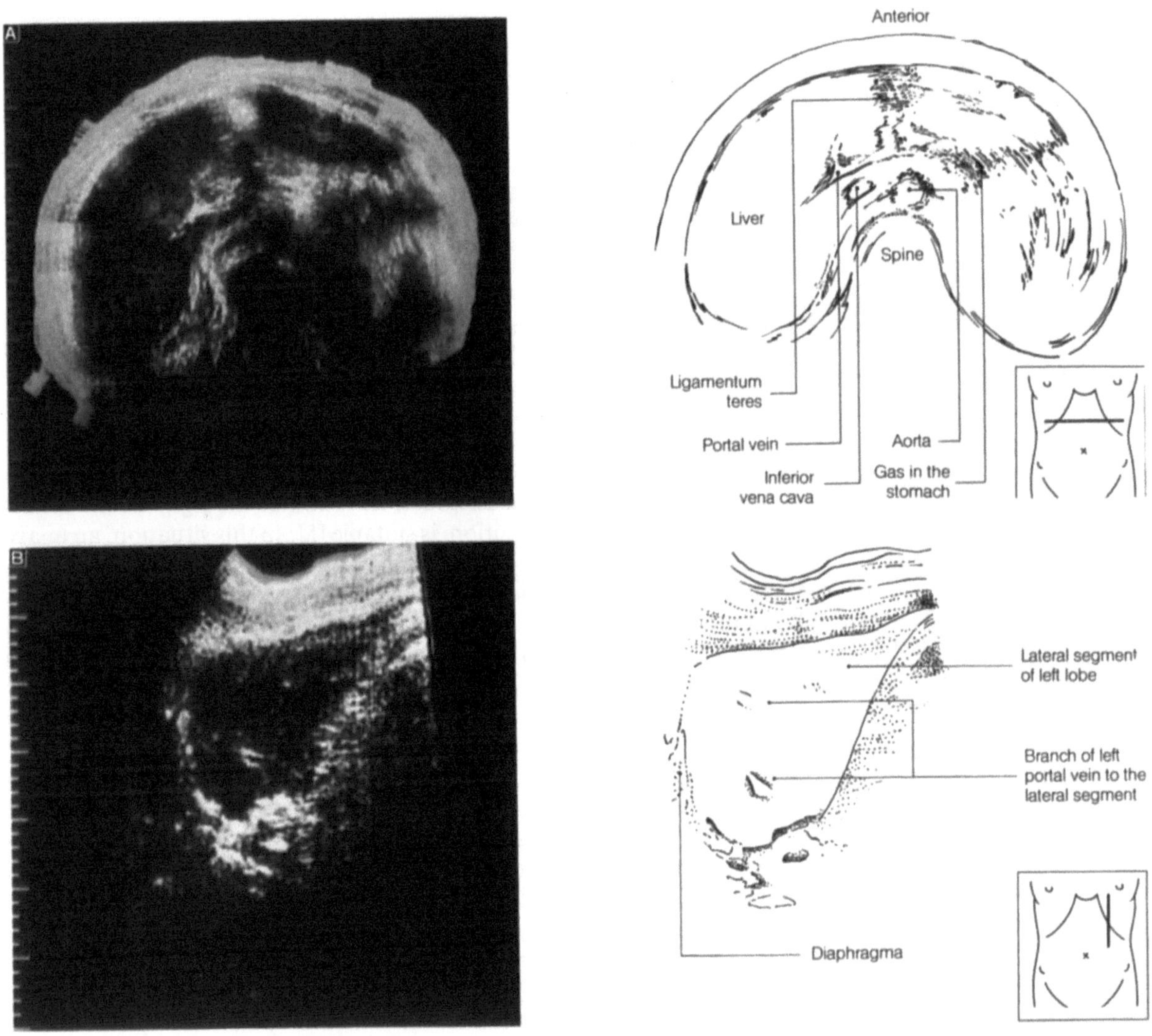

Fig. 2.4. A–D. Ultrasonogram of the normal liver

2.3 Liver

Figure 2.4 consists of ultrasonograms of the normal liver; these images were photographed under optimum conditions with a transverse and sagittal scan. Unlike X-ray CT, ultrasound imaging is not limited to transverse scan so that three-dimensional information can be obtained. On the other hand, knowledge of the anatomical relationship of the abdominal organs should be secured for an accurate diagnosis [59, 86, 87].

During ultrasonic diagnosis of the liver, it is important to understand the relationship between the portal and hepatic veins. With these intrahepatic vessels, the hepatic segment can be approximately determined [24].

Cantlie's line separating the right and left hepatic lobe corresponds to the main lobar fissure. This line connects the fossa of the gallbladder and sulcus of the vena cava. The middle hepatic vein runs in this fissure. Aiming at the middle hepatic vein, the left and right hepatic lobes can be recognized (Fig. 2.5). The right hepatic vein runs in the right segmental fissure which separates the anterior and posterior segments of the right hepatic lobe (Fig. 2.6).

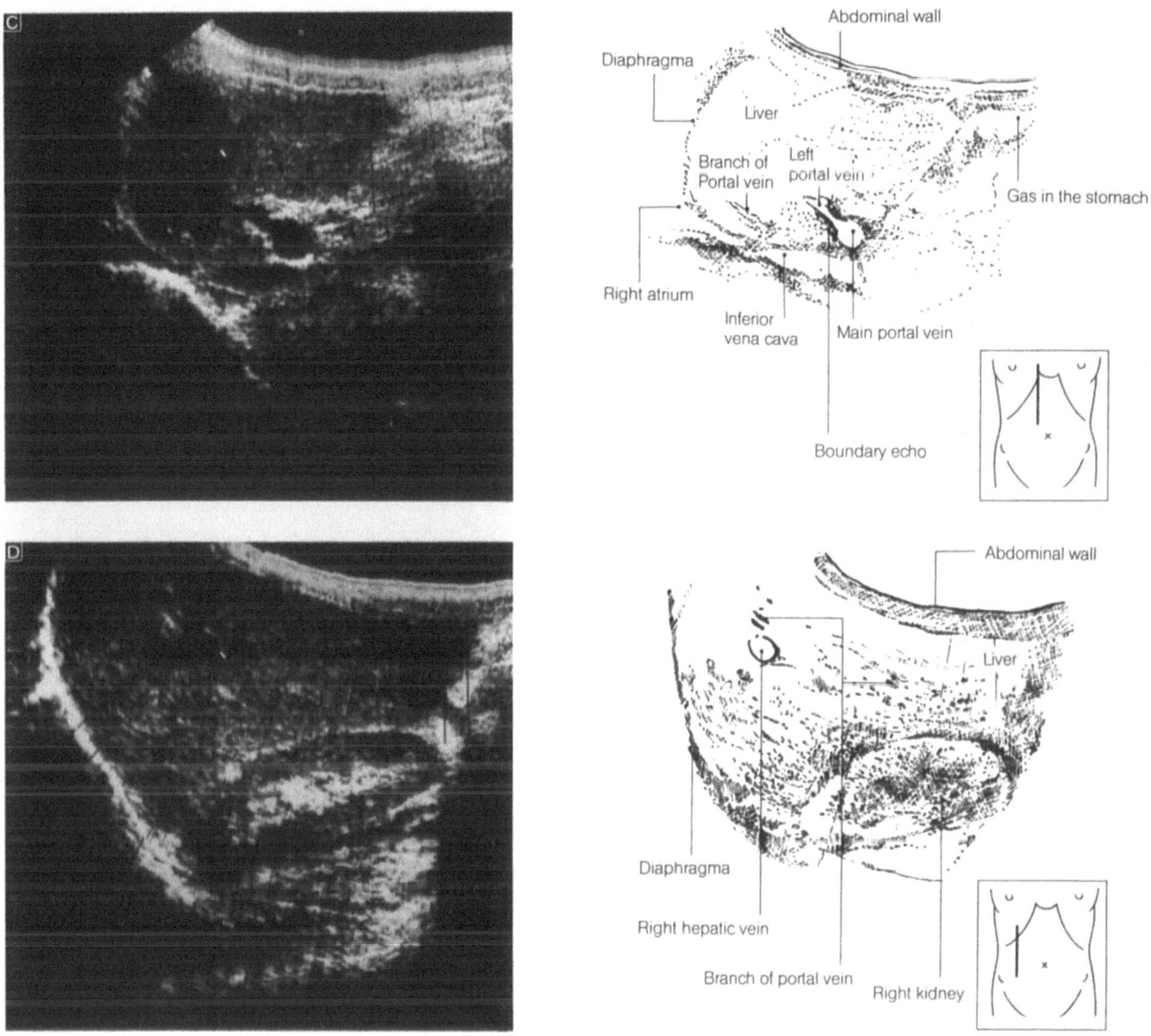

Fig. 2.4. A–D. (continued)

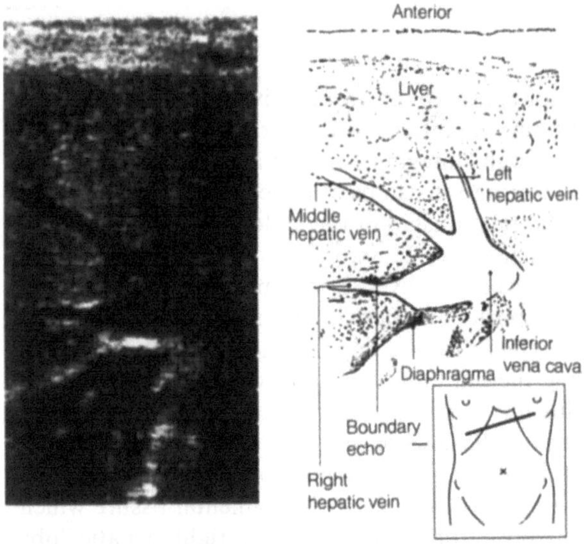

Fig. 2.5. Normal hepatic vein

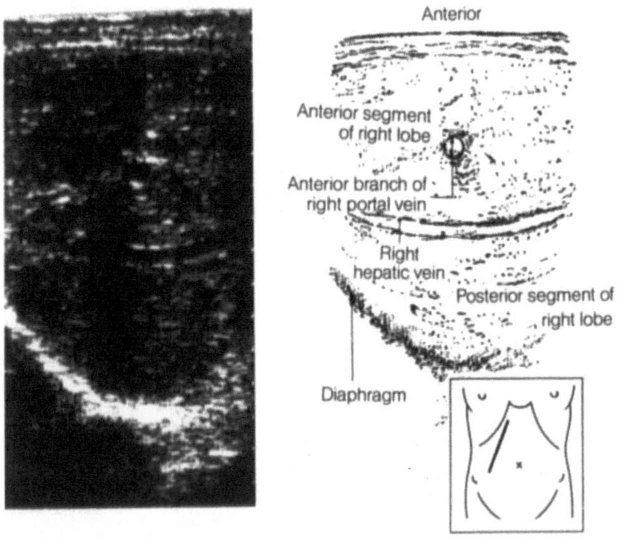

Fig. 2.6. Right hepatic vein

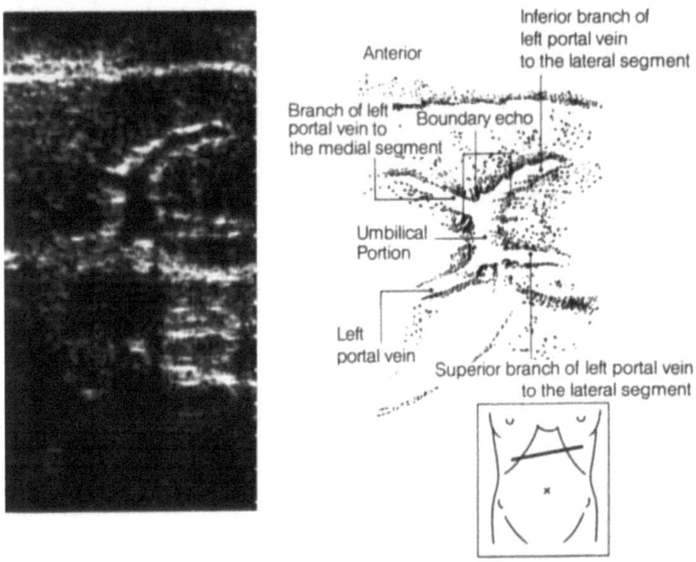

Fig. 2.7. Left branch of intrahepatic portal vein

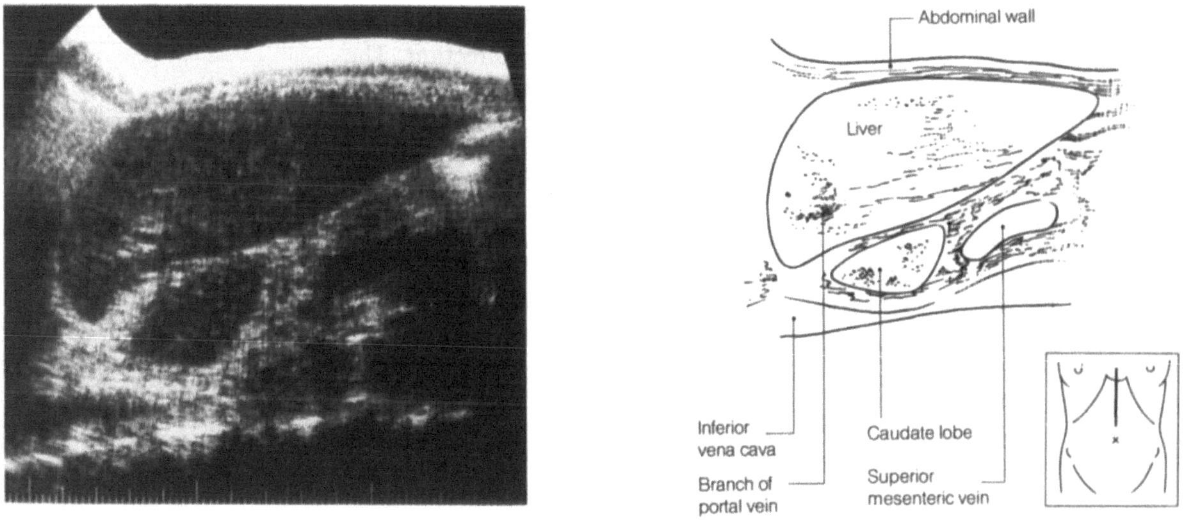

Fig. 2.8. Caudate lobe

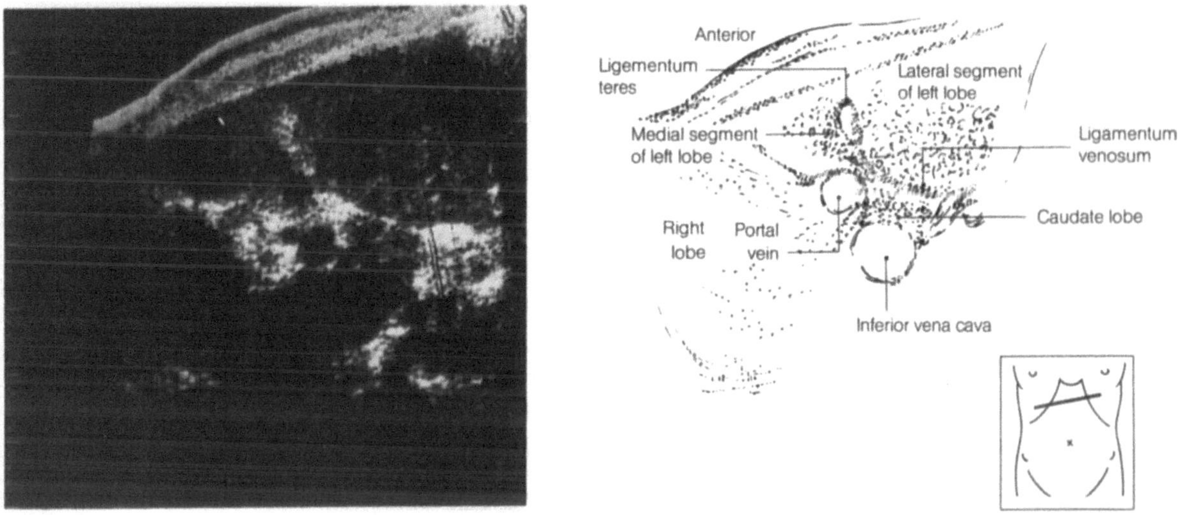

Fig. 2.9. Ligamentum venosum

To distinguish the lateral and medial segments of the left hepatic lobe, which are separated by the left segmental fissure, transverse scan images are desirable. The recognition point is obtained by finding the left hepatic vein running in the upper portion of the fissure and umbilical portion of the left portal vein positioned at the middle portion of the fissure (Fig. 2.7), and the round or oval echogenic image produced by the ligamentum teres is viewed at the lower portion of the fissure (Fig. 2.4a).

In sagittal scanning, the caudate lobe is observed between the main portal vein and the inferior vena cava (Fig 2.8). The caudate lobe and lateral segment of the left hepatic lobe can be distinguished by the vivid line which is the fissure for the ligamentum venosum displayed on the transverse scan image [69] (Fig. 2.9). In other words, the caudate lobe exists between the inferior vena cava and fissure for the ligamentum venosum.

The intrahepatic vessels are observed as an unechoic image. They become tubular, circular, or oval according to the scanning direction. The intrahepatic portal vein, which normally has rich surrounding connective tussues, is usually observed as a bright echo (the boundary echo) [14] (Figs. 2.5–2.7). However, depending upon the direction of the ultrasound beam, the boundary echo does not always appear. Using the real-time scanner, images of the vessels can be followed from the inferior vena cava and the superior mesenteric vein to the intrahepatic vein and the portal vein by moving the transducer; thus, distinguished the hepatic vein or the portal vein from the existence of the boundary echo is not always necessary.

2.3.1 Ambiguous Image from a Pathological Lesion. An ambiguous image from the pathological lesion is frequently seen because of reflection and absorption of ultrasound. On the transverse scan, a bright round or oval focal echo is often apparent in the right of the midline, owing to ultrasonic reflection at the fissure of the ligamentum teres [42, 83]. This is not image of a pathological lesion [72]. Although the pathological lesion can be observed on the sagittal scan image, the ligamentum teres cannot (Fig. 2.4a).

On the sagittal scan image, a masslike image below the left hepatic lobe may be observed. This is the cross-section image of the caudate lobe of the liver (Fig. 2.8). On the transverse scan, the image due to ultrasound reflected by the lung and ribs may appear as an intrahepatic lesion (Fig. 2.10). Scanning from at least two different directions is necessary to avoid these ambiguous findings caused by these artifacts.

Another example is the connective tissue surrounding the left portal vein, which may be confused for the posterior margin of the left hepatic lobe and also the parenchymal image behind it for a mass lesion because of the glitter [9]. Figure 2.11 shows an example of the stomach filled with food and gastric juices mixed together (observed as a liver tumor).

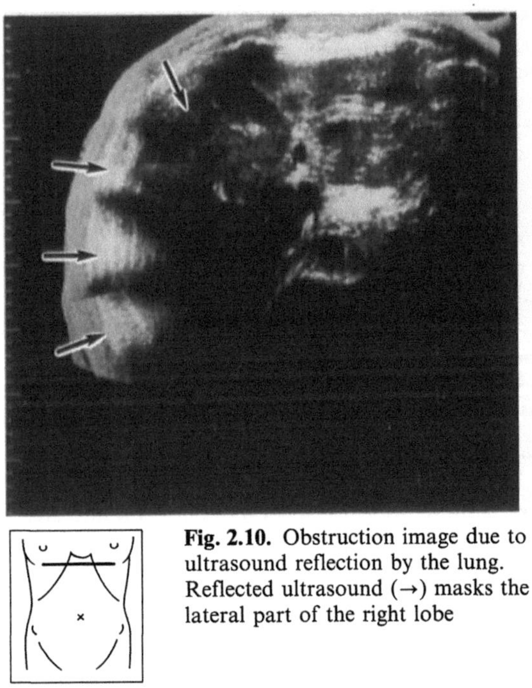

Fig. 2.10. Obstruction image due to ultrasound reflection by the lung. Reflected ultrasound (→) masks the lateral part of the right lobe

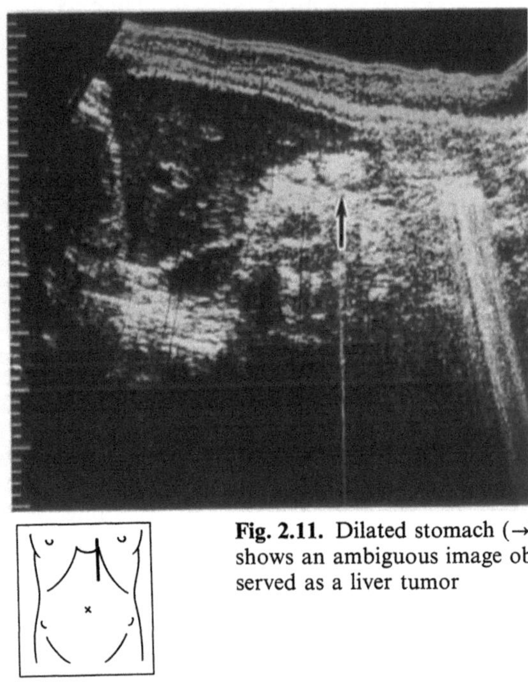

Fig. 2.11. Dilated stomach (→) shows an ambiguous image observed as a liver tumor

2.3.2 Pathological Conditions. There are numerous grades of pathological conditions in the liver showing findings from the cystic pattern with no internal echo to a solid mass pattern with an echo stronger than hepatic parenchyma.

Ultrasonic findings of a liver cyst are charcterized by its smooth contour and unechoic image with a strong bright echo on the posterior wall where the ultrasonic beam penetrates [84] (Fig. 2.12). The parasitic inflammation causes various echo patterns in the cyst; occasionally, complicated echoes such as septum in the cyst or daughter satellites may be seen [39]. In the case of a liver abscess, an echo is sometimes unobserved (Fig. 2.13); normally, fine echo patterns of debris are visualized in the cyst. Thick walls, irregular outlines, and usually complex forms are characteristics of this [65] (Fig. 2.14). Echoes may appear as a tumor pattern of the bull's-eye type in

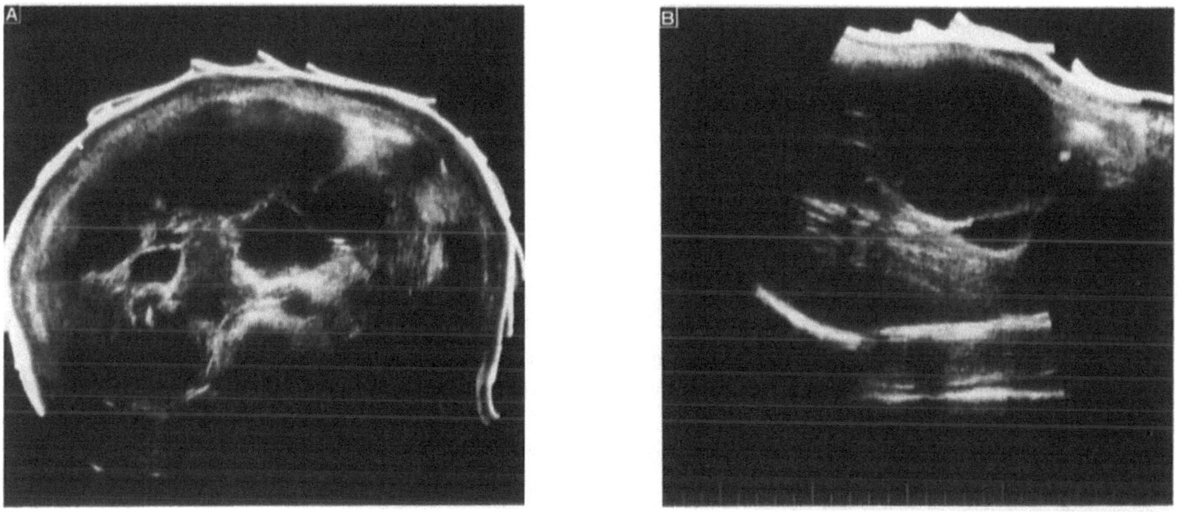

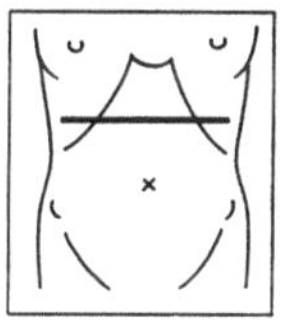

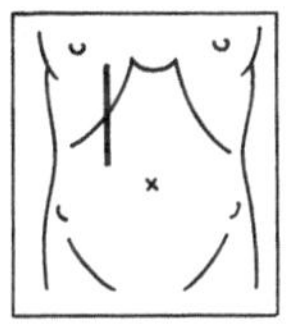

Fig. 2.12 A, B. Liver cysts. Multiple cysts with septum in the liver and echo enhancement at posterior of the cysts. Same case as shown in Figs. 4.11 and 5.14

Fig. 2.13. Liver abscess with cystic echo 3.5 × 4 cm in the right lobe and surrounding solid echoes

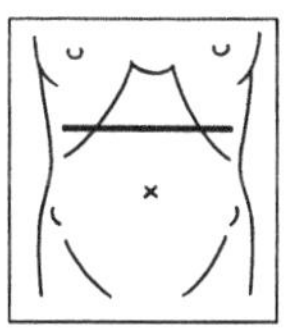

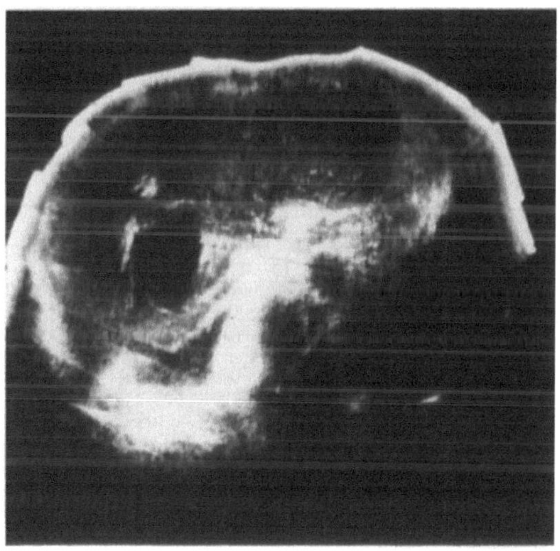

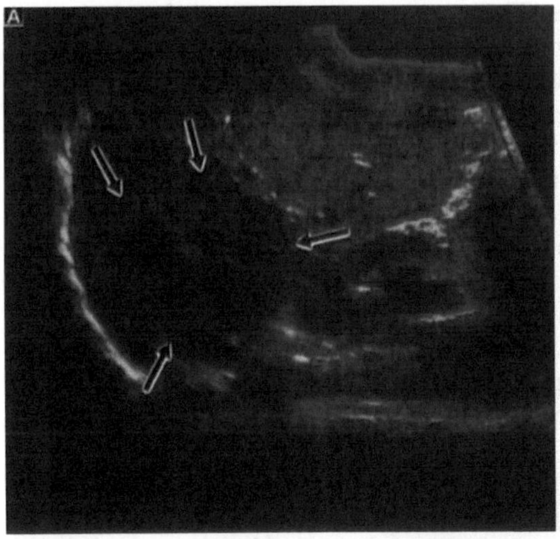

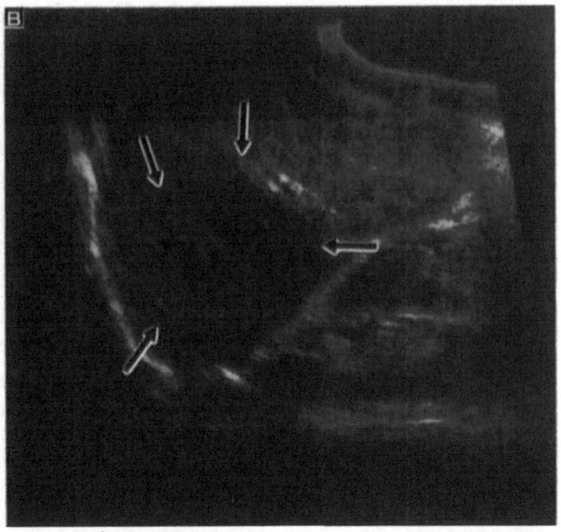

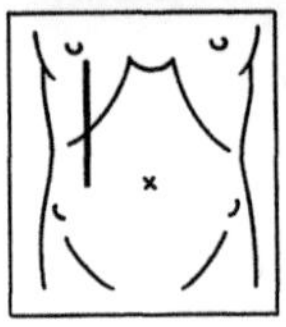

Fig. 2.14 A, B. Liver abscess with a lower echo level (→) than in liver parenchyma with an internal unechoic part. Same case as shown in Fig. 4.13

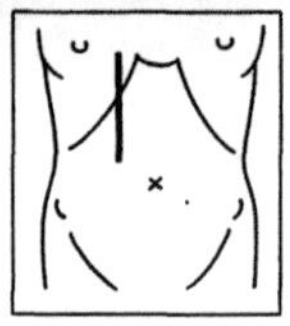

the case of a microabscess [11]. In the case of primary tumor and metastatic carcinoma of the liver, various internal echoes are visible [45, 61]. Its echo level is higher or lower than that of liver parenchyma in most cases, but sometimes similar. A sonolucent zone surrounding the tumor image can also be observed (bull's-eye type) [80] (Figs. 2.15–2.17).

It is impossible to differentiate between benign or malignant, primary or metastatic tumors by ultrasonographic examinations alone [15, 36, 101]. Tables 2.1 and 2.2 support this fact, exhibiting the classification of 40 examples of primary hepatocellular carcinoma and 23 examples of metastatic tumors of the liver according to their echo patterns. No characteristic information can be obtained from these various ultrasonographic images.

Sometimes, space-occupying lesions are not visible when they have diffuse inhomogeneous echo patterns and obscure outlines. On the ultrasonic

Table 2.1. Differences in echo patterns cannot be observed in various types of tumors

Tumor type / Pattern of echo level	Cholangio-carcinoma	Hepatocellular carcinoma	Metastatic carcinoma
High	0	5	5
Ortho	0	2	1
Low	0	0	2
Mixed	2	31	15

Table 2.2. Major differences cannot be found in the appearance rate of the bull's-eye type

Cholangiocarcinoma	Hepatocellular carcinoma	Metastatic carcinoma
1/2	12/38	8/23

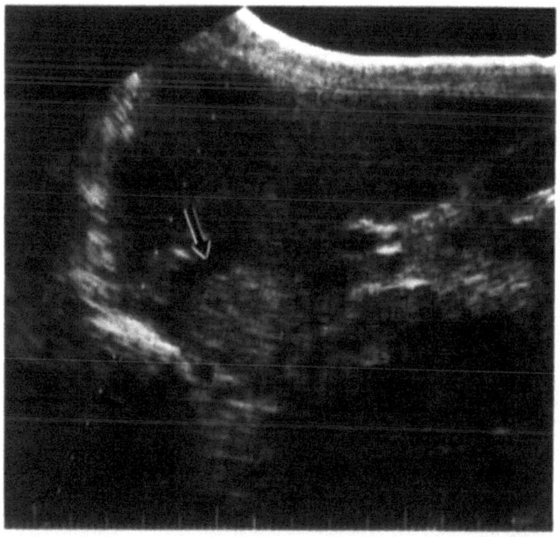

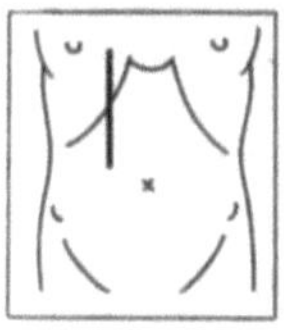

Fig. 2.15. Hepatocellular carcinoma with an echogenic mass at the posterior portion of the right lobe with surrounding sonolucent zone (→), the so-called bull's-eye type

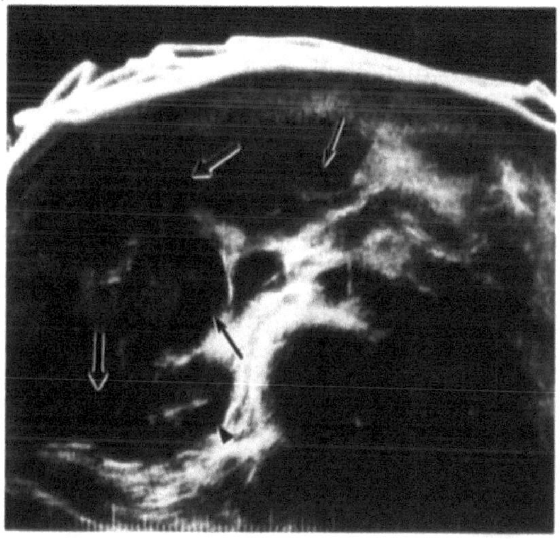

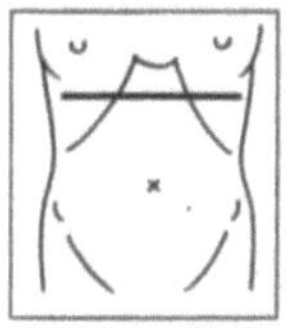

Fig. 2.16. Metastatic liver tumor (malignant lymphoma): multiple low level echo (→), bull's-eye type pattern (→), and right kidney (▶). Same case as shown in Figs. 3.9 and 4.17

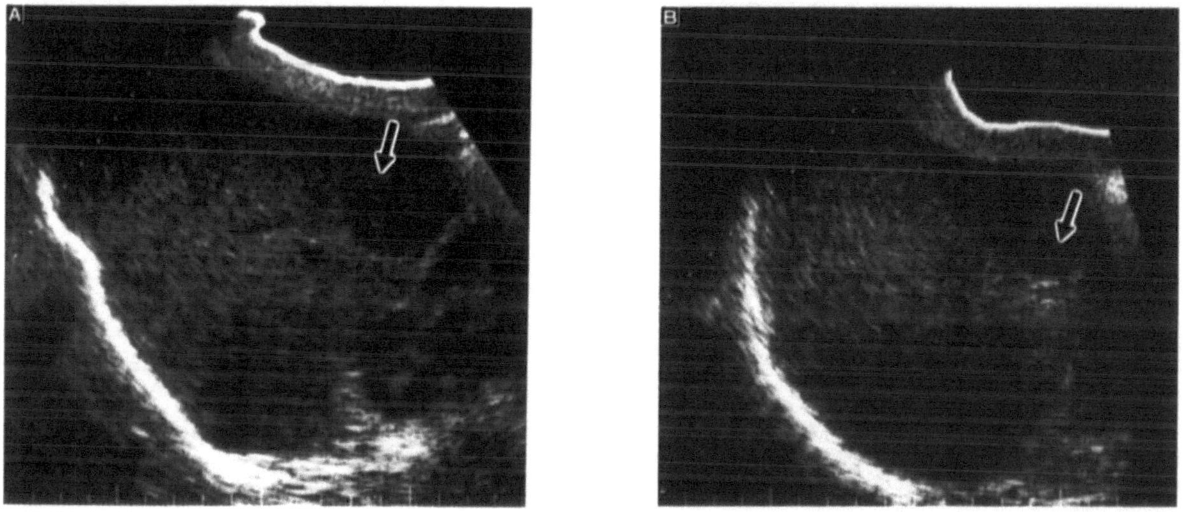

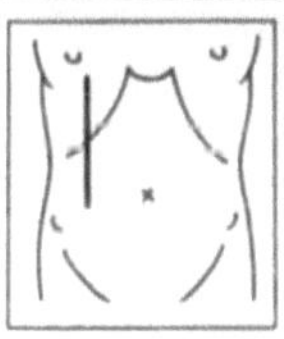

Fig. 2.17 A, B. Metastatic liver carcinoma (laryngeal carcinoma). **A** Low level echos of the bull's-eye type are in the right lobe (→). **B** After 14 months of chemotherapy, diminishing tumor and internal necrotic area are seen as cyst (→)

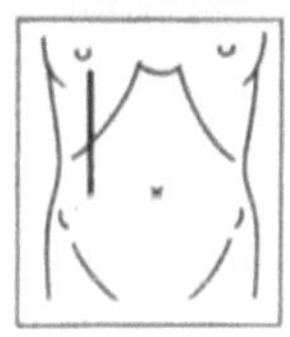

image of a malignant neoplasm, necrosis causes an echo-free area to expand due to chemotherapy [7] (Fig. 2.17). As the necrotic area expands, it becomes difficult to differentiate the cyst and abscess from the solid mass as carcinoma [91, 103].

Hemangioma is one of the main benign tumors of the liver. It may be observed as a mass with strong internal echoes (Fig. 2.18), an echo pattern with a level lower than hepatic parenchyma (Fig. 2.19), or mixed types.

With diffuse hepatocellular lesions, such as advancement of fatty infiltration in fatty livers or growth of fibrotic tissue in liver cirrhosis, the attenuation of the ultrasound increases at the point far from the ultrasonic probe, and then the echo level decreases. Advanced liver cirrhosis may make the diaphragm image impossible to obtain even if the far gain (echo amplifier which strengthens the reflected ultrasound at a distance from the probe) is increased.

This condition of the liver is observed as entirely bright due to the intrahepatic strong echo and is called bright liver [44]. To diagnose bright

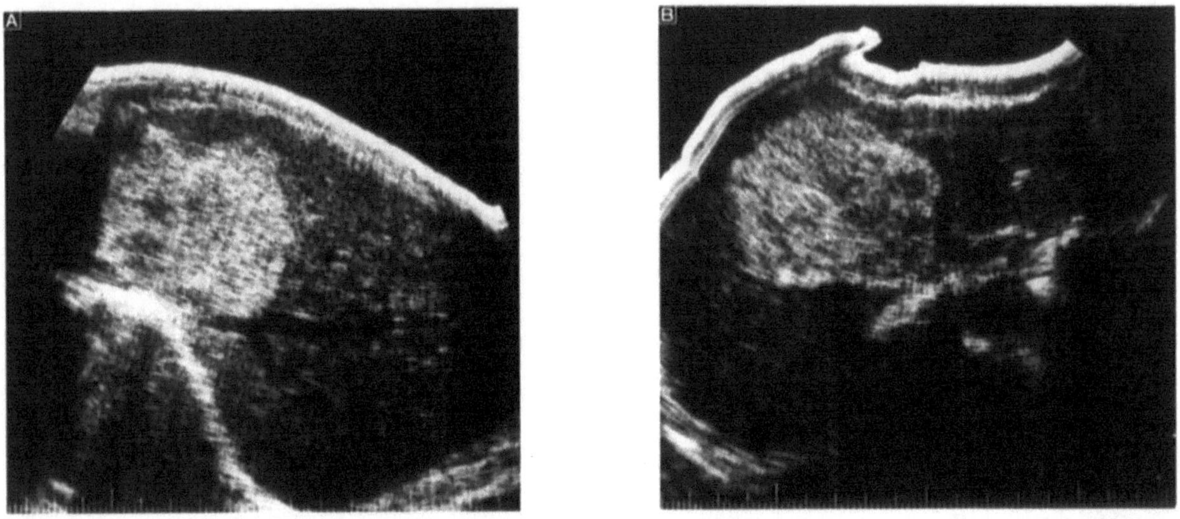

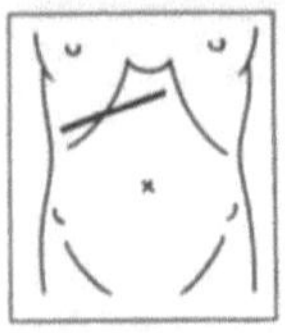

Fig. 2.18 A, B. Hemangioma of the liver. There are higher echo patterns with irregular contour and a partial low internal echo in the anterior segment of the right lobe

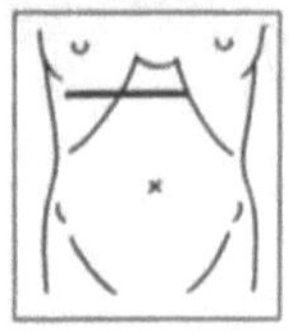

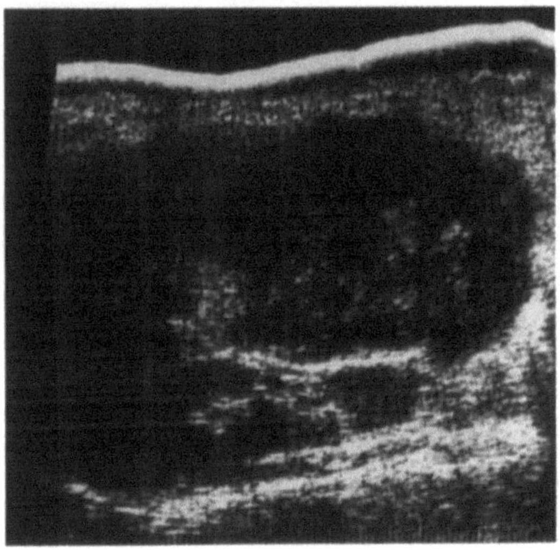

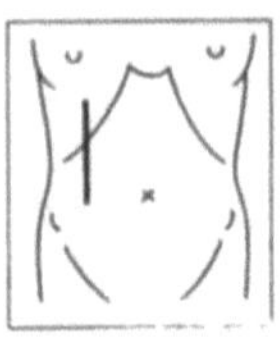

Fig. 2.19. Hemangioma of the liver. A giant hemangioma occupies the right lower lobe of the liver with echoes showing several grades lower than in liver parenchyma. Same case as shown in Fig. 4.14

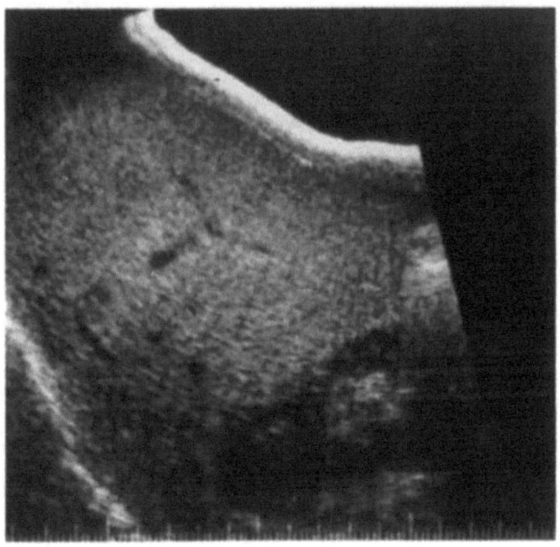

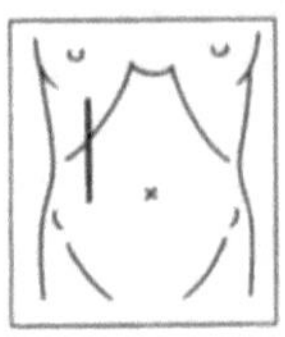

Fig. 2.20. The fatty liver shows a higher level of echo than the right kidney, the so-called bright liver. Same case as shown in Fig. 4.23

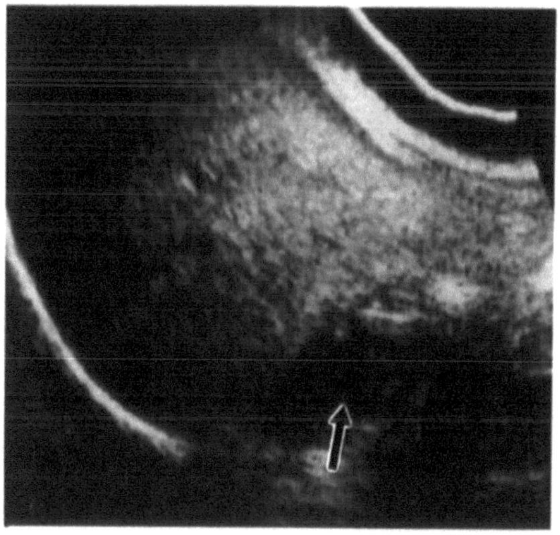

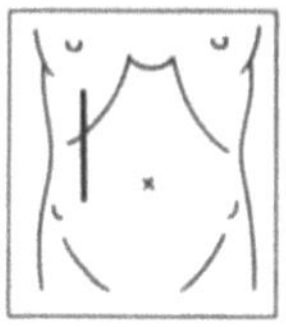

Fig. 2.21. Liver cirrhosis. There is a bright liver compared with low level echo of right kidney (→)

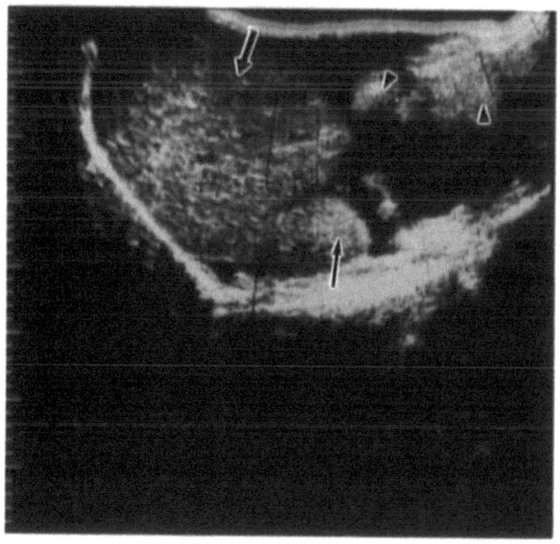

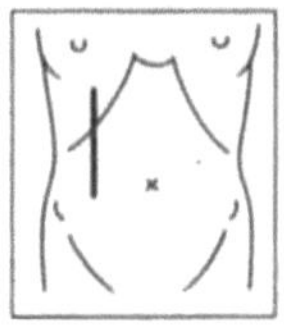

Fig. 2.22. Ascites (liver cirrhosis). The unechoic pattern corresponds to ascites. Liver (→), kidney (→), and intestine (▶)

liver, the echo level of the right kidney is invaluable as a reference. A blurring of the echo image of the wall of the intrahepatic portal vein, which normally appears bright, and decreased vascularity can also be useful in diagnosis [32] (Figs. 2.20 and 2.21).

Although diagnosis of diffuse hepatocellular lesions of the liver may be obtained with ultrasonic techniques, quality diagnosis cannot be expected from ultrasound at present.

Ultrasonic diagnosis of ascites with liver cirrhosis is easily possible (Fig. 2.22). On the other hand, recanalization of the umbilical vein by portal hypertension may cause a bull's-eye pattern in the falciform ligament [79]. With acute hepatitis, the echo level in the whole liver becomes lower, and accordingly the echo of the wall of the portal vein is brightly visualized, and the observable range of the portal vein becomes broadened. Conversely, chronic hepatitis is characterized by a weak echo in the wall of the portal vein, the ultrasonically visible portal vein fades, and a rough and moderately enhanced echo in the liver parenchyma can be visualized [48].

2.4 Gallbladder and Bile Duct

A normal finding observes the gallbladder as an unechoic eggplant-shaped image (Fig. 2.23) above the right kidney at the lower posterior side of the right hepaitc lobe with a longitudinal scanning direction of 4–5 cm from the right of the midline.

Without contraction, it is normally 3–4 cm in the short axis and 8–9 cm in the long axis. Generally, the gallbladder cannot be determined because its location, shape, and size differs individually, and its size varies with time from patient to patient.

Normally, the wall of the gallbladder is less than 2–3 mm thick [27]. The cystic duct is generally difficult to visualize although it is occasionally

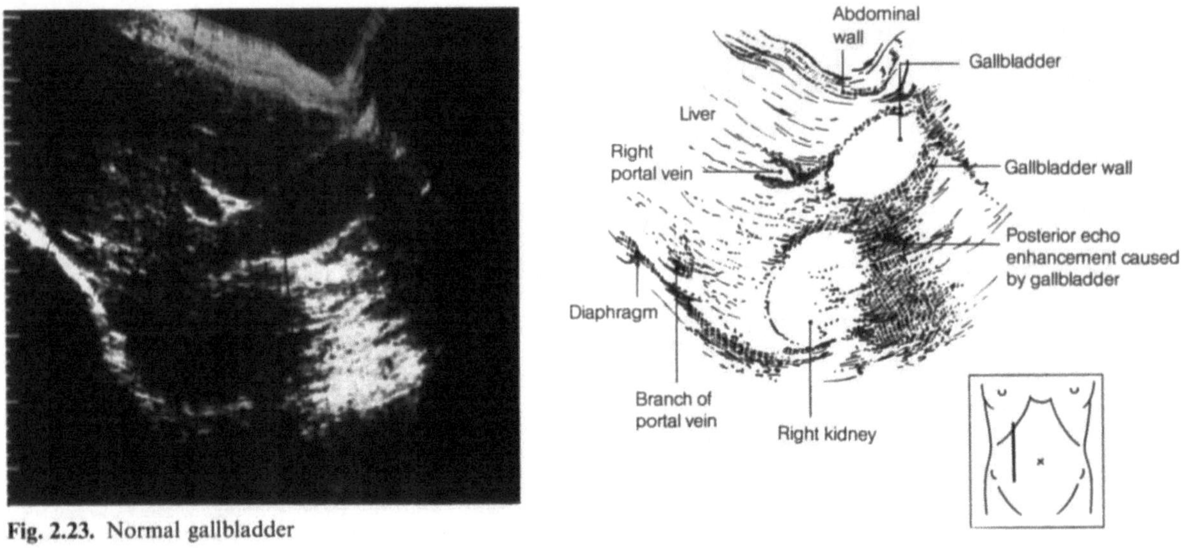

Fig. 2.23. Normal gallbladder

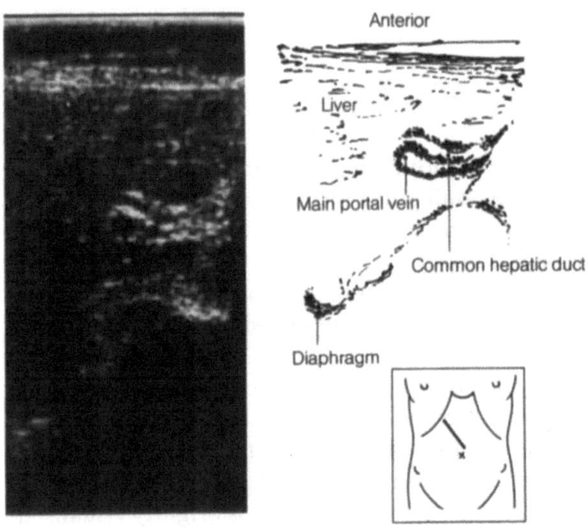

Fig. 2.24. Common hepatic duct

displayed as a thin tubular structure. The spiral valve in the cystic duct caused by abundant reflection of the ultrasound sometimes may be observed as a bright echo. The bright echo and acoustic shadow behind it is frequently incorrectly recognized as a gallstone.

The common bile duct and the common hepatic duct can be observed as a tubular structure on the image obtained with a sagittal scan. The common hepatic duct is readily visible with the landmark of the portal vein because it runs parallel to the right anterior side of the portal vein in the porta hepatis or the gastrohepatic ligament [71]. With contact scanning, demonstrating the portal vein and the bile duct on the same section by elevating the right side of a patient, the image of the thin common hepatic ducts is visualized anterior to the thick portal vein (Fig. 2.24). However, the lower part of the common bile duct frequently cannot be easily observed because of the removal of the running direction of the duct from the ultrasonic beam and obstruction by bowel gas. Conversely, with real-time scan-

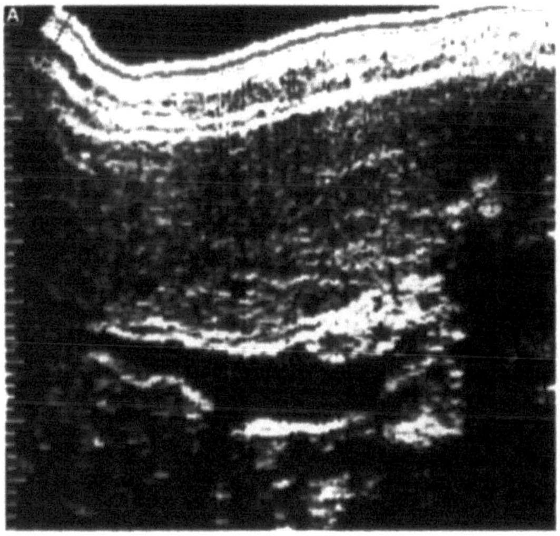

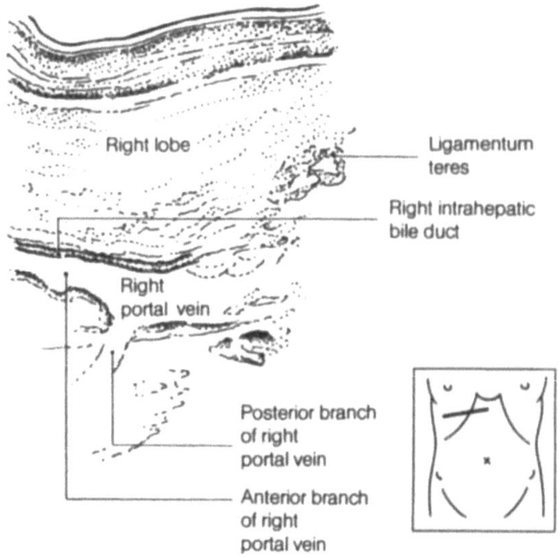

Fig. 2.25. Intrahepatic bile duct and portal vein

ning, the whole image of the common bile duct can be obtained quite easily by means of free operation of the ultrasonic probe.

Observed with the ultrasonic image, the normal inside diameter of the common bile duct never exceeds 5–7 mm [70, 77]. The sonolucent ring structure image of the common hepatic duct can be observed anterior to the right portal vein prior to branching with sagittal scanning. In normal cases, the inside diameter does not exceed 4 mm [19]. Sometimes, the intrahepatic bile ducts of the right lobe can be displayed anterior to the portal vein by scanning along the right portal vein (Fig. 2.25). The intrahepatic bile ducts of the left lobe can be observed in the same manner as above.

If dilatation in the common bile duct is observed, it is necessary to determine its cause. In a postcholecystectomy patient, the common bile duct may dilate even by around 10 mm without abnormality. However, if diameters of over 8 mm for the common bile duct and over 6 mm for the common hepatic ducts are observed in a postcholecystectomy patient, it is considered abnormal and further examination is required [34, 35, 63, 98].

The image of the transverse section of the right hepatic artery is sometimes visible between the portal vein and the right hepatic duct, with a longitudinal image of the portal vein and the right hepatic ducts [19, 102] (Fig. 2.35). Generally, ultrasonic images of the portal vein and bile duct are obtained by following these structures with a flexible transducer operation so that a real-time scanner is more valuable than a contact compound scanner. However, since they run very closely to each other, it is sometimes impossible to distinguish between them, and they appear as one tube because of obstruction of the beam width artifact.

2.4.1 Pathological Conditions. For the diagnosis of a gallstone, the finding of a strong echo in the gallbladder, which is caused by the reflection of the echo created by the stones, and no transmission of sound beyond the stone (so-called acoustic shadow) are valuable determining signs in ultrasonographic examinations (Figs. 2.26 and 2.27).

Nowadays, the accuracy of sonographic diagnosis of gallstones is 88%–100%, and it is regarded as the diagnostic examination of choice, which can be used in place of cholecystography [41].

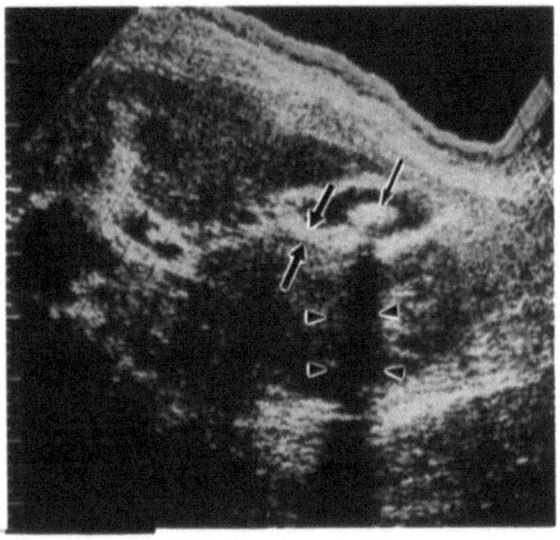

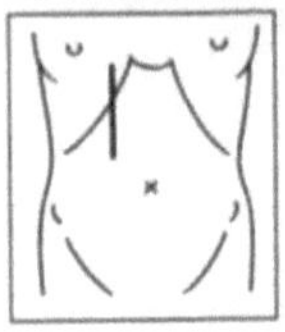

Fig. 2.26. Cholecystolithiasis with colecystitis; thickened gallbladder wall (1 cm) (→) and gallstone (1.5 cm) (→) with acoustic shadow (▶)

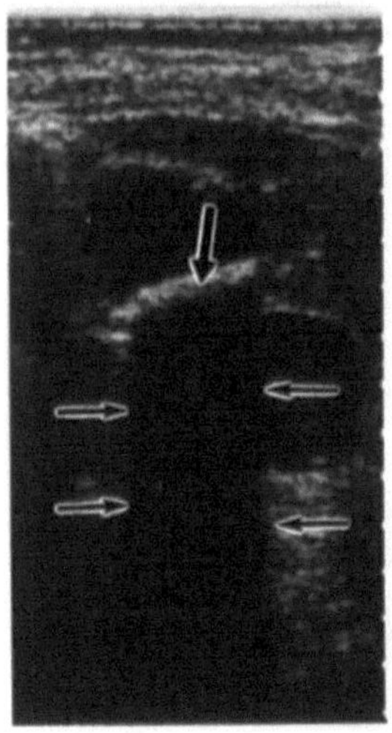

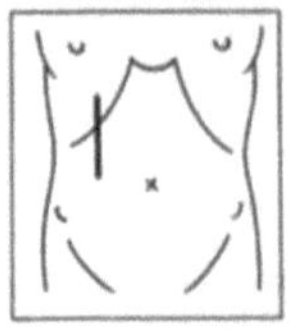

Fig. 2.27. multiple gravels with band-shaped strong echo (→) at posterior wall of the gallbladder with acoustic shadow (→). Same case as shown in Figs. 1.14 and 4.32

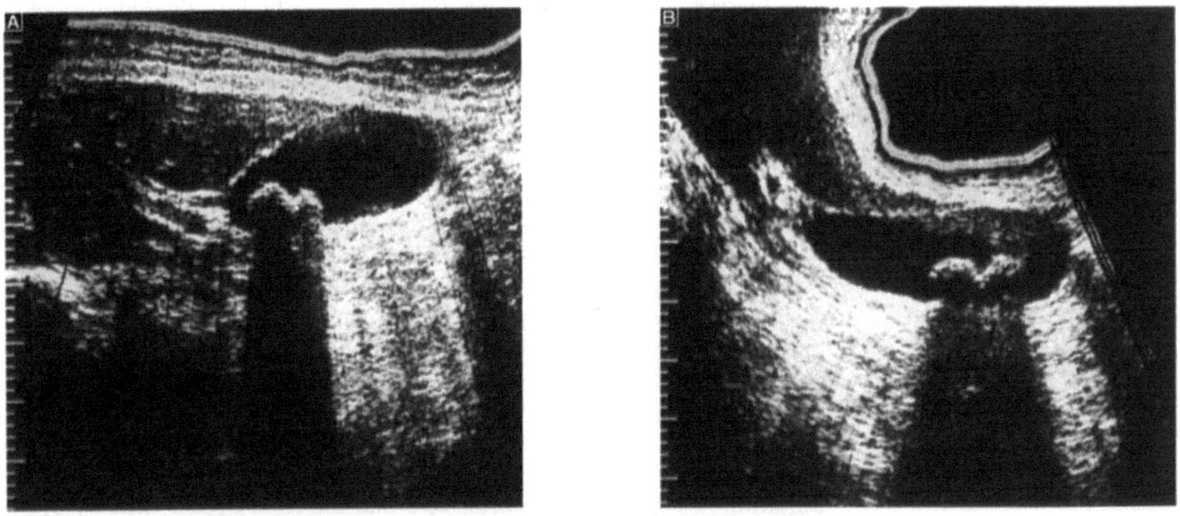

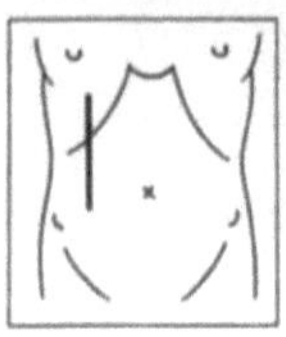

Fig. 2.28 A, B. Cholecystolithiasis. **A** Supine position: a strong echo in the gallbladder and a posterior acoustic shadow are seen. **B** Sitting position: by changing the patient's position from the supine to a sitting position, the strong echo shifts downward in the gallbladder

The most valuable diagnostic information is the acoustic shadow. It is said to be consistently demonstrated irrespective of the specific properties of the gallstones in in vitro investigations [26]. However, in some clinical cases the acoustic shadow may be unobservable [37, 43, 82, 88], for example, tiny stones in comparison with the beam width, an inadequate angle of the beam to the stone, an inadequate frequency of ultrasound, an inadequate focal length, and an inappropriate gain setting of the amplifier. Purdom et al. [73] have shown that the intrinsic attenuation of a stone is an important factor in making the acoustic shadow. Stones with higher attenuation show the most acoustic shadow. In addition, attenuation can be correlated with physical structure: more highly attenuating stones tend to have the largest percentage of crystalline material, a larger average crystal size, and a more rigid structure. Even in cases of a lack of an acoustic shadow, only the bright shining echo reflected on the surface of the stone can be seen so that the gallstone can be diagnosed if it is proven that the echo will move by changing the patient's position (Fig. 2.28).

This rescanning in a different position is an important operation to differentiate between the gravel and the biliary sludge. By changing the position, the gravel moves instantly and the biliary sludge moves slowly [1, 8] (Fig. 2.29). In the case of a gallbladder filled with numerous small stones or contracted and thickened with cholecystitis, the anterior wall of the gallbladder and the strong acoustic shadow behind its wall are observed, but the posterior wall is invisible due to obstruction by a markedly strong acoustic shadow (Fig. 2.30). Sometimes, only a strong echo and acoustic shadow are observed [49]. A pseudoimage of the gallstone is occasionally obtained due to obstruction from intestinal gas. In this case, it is necessary to change the scanning direction of the ultrasonic beam or to reexamine at another time.

Except for a gallbladder filled with numerous stones, a fluid-filled gallbladder is normally observed as a well-defined acoustic outline with a homogeneous sonolucent interior. However, when the gallbladder is greatly obscured by gas in the intestine, it cannot be visualized. When the gallbladder is filled with a high concentration of bile juice [18] or filled with tumors (gallbladder carcinoma), the cavity may be observed as a solid mass.

In particular cases such as agenesis or dislocation of the gallbladder, it is not possible to visualize the gallbladder [4]. If the image of the gallbladder is invisible or ambiguous, it may be found from the landmark of the main lobar fissure, which is a linear echo extending from the gallbladder to the right or the main portal vein [10].

If a fungating echo pattern on the wall of the gallbladder can be visualized and not removed by changing the body position, polyps [75], tumor, adenoma [13], or gallstone buried in the wall should be presumed. Occasionaly, partly raised mucosal folds may be seen as such lesions [3, 85].

In the case of cholecystitis, a wall more than 5 mm thick without the contraction of the gallbladder [57, 62] (Fig. 2.26) or a sonolucent zone in the wall (Fig. 2.31) may be observed. For the diagnosis of acute cholecystitis, the finding of a sonolucent zone in the gallbladder wall is a helpful sign [46, 58]. This sonolucent zone is also observed in cases of pericholecystic abscesses [6]. Consequently, although thickening of the gallbladder wall can be useful information [40], it is not adequate in itself to make a definite diagnosis of cholecystitis [23, 81].

Carcinoma of the gallbladder may be observed as an image protruding from the wall into the cavity [67] (Fig. 2.32). However, in an advanced stage, the echo of the gallbladder cavity appears at various levels because it is filled with the tumor [105] (Fig. 2.33). Generally, advanced carcinoma of the gallbladder is defined as a tumor image at the porta hepatis, and distinguishing it from carcinoma of the bile duct is often difficult.

The real-time scanner is superior to the contact compound scanner in the examination of contractibility of the gallbladder by administering a drug to the patient [68] (Fig. 2.34). For instance, the superiority of ultrasound is exhibited in the differential diagnosis of obstructive jaundice [20, 29, 47, 56, 64, 94, 106], as its accuracy is supposed to be 90%–97%

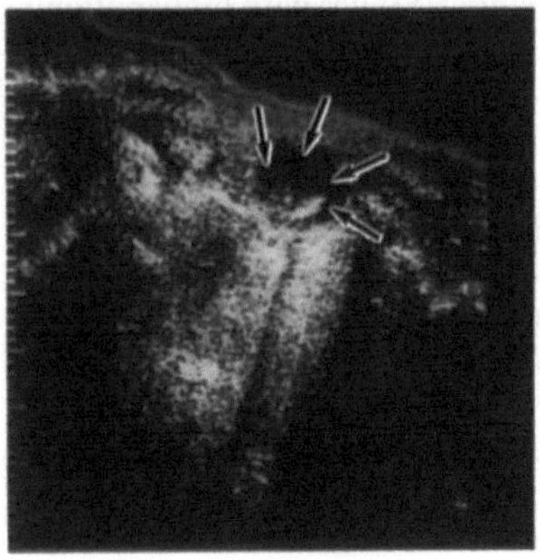
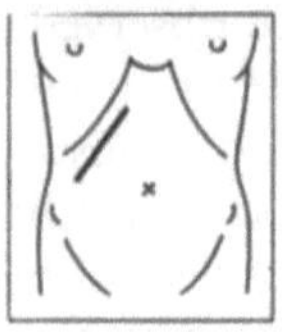

Fig. 2.29 A–C. Sludge. **A** Solid echo image (→) and a small stone are observed in the gallbladder.

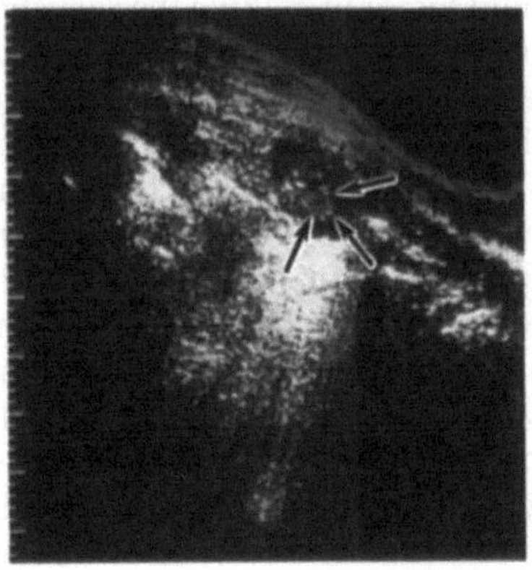
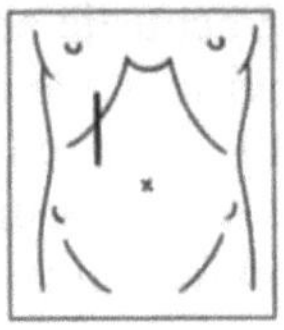

B Sitting position: this image (→) does not shift quickly by changing to the sitting position.

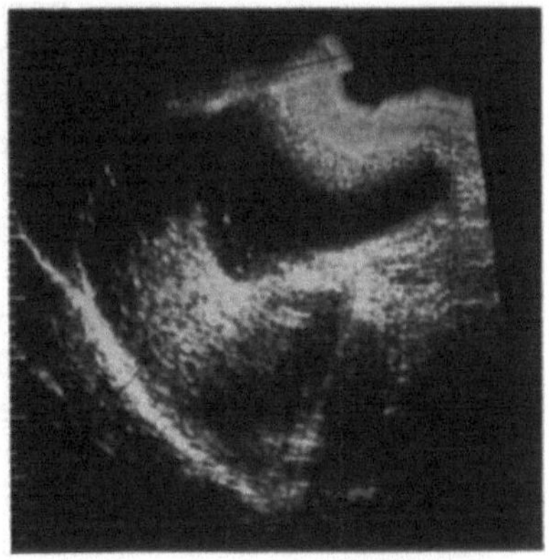
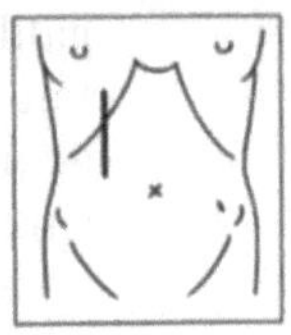

C After 10 days, no solid image is observed although from another scanning level a small stone is seen

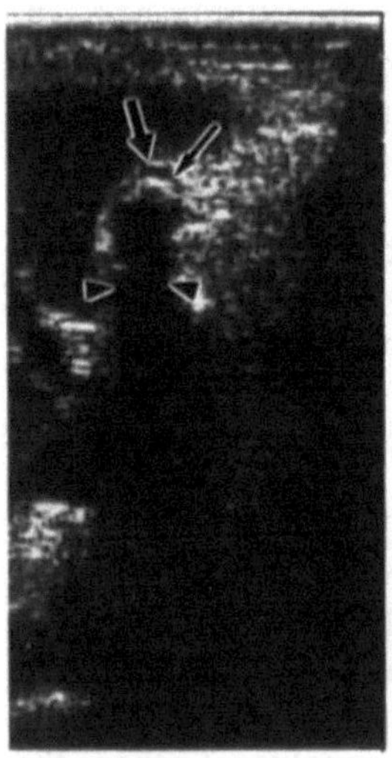
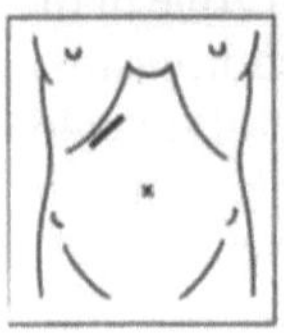

Fig. 2.30. Cholecystolithiasis. Only a part of the gallbladder wall (→) can be visualized with gallstone (→) and acoustic shadow (▶)

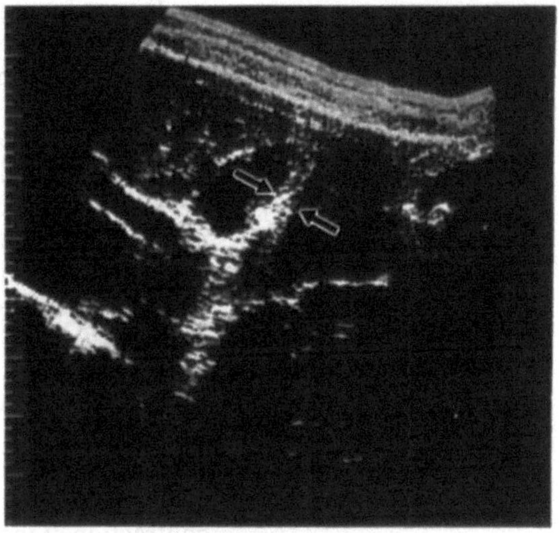
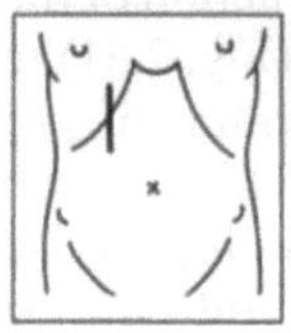

Fig. 2.31. Cholecystitis. A thickened gallbladder wall (→) and sonolucent zone in the wall can be seen

(Fig. 2.35), based on finding dilatation of the intra- and extrahepatic bile duct. Dilatation of the bile ducts is inferred when the diameter of the extrahepatic bile duct exceeds 6–8 mm. The bile duct may be observed to be as thick as the portal vein due to dilatation and is called the parallel-channel [17], the double-barrel [50], or the shotgun sign [95].

In obstructive jaundice caused by a stone, dilatation sometimes occurs not in the intrahepatic but only in the extrahepatic bile duct. Depending on the time of the examination, dilatation of the bile duct may remain unobserved even if jaundice exists, and conversely dilatation may be observed without jaundice [100]. If jaundice and dilatation of the bile duct are visualized, examination is needed to determine whether the causes are stones

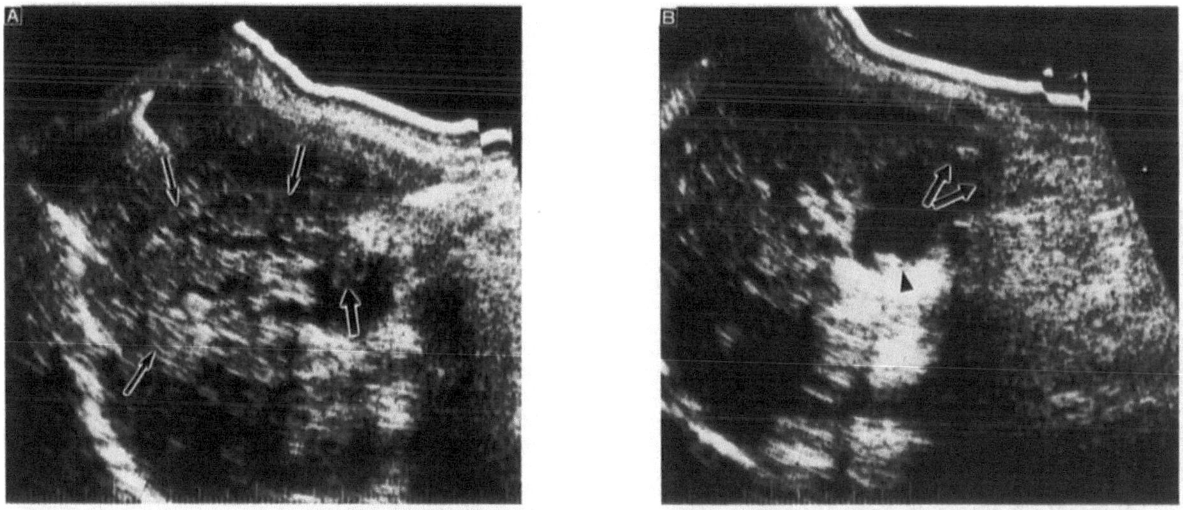
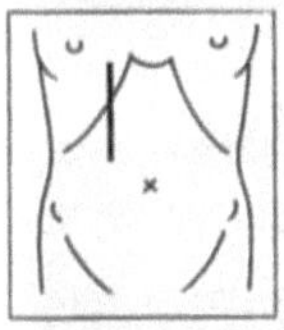

Fig. 2.32 A, B. Gallbladder carcinoma. A gallstone with a diameter of 5 mm (▶), a cancer occupying a part of the gallbladder cavity (→), and infiltration into the liver (→) can be seen. Same case as shown in Figs. 4.36 and 5.22

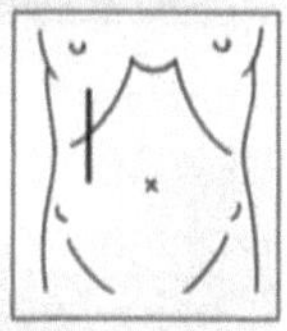

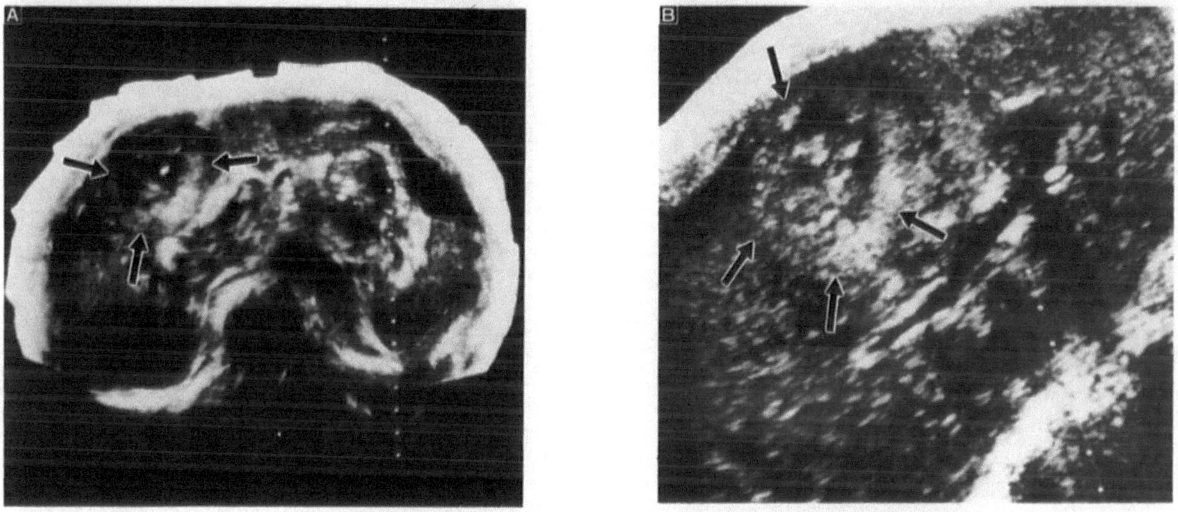
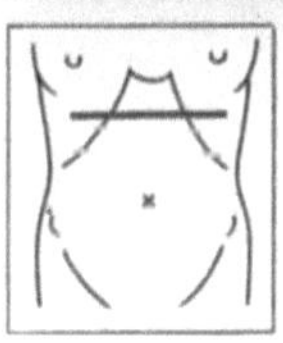

Fig. 2.33 A, B. Gallbladder carcinoma. There is a marked thickening of the gallbladder wall (→) and a solid echo extending upward into the cavity

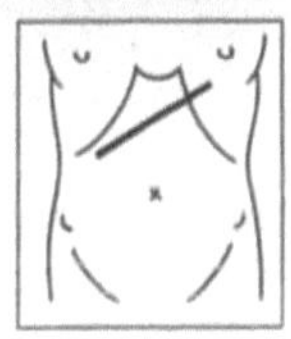

(Figs. 2.36 and 2.37), tumors (Fig. 2.38) or extrinsic compressions. Causes of diseases originating in the extrahepatic bile duct are diagnosed in only 50%–82% of cases [20, 47, 77] because of obstruction by bowel gas. If dilatation is observed in both bile and pancreatic ducts, disease of the papilla of Vater may be suspected.

Choledocholithiasis with marked dilatation of the biliary tract can easily be diagnosed by ultrasonography, as can gallstones using information from characteristic ultrasonic findings of stones (Fig. 2.36). Ultrasonic diagnosis must be performed using the landmark of the strong echo of the

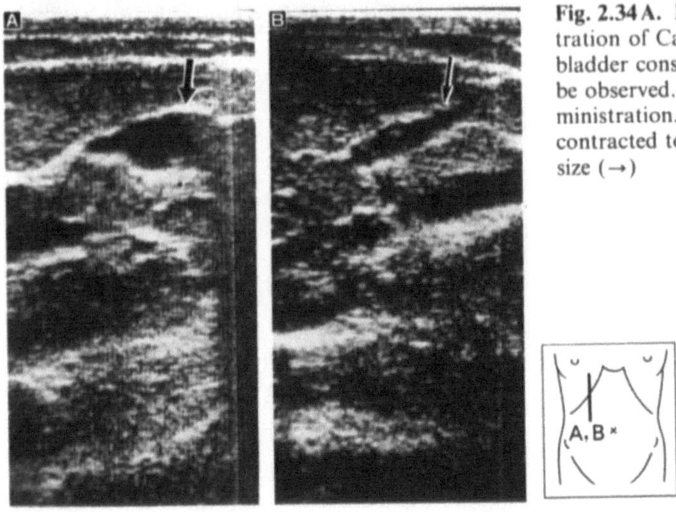

Fig. 2.34 A. Before administration of Caerulein. Gallbladder constriction cannot be observed. (→) **B** After administration, the gallbladder contracted to one-third in size (→)

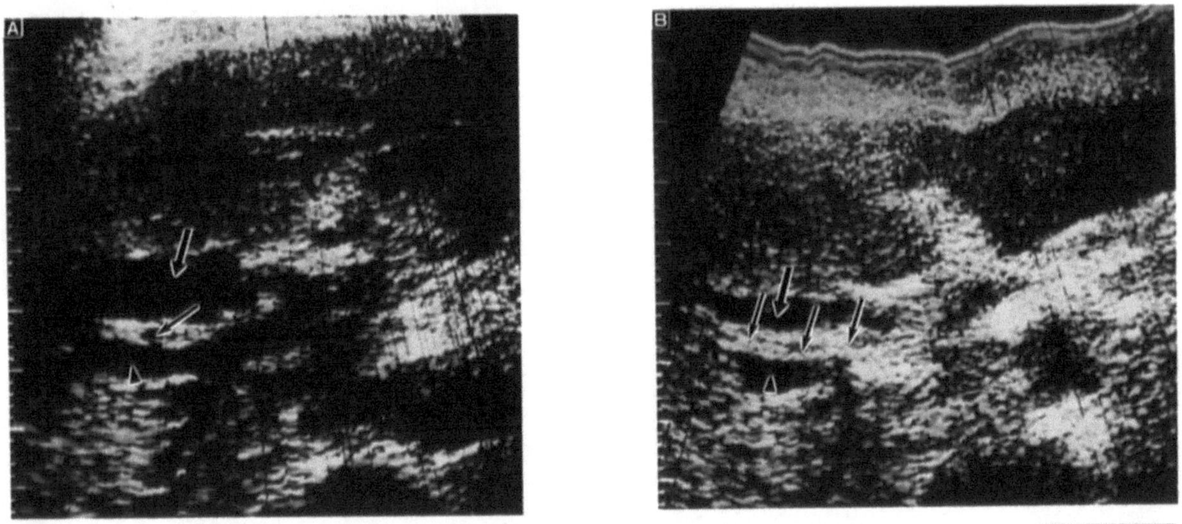

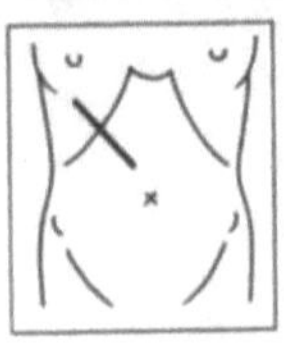

Fig. 2.35 A, B. Dilated right hepatic duct (→), right hepatic artery (→), and portal vein (▶)

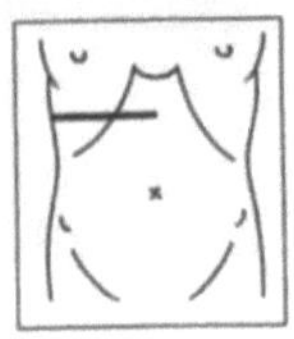

stone and distal acoustic shadow without dilatation of the bile duct. There may be common bile ducts stones which do not show the acoustic shadow and thus may be misdiagnosed as tumor masses [21]. Careful diagnosis is required in postcholecystectomy patients because a stone may be mistaken for the surgical clip or postoperative scar in the gallbladder bed [74].

Hepatolithiasis can be recognized with the landmark of the strong echo and the acoustic shadow (Fig. 2.37). Findings similar to those of hepatolithiasis may be obtained in calcified granuloma, air in the biliary tree, calcified metastatic foci, and foreign bodies in the liver [92].

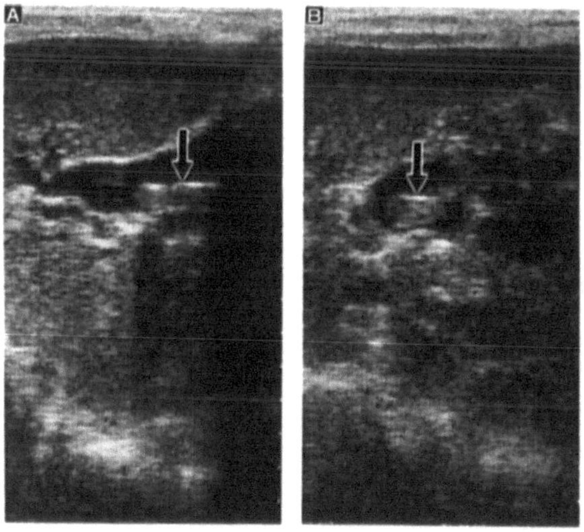

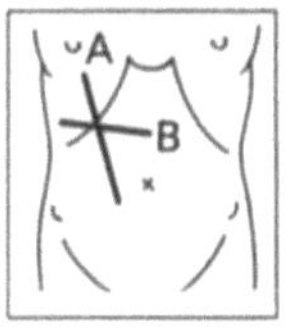

Fig. 2.36 A, B. Choledocholithiasis: common bile duct dilated to 2 cm in size in a case of postcholecystectomy and a 2 × 1 cm stone in the common bile duct (→) with acoustic shadow

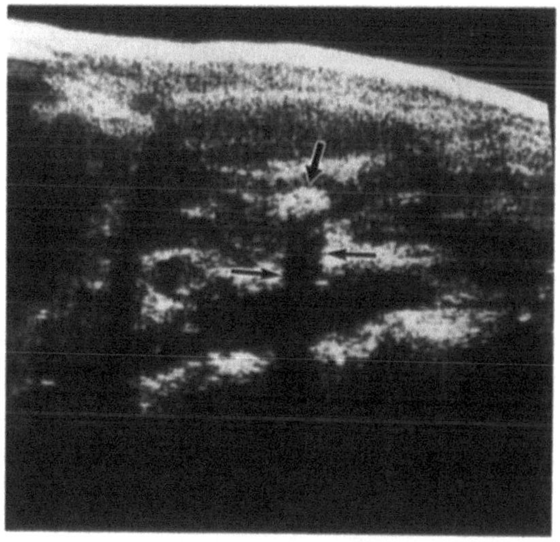

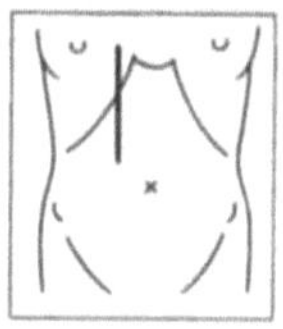

Fig. 2.37. Hepatolithiasis: 15 × 10 mm stone in left lobe with strong echo (→) associated with acoustic shadow (→). Same case as shown in Fig. 4.30

Fig. 2.38. Carcinoma of the common bile duct with markedly dilated intrahepatic bile duct (→) obstructed at the porta hepatitis (→)

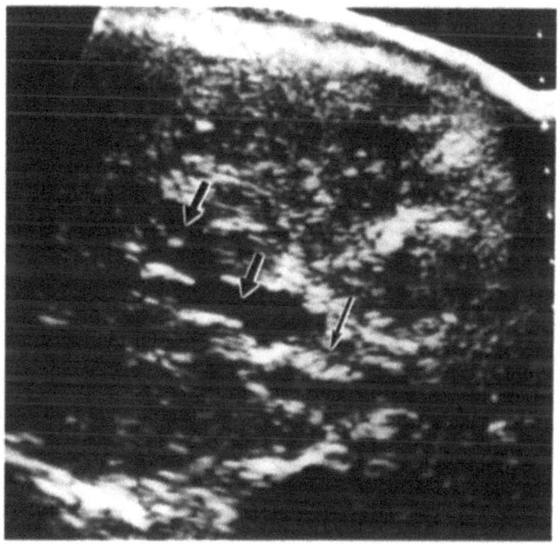

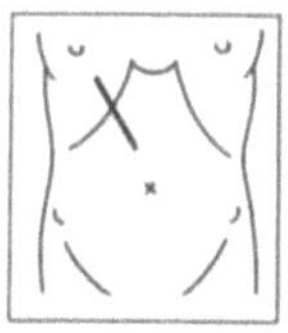

2.5 Pancreas

2.5.1 Normal Conditions. The pancreas is a rather difficult organ to visualize, and its visualization rate is supposed to be between 60% and 90% [2]. In particular, the tail of the pancreas can only be visualized 10% of the time using conventional contact scanning techniques in the supine position [55]. To obtain a fine image of the pancreas, it is generally necessary for the patient to be in the sitting position and to take 500 ml of degassed water or methylcellulose to form an acoustic window [55, 90, 93]. Even with this technique, observation of the tail of the pancreas is still not easy.

To identify the pancreas, it is important to scan the entire area using the relation of the surrounding vascular structure as aim [52, 76, 78] (Fig. 2.39). The aorta, the inferior vena cava, the superior mesenteric artery, the superior mesenteric vein, and the splenic vein are vessels used as landmarks to identify the pancreas. Ultrasonic findings of the common bile duct and the descending portion of the duodenum filled with water can also be used as fine landmarks.

The pancreas is visualized as a homogenous internal echo with the echogenicity equal to or greater than that of the liver [25] (Figs. 2.40–2.41). The echo level of pancreas depends on the grade of fatty infiltration [25, 60]. The anterior-posterior diameter of the pancreas may not exceed 18–20 mm, although this may vary according to the region [2, 33, 38, 54, 95].

The main pancreatic duct is observed as a well-defined contour with a strong echo on the long axis image of the pancreas [22]. Under normal conditions 50%–60% of the main pancreatic duct is observed (Fig. 2.42). In normal cases, the ability to visualize the duct is elevated to 84% by using secretin [66]. In cases of pancreatic carcinoma and chronic pancreatitis, the main pancreatic duct is more visible. The diameter of the main pancreatic duct is below 0.8 mm in normal cases.

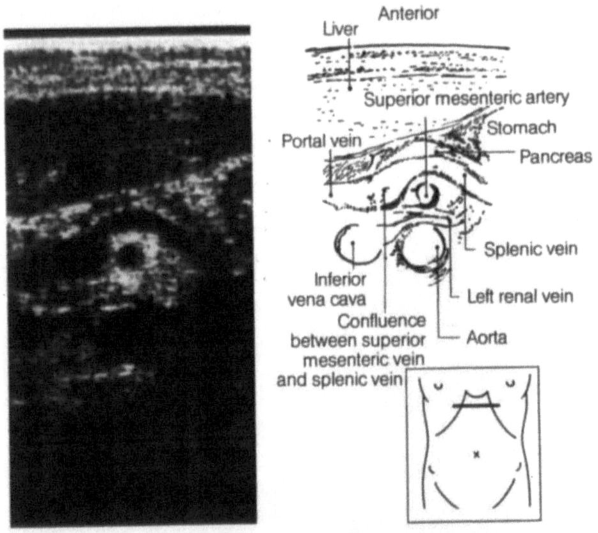

Fig. 2.39. Vasculature surrounding the pancreas

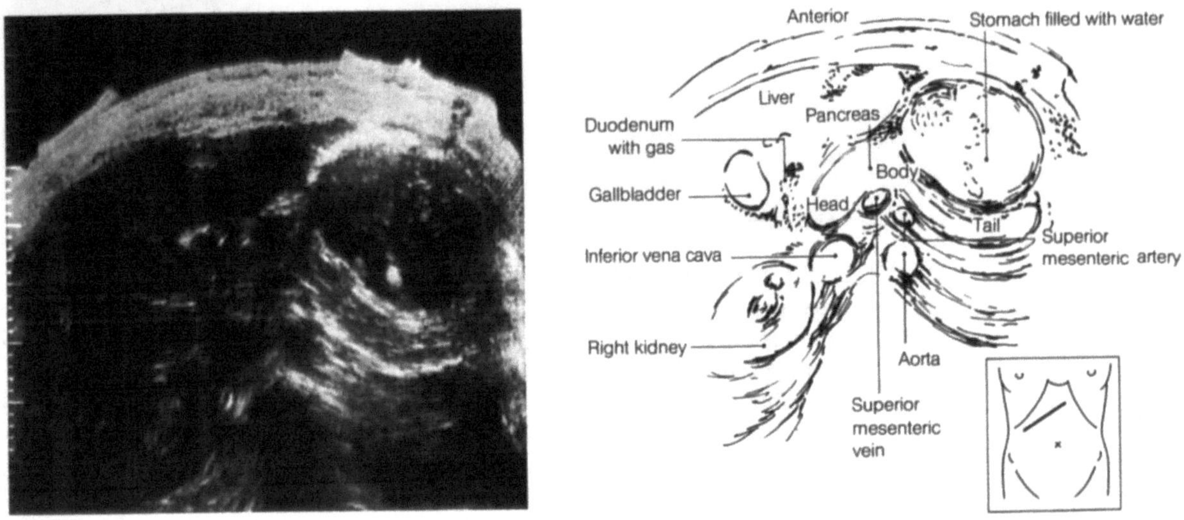

Fig. 2.40. Normal pancreas with strong echo in the pancreatic tail due to posterior enhancement from water in the stomach

Fig. 2.41. Normal pancreas

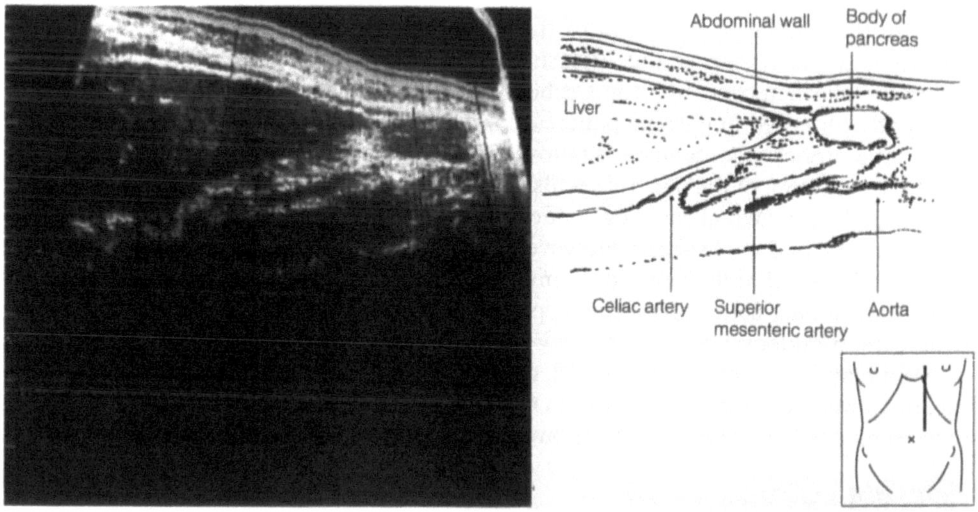

Fig. 2.42. Normal pancreatic duct: main pancreatic duct with tubular image (→) in the body of pancreas (→)

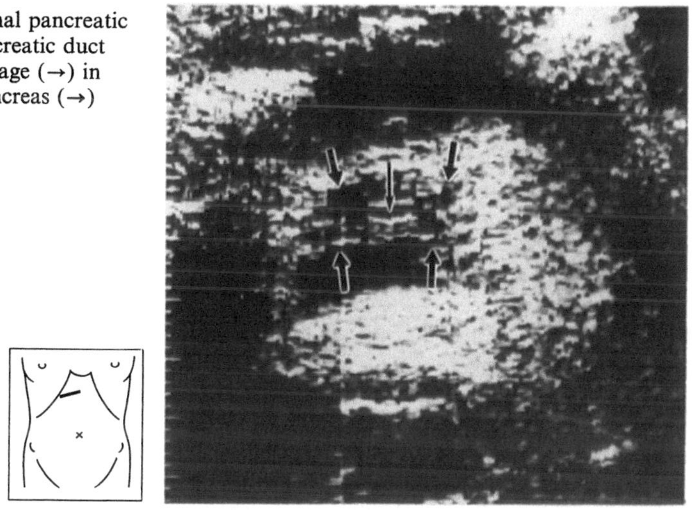

Unfamiliarity with ultrasonic diagnosis may result in confusing the splenic vein running parallel to the pancreas with the main pancreatic duct. The fat pad surrounding the pancreas and the posterior wall of the stomach may be visualized as a tubular image and is also apt to be confused with the main pancreatic duct so that much care is needed.

Valuable information in diagnosing the pancreas is provided by its diameter, shape, the condition of the internal echo, and the image of the main pancreatic duct. This information makes screening examinations possible in 87% of cases [54].

2.5.2 Pathologcial Conditions. In the case of acute pancreatitis, a swollen and edematous pancreas is visualized, and the level of the internal echo decreases (Fig. 2.43). An adequate examination is often impossible because of obstruction by intestinal gas caused by the pancreatitis.

In the case of chronic pancreatitis, swelling may be visible and sometimes irregular contours can also be observed. Chronic pancreatitis may result in the finding of dilatation of the main pancreatic duct, which frequently is the only sign of this disease [99] (Fig. 2.44). Pancreatic stones, which are characterized by bright echoes and acoustic shadows [97], are frequently observed in chronic pancreatitis. However, in the case of small pancreatic stones, the acoustic shadow may occasionally remain unobserved. Pseudocyst of the pancreas is also a fine indicator for ultrasographic diagnosis. The typical ultrasonographic appearance is sharply defined with a smooth wall and ovoid shape. However, atypical findings may be encountered, such as multiple septations, multiple echoes within a sonolucent mass, and nonacoustic enhancement posterior to pseudocyst [51]. Extrapancreatic pseudocyst may be misdiagnosed as other disorders [17].

Pancreatic carcinoma, if advanced, can also be diagnosed at quite a high rate on ultrasonographic examination. Characteristic findings of pancreatic carcinoma are the image of focal enlargement and irregular contours with

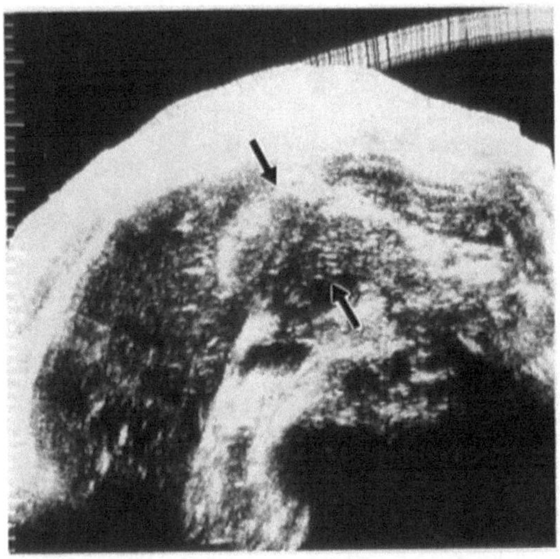

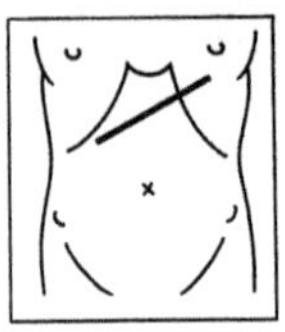

Fig. 2.43. Acute pancreatitis: the anteroposterior width of the head of the pancreas is swollen to 25 mm (→) with a lower echo level than in liver parenchyma 12 days after attack

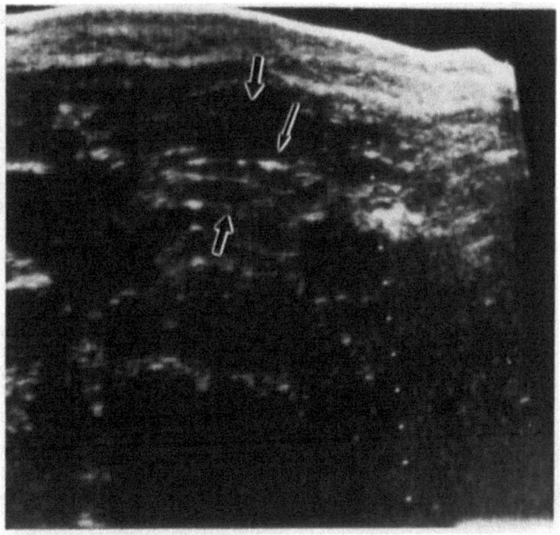

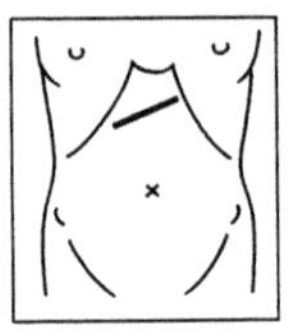

Fig. 2.44. Chronic pancreatitis: swelling in the body of the pancreas (→) and dilated main pancreatic duct (→)

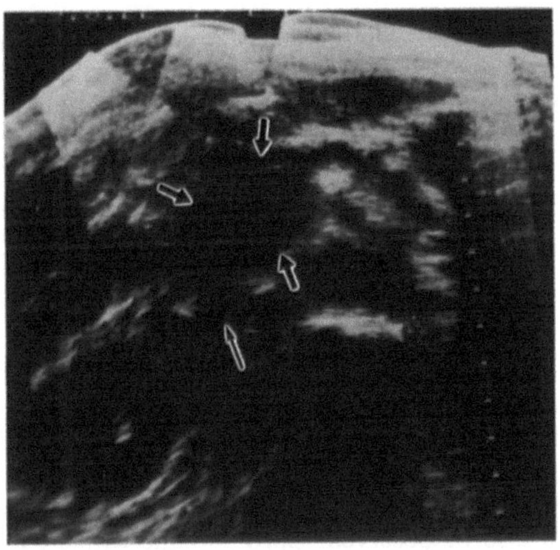

Fig. 2.45. Carcinoma of the head of the pancreas: swelling with uneven inner echo (→) lower than in the body of the pancreas and displacement of the inferior vena cava (→)

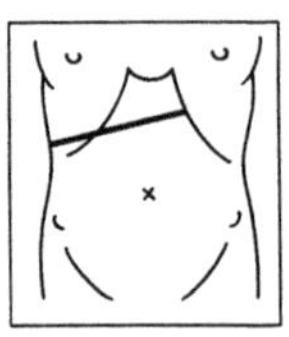

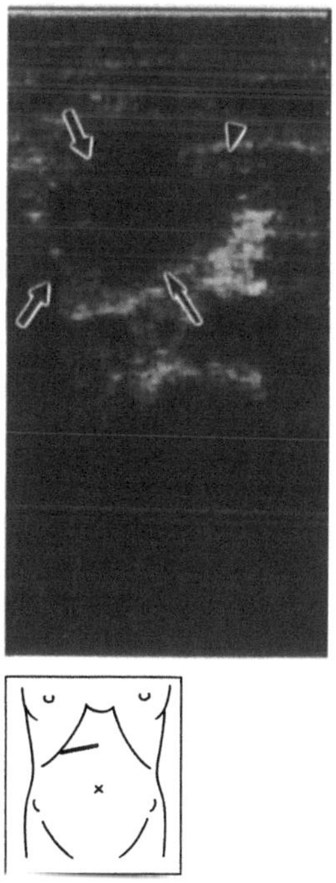

Fig. 2.46. Carcinoma of the head of the pancreas: swelling of the head of the pancreas (→) with coarse uneven echo slightly lower than in the normal portion. Displacement of the vena cava (→) and the main pancreatic duct (▶) can be seen. Same case as shown in Fig. 4.42

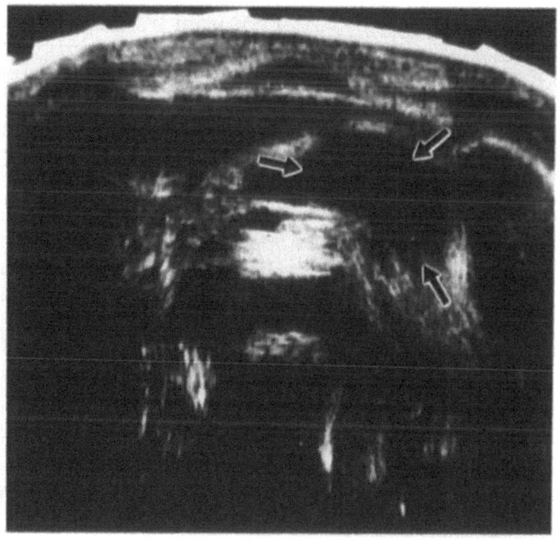

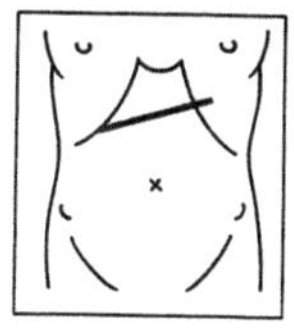

Fig. 2.47. Carcinoma of the body and tail of the pancreas: mass echo between the body and tail of the pancreas (→) with swelling and a slightly lower level and coarser internal echo than in the normal portion

inhomogeneous internal echoes and a low echo level mass lesion in some cases [89, 104] (Figs. 2.45–2.47). If ultrasonographic mass lesions are absent, pancreatic carcinoma may be suspected indirectly if dilatation is found in the intra- and extrahepatic bile duct and the main pancreatic duct [31, 99].

Cystadenoma and cystadenocarcinoma of the pancreas may be observed as a cystic mass with septum [28] or, if the cystic area is small, as a hyperechoic mass [12, 53]. In ultrasonic diagnosis, tumor of the pancreas is occasionally difficult to distinguish from the swelling of the lymph node in the retroperitoneum.

References

Ultrasonography

1. Anderson JC, Harned RK (1977) Gray scale ultrasonography of the gallbladder: An evaluation of accuracy and report of additional ultrasound signs. AJR 129:975–977
2. Arger PH, Mulhern CB, Bonavita JA, Stauffer DM, Hale J (1979) An analysis of pancreatic sonography in suspected pancreatic disease. JCU 7:91–97
3. Arnon S, Rosenquist CJ (1976) Gray scale cholecystosonography: an evaluation of accuracy. AJR 127:817–818
4. Azimi F, Marangola JP, Bryan PJ (1977) Ultrasound evaluation of the nonvisualized gallbladder. Gastrointest Radiol 1:293–299
5. Behan M, Kazam E (1978) Sonography of the common bile duct: value of the right anterior oblique view. AJR 130:701–709
6. Bergman AB, Neiman HL, Kraut B (1979) Ultrasonographic evaluation of pericholecystic abscesses. AJR 132:201–203
7. Bernardino ME, Green B (1979) Ultrasonographic evaluation of chemotherapeutic response in hepatic metastases. Radiology 133:437–441
8. Buschi AJ, Brenbridge ANAG, Cochrane JA, Teates CD (1979) A further observation on gallbladder debris. JCU 7:152–153

9. Callen PW, Filly RA,. DeMartini WJ (1979) The left portal vein: a possible source of confusion on ultrasonograms. Radiology 130:205–206
10. Callen PW, Filly RA (1979) Ultrasonographic lacalization of the gallbladder. Radiology 133:687–691
11. Callen PW, Filly RA, Marcus FS (1980) Ultrasonography and computed tomography in the evaluation of hepatic microabscesses in the immunosuppressed patient. Radiology 136:433–434
12. Carroll B, Sample WF (1978) Pancreatic cystadenocarcinoma: CT body scan and gray scale ultrasound appearance. AJR 131:339–341
13. Carter SJ, Rutledge J, Hirsch JH, Vracko R, Chikos PM (1978) Papillary adenoma of the gallbladder: ultrasonic demonstration. JCU 6:433–435
14. Chafetz N, Filly RA (1979) Portal and hepatic veins: accuracy of margin echoes for distinguishing intrahepatic vessels. Radiology 130:725–728
15. Cimmino CV, Scott DW III (1978) Case report: benign liver tumor with central necrosis. JCU 6:119–120
16. Conrad MR, Landy MJ, Khoury M (1978) Pancreatic pseudocysts: Unusual ultrasound features. AJR 130:265–268
17. Conrad MR, Landy MJ, Janes JO (1978) Sonographic "parallel channel" sign of biliary tree enlargement in mild to moderate obstructive jaundice. AJR 130:279–286
18. Conrad MR, Janes JO, Dietchy J (1979) Significance of low level echoes within the gallbladder. AJR 132:967–972
19. Cooperberg PL (1978) High-resolution real-time ultrasound in the evaluation of the normal and obstructed biliary tract. Radiology 129:477–480
20. Dewbury, KC, Joseph AEA, Hayes S, Murray C (1979) Ultrasound in the evaluation and diagnosis of jaundice. Br J Radiol 52:276–280
21. Dewbury KC, Smith CL (1983) The misdiagnosis of common bile duct stones with ultrasound. Br J Radiol 56:625–630
22. Eisenscher A, Weill F (1979) Ultrasonic visualization of Wirsung's duct: dream or reality? JCU 7:41–44
23. Engel JM, Deitch EA, Sikkema W (1980) Gallbladder wall thickness: Sonographic accuracy and relation to disease. AJR 134:907–909
24. Filly RA, Laing FC (1978) Anatomic variation of portal venous anatomy in the porta hepatis: Ultrasonographic evaluation. JCU 6:83–89
25. Filly RA, London SS (1979) The normal pancreas: acoustic characteristics and frequency of imaging. JCU 7:121–124
26. Filly RA, Moss AA, Way LW (1979) In vitro investigation of gallstone shadowing with ultrasound tomography. JCU 7:255–262
27. Finberg HJ, Birnholz JC (1979) Ultrasound evaluation of the gallbladder wall. Radiology 133:693–698
28. Freeny PC, Weinstein CJ, Taft DA, Allen FH (1978) Cystic neoplasm of the pancreas: new angiographic and ultrasonographic findings. AJR 131:795–802
29. Goldberg BB (1976) Ultrasonic cholangiography. Radiology 118:401–404
30. Goldstein HM, Katragadda CS (1978) Prone view ultrasonography for pancreatic tail neoplasms. AJR 131:231–234
31. Gosink BB, Leopold GR (1978) The dilated pancreatic duct: ultrasonic evaluation. Radiology 126:475–478
32. Gosink, BB, Lemon, SK, Scheible W, Leopold GR (1979) Accuracy of ultrasonography in diagnosis of hepatocellular disease. AJR 133:19–23
33. De Graaff CS, Taylor KJW, Simonds BD, Rosenfield AJ (1978) Gray-scale echography of the pancreas. Radiology 129:157–161
34. Graham MF, Cooperberg, PL, Cohen MM, Burhenne HJ (1980) The size of the normal common hepatic duct following cholecystectomy: an ultrasonographic study. Radiology 135:137–139
35. Graham MF, Cooperberg PL, Cohen MM, Burhenne HJ (1981) Ultrasonographic screening of the common hepatic duct in symptomatic patients after cholecystectomy. Radiology 138:137–139
36. Green B, Bree RL, Goldstein HM, Stanley C (1977) Gray scale ultrasound evaluation of hepatic neoplasms: patterns and correlations. Radiology 124:203–208
37. Grossman, M (1978) Cholelithiasis and acoustic shadowing. JCU 6:182–184
38. Haber K, Freimanis AK, Asher WM (1976) Demonstration and dimensional analysis of the normal pancreas with gray-scale echography. AJR 126:624–628
39. Hadidi A (1979) Ultrasound findings in liver hydatid cysts. JCU 7:365–368
40. Handler, SJ (1979) Ultrasound of gallbladder wall thickening and its relation to cholecystitis, AJR 132:581–585

41. Hessler PC, Hill DS, Detorie FM, Rocco AF (1981) High accuracy sonographic recognition of gallstones. AJR 136:517–520
42. Hillman BJ, D'Orsi CJ, Smith EH, Bartrum RJ (1979) Ultrasonic appearnce of the falciform ligament. AJR 132:205–206
43. Jaffe CC, Taylor KJW (1979) The clinical impact of ultrasonic beam focusing patterns. Radiology 131:469–472
44. Joseph AEA, Dewbury KC, McGuire PG (1979) Ultrasound in the detection of chronic liver disease (the "bright liver"). Br J Radiol 52:184–188
45. Kamin PD, Bernardino ME, Green B (1979) Ultrasound manifestations of hepatocellular carcinoma. Radiology 131:459–461
46. Kane RA (1980) Ultrasonographic diagnosis of gangrenous cholecystitis and empyema of the gallbladder. Radiology 134:191–194
47. Koenigsberg M, Wiener SN, Walzer A (1979) The accuracy of sonography in the differential diagnosis of obstructive jaundice: a comparison with cholangiography. Radiology 133:157–165
48. Kurtz AB, Rubin CS, Cooper HS, Niesenbaum HL, Cole-Beuglet C, Medoff J, Goldberg BB (1980) Ultrasound findings in hepatitis. Radiology 136:717–723
49. Laing FC, Gooding GAW, Herzog KA (1977) Gallstones preventing ultrasonographic visualization of the gallbladder. Gastrointest Radiol 1:301–303
50. Laing FC, London LA, Filly RA (1978) Ultrasonographic identification of dilated intrahepatic bile ducts and their differentiation from portal venous structures. JCU 6:90–94
51. Laing FC, Gooding GAW, Brown T, Leopold GR (1979) Atypical pseudocysts of the pancreas: an ultrasonographic evaluation. JCU 7:27–33
52. Leopold, GR (1975) Gray scale ultrasonic angiography of the upper abdomen. Radiology 117:665–671
53. Lloyd TV, Antonmattei S, Freimanis AK (1979) Gray scale sonography of cystadenoma of the pancreas: report of two cases. JCU 7:149–151
54. Lowson TL (1978) Sensitivity of pancreatic ultrasonography in the detection of pancreatic disease. Radiology 128:733–736
55. MacMahon HR, Bowie JD, Beezhold C (1979) Erect scanning of pancreas using a gastric window. AJR 132:587–591
56. Malini S, Sabel J (1977) Ultrasonography in obstructive jaundice. Radiology 123:429–433
57. Marchal G, Crolla D, Baert AL, Fevery J, Kerremans R (1978) Gallbladder wall thichening: a new sign of gallbladder disease visualized by gray scale cholecystosonography. JCU 6:177–179
58. Marchal GJF, Casaer M, Baert AL, Goddeeris PG, Kerremans R, Fevery J (1979) Gallbladder wall sonolucency in acute cholecystitis. Radiology 133:429–433
59. Marks WM, Filly RA, Callen PW (1979) Ultrasonic anatomy of the liver: a review with new applications. JCU 7:137–146
60. Marks WM, Filly RA, Callen PW (1980) Ultrasonic evaluation of normal pancreatic echogenicity and its relationship to fat deposition. Radiology 137:475–479
61. McArdle, CR (1976) Ultrasonic diagnosis of liver metastases. JCU 4:265–268
62. Mindell HJ, Ring BA (1979) Gallbladder wall thickening: ultrasonic findings. Radiology 133:699–701
63. Mueller PR, Ferrucci JT Jr, Simeone JF, Wittenberg J, Van Sonnenberg E, Polansky A, Isler RJ (1981) Postcholecystectomy bile duct dilatation: myth or reality? AJR 136:355–358
64. Neiman HL, Mintzer RA (1977) Accuracy of biliary duct ultrasound: comparison with cholangiography. AJR 129:979–982
65. Newlin N, Silver TM, Stuck KJ, Sandler MA (1981) Ultrasonic features of pyogenic liver abscesses. Radiology 139:155–159
66. Ohto M, Saotome N, Saisho H, Tsuchiya Y, Ono T, Okuda K, Karasawa E (1980) Real-time sonograpy of the pancreatic duct: application to percutaneous pancreatic ductography. AJR 134:647–652
67. Olken, SM, Bledsoe R, Newmark H III (1978) The ultrasonic diagnosis of primary carcinoma of the gallbladder. Radiology 129:481–482
68. Palframan A (1979) Real-time ultrasound. A new method for studying gall-bladder kinetics. Br J Radiol 52:801–803
69. Parulekar SG (1979) Ligaments and fissures of the liver: sonographic anatomy. Radiology 130:409–411
70. Parulekar SG (1979) Ultrasond evaluation of common bile duct size. Radiology 133:703–707
71. Perlmutter GS, Goldberg BB (1976) Ultrasonic evaluation of the common bile duct. JCU 4:107–111

72. Prando A, Goldstein HM, Bernardino ME, Green B (1979) Ultrasonic pseudolesions of the liver. Radiology 130:403–407
73. Purdon RC, Thomas SR, Kereiakes JG, Spitz HB, Goldenberg NJ, Krugh KB (1980) Ultrasonic properties of biliary calculi. Radiology 136:729–732
74. Raptopoulos VD (1980) Ultrasonic pseudocalculus effect in postcholecystectomy patients. AJR 134:145–148
75. Ruhe AH, Zachman JP, Mulder BD, Rime AE (1979) Cholesterol polyps of the gallbladder: ultrasound demonstration. JCU 7:386–388
76. Sample WF (1977) Techniques for improved delineation of normal anatomy of the upper abdomen and high retroperitoneum with gray-scale ultrasound. Radiology 124:197–202
77. Sample WF, Sarti DA, Goldstein LI, Weiner M, Kadell BM (1978) Gray-scale ultrasonography of the jaundiced patient. Radiology 128:719–725
78. Sanders RC, Conrad MR, White RI Jr (1977) Normal and abnormal upper abdominal venous structures as seen by ultrasound. AJR 128:657–662
79. Schabel, SI, Rittenberg, GM, Javid LH, Cunningham J, Ross P (1980) The "bull's-eye" falciform ligament: a sonographic finding of portal hypertension. Radiology 136:157–159
80. Scheible W, Gosink BB, Leopold GR (1977) Gray scale echographic patterns of hepatic metastatic disease. AJR 129:983–987
81. Shlaer WJ, Leopold GR, Scheible FW (1981) Sonography of the thickened gallbladder wall: a nonspecific finding. AJR 136:337–339
82. Simeone JF, Mueller PR, Ferrucci JT Jr, Harbin WP, Wittenberg J (1980) Significance of nonshadowing focal opacities at cholecystosonography. Radiology 137:181–185
83. Sones, PJ Jr, Torres WE (1978) Normal ultrasonic appearance of the ligamentum teres and falciform ligament. JCU 6:392–394
84. Spiegel, RM, King DL, Green WM (1978) Ultrasonography of primary cysts of the liver. AJR 131:235–238
85. Sukov RJ, Sample WF, Sarti DA, Whitcomb MJ (1979) Cholecystosonography – The junctional fold. Radiology 133:435–436
86. Taylor KJW, Carpernter DA (1975) The anatomy and pathology of the porta hepatis by gray scale ultrasonography. JCU 3:117–119
87. Taylor KJW, Carpenter DA, Hill CR, McCready VR (1976) Gray scale ultrasound imaging. The anatomy and pathology of the liver. Radiology 119:415–423
88. Taylor KJW, Jacobson P, Jaffe CC (1979) Lack of an acoustic shadow on scans of gallstones: a possible artifact. Radiology 131:463–464
89. Walls WJ, Templeton AW (1977) The ultrasonic demonstration of inferior vena caval compression: a guide to pancreatic head enlargement with emphasis on neoplasm. Radiology 123:165–167
90. Waren PS, Garrett WJ, Kosoff G (1978) The liquid-filled stomach – An ultrasonic window to the upper abdomen. JCU 6:315–320
91. Weaver RM Jr, Goldstein HM, Green B, Perkins C (1978) Gray scale ultrasonographic evaluation of hepatic cystic desease. AJR 130:849–852
92. Weeks LE, McCune BR, Martin JF, O'Brien TF (1978) Differential diagnosis of intrahepatic shadowing on ultrasound examination JCU 6:399–401
93. Weighall SL, Wolfman NT, Watson N (1979) The fluid-filled stomach: a new sonic window. JCU 7:353–356
94. Weill F, Eisenscher A, Aucant D, Bourgoin A, Gallinet D (1975) Ultrasonic study of venous patterns in the right hypochondrium: an anatomical approach to differential diagnosis of obstructive jaundice. JCU 3:23–28
95. Weill F, Schraub A, Eisenscher A, Bourgoin A (1977) Ultrasonography of the normal pancreas. Radiology 123:417–423
96. Weill F, Eisencher, A, Zeltner F (1978) Ultrasonic study of the normal and dilated biliary tree. The "Shotgun" sign. Radiology 127:221–224
97. Weinstein BJ, Weinstein DP, Brodmerkel GJ (1980) Ultrasonography of pancreatic lithiasis. Radiology 134:185–189
98. Weinstein BJ, Weinstein DP (1980) Biliary tract dilatation in the nonjaundiced patient. AJR 134:899–906
99. Weinstein DP, Weinstein BJ (1979) Ultrasonic demonstration of the pancreatic duct: an analysis of 41 cases. Radiology 130:729–734
100. Weinstein DP, Weinstein BJ, Brodmerkel GJ (1979) Ultrasonography of biliary tract dilatation without jaundice. AJR 132:729–734
101. Whitley NO, Cunningham JJ (1978) Angiographic and echographic findings in avascular focal nodular hyperplasia of the liver. AJR 130:777–779

102. Willi UV, Teele RL (1979) Hepatic arteries and the parallel-channel sign. JCU 7:125–127
103. Wooten WB, Green B, Goldstein HM (1978) Ultrasonography of necrotic hepatic metastases. Radiology 128:447–450
104. Wright CH, Maklad F, Rosenthal SJ (1979) Grey-scale ultrasonic characteristics of carcinoma of the pancreas. Br J Radiol 52:281–288
105. Yeh HC (1979) Ultrasonograhy and computed tomography of carcinoma of the gallbladder. Radiology 133:167–173
106. Zeman RK, Dorfman GS, Burrell MI, Stein S, Berg GR, Gold JA (1981) Disparate dilatation of the intrahepatic and extrahepatic bile ducts in surgical jaundice. Radiology 138:129–136

3 Nuclear Examination

3.1 Colloid Liver Scintigraphy

Nowadays, about one-third of examinations by radioisotopic imaging are accounted for by colloid liver scintigraphy. Even though this method is used at a high rate of frequency, some believe it to be less efficient for detecting lesions. Scintigraphy is noninvasive, and undoubtedly this technique is easy if complete equipment is available.

Detectable mass lesions situated deep in the right lobe of the liver are regarded to exceed 3–4 cm in size, although smaller lesions such as 1 cm can be detected in the thin portion of the liver. Accordingly, liver scintigraphy is frequently used with X-ray computed tomography (CT) or ultrasonography rather than independently.

At present, the diagnostic accuracy of liver scintigraphy is considered to be 75%–80%; the false-positive rate is 15%–25% and the false-negative rate 6%–25% [13, 20, 26]. To improve the diagnostic accuracy of liver scintigraphy, it is advisable to use tomography scanning simultaneously [18, 30]. Examples of this method are the collimator shifting method, the seven pinhole collimator method [29], and single photon emission CT [15] (Fig. 3.1).

3.1.1 Examination Procedures. The image quality of scintigraphy depends upon the performance of the scinticamera. Nowadays, the Anger-type gamma camera has been improved to obtain a wide field, the efficient viewing field has been enlarged up to 39–42 cm, and because of the increased resolution power of 1.4–2 mm of the scinticamera, the image quality has been greatly improved. A higher diagnostic image quality of scintigrams can be obtained not only by using the high-quality scinticamera but also by choosing an adequate collimator and appropriate setting of the distance between organs and the collimator and the pulse-height analyzer window setting according to the energy of the radiopharmaceuticals used.

The colloid liver scintigram utilizes the isotope injected intravenously and phagocyted by the reticuloendothelial cell (Kupffer's cell) in the liver. In other words, it shows the distribution of Kupffer's cells in the liver. In the normal liver, dense homogeneous scintigrams can be obtained because cells are invariably disposed homogeneously and the phagocyted radiocolloids on the Kupffer's cells are seldom excreted. However, in the case of space-occupying lesions, such as tumors, abscesses, and cysts of the liver, the Kupffer's cells are nonexisitent, and this corresponding area causes a defected image on the scintigram.

In diffuse parenchymal liver disease, such as liver cirrhosis, which has an abnormal distribution of reticuloendothelial cells, the configuration or distribution of the radiocolloids may be informative for diagnosis.

Formerly, ^{198}Au was used as a radiocolloid. Recently, short half-life ^{99m}Tc-labeled colloids, such as ^{99m}Tc-sulfur colloid and ^{99m}Tc-tin colloid, have been used [8]. Colloidizing in the blood can be performed by administering ^{99m}Tc-phytate, which is another method. Advantages of ^{99m}Tc are a short half-life and low gamma ray energy. In comparison to 0.41 MeV of gamma rays radiated from ^{198}Au, the gamma ray energy is only 0.14 MeV with ^{99m}Tc. High-quality images in resolution can be obtained due to the fact that the short half-life of 6 h can increase the dose to 1–3 mCi in comparison to the 150–400 μCi of ^{198}Au. In addition, the dose absorbed

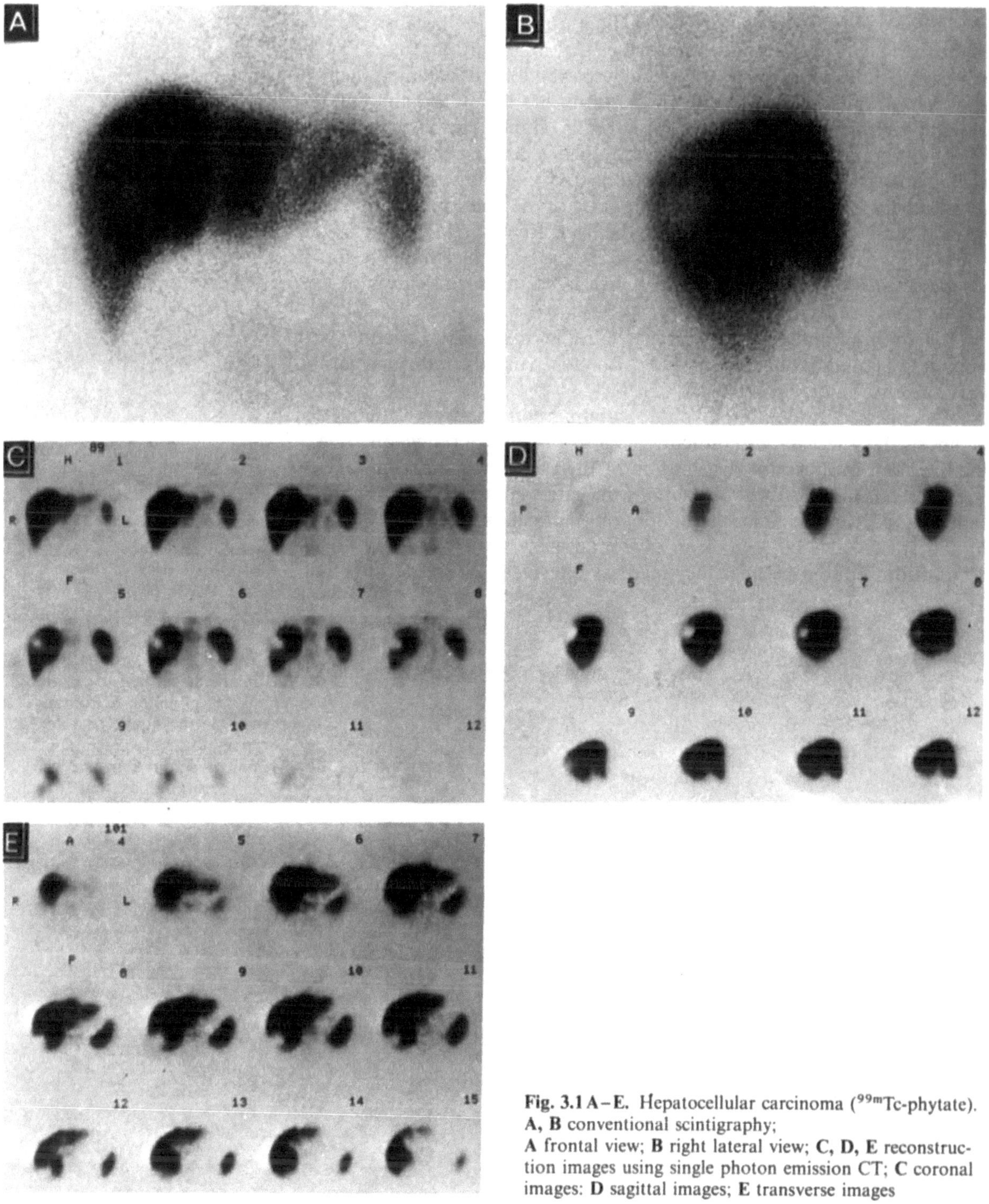

Fig. 3.1 A–E. Hepatocellular carcinoma (^{99m}Tc-phytate). **A, B** conventional scintigraphy; **A** frontal view; **B** right lateral view; **C, D, E** reconstruction images using single photon emission CT; **C** coronal images: **D** sagittal images; **E** transverse images

of only 0.7–1 rad is small (1/6–1/25) while it is 6–24 rad using the ^{198}Au colloid.

Photographing must be done 10–20 min after intravenous injection when the colloid has sufficiently accumulated in the liver. It is appropriate to photograph after 30–60 min in patients with cardiac failure or lowered liver clearance due to liver dysfunction. Delayed photographing will decrease efficiency because of the short half-life of ^{99m}Tc.

The erect or sitting position is convenient for imaging because the area of the liver facing the camera widens with the sitting position (Fig. 3.2). The scinticamera must be set up to view the upper abdomen including the liver and spleen. The photographing projections are frontal, right anterior oblique, right lateral, left lateral, left anterior olique, and posterior views. The photographing conditions are determined according to the amount of radiopharmaceuticals injected and the sensitivity of the scinticamera. The scinticamera must be set under consideration of the relation with the background count and maximum count in the liver. Removing the background count allows a fine image to be obtained, but too much removal results in disappearance of the bone marrow, which is useful for diagnosis of liver cirrhosis.

Liver scintigraphy is often ineffective in the diagnosis of patients with obstructive jaundice or hepatitis, and it is better to use (excretory) hepatobiliary scintigraphy (see Sect. 3.3.).

Awareness of the different photographing conditions is valuable for diagnosis. It is necessary to estimate the position, morphology, and size of the liver and intrahepatic distribution of the radioisotope and uptake by organs other than the liver. To examine the extrahepatic distribution of the radioisotope, careful choice of radiopharmaceuticals is required. The image of the spleen can be seen from a frontal view with the ^{99m}Tc-tin or ^{99m}Tc-sulfur colloid because they increase the spleen uptake. Conversely,

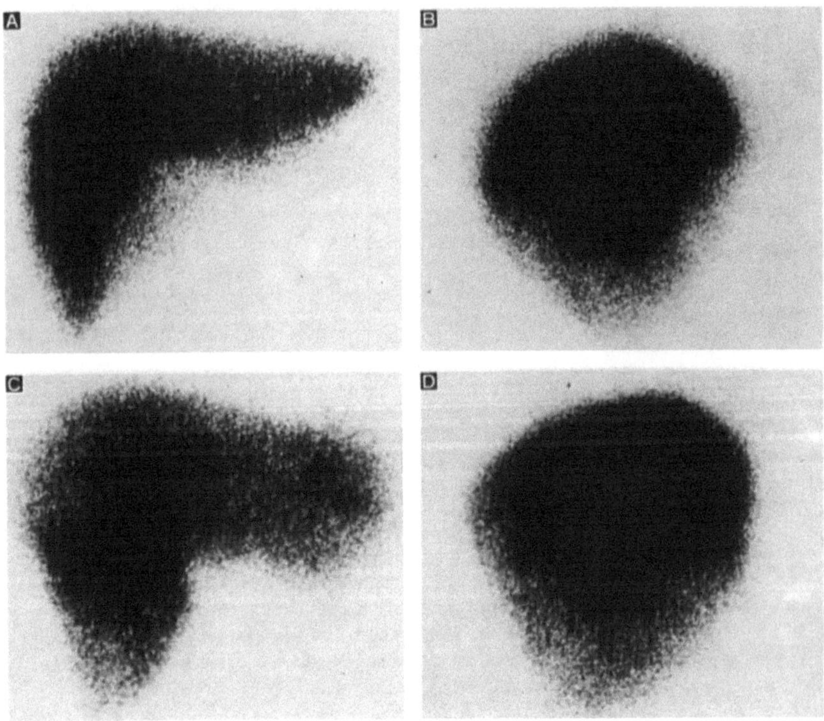

Fig. 3.2 A–D. Differences of images according to position (^{99m}Tc-phytate). **A** frontal view in the supine position; **B** right lateral view in the supine position; **C** frontal view in the sitting position; **D** right lateral view in the sitting position

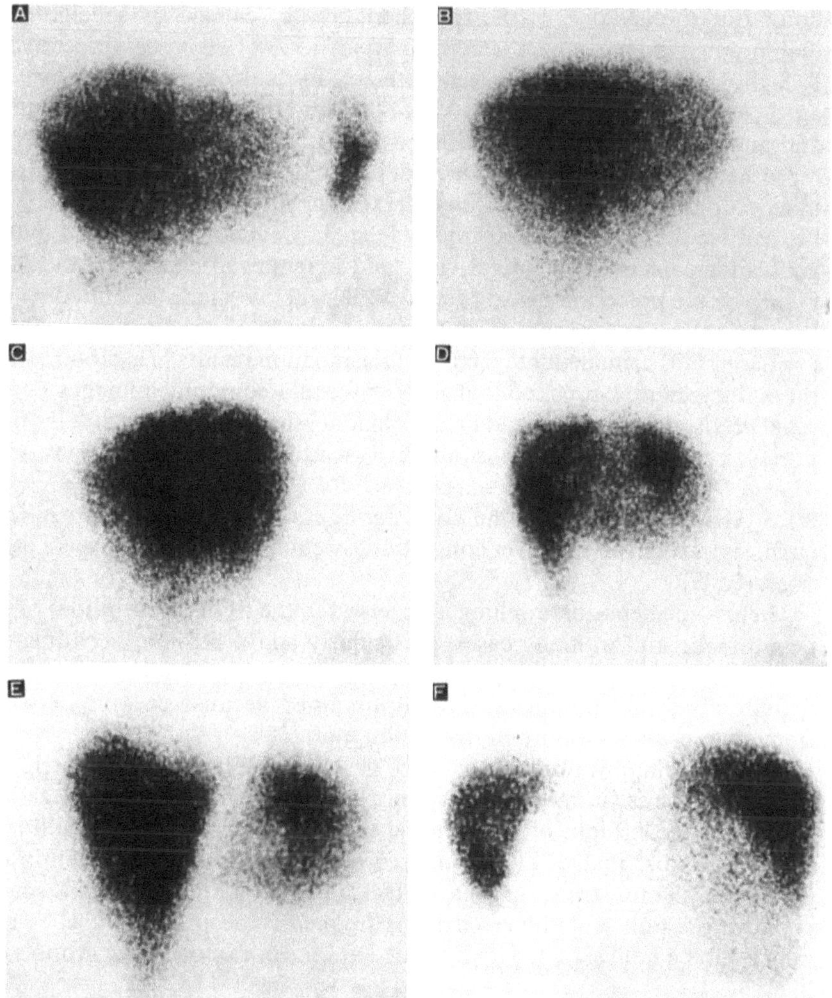

Fig. 3.3 A–F. Normal liver (sitting position) (^{99m}Tc-Sn colloid). **A** frontal view; **B** right anterior oblique view; **C** right lateral view; **D** left lateral view; **E** left anterior oblique view; **F** posterior view

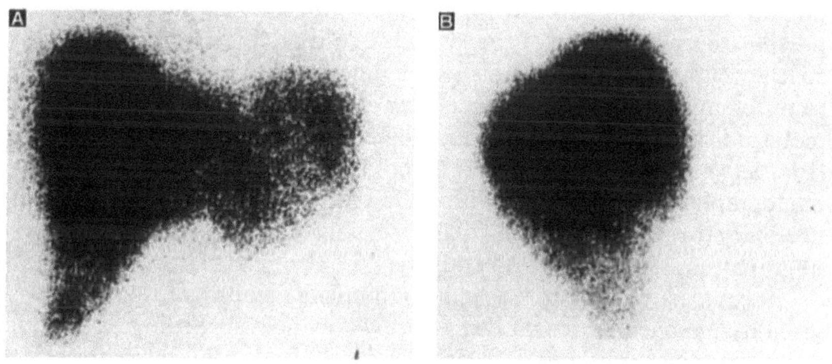

Fig. 3.4 A, B. Expansion of the right lobe to the intrathoracic cavity (^{99m}Tc-phytate). **A** frontal view; **B** right lateral view

with the ^{99m}Tc-phytate or the ^{198}Au colloid, the image of the spleen is normally invisible and if observable can be diagnosed as an abnormal finding [1].

3.1.2 Normal Findings in the Liver. Figure 3.3 shows a scintigram of a normal liver. Images of the normal liver vary [21, 23] and are observed as triangular in about 40% of cases. Other types of liver morphology are a notable indentation at the porta hepatis, a square shape, and a prominent dome due to elevation of the right hepatic lobe caused by a heightened diaphragm, which can be observed in about 15% of all cases, respectively. A high dome in the liver is often observed in females and particularly in aged patients (Fig. 3.4). About 40% of the right lateral views are triangular and another 40% are diamond shaped.

Other examples of various forms of normal findings of the liver [3, 6] are indentations caused by the gallbladder, the porta hepatis, hepatic vein, or the cardiac fossa on the frontal view (Fig. 3.5), indentation caused by the gallbladder on the right lateral view, and indentation caused by the right kigney on the posterior view. In females, obstructive shadows caused by the breasts may be recognized on images photographed in the sitting position.

Using ^{99m}Tc, inadequate mixing of the medium results in excretion from the kidney caused by uncolloidized ^{99m}Tc, and sometimes images of the renal pelvis, urinary tract, and urinary bladder may be visualized. It is of the utmost importance to diagnose the liver scintigram adequately.

3.1.3 Abnormal Findings in the Liver. In the cases of chronic hepatitis, liver cirrhosis, fatty liver, and liver congestion, swelling of the entire liver is often observed [7].

In chronic hepatitis, swelling is observed in the right or both sides of the hepatic lobe and in many cases, particularly active chronic hepatitis, the uptake of the radioisotope into the spleen increases. In general, however, definite abnormal findings are rarely obtained because chronic hepatitis frequently presents a normal liver scintigram.

Focal swelling is observed in cases of Riedel's lobe [19], liver cirrhosis, tumor, or abscess in the liver. Liver cirrhosis (Fig. 3.6) is characterized by swelling in the left lobe of the liver and the spleen, atrophy of the right lobe of the liver, and images of bone marrow. Radiocolloid distribution in the liver often demonstrates uneven images and may be misread as a space-occupying lesion [16]. Liver cirrhosis frequently occurs with ascites and may exhibit a halo sign due to decreased uptake of radioactivity around the liver.

On the other hand, in cases of tumor or abscess in the liver, the cold area (area of decreased uptake of radiocolloids) on the image is visualized proportionate to the extent of the lesion. A cold area is observed not only in space-occupying lesions but also sometimes in liver cirrhosis. It is difficult to differentiate between hepatocellular carcinoma (Figs. 3.1, 3.7, and 3.8), metastatic liver carcinoma (Fig. 3.9), liver abscess (Fig. 3.10), and liver cyst (Fig. 3.11), which are observed as cold area images [22]. Radioisotope angiography or scintigraphy with ^{67}Ga-citrate or ^{75}Se-selenomethionine is necessary for these differential diagnoses. In addition, X-ray CT or ultrasonography must be used consecutively.

In contrast to the entire swelling, complete atrophy of the liver is often visualized in aged patiens. Liver atrophy advances according to age due to decreasing liver cells and is sometimes recognized in liver cirrhosis.

3.2 Radioisotope Angiography of the Liver

Radioisotope angiography is also helpful for examination of the liver. It is performed by photographing the serial liver scintigram after an intravenous injection of ^{99m}Tc-labeled human serum albumin or ^{99m}Tc colloid [4]. To acquire these sequential scintigrams of the liver, it is necessary to photograph continuously using a multiformat camera or recording with a video

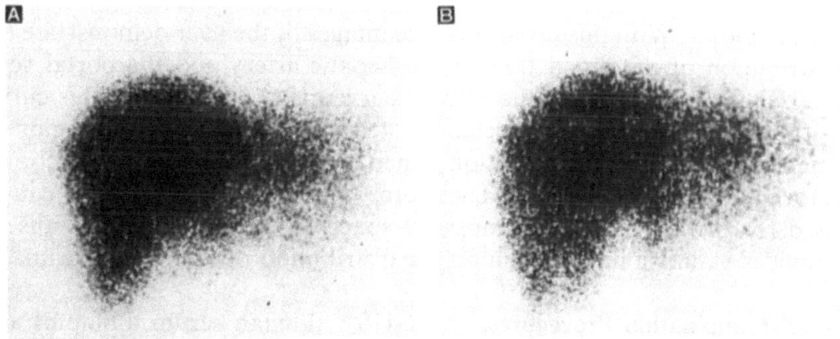

Fig. 3.5 A, B. Gallbladder indentation and cardiac fossa (^{99m}Tc-phytate). **A** frontal view; **B** right anterior oblique view

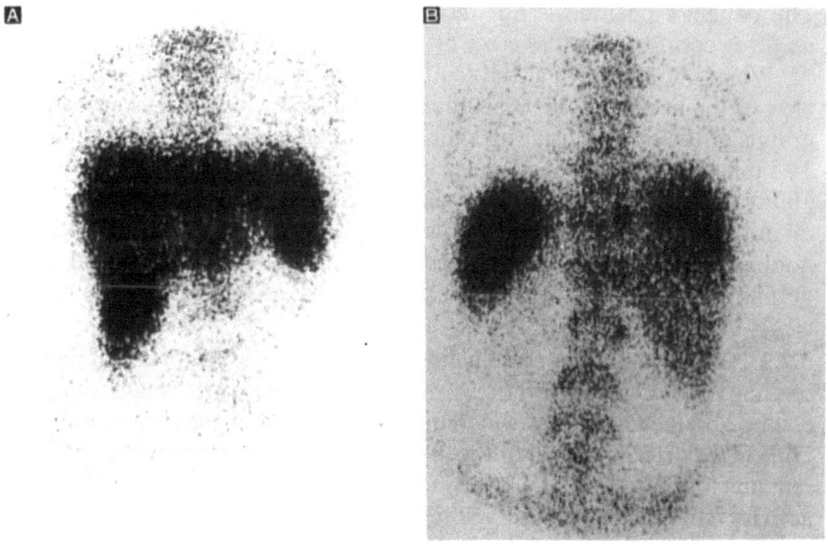

Fig. 3.6 A, B. Liver cirrhosis (^{99m}Tc-phytate). **A** frontal view; **B** posterior view

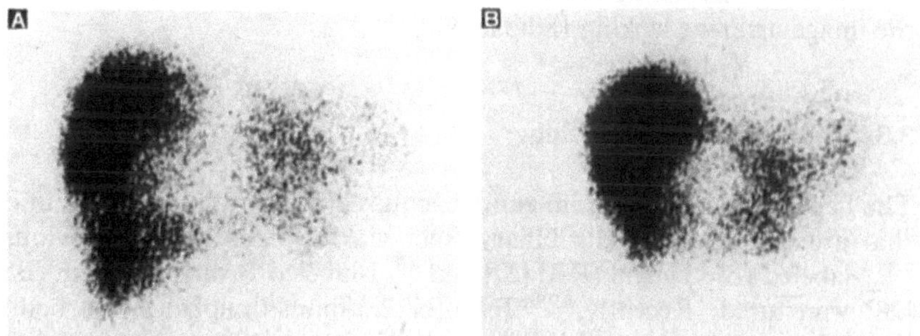

Fig. 3.7 A, B. Hepatocellular carcinoma (^{99m}Tc-phytate). **A** frontal view; **B** right anterior oblique view

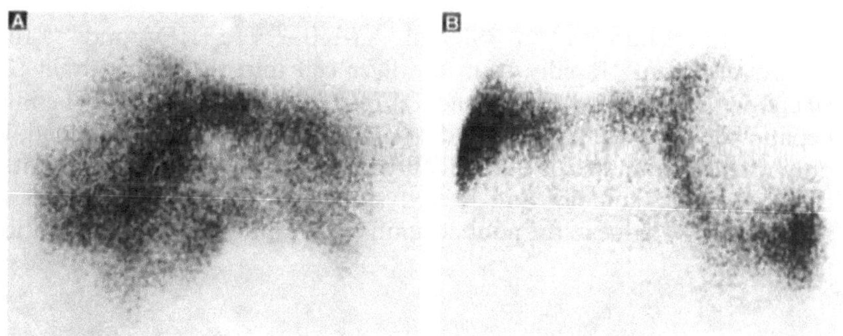

Fig. 3.8 A, B. Hepatocellular carcinoma (^{99m}Tc-phytate). **A** frontal view; **B** posterior view

tape recorder. With this procedure, the images of the liver demonstrate the distribution of the blood flow of the hepatic artery and the portal vein.

Using a computer, a time-activity curve may be obtained. This curve, with time, demonstrates the change of isotope activity of the region of interest and exhibits the condition of hepatic blood flow so that functional information can be obtained. Therefore, radioisotope angiography can be used for the differential diagnosis of space-occupying lesions because it provides valuable information on the distribution of the bloodstream.

3.2.1 Examination Procedures. ^{99m}Tc-HSA (human serum albumin) and ^{99m}Tc-sulfur colloid are used as radiopharmaceuticals. They may be intravenously injected at a normal speed, and bolus injection is not necessary. The patient's position is not restricted; the supine position is frequently used for comfort, but the erect or sitting position is also suitable.

While photographing, the scinticamera must be set to cover the entire view of the liver, and the heart must be shielded with a lead screen. Photographs of the liver scintigram should be taken every 1–3 s consistently for 3–4 min. Using the ^{99m}Tc-labeled colloid, a static image must also be taken about 10 min after the injection when the colloid has been sufficiently taken up into the reticuloendothelial cells in the liver. Using ^{99m}Tc-HSA, the liver pool scintigram can be obtained 6–7 min after routine serial photographing, which is often useful for the diagnosis of hemangioma of the liver.

3.2.2 Normal and Abnormal Findings. The image of the aorta can be visualized 2–5 s after the intravenous injection, and the entire image of the liver can be obtained after 4–5 s including the small intestinal tract and kidney. During the arterial phases of the liver image, the radioactivity of the isotope remains low. In cases of a hypovascular lesion, the areas devoid of radioactivity can be clearly observed.

The concentration of the isotope in the liver greatly increases on the image during the venous phase 10–20 s after the injection. During the venous phase, hypovascular lesions often cannot be observed distinctly on the image as areas lacking radioactivity.

3.3. Hepatobiliary Scintigraphy

The hepatobiliary scintigram can be acquired using radiopharmaceuticals that are excreted into the biliary tract via the hepatic cell. Previously, ^{131}I-labeled rose bengal (RB) [27] and ^{131}I-labeled Bromsulphalein (BSP) [28] were used. Recently, ^{99m}Tc-N-[N'(2,6-diamethylphenyl) carboamyl methyl] iminodiacetic acid (HIDA) [11] and ^{99m}Tc-pyridoxylideneiso-leucine (PI) [17] have almost always been used. ^{99m}Tc-HIDA is similar to ^{131}I-BSP and ^{99m}Tc-PI is close to ^{131}I-RB regarding biological dynamics.

In comparison with ^{131}I-BSP and ^{131}I-RB, ^{99m}Tc-HIDA and ^{99m}Tc-PI are excreted more rapidly from the liver cell into the biliary tract [24]. Therefore, using ^{99m}Tc-HIDA and ^{99m}Tc-PI, superior images of the intrahepatic bile duct, gallbladder, and common bile duct can be obtained, but only when no jaundice or other disturbance of liver function is present. In cases of severe jaundice and liver dysfunction, high-quality images are seldom achieved due to the poor accumulation of the radiopharmaceuticals in the liver.

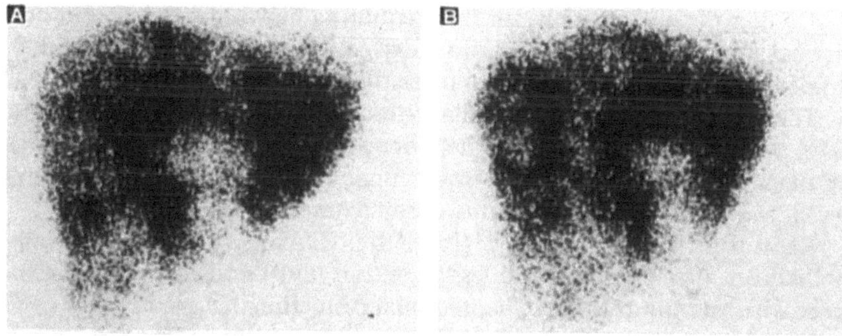

Fig. 3.9 A, B. Metastatic carcinoma from malignant lymphoma (^{99m}Tc-phytate). **A** frontal view; **B** right anterior oblique view. Same case as shown in Figs. 2.16 and 4.17

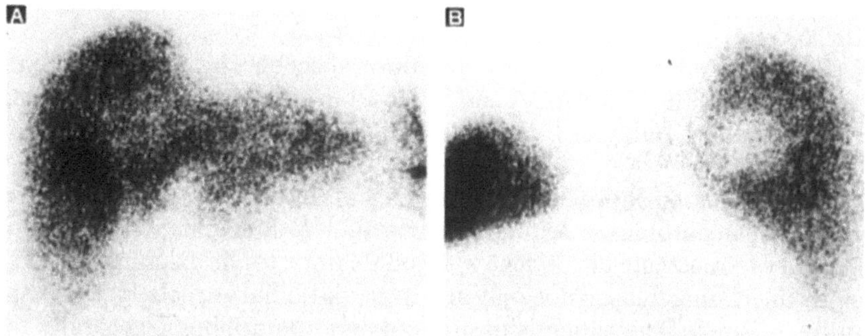

Fig. 3.10 A, B. Liver abscess (^{99m}Tc-phytate). **A** frontal view; **B** posterior view

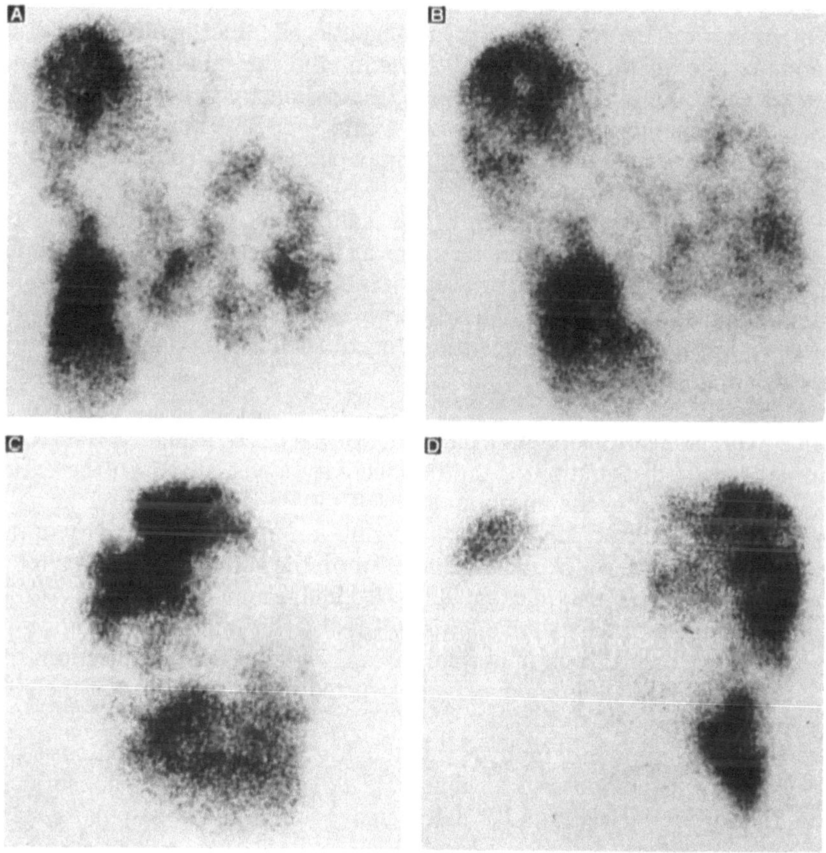

Fig. 3.11 A–D. Polycystic disease of the liver (^{99m}Tc-phytate). **A** frontal view; **B** right anterior oblique view; **C** right lateral view; **D** posterior view

^{99m}Tc is disadvantageous for differentiating between surgical and nonsurgical jaundice, which requires a long period of time, because the 6 h physical half-life of ^{99m}Tc is far shorter than the 8 days of ^{131}I.

The excretion rate into the biliary tract of ^{99m}Tc-HIDA is as high as 60%; about 20% excretion into the kidney may be an obstacle in diagnosing the scintigram. In cases of liver dysfunction, the isotope excretion into the kidney increases rendering this obstacle more serious.

Recently, ^{99m}Tc-E-HIDA (^{99m}Tc-diethyl-IDA) [31], which is absorbed by the liver at a high rate with less excretion into the urinary system, has been used, and the analysis of hepatobiliary function has greatly improved.

Furthermore, the time-activity curve of the region of interest can be obtained with a computer by memorizing the time-sequential scintigram, the so-called blood-clearance curve. The residual rate of ^{99m}Tc-HIDA in the blood 5 min after the injection is about $32\% \pm 4.9\%$ and $5.1\% \pm 2.8\%$ after 60 min.

In hepatobiliary scintigraphy, the dose absorbed by the liver is only 0.06–0.7 rad with ^{99m}Tc-HIDA and ^{99m}Tc-PI in comparison to 0.5 rad with ^{131}I-RB and 0.2 rad with ^{131}I-BSP.

3.3.1 Examination Procedures. Isotopic agents should be injected intravenously. In hepatobiliary scintigraphy using ^{131}I-RB and ^{131}I-BSP, it is necessary to medicate the patient with iodide prior to the examination. The scinticamera must cover not only the liver and biliary tracts but also the entire abdomen. The patient's position for photographing is generally the frontal projection, but in some cases the right anterior oblique or right lateral projection may be required. The duration of photographing depends upon the type and quality of the radiopharmaceuticals.

Using ^{99m}Tc-HIDA (Fig 3.12), the image of the liver is visualized 3–15 min after the injection; the intrahepatic bile duct, gallbladder, and common bile duct appear after 10–30 min, and the small intestine is observed after 30 min. After 90–120 min, the radioactivity is almost entirely excreted from the liver parenchyma. Using ^{131}I-BSP and ^{131}I-RB with nonexcreting function, the scintigram may occasionally be obtained 24 or 48 h after the injection.

In addition, the contraction of the gallbladder can be examined by administering a cholecystokinetic agent at the time when the gallbladder image is clearly visualized. In this case, it is necessary to photograph 60 min after administration of yolk or a drug with a similar function or 10–15 min after an intravenous injection with an agent such as Caerulein (ceruletide diethylamine).

3.3.2 Normal and Abnormal Findings. In normal cases, using ^{99m}Tc-HIDA, homogeneous distribution of the radioactivity is visualized on the entire liver 3–15 min after the injection; after 10–30 min, the image of the gallbladder can be observed with dense distribution of the radioactivity in the porta hepatis. After a period of 20–120 min, the radioactivity is excreted into the small intestinal tract, and a banded image may be observed. At this time, the image of the gallbladder is still visible without administration of a contractive agent. Even in normal cases, 2–4 min after the injection, the diagnosis of the scintigram may be obstructed by visualization of the kidney.

Hepatobiliary scintigraphy is valuable for the differential diagnosis between surgical and nonsurgical jaundice [5, 9, 10]. In the case of nonsurgical jaundice, using ^{131}I-BSP and ^{131}I-RB, images of the cardiovascular system

Fig. 3.12 A–F. Excretory hepatobiliary scintigram by ^{99m}Tc-HIDA (normal case). **A** after 3 min; **B** after 10 min; **C** after 20 min; **D** after 30 min; **E** after 40 min; after 60 min

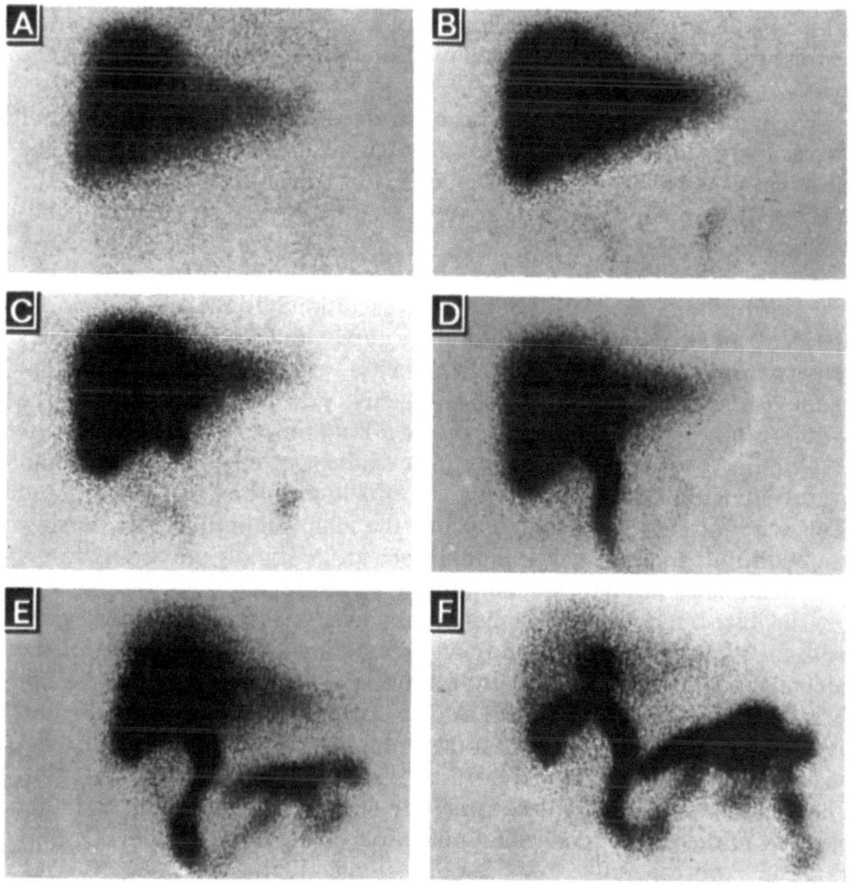

Fig. 3.13 A–D. Obstructive jaundice caused by choledocholithiasis. Excretory hepatobiliary scintigram by ^{99m}TC-HIDA. No excretion to the biliary tract.
A after 3 min; **B** after 15 min; **C** after 60 min; **D** after 150 min

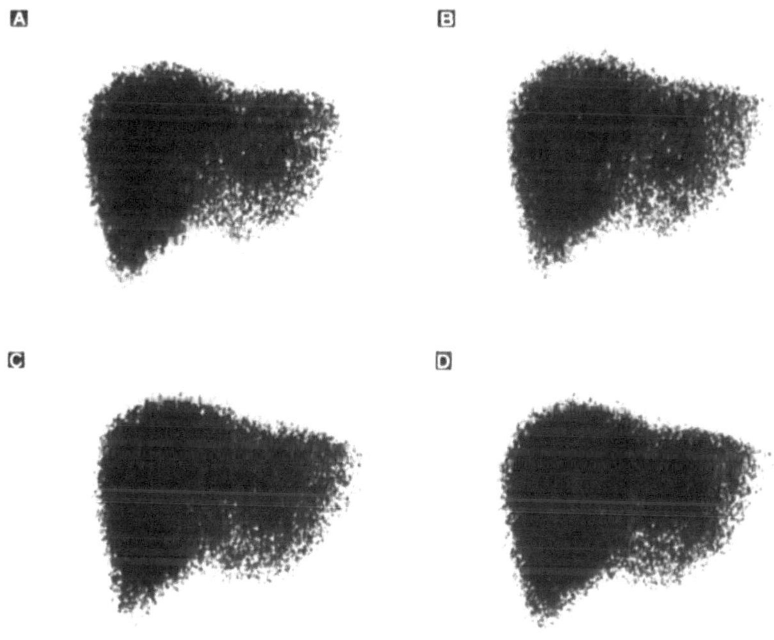

caused by the cardiac blood pooling are observable for rather a long period because the radioactivity remains in the blood due to the slow uptake by the liver.

Excretion from the liver is also obstructed, and the accumulation of radioactivity in the liver endures for a long time; usually, excretion into the intestinal tract can be observed on images photographed 24 or 48 h after the injection. However, this excretion may be unobserved with advanced cholestasis.

On the other hand, in the case of surgical jaundice with complete obstruction of the extrahepatic bile duct, no excretion into the intestine can be observed, and dense images of the kidney appear due to excretion of radioactivity from the urinary system. In this case, with secondary dysfunction of the liver, decreasing uptake of radioactivity by the liver results in the cardiac blood pool remaining for rather a long time.

With incomplete obstruction of the extrahepatic bile duct and without liver dysfunction, the radioactivity is normally absorbed by the liver, and slow excretion into the intestine will be the main finding. Even with slow excretion into the intestine, a finding of cardiac blood pooling is rarely observed due to normal excretion into the liver.

The distribution of radioactivity in the liver is visualized as decreasing from the peripheral region and finally remaining as a dense image of the porta hepatis, the so-called centralization image. This finding can be observed identically with ^{99m}Tc-HIDA (Fig. 3.13), but in the case of obstructive jaundice with over 10 mg/dl total serum bilirubin, more valuable diagnostic information can be obtained by using ^{131}I-BSP and ^{131}I-RB [14]. This examination is helpful not only for diagnosing obstructive jaundice but also in the case of congenital dilatation of the biliary tract. Bile flow patterns in postoperative cases can also studied [25].

In addition, it is valuable for the differential diagnosis of Dubin-Johnson, Rotor's, and Gilbert's syndromes using only the radiopharmaceuticals of ^{131}I-BSP, ^{99m}Tc-HIDA, or ^{99m}Tc-PI [2, 12].

The findings for the differential diagnosis of Dubin-Johnson syndrome are normal uptake by and slow excretion from the liver. Rotor's syndrome can be distinguished by the findings of slow uptake by the liver and notable delay of blood clearance; Gilbert's syndrome is charcterized by normal clearance.

References

Nuclear Examination

1. Aburano T, Ueno K, Watanabe H, Hisada K (1974) Liver scintigraphy with ^{99m}Tc-sn-colloid and ^{99m}Tc-phytate (Comparison with ^{198}Au-colloid and ^{99m}Tc-sulfur colloid) (in Japanese). Jpn J Nucl Med 11:617–623
2. Bar-Meir S, Baron J, Seligson U, Gottesfeld, F, Levy R, Gilat T (1982) ^{99m}Tc-HIDA cholescintigraphy in Dubin-Johnson and Rotor syndrome. Radiology 142:743–746
3. Covington EE (1970) Pitfalls in liver photoscans. AJR 109:745–748
4. DeNardo GL, Stadalnik RC, DeNard SJ, Raventos A (1974) Hepatic scintigraphic patterns. Radiology 111:135–141
5. Eyler WR, Schuman BM, DuSault LA, Hinson RE (1965) The radioiodinated rose bengal liver scan as an aid in the differential diagnosis of jaundice. AJR 94:496–476

6. Freeman L, Meng C, Johnson P, Bernstein R, Bosniac M (1969) False positive liver scans caused by disease processes in adjacent organs and structures. Br J Radiol 42:651–656
7. Geslien GE, Pinsky SM, Poth RK, Johnson MC (1976) The sensitivity and specificity of ^{99m}Tc-sulfur colloid liver imaging in diffuse hepatocellular disease. Radiology 118:115–119
8. Gottschalk A (1966) Radioisotope scintigraphy with technetium 99m and the gamma scintilation camera. AJR 97:860–868
9. Greene AG, Sadowsky NL (1972) A radiologic approach to the differential diagnosis of surgical and non-surgical jaundice. AJR 116:368–374
10. Handmaker H (1975) Nuclear medicine in the evaluation of the patient with jaundice. JAMA 231:1172–1176
11. Harvey E, Loberg M, Cooper M (1975) Tc-99m-HIDA: a new radiopharmaceutical for hepato-biliary imaging (Abstract). J Nucl Med 16:533
12. Iio M, Yamada H, Chiba K, Kameda H, Ueda H (1970) Studies on the contitutional hyperbilirubinemia using I-131-BSP sequential scanning method (in Japanese). Jpn J Nucl Med 7:189–200
13. Ishikawa T, Kakehi H, Uchiyama G, Sono F (1978) Evaluation on the diagnostic capability of hepatoscintigraphy on liver metastasis, in comparison with the operative findings (in Japanese). Jpn J Nucl Med 15:523–531
14. Itoh K, Nasuhara K, Koshiba R, Saito C, Furudate M (1979) Analysis of hepatobiliary scintigraphy with ^{99m}Tc-HIDA in various diseases (in Japanse). Jpn J Nucl Med 16:1379–1394
15. Jaszczak RJ, Murphy PH, Huard D, Burdine JA (1977) Radionuclide emission computed tomography of the head with ^{99m}Tc and a scintillation camera. J Nucl Med 18:373–380
16. Johnson PM, Sweeney WA (1967) The false-positive hepatic scan. J Nucl Med 8:451–460
17. Kato M, Hazue M (1978) Tc-99m(Sn)pyridoxylideneaminates: preparation and biologic evaluation. J Nucl Med 19:397–406
18. Katsuyama N (1979) Radionuclide tomographic scan of the liver (in Japanese). Jpn J Nucl Med 16:127–139
19. Lipchik EO, Schwartz SI (1976) Angiographic and scintillographic identification of Riedel's lobe of the liver. Radiology 88:48–50
20. Lunia S, Parthasarathy KL, Bakshi S, Bender MA (1975) An evaluation of ^{99m}Tc-Sulfur colloid liver scintiscans and their usefulness in metastatic workup: a review of 1424 studies. J Nucl Med 16:62–65
21. McAfee JG, Ause RG, Wagner HN Jr (1965) Diagnostic value of scintillation scanning of the liver. Follow-up of 1,000 studies. Arch Intern Med 116:95–110
22. McCready VR (1972) Scintigraphic studies of space-occupying liver disease. Semin Nucl Med 2:108–127
23. Mould RF (1972) An investigation of the variations in normal liver shape. Br J Radiol 45:586–590
24. Rosenthall L, Shaffer EA, Lisbona R, Pare P (1978) Diagnosis of hepatobiliary disease by ^{99m}Tc-HIDA cholescintigraphy. Radiology 126:467–474
25. Rosenthall L, Fonseca C, Arzoumanian A, Hernandez M, Greenberg D (1979) ^{99m}Tc-IDA hepatobiliary imaging following upper abdominal surgery. Radiology 130:735–739
26. Snow JH Jr, Goldstein HM, Wallace S (1979) Comparison of scintigraphy, sonography, and computed tomography in the evaluation of hepatic neoplasms. AJR 132:915–918
27. Taplin VG, Meredith OM Jr, Kade II (1955) The radioactive (^{131}I-tagged) rose bengal uptake-excretion test for liver function using external gamma-ray scintillation counting techniques. J Lab Clin Med 45:665–678
28. Tubis M, Nordyke RA, Posnick E, Blahd WH (1961) The preparation and use of I^{131} labeled sulfobramophthalein in liver function testing. J Nucl Med 2:282–288
29. Vogel RA, Kirch D, LeFree M, Steele P (1978) A new method of multiplanar emission tomography using a seven pinhole collimator and an Anger scintillation camera. J Nucl Med 19:648–654
30. Volpe JA, McRae J, Anger HO (1971) Clinical experience with the multiplane tomographic scanner. J Nucl Med 12:101–106
31. Wistow BW, Subramanian G, Van Heertum RL, Henderson RW, Gagne GM, Hall RC, McAfee JG (1977) An evaluation of ^{99m}Tc-labeled hepatobiliary agents. J Nucl Med 18:455–461

4 X-ray Computed Tomography

X-ray computed tomography (CT) is remarkably helpful in the diagnosis of diseases of the upper abdominal organs, particularly the liver, biliary tract, and pancreas. However, CT examination has not been established as reliable pathognomonic method due to the rapid development of technique and equipment. Therefore, when diagnosing with tomograms, it is necessary to have sufficient knowledge of the characteristics of the equipment.

4.1 Equipment

In 1973, when the CT scanner was first developed, image quality was not sufficiently high due to the artifacts caused by respiration, as the equipment required about 4 min for one tomogram.

Nowadays, as a remarkable improvement, equipment taking only 1–2 s scanning time has been developed.

This advance has been achieved by improvement of the scanning method.

The progress of scanning systems may be divided into four generations; recently, whole body scanners of the third and fourth generations have been frequently used.

With these developments, CT can be performed with hardly any artifacts from respiratory movement or peristalsis of the intestine. In addition, the reconstruction time of the image has been shortened by high-speed computers in conjunction with the development of high-speed scanning techniques so that tomograms can be achieved instantaneously. Furthermore, some equipment can display the image instantly after mechanical scanning.

4.2 Premedication

Testing of sensitivity to the contrast medium is necessary prior to examination because contrast enhancement, which increases the image contrast by intravenous injection of contrast media, may be required at any time during examination. Emptying the patient's stomach is required to avoid vomiting

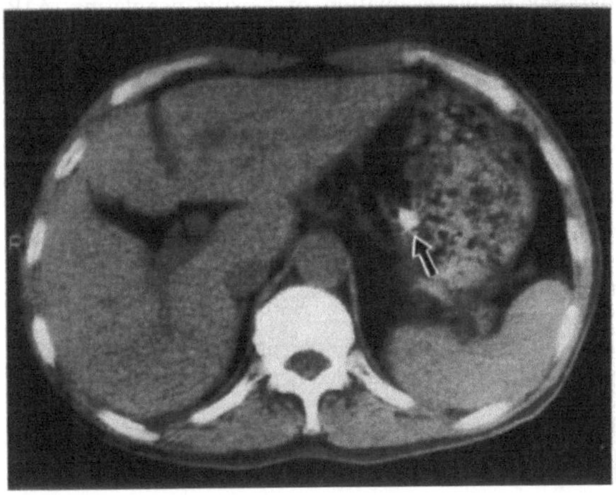

Fig. 4.1. Higly dense image due to tablet (→) mixed with residual food in the stomach

from toxicity of the contrast medium. Overnight fasting is basically important to obtain a good quality image.

Images constructed by residual foods in the stomach may be confused ambiguously with disease of the pancreas, and drugs may appear as pathological findings (Fig. 4.1). Gas in the stomach sometimes causes artifacts. In cases using CT equipment requiring a long scanning time, the artifacts caused by peristaltic motion must be excluded by antiperistalitic agents [48].

4.3 Examination Procedures

Generally, the patient should be in the supine position; the prone or side position may be used depending on the case. Scanning must be carried out at right angles to the longitudinal axis of the body. After positioning, the patient must remain motionless.

The scanning level must be properly determined by utilizing the plain radiograms previously made. Recently, the procedures for determining the scanning level have become much easier due to improved equipment employing slit scanography using the X-ray tube of the CT (Fig. 4.2).

Holding respiration is always required during the scanning, and appropriate training of respiration stoppage is necessary because scanning levels on the skin differ from the organ levels, particularly as respiratory movement is noticed not only on the liver and gallbladder but also on the pancreas.

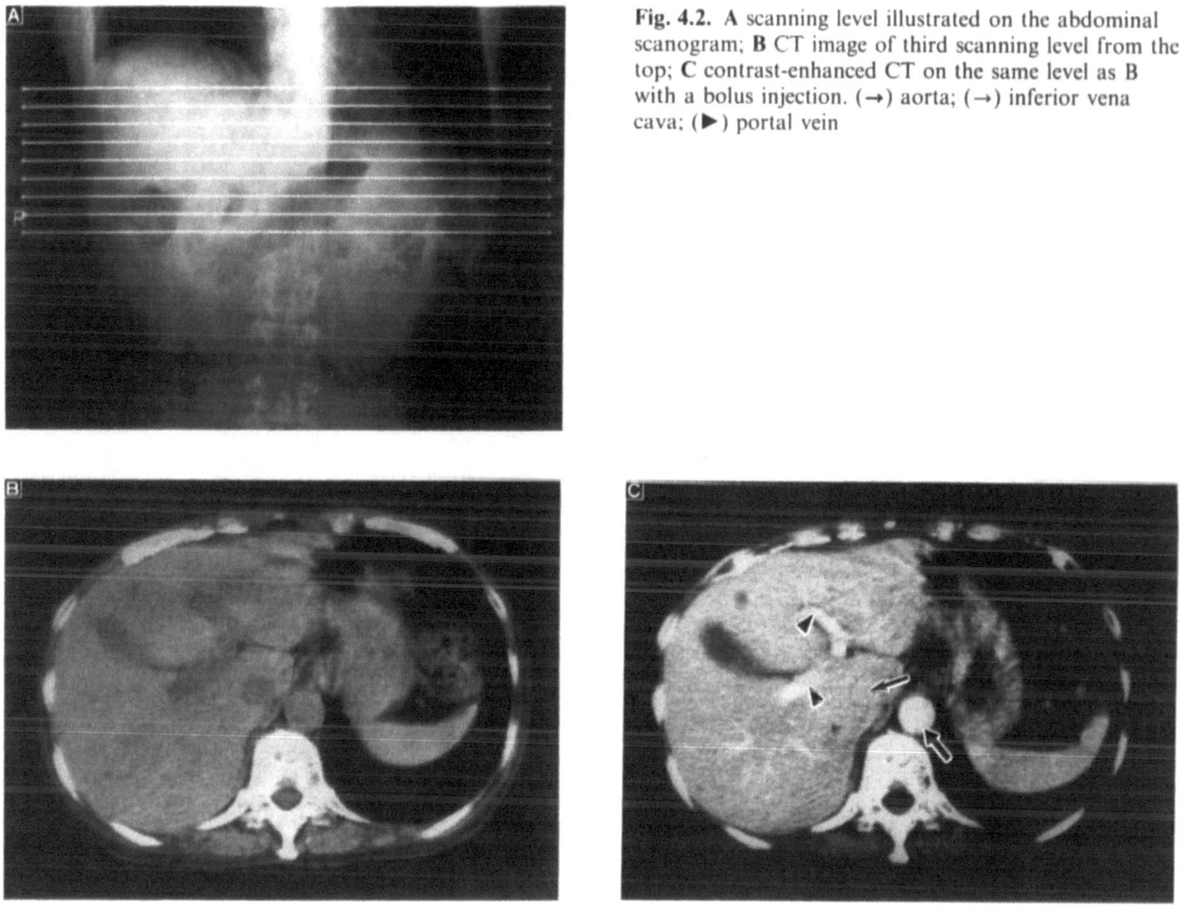

Fig. 4.2. A scanning level illustrated on the abdominal scanogram; **B** CT image of third scanning level from the top; **C** contrast-enhanced CT on the same level as B with a bolus injection. (➞) aorta; (→) inferior vena cava; (▶) portal vein

4.4. Contrast Medium Administration

With oral administration, to avoid artifacts, the patient must be given 300–400 ml of 2%–3% solution of meglumine diatrizoate (Gastrografin) 30–60 min prior to examination, and it is necessary to avoid air intake during administration. Thereafter, ejecting the media smoothly from the duodenum into the small intestine by changing the patient's position is important in order to photograph the upper gastrointestinal tracts as images with a higher attenuation value.

For intravenous injections of the contrast media, water-soluble contrast agents for angiography or urography such as meglumine diatrizoate 65% (Angiografin), meglumine iothalamate 30%–60% (Conray), and meglumine iodamide 65% (Renovue-65) are normally used. The contrast medium is given intravenously as a 200 ml drip infusion, a 50 ml bolus injection (Fig. 4.2), or a combination of these [41]. Selective arterial infusion allows a pathological lesion to be more clearly demonstrated [59].

Recent technological developments have made it possible to perform dynamic CT (Figs. 4.3–4.5). Serial CT images at a single level or various levels can be obtained by rapid intravenous injection in 5–6 s with 50–60 ml of contrast medium. By employing this new technique, not only has more detailed analysis of the vascular construction of the tumor been made possible [26, 72], but also hemodynamic information about the tumor itself is now obtainable [1, 25]. Diagnosis with CT has been greatly enhanced by this technical development [4, 5, 25, 30].

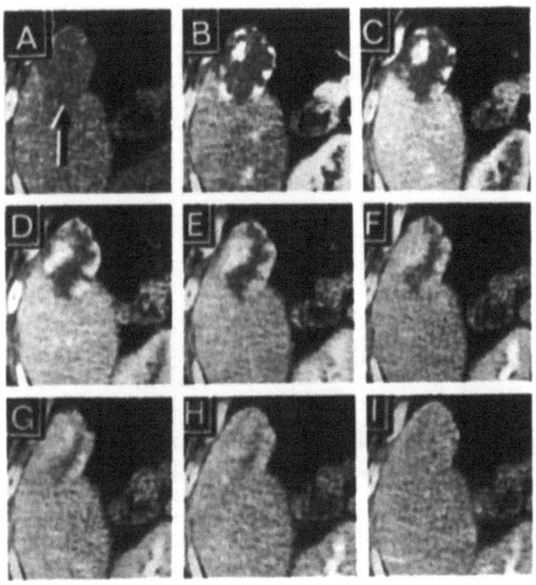

Fig. 4.3 A–I. Hemangioma of the liver seen with dynamic CT scanning. **A** before administration of the contrast medium; **B–I** dynamic serial scanning, 14 (**B**), 29 (**C**), 49 (**D**), 90 (**E**) s, 3 (**F**), 5 (**G**), 8 (**H**), and 12 (**I**) min after bolus injection of the contrast medium. A low-density mass (→) in the phase before contrast enhancement becomes gradually stained from the peripheral area to the center after the administration of the contrast medium, and complete staining is obtained after 12 min (**I**)

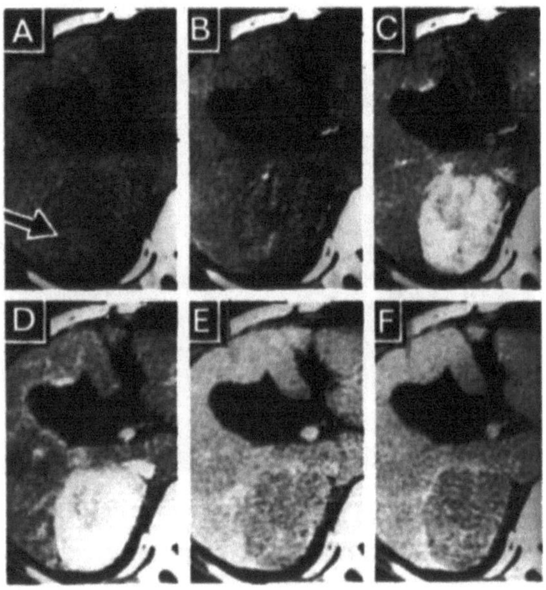

Fig. 4.4 A–F. Hepatocellular carcinoma seen with dynamic CT scanning. **A** before administration of the contrast medium; **B–F** dynamic serial scanning, 8 (**B**), 15 (**C**), 22 (**D**), 70 (**E**), and 120 (**F**) s after bolus injection of the contrast medium. A slight low-density mass (→) in the phase before contrast enhancement appears as a densely stained tumor in the arterial phase after the administration of the contrast medium (**C, D**). In a later phase (**E, F**), the tumor with a rim enhancement is lower in density than normal liver parenchyma

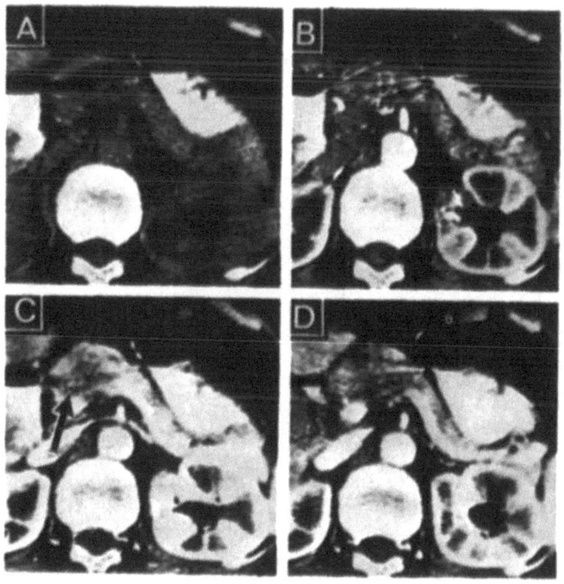

Fig. 4.5 A–D. Carcinoma of the head of the pancreas seen with dynamic CT scanning. **A** before administration of the contrast medium; **B–D** 8 (**b**), 15 (**c**), and 22 (**d**) S, after administration of the contrast medium. A tumor is clearly demonstrated in the arterial phase (**C**→)

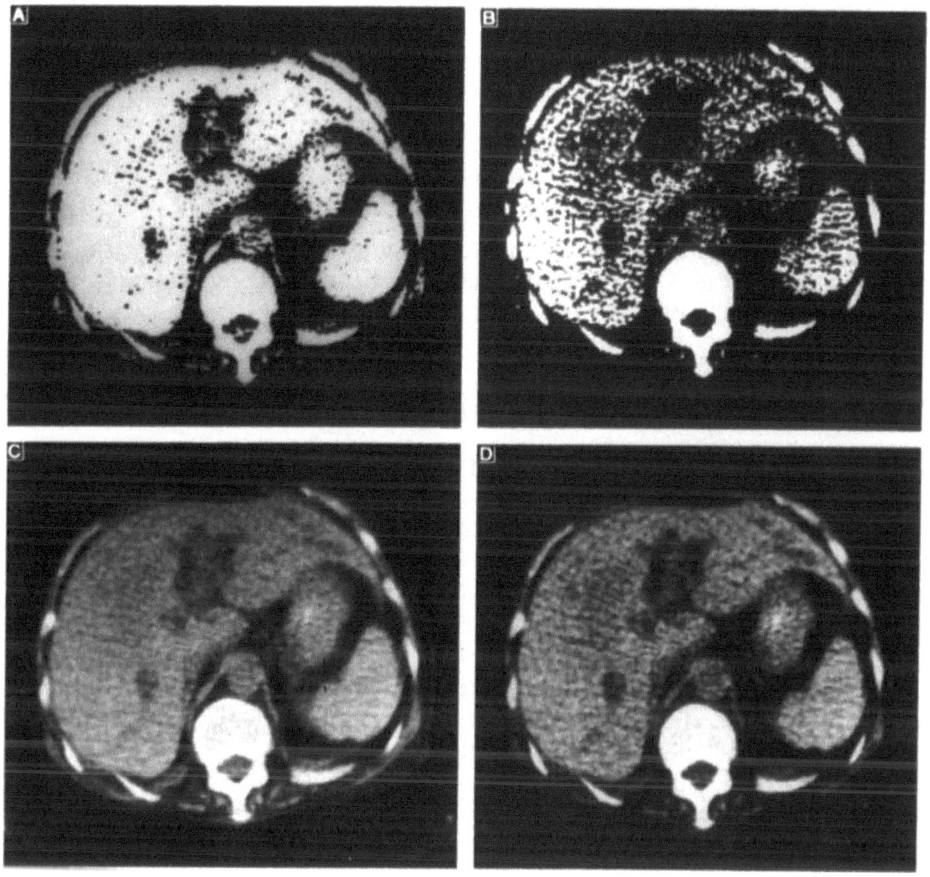

Fig. 4.6 A–D. Different images with different window settings. In **A, B**, the window width is zero, so the value for window level shows the CT number at the border between white and black images

	Window level	Window width
A	34	0
B	61	0
C	51	+251 ~ −149
D	51	+154 ~ − 46

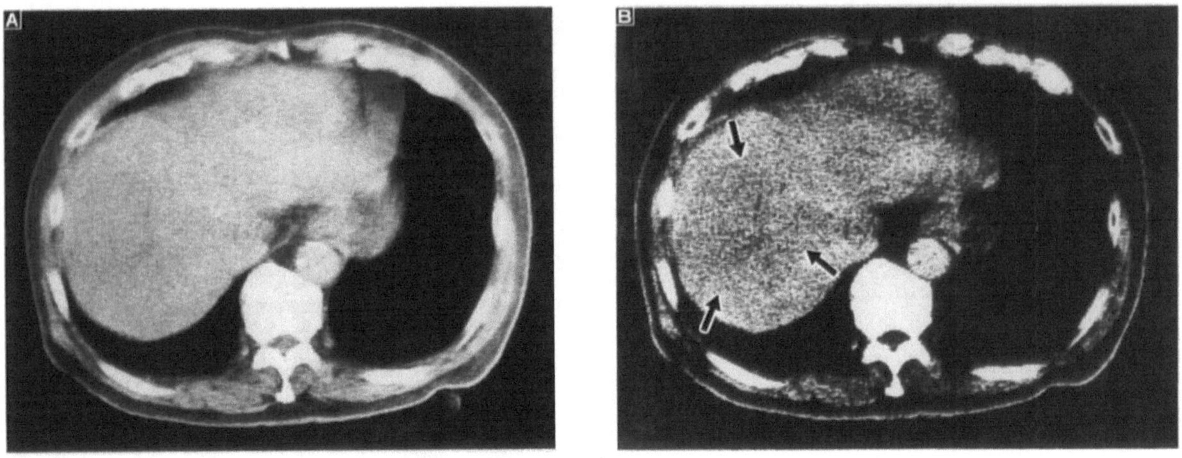

Fig. 4.7 A, B. Liver metastasis from carcinoma of the stomach. A window level + 16, width + 216 ~ − 184; B window level + 76, width + 133 ~ + 19. Useful diagnostic sign clearly seen (B →) by adjusting the level and width of the window setting

4.5 Viewing of the Images

During diagnosis, it is necessary to check the following points while examining the CT images displayed on the cathode ray tube (CRT):

1. The proper images of interest are displayed
2. Contrast enhancement with contrast medium is required
3. The window setting is adequately adjusted

In particular, the width and level of the window must be precisely adjusted in case of small differences in X-ray absorption between the normal and pathological regions (Figs. 4.6 and 4.7).

4.6 CT Images of the Normal Liver, Biliary Tract, and Pancreas

Figure 4.8 shows CT images of the normal upper abdomen and corresponding schematic illustrations. Figure 4.9 illustrates the intrahepatic vascular system.

The liver is observed as a smooth contoured image, and the parenchyma is homogeneous in density. The intrahepatic vasculature is visualized as a tubular, round, or oval image of low-density structure, and the portal vein is visible quite distinctly in the porta hepatis.

The right and left lobes of the liver are anatomically separated slightly to the right of the midline. These lobes are separated anteriorly by the falciform ligament and posteriorly by the ligamentum venosum. These ligaments are also low-density structures demonstrated as images.

The caudate lobe of the liver can be visualized projecting into the right lobe between the inferior vena cava and fissure of the ligamentum venosum. The quadrate lobe is observed superior to the caudate lobe between the gallbladder fossa and ligamentum teres [71].

Attenuation values of normal liver parenchyma are +40 to +70 HU, which is generally higher than those in the spleen, kidney, pancreas, and muscles [45]. The normal liver parenchyma appears homogenous in attenuation values.

To identify the hepatic segment, the hepatic vein is a good indicator because the hepatic segment corresponds with the branching of the hepatic vein.

Depending on the viscosity of the bile juice, the attenuation value of CT of the gallbladder is 0–20 HU. The image of the gallbladder is seen as an oval shape and observed medial to the right lobe and lateral to the main lobar fissure; it may rarely be located medial to the main lobar fissure or entirely in the liver if the quadrate lobe is absent [24]. The entire image of the intrahepatic bile duct cannot be observed as a tubular or a round cross-sectional image without dilatation of the bile duct. The normal common bile duct can be observed as a 3–6 mm ringlike structure in about 30% of cases [18].

The pancreas is located obliquely from the tail, which is close to the hilum of the spleen, down to the head. Then, it is difficult to secure the entire image of the pancreas on a single slice plane of a CT image so that several CT images are required, especially to visualize the distal portion of the pancreatic tail and uncinate process of the pancreas. The tail of the pancreas is located anterior or anterolateral to the left kidney. In patients with an absent kidney, the pancreatic tail lies dorsomedial, adjacent to the spine, and bowel and spleen occupy the empty renal fossa [53].

The inferior vena cava is observed posterior to the head of the pancreas, the descending portion of the duodenum is observed outside, and the gastric antrum is observed anteriorly.

In several cases, images of the uncinate process of the pancreas, situated posterior to the superior mesenteric artery, require differential diagnosis from the horizontal portion of the duodenum.

The body of the pancreas is visualized posterior to the region from the gastric antrum to the body of the stomach. The abdominal aorta is located posterior to the body of the pancreas, and the superior mesentric artery and vein can be observed between the abdominal aorta and body of the pancreas [68].

The region from the body to the tail of the pancreatic parenchyma occasionally cannot be distinguished from the parallelly running splenic vein, posterior to the pancreas.

Particularly in thin patients lacking fat layers between the splenic vein and the pancreas, differential observation is impossible without elevating the attenuation value of the splenic vein with contrast enhancement.

With sufficient fat layers between the splenic vein and body of the pancreas, the pancreas can be observed distinctly apart from the splenic vein. Exhibiting a low-density area, this fat layer may be misdiagnosed for a dilated pancreatic duct [64]. Thus, the fat layer is a significant structure for distinguishing the pancreas from the splenic vein and other neighboring structures.

In the case of thin patients, the position of the pancreas is more easily defined by opacification of the stomach and small intestine by means of oral administration of contrast media. The head of the pancreas can be easily differentiated by moving the contrast media into the duodenum by changing the patient's position to right lateral and taking scans under these conditions (Fig. 4.10).

For differentiation of the surrounding vessels from the pancreas, intravenous injection of contrast medium is useful. The dilated pancreatic duct can be better demonstrated by scanning with a slice less than 5 mm thick and increasing X-ray dosage [9].

The anterior-posterior diameter of the pancreas decreases from the head to the tail.

Fig. 4.8 A–F. CT image of the normal liver, biliary tract, and pancreas compared with schematic diagram

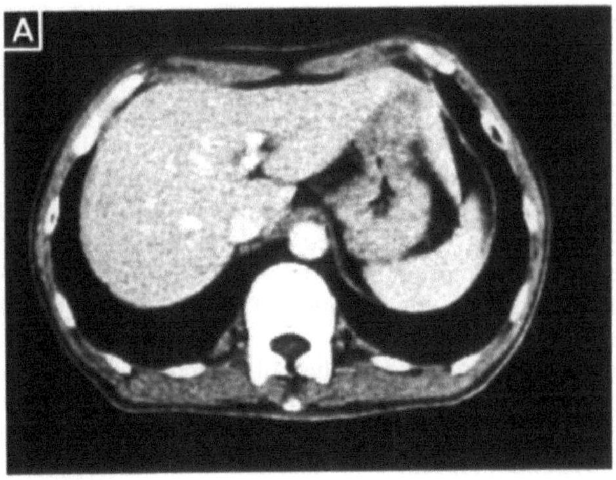

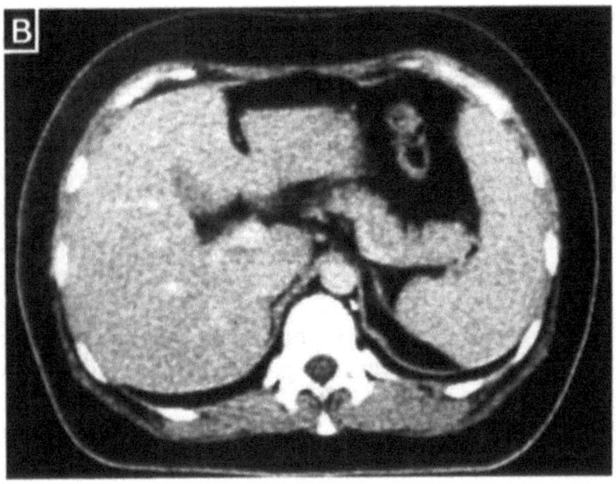

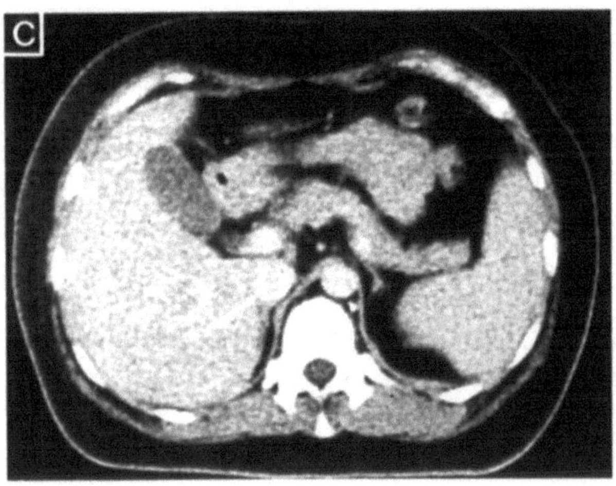

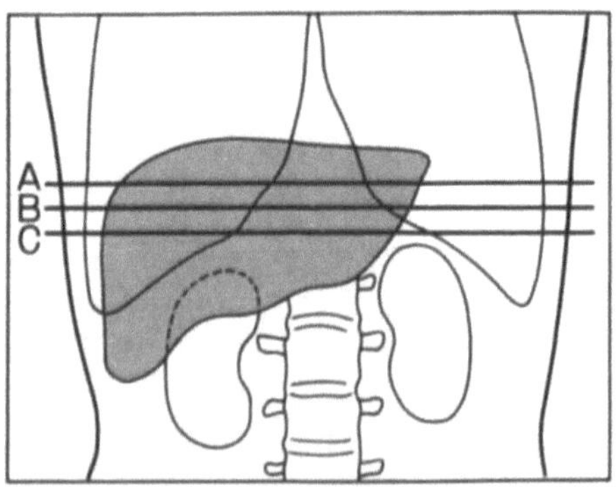

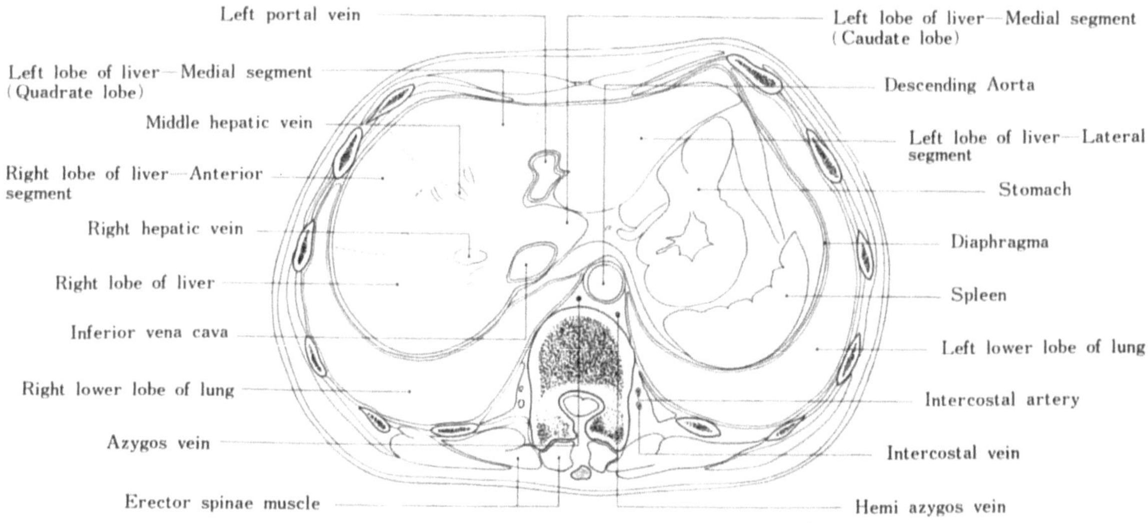
Left portal vein
Left lobe of liver—Medial segment (Caudate lobe)
Left lobe of liver—Medial segment (Quadrate lobe)
Descending Aorta
Middle hepatic vein
Left lobe of liver—Lateral segment
Right lobe of liver—Anterior segment
Stomach
Right hepatic vein
Diaphragma
Right lobe of liver
Spleen
Inferior vena cava
Left lower lobe of lung
Right lower lobe of lung
Intercostal artery
Azygos vein
Intercostal vein
Erector spinae muscle
Hemi azygos vein

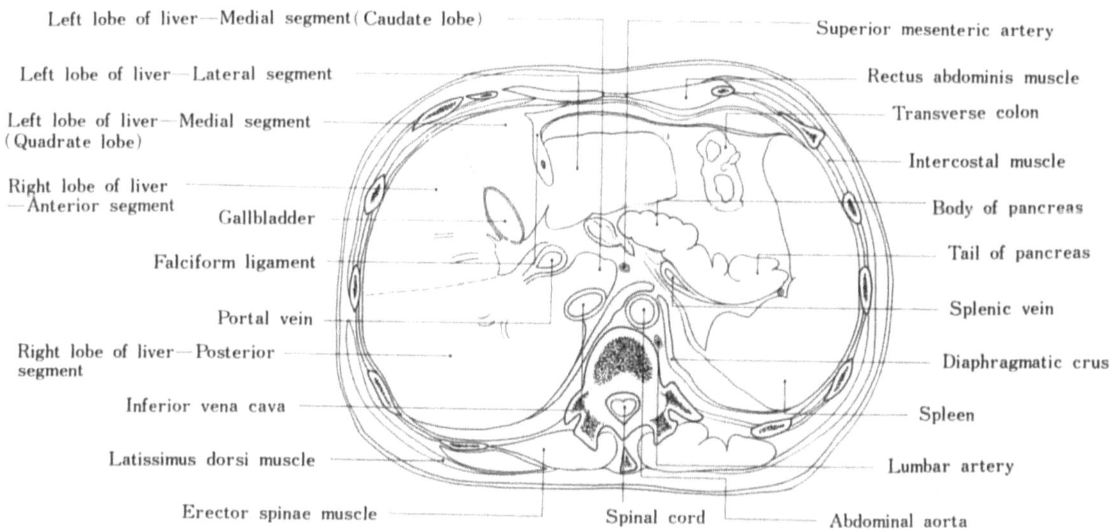
Left lobe of liver—Medial segment (Caudate lobe)
Superior mesenteric artery
Left lobe of liver—Lateral segment
Rectus abdominis muscle
Left lobe of liver—Medial segment (Quadrate lobe)
Transverse colon
Intercostal muscle
Right lobe of liver—Anterior segment
Gallbladder
Body of pancreas
Tail of pancreas
Falciform ligament
Portal vein
Splenic vein
Right lobe of liver—Posterior segment
Diaphragmatic crus
Inferior vena cava
Spleen
Latissimus dorsi muscle
Lumbar artery
Erector spinae muscle
Spinal cord
Abdominal aorta

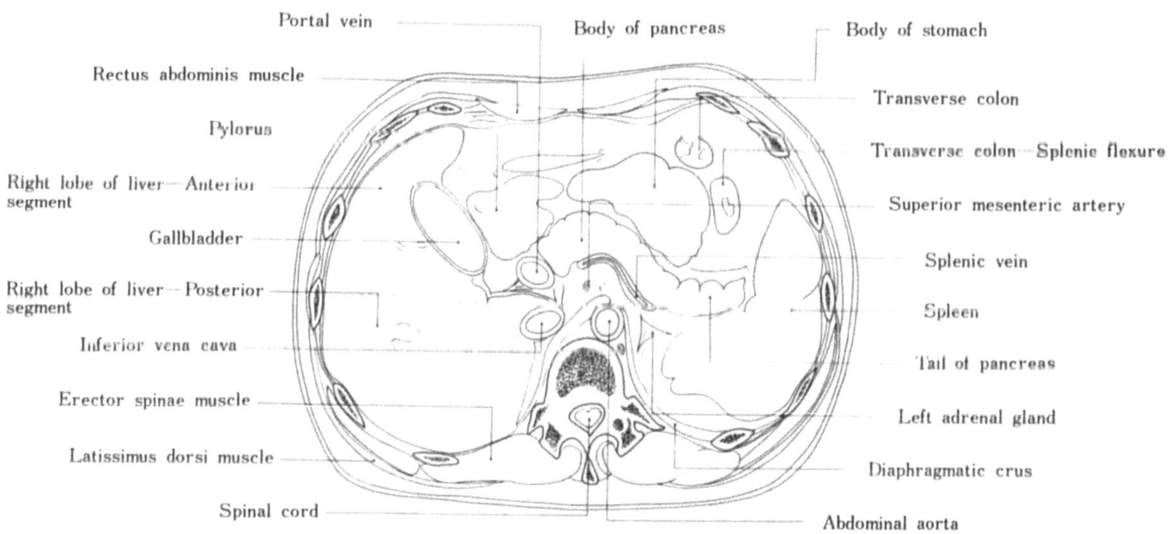
Portal vein
Body of pancreas
Body of stomach
Rectus abdominis muscle
Transverse colon
Pylorus
Transverse colon—Splenic flexure
Right lobe of liver—Anterior segment
Superior mesenteric artery
Gallbladder
Splenic vein
Right lobe of liver—Posterior segment
Spleen
Inferior vena cava
Tail of pancreas
Erector spinae muscle
Left adrenal gland
Latissimus dorsi muscle
Diaphragmatic crus
Spinal cord
Abdominal aorta

Fig. 4.8 (continued)

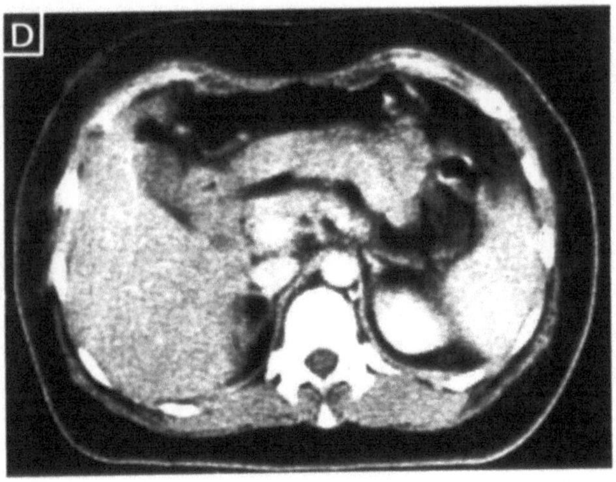

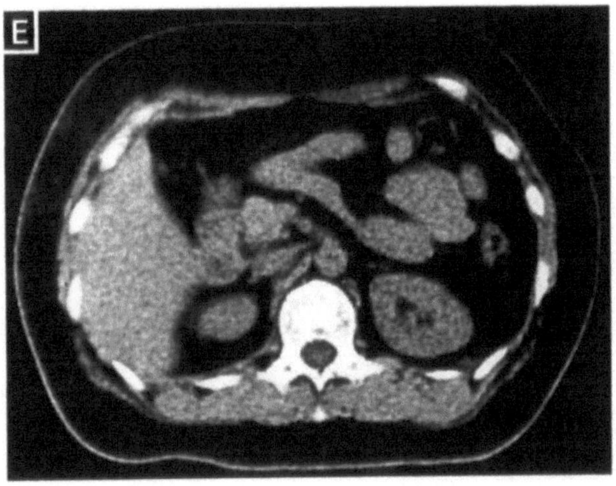

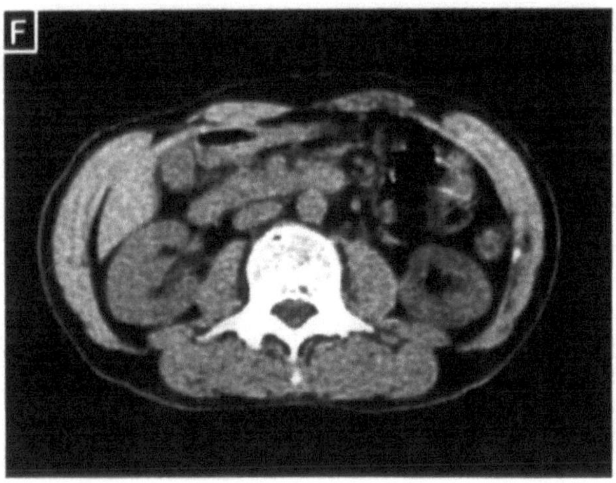

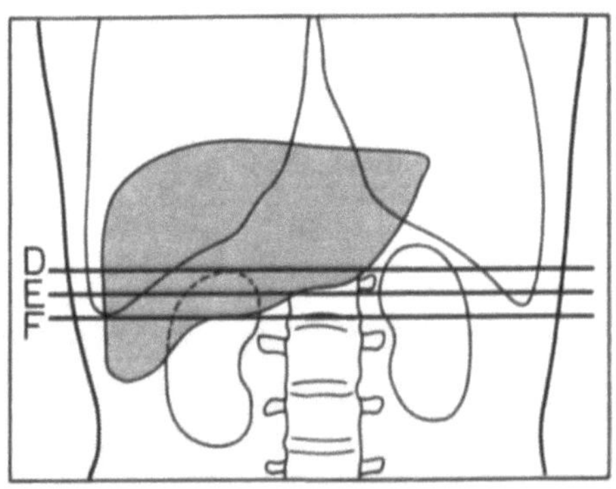

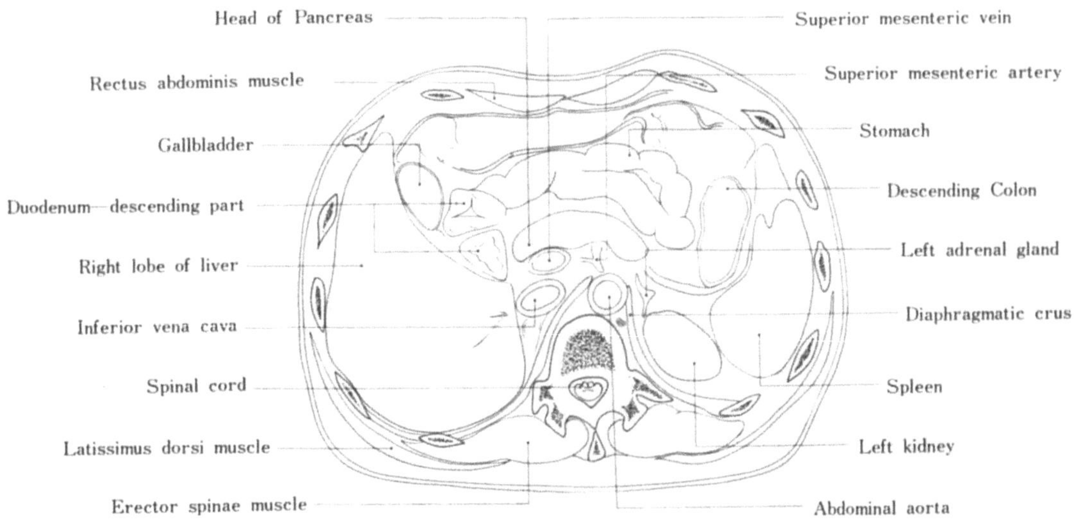
Head of Pancreas
Rectus abdominis muscle
Gallbladder
Duodenum—descending part
Right lobe of liver
Inferior vena cava
Spinal cord
Latissimus dorsi muscle
Erector spinae muscle
Superior mesenteric vein
Superior mesenteric artery
Stomach
Descending Colon
Left adrenal gland
Diaphragmatic crus
Spleen
Left kidney
Abdominal aorta

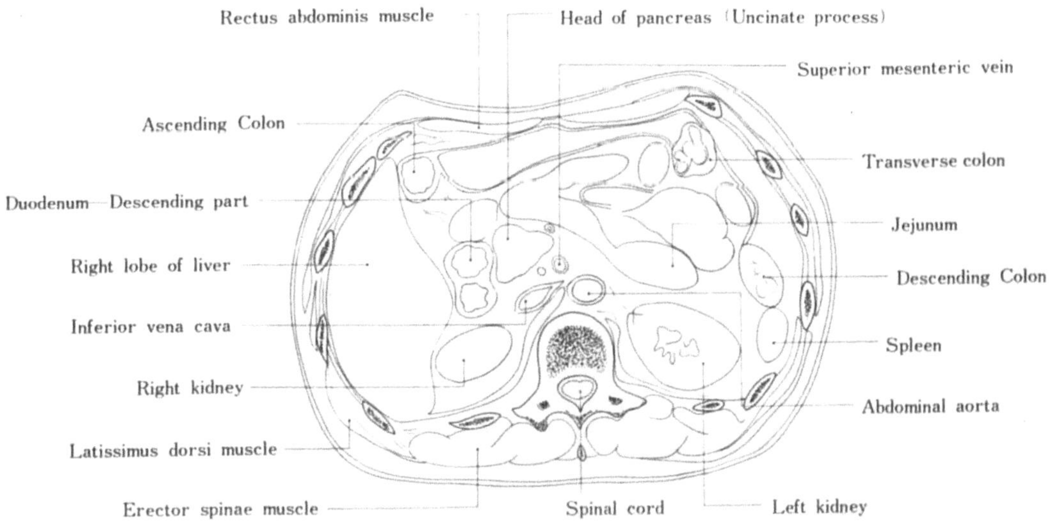
Rectus abdominis muscle
Head of pancreas (Uncinate process)
Superior mesenteric vein
Ascending Colon
Duodenum—Descending part
Right lobe of liver
Inferior vena cava
Right kidney
Latissimus dorsi muscle
Erector spinae muscle
Transverse colon
Jejunum
Descending Colon
Spleen
Abdominal aorta
Spinal cord
Left kidney

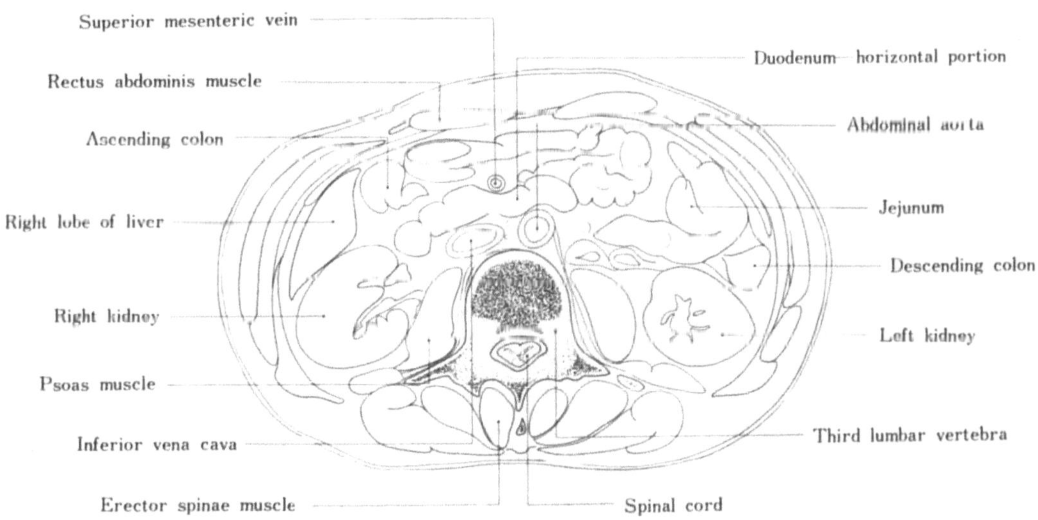
Superior mesenteric vein
Rectus abdominis muscle
Ascending colon
Right lobe of liver
Right kidney
Psoas muscle
Inferior vena cava
Erector spinae muscle
Duodenum—horizontal portion
Abdominal aorta
Jejunum
Descending colon
Left kidney
Third lumbar vertebra
Spinal cord

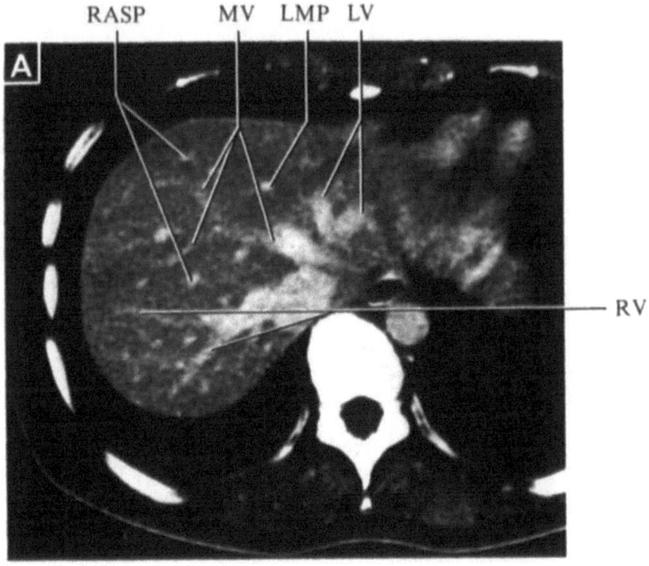

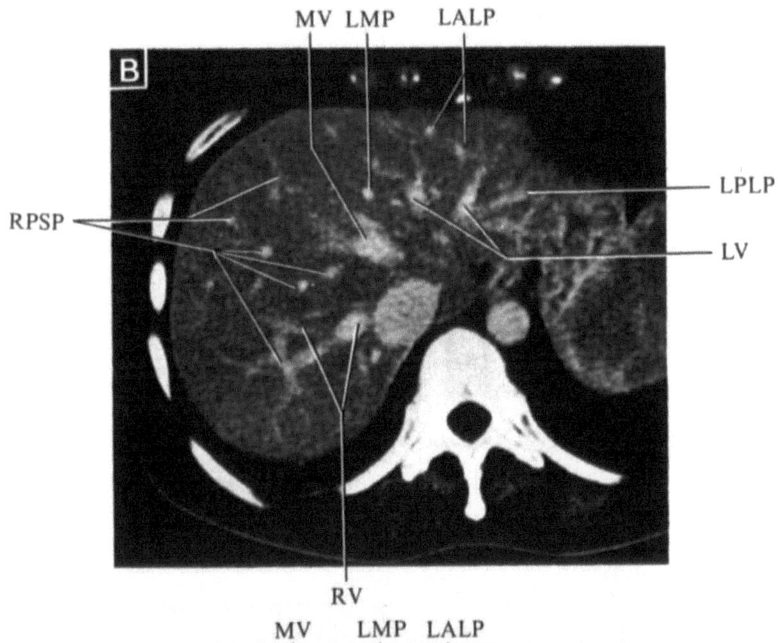

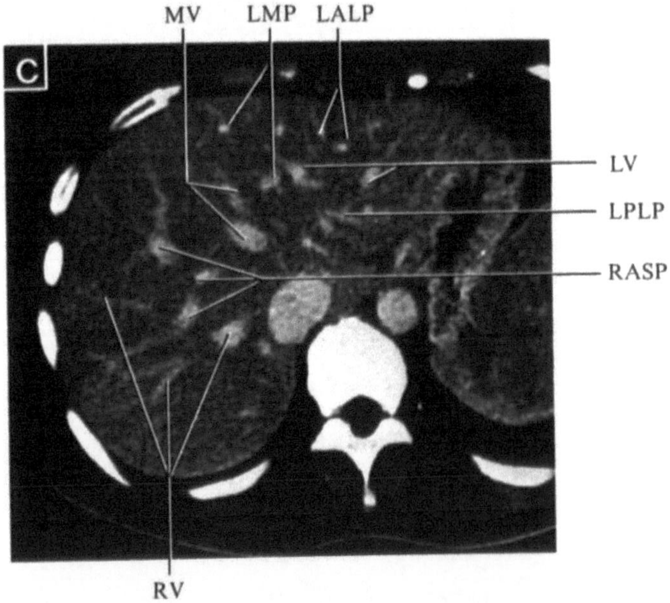

Fig. 4.9 A–H. Intrahepatic vascular CT anatomy.
RV = right hepatic vein;
MV = middle hepatic vein;
LV = left hepatic vein;
SV = short hepatic vein;
MPV = main portal vein;
RMP = right main portal branch;
RPP = right posterior portal branch;
LMP = left medial portal branch;
LPLP = left posterolateral portal branch;
LALP = left anterolateral portal branch;
RASP = right anterosuperior portal branch;
RAIP = right anteroinferior portal branch;
RPSP = right posterosuperior portal branch;
RPIP = right posteroinferior portal branch

Fig. 4.9 (continued)

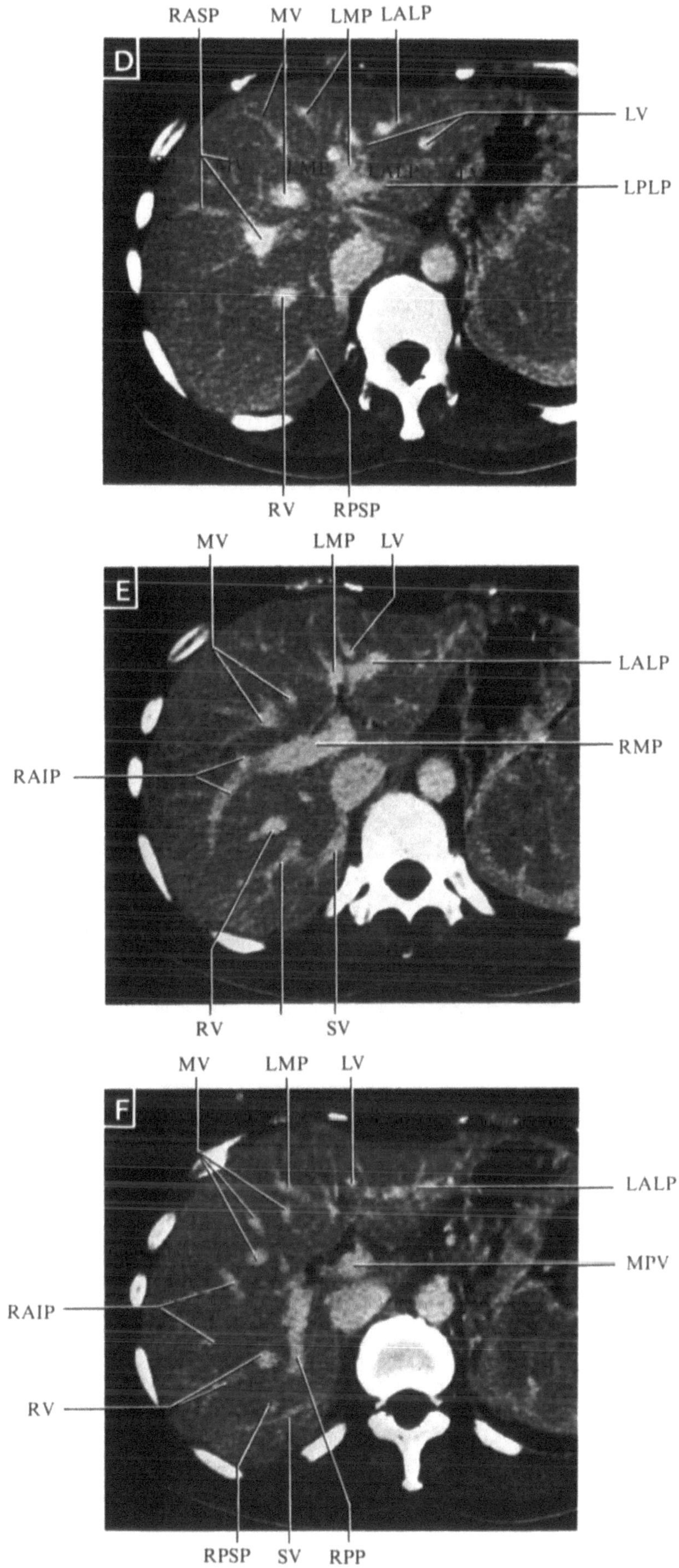

Fig. 4.9 (continued)

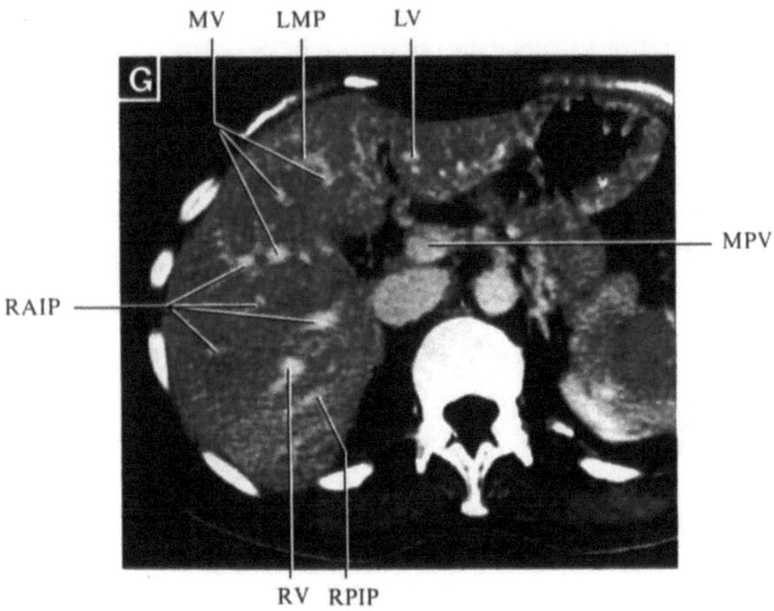

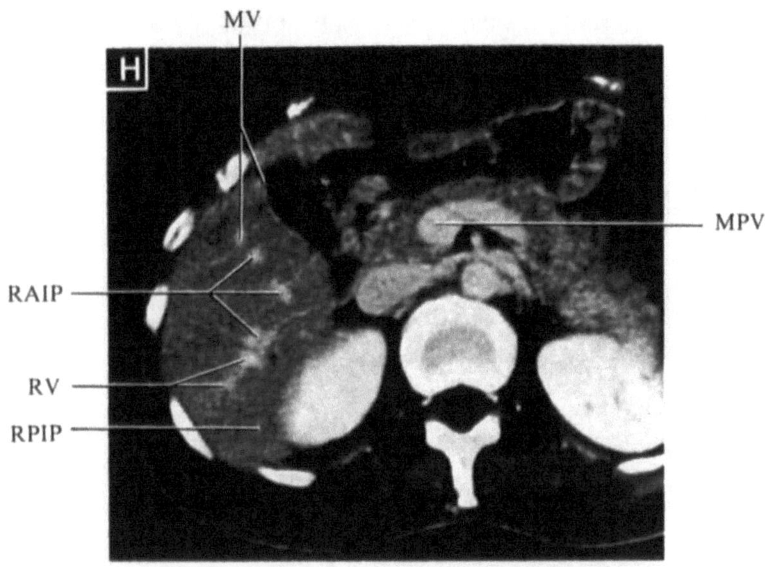

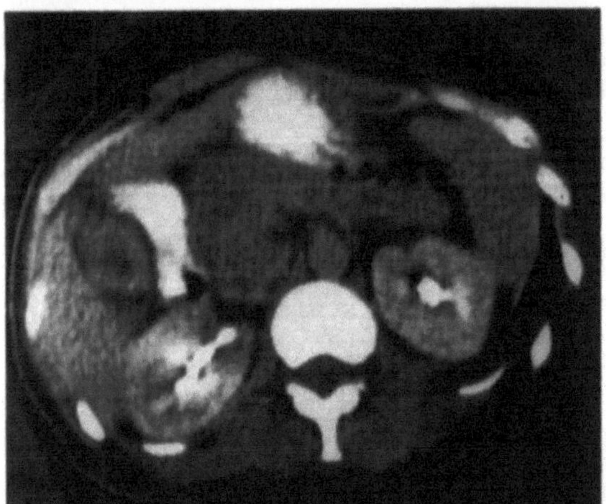

Fig. 4.10. A clear boundary between the duodenum and the head of the pancreas can be seen in the right latera position after transoral administration of Gastrografin

Standardizing the transverse diameter of the adjacent lumbar vertebra as 1, the head of the pancreas shows normally a pancreatic-vertebral ratio of 0.6 ± 0.1, the body and the tail of the pancreas 0.5 ± 0.1, the upper limit of the head 1, and the body and tail 2/3 [70].

On the other hand, some reports state the normal range of the head of the pancreas to be 23 ± 3 mm, the body 20 ± 3 mm, and the tail 15 ± 2.5 mm and the upper limit to be 30 mm in the head, 25 mm in the body, and 20 mm in the tail [42].

Although the pancreas exhibits a CT number of 30–45 HU, being smaller than the liver in size, the reliability of the CT number of the pancreas remains inferior due to the strong influence of the partial volume effect. The CT number tends to decrease with aging.

4.7 CT Images of the Diseased Liver

4.7.1 Space-Occupying Lesions of the Liver. With CT scanning, the accuracy of diagnosing space-occupying lesions of the liver is about 90%; this rate increases for lesions with a diameter of over 2 cm [61, 69]. Detectability of space-occupying lesions increases with the size of the lesions. In in vitro CT studies, the smallest lesions detectable on CT were 0.5 cm in diameter, but CT disclosed focal lesions of this small size in only 15% of the cases [62]. It depends on the CT scanner, on the difference between the density of the lesion and the adjacent structures, and on its position relative to the respective CT slice.

Among space-occupying lesions, the image of a liver cyst is characterized by smooth contours and clear boundaries. Its CT number exhibits 0–15 HU; this is close to water and lower than that of the hepatic parenchyma. Small cysts, however, may cause higher CT value due to the so-called partial volume effect. The contrast enhancement causes no change in the CT number of a liver cyst (Figs 4.11 and 4.12).

In contrast, although also visualized as a low-density structure of 0–25 HU, the image of a liver abscess is characterized by a thick and irregular contour of the wall whose CT number may be elevated by contrast enhancement (Fig. 4.13).

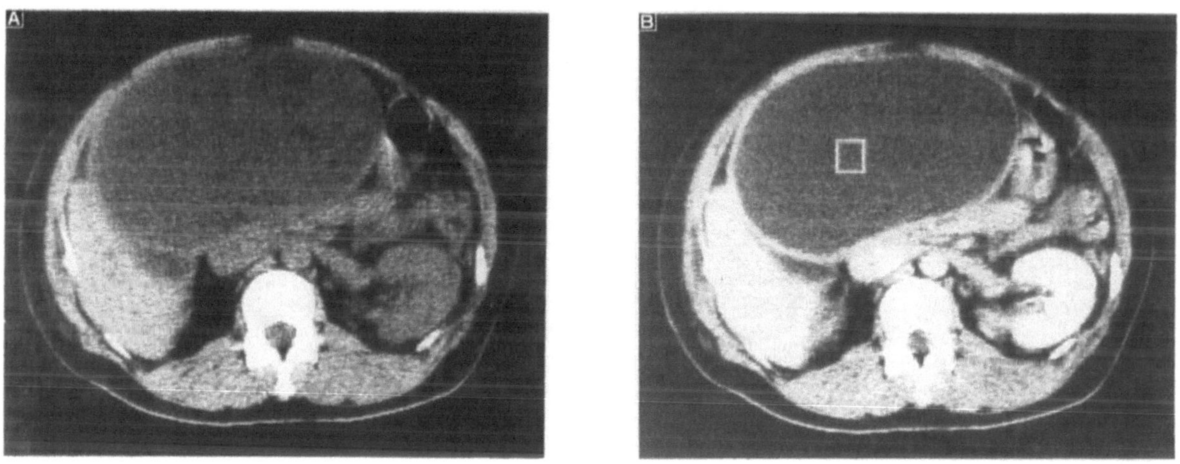

Fig. 4.11 A, B. Liver cyst. **A** before administration of the contrast medium (CT number of the liver parenchyma = 51.9 HU); **B** after administration of the contrast medium (CT number of the liver parenchyma is increased to 68.7 HU, but CT number of the cyst does not change and is 8.3 HU)

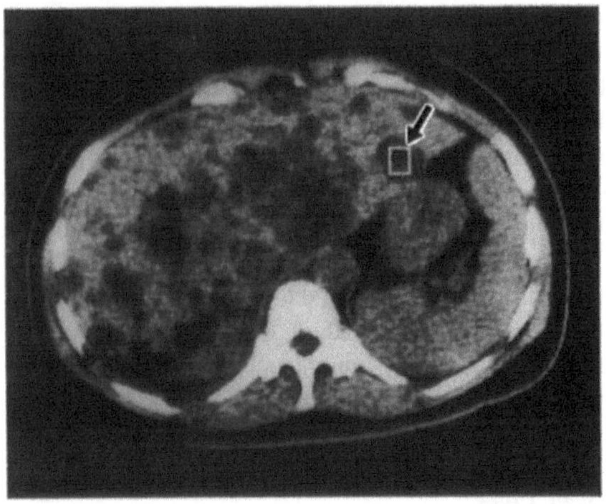

Fig. 4.12. Multiple cysts of the liver. The CT number of the cyst at the lateral segment of the left lobe is 5.9 HU obtained (→) by setting of ROI

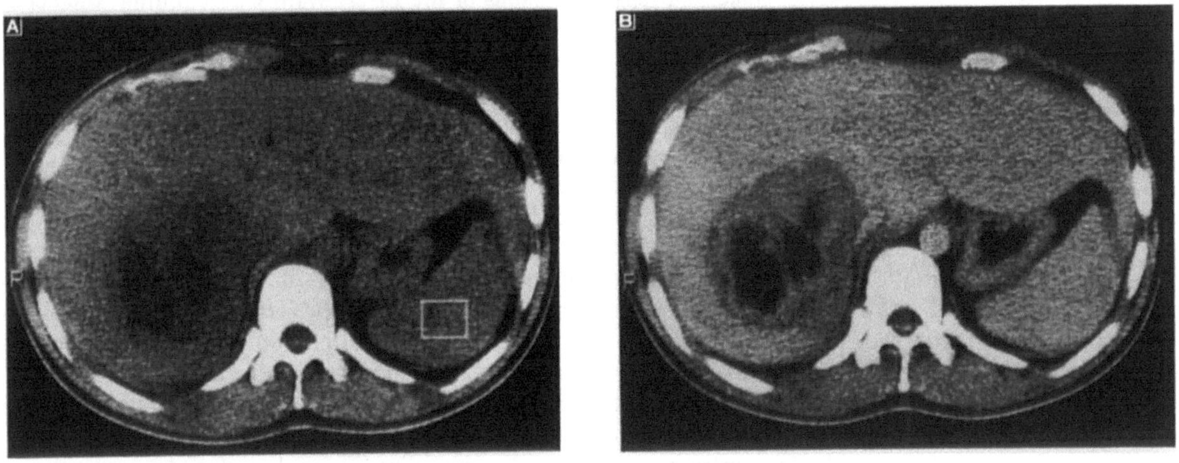

Fig. 4.13 A, B. Liver abscess. **A** before administration of the contrast medium; **B** after administration of the contrast medium with a bolus injection. The wall of the abscess and necrotic region are clarly seen. Same case as shown in Fig. 2.14

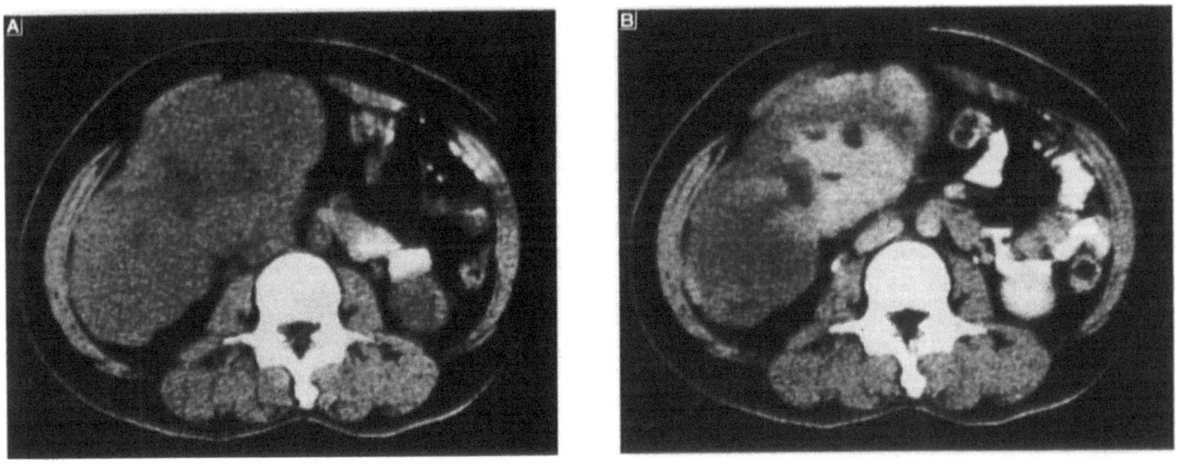

Fig. 4.14 A, B. Hemangioma of the liver occupying the lower part of the right lobe. **A** before administration of the contrast medium (low-density image of hemangioma with lower density of internal regions); **B** after a bolus injection (periphery of the hemangioma is opacified irregularly). Same case as shown Fig. 2.19

Before the administration of contrast medium, the liver hemangioma image sometimes exhibits a homogeneous low density with an even lower density area within [19]. After administration, the peripheral area of the mass gradually increases in density, and finally the small low-density area may remain in the center [33, 38]. In these cases, the contrast-enhanced effect does not always become circular, but sometimes shows partially defected patterns and is inhomogeneous; also, the remaining central low-density part is lower in CT number than in the enhanced liver parenchyma (Fig. 4.14).

In a scanning image 20–30 min after bolus injection of contrast medium, various levels of high-density area are also visualized in the central low-density area, the so-called delayed central enhancement [2]. However, as far as the authors' experience with dynamic CT studies is concerned, cases of complete staining of the tumor with contrast medium have been frequent although they have depended upon the size of the tumor (Fig. 4.3).

Figure 4.15 is a case of hepatocellular carcinoma. The CT number of the tumor in the precontrast phase is lower than the surrounding normal liver parenchyma and higher than in cysts and abscesses. In cases with a slight

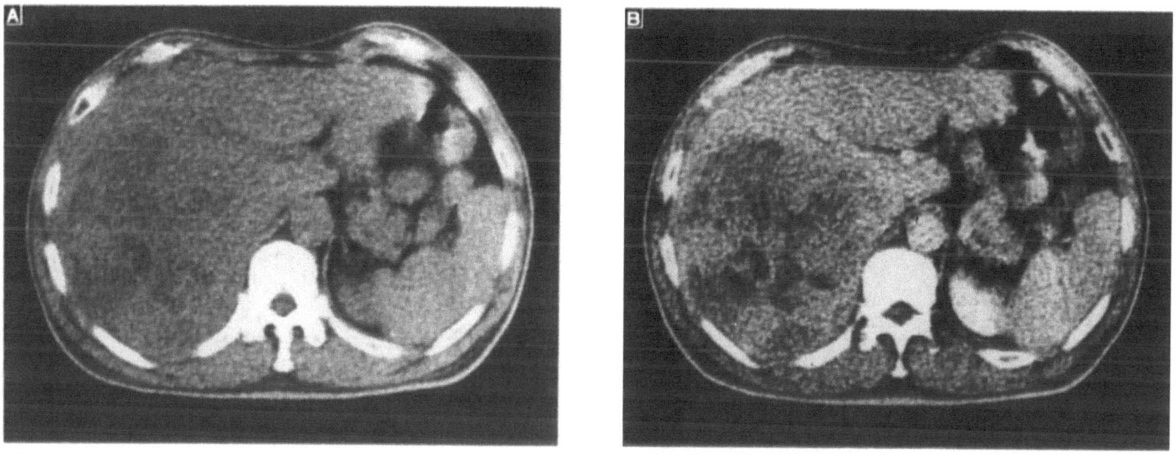

Fig. 4.15 A, B. Hepatocelullar carcinoma. **A** before administration of the contrast medium; **B** after administration of the contrast medium. The boundary of the tumor and necrotic condition are clearly visualized

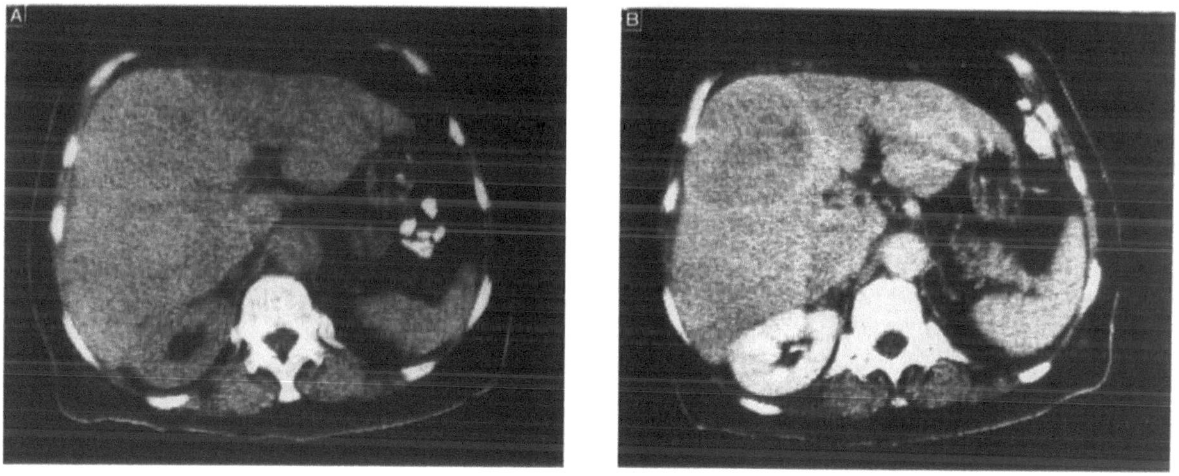

Fig. 4.16 A, B. Hepatocelullar carcinoma. **A** before administration of the contrast medium; **B** after administration of the contrast medium (clearly visualized tumor)

difference in CT number between the parenchyma and tumor, contrast enhancement by injection of contrast medium is required since the tumor cannot be recognized merely by an adequate window setting (Fig. 4.16). In dynamic CT studies, a tumor shows homogeneous enhancement in the arterial phase and lower density than the liver parenchyma in the venous phase [1, 30] (Fig. 4.4). Dynamic CT is valuable for diagnosis of a small hepatocellular carcinoma [29].

If the portal vein is obstructed by tumors, noncancerous areas supplied by obstructed portal veins have a lower density than normally supplied areas, and these density relationships are not changed by contrast enhancement [28].

A well-defined round cystic mass with internal papillary projections or dilatation of the intra- and extrahepatic ducts are important clues leading to a diagnosis of primary intrahepatic biliary malignancy [36].

A solitary metastatic tumor in the liver may be indistinguishable from hepatocellular carcinoma (Fig. 4.7). With necrosis in metastatic carcinoma, if the attenuation value of the necrotic area approaches that of water, differential diagnosis from cysts and abscesses become difficult (Fig. 4.17). Ultrasonography may depict the true morphology of these lesions more clearly than CT [14]. Sometimes, the CT number of the tumor is higher than in liver parenchyma in the case of calcified metastatic lesions [6] (Fig. 4.18) or rarely hepatocellular carcinoma [61]. In dynamic CT studies, metastatic tumors have a rim enhancement in the arterial phase [30, 51] (Fig. 4.19).

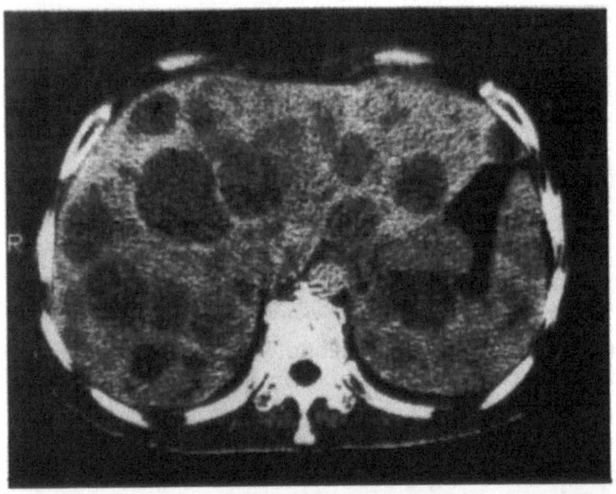

Fig. 4.17. Metastatic liver and spleen carcinoma from malignant lymphoma. After administration of the contrast medium, multiple low-density images in the liver and spleen. Same case as shown in Figs. 2.16 and 3.9

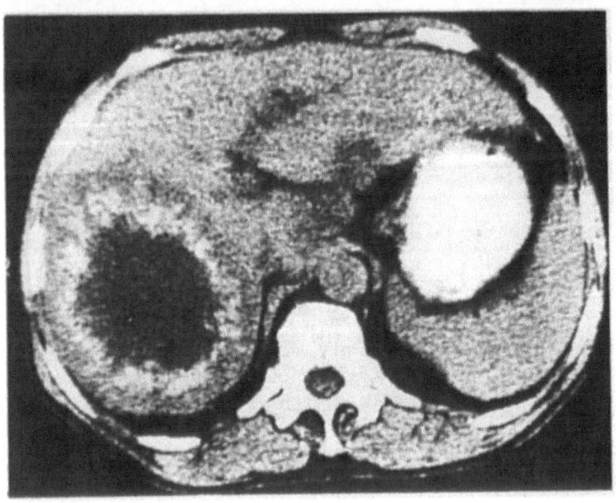

Fig. 4.18. Metastatic liver carcinoma associated with calcification (large cell carcinoma)

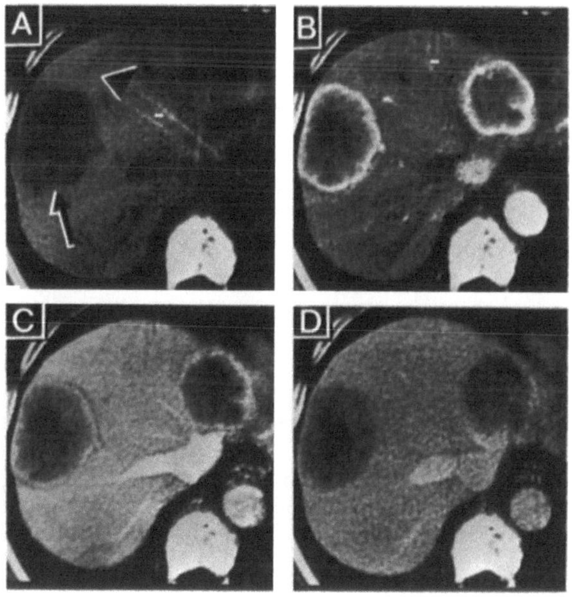

Fig. 4.19 A–D. Hepatic metastasis from carcinoma of the sigmoid colon seen with dynamic CT scanning. **A** before administration of the contrast medium; **B–D** dynamic serial scanning 15 (**B**), 30 (**C**), and 90 (**D**) s after administration of the contrast medium with a bolus injection. Low-density masses in the right lobe (→) and medial segment (►) in the phase before contrast enhancement show rim enhancement in the arterial phase (**B, C**)

Whether the carcinoma of the liver is primary or secondary, contrast enhancement must be performed for diagnosing the liver tumor. The effect of contrast enhancement varies depending on tumor vascularity, concentration of the contrast medium, quantity and method of medication, and timing of scanning after administration [75]. Occasionally, the tumor may exhibit no difference in contrast from parenchyma [32] (Fig. 4.20).

Generally, drip infusion of contrast medium is almost ineffective in contrast enhancement of liver carcinoma [49]. The liver blood supply is usually 25% from the hepatic artery and 75% from the portal vein. However, the blood supply to the tumor is limited from the hepatic artery. Therefore, bolus injections (Fig. 4.21) or arterial infusions are necessary for effective contrast enhancement of liver tumors [51, 59]. Dynamic scanning by means of a bolus injection can provide much better diagnostic information.

Hypervascular tumors are visualized as images of high-density structures by bolus injections of contrast medium. However, hypovascular tumors are observed as images less dense than liver parenchyma.

In the case of hypervascular tumors, the best quality images can be obtained about 20 s after the bolus injection; only at this point does the arterial blood contribute to liver opacification (Fig. 4.4). To obtain the finest image, a hypovascular tumor is scanned about 45 s after injection when the portal blood also contributes to liver opacification [30, 44, 51].

Differential diagnosis is necessary between liver carcinoma, hepatic adenoma, focal fatty metamorphosis, and focal nodular hyperplasia because they may exhibit similar CT findings. Focal nodular hyperplasia often presents as a well-defined lesion with a central, stellate, fibrous scar and hepatic adenoma, which is associated with the use of oral contraceptives, is a smooth-bordered mass with foci of acute hemorrhage [17].

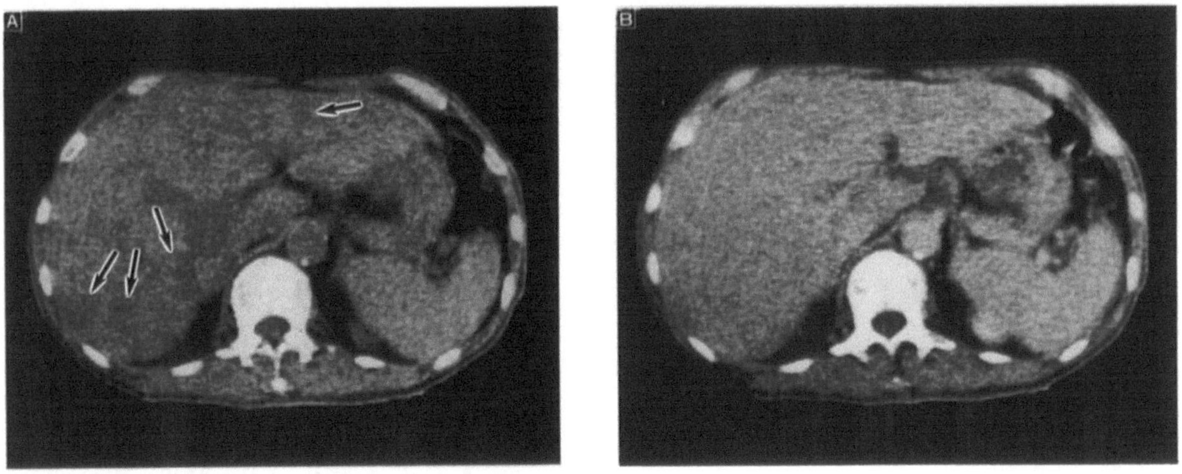

Fig. 4.20 A, B. Hepatocellular carcinoma. **A** before administration of the contrast medium: multiple low-density lesions in entire liver (→); **B** after administration of the contrast medium by a drip infusion. The liver is stained uniformly and lesions cannot be seen

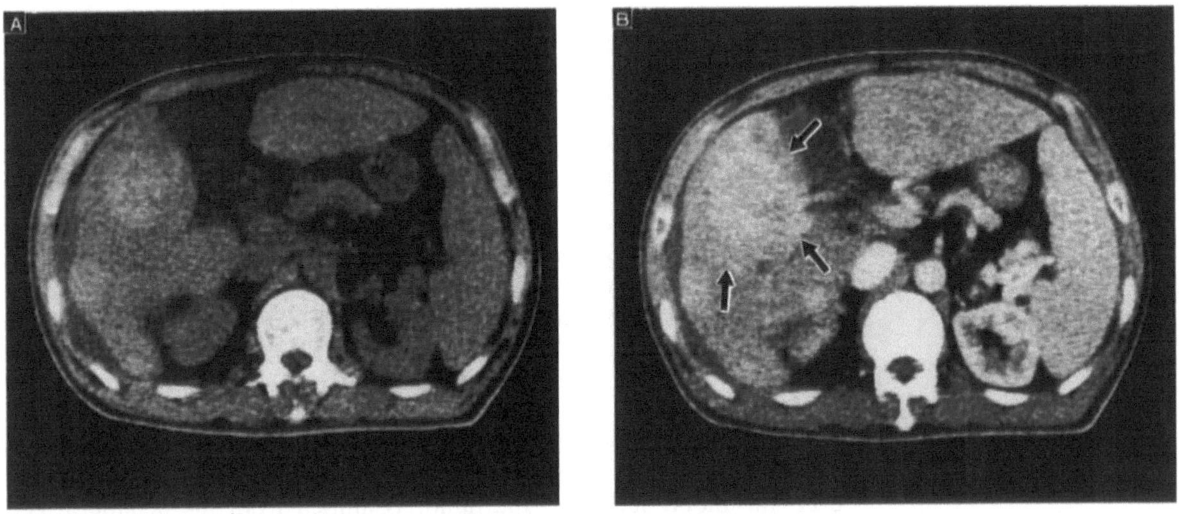

Fig. 4.21 A, B. Hepatocelullar carcinoma. **A** before administration of the contrast medium; **B** after administration of the contrast medium by a bolus injection; more clearly visualized tumor (→) in **B** than in **A**

4.7.2 Diffuse Liver Disease. In the fatty liver, partial or entire liver parenchyma with a decreased CT number is observed, the so-called gray liver. In this case, the CT number of the liver parenchyma is lower than the spleen [57], and in advanced stages with a minimum of 70% fatty infiltration, the CT number is decreased further. As a result, the hepatic vasculature can be observed as images of higher density than the liver parenchyma [62] (Fig. 4.22). With focal fatty infiltration, differentiation from an intrahepatic space-occupying lesion is necessary [52, 63] (Fig. 4.23).

In the case of iron deposits, such as in hemochromatosis and hemosiderosis, the CT number of the liver parenchyma may exceed the normal range and occasionally elevates to more than 90 HU, the so-called white liver. In this case, as opposed to the fatty liver, the vasculature is observed as a low-density tubular structure (Fig. 4.24).

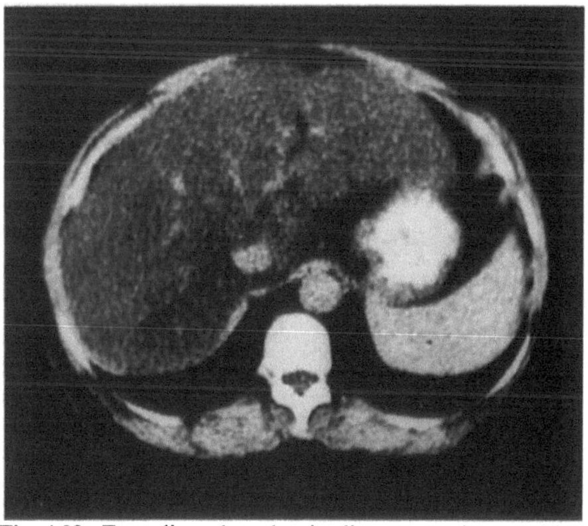

Fig. 4.22. Fatty liver: low-density liver parenchyma with a high-density image of the intrahepatic portal vein and hepatic vein, characteristic of fatty liver

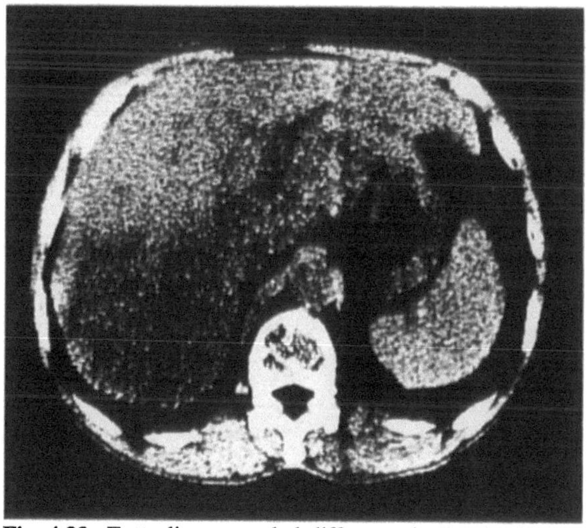

Fig. 4.23. Fatty liver: mottled difference in density in the liver, suggesting inhomogeneous fatty deposit. Same case as shown in Fig. 2.20

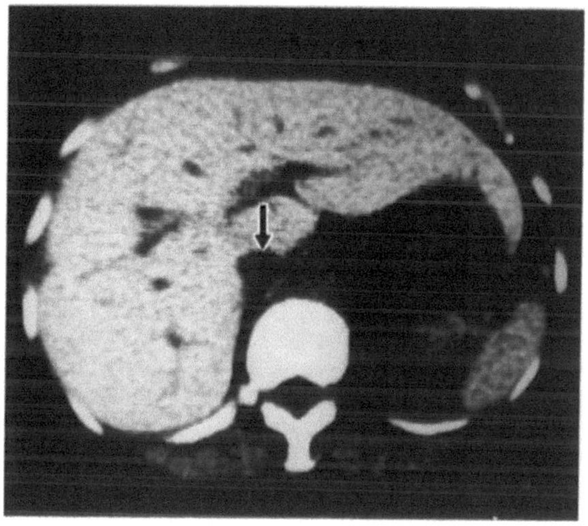

Fig. 4.24. Hemosiderosis: the liver parenchyma has a high CT number of about 119 HU, and the intrahepatic vessels, bile duct, and inferior vena cava (→) are less dense than the liver parenchyma

Table 4.1. CT findings of diffuse hepatocellular disease

CT finding \ Disease	Fatty liver (13 cases)	Chronic hepatitis (56 cases)	Liver cirrhosis (82 cases)
Swelling of left lobe	12 (92%)	34 (61%)	58 (71%)
Atrophy of right lobe	1 (8)	19 (34)	56 (68)
Swelling of caudate lobe	11 (85)	18 (32)	30 (37)
Atrophy of quadrate lobe	5 (38)	42 (75)	74 (90)
Nodular formation			
Caudate lobe	3 (23)	16 (29)	71 (87)
Other lobe	1 (8)	0 (0)	48 (59)
Varices	0 (0)	0 (0)	52 (63)
Splenomegaly	6 (46)	30 (54)	68 (83)
Ascites	0 (0)	0 (0)	12 (15)

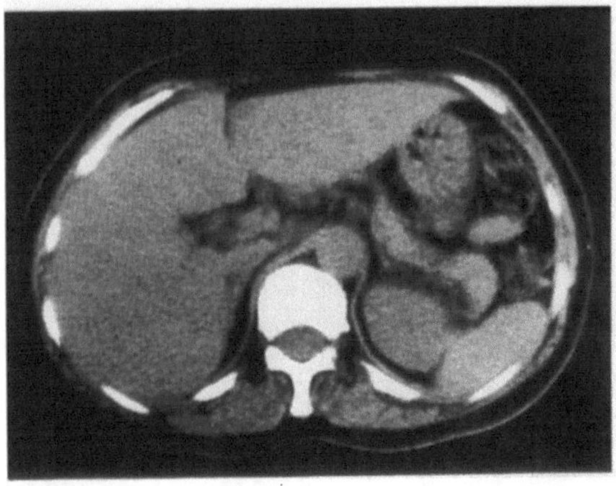

Fig. 4.25. Chronic hepatitis: the tip of the lateral segment of the liver shows beak formation. The tip angle is less than 30°, the tangential line of the posterior medial border of the right lobe is parallel with the sagittal plane, and there is a wide space between the right diaphragmatic crus and posterior medial border of the right lobe

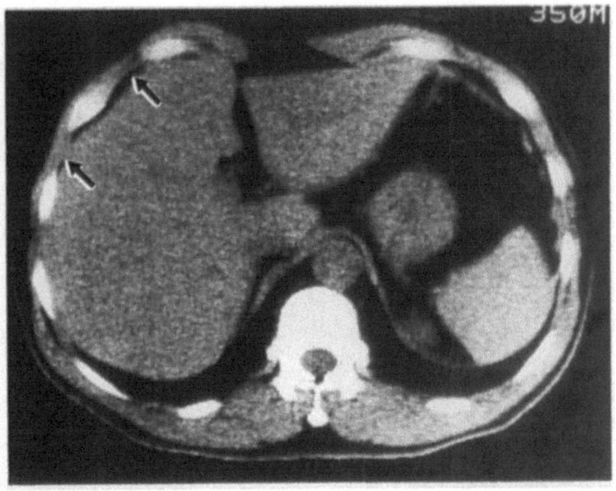

Fig. 4.26. Chronic hepatitis: wide rib compression (→) indicates progressive fibrosis of the liver

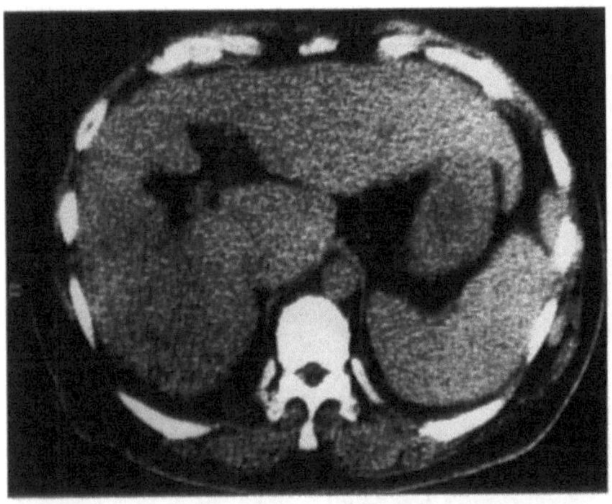

Fig. 4.27. Liver cirrhosis (compensatory stage): there is advanced compensatory swelling, and the tip of the lateral segment extends far to the left with a beak-formation angle of less than 30°. There is marked atrophy of the right lobe, Cantlie's line is horizontal, and the tangential line of the posterior medial border of the right lobe rotates counterclockwise. Also, there is swelling in the caudate lobe, atrophy in the quadrate lobe, and a deep incision of the porta hepatis

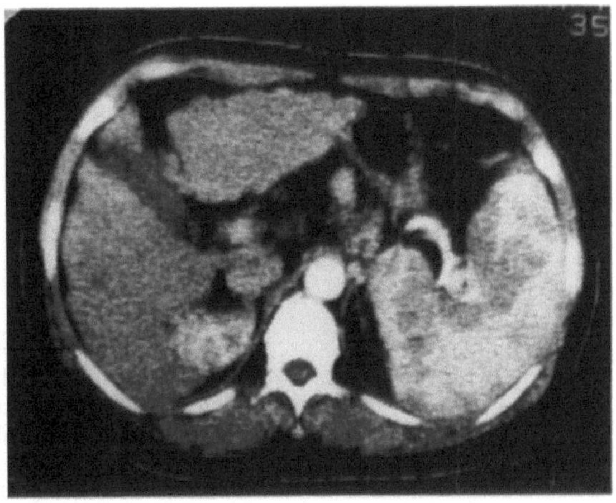

Fig. 4.28. Liver cirrhosis (noncompensatory stage): there is loss of liver contour smoothness and formation of coarse nodulation. No findings are as characteristic as in the compensatory stage, and there is marked swelling of the spleen

In chronic hepatitis and liver cirrhosis, diagnostic information cannot be obtained from the CT number of the liver parenchyma [13]. However, some information is provided by morphological abnormalities of the liver [22] (Table 4.1). For example, with the liver in the early stages of chronic hepatitis and cirrhosis, swelling of the lateral segment, atrophy of the quadrate lobe, and progression of fibrosis can be observed.

A characteristic CT finding of the swollen lateral segment of the liver is a beaked appearance extending to the left side forming an acute angle of less than 30° (Fig. 4.25). In our experience, this finding could be seen in 70% of cases of chronic hepatitis and liver cirrhosis.

On the other hand, progression of fibrosis is characterized by the finding of a rib compression of the liver contour caused by a compression of long duration. Although the rib compression sign may also be observed in normal cases, it is restored if the compression is removed. However, in the case of a liver lacking elasticity with advanced fibrosis, the finding of a rib compression is always visible because there is no restoration and is observed gradually expanding to a wide range exceeding one intercostal space (Fig. 4.26)

In the case of liver cirrhosis, the caudate lobe swells as its stages progress (Fig. 4.27). So far from our experience, the caudate lobe swells to more than two-thirds of the transverse diameter of the vertebral body and is observable in 37% of cases of liver cirrhosis. This finding of swelling of the caudate lobe can also be observed in chronic active hepatitis. In liver cirrhosis, in addition to this finding, dilatation of the gastric coronary vein can be frequently observed.

Complete liver cirrhosis is characterized by swelling of the caudate lobe, atrophy of the quadrate lobe, and loss of liver contour smoothness and the forming of nodulation (Fig. 4.28). Furthermore, atrophy of the right lobe of the liver is marked. The CT findings are characterized by the main lobar fissure shifting to the right side of the right edge of the body of the vertebra, Cantlie's line leveling horizontally, the tangential line of the posterior medial border of the right lobe becoming parallel to the sagittal plane and, furthermore, rotating counterclockwise, and the space between the diaphragmatic crus and posterior medial border of the right lobe widening (Fig. 4.27).

These CT findings are all caused secondary to the decreasing capacity of the right lobe of the liver due to atrophy.

4.8 CT Images of Gallbladder and Biliary Tract Diseases

The attenuation value of the gallstone is higher, lower, or the same as that of the bile juice depending on the substance of the gallstone [24, 50] (Fig. 4.29). Calcified gallstones as small as 2 mm can be detected easily [50].

The accuracy of CT diagnosis of a gallstone is 80%–90%, and, concerning stones in the gallbladder, ultrasonograhy is superior to CT in diagnostic ability. However, in the case of intrahepatic stones and choledocholithiasis, if the stone is calcified, CT is superior to ultrasonography (Figs. 4.30 and 4.31). The superiority of CT can also be confirmed in the diagnosis of emphysematous cholecystitis [58] and milk of calcium bile (Fig. 4.32).

For the differential diagnosis of obstructive jaundice, dilatation of the bile duct can be a useful indicator. The accuracy of CT diagnosis for differentiating the causes of jaundice is 86%–96%, which is almost the same rate of accuracy as for ultrasonography [20, 23] (Fig. 4.23). However, CT is superior to ultrasonography in the diagnosis of the cause or site of an obstruction because CT is not obstructed by images of intestinal gas, while ultrasound is frequently obstructed by the gas overlying the common bile duct. Nevertheless, the common bile duct can be visualized with CT only on the transverse image so that in some cases ultrasonography may be superior because it demonstrates the longitudinal section image along the common bile duct.

In the case of obstructive jaundice, the common bile duct may be dilated without dilatation of the intrahepatic bile duct. Therefore, the biliary tract requires continuous observation extending to the distal portion [65].

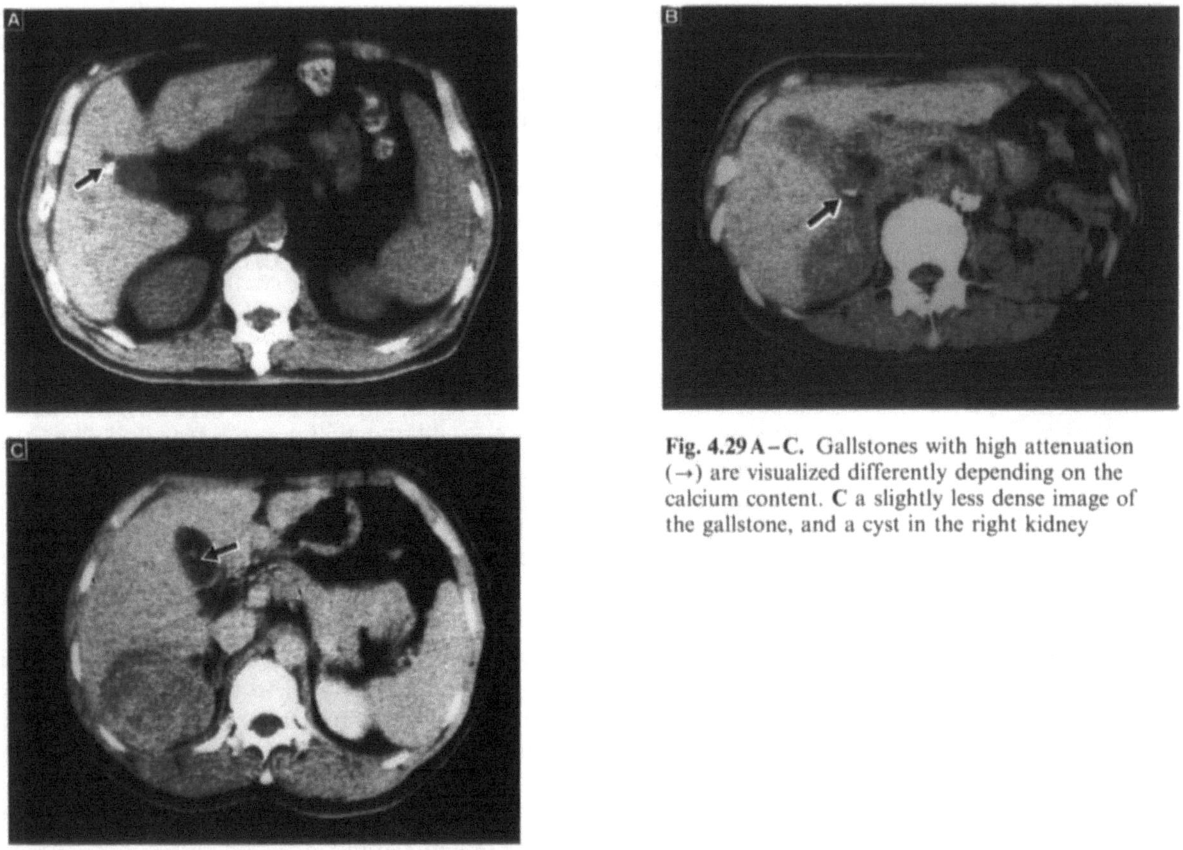

Fig. 4.29 A–C. Gallstones with high attenuation (→) are visualized differently depending on the calcium content. **C** a slightly less dense image of the gallstone, and a cyst in the right kidney

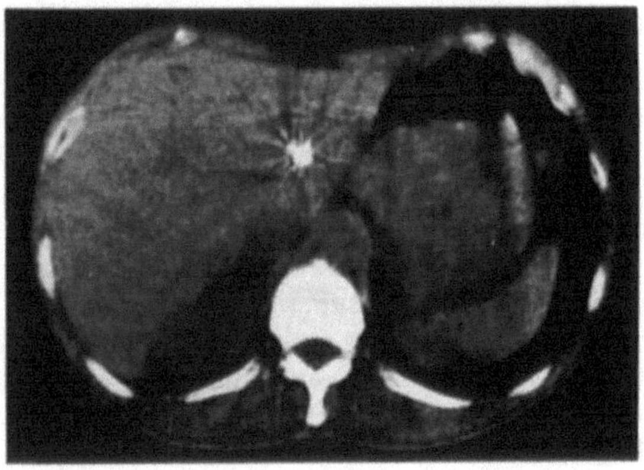

Fig. 4.30. Hepatolithiasis: calculus with high attenuation in the left lobe of the liver. Same case as shown in Fig. 2.37

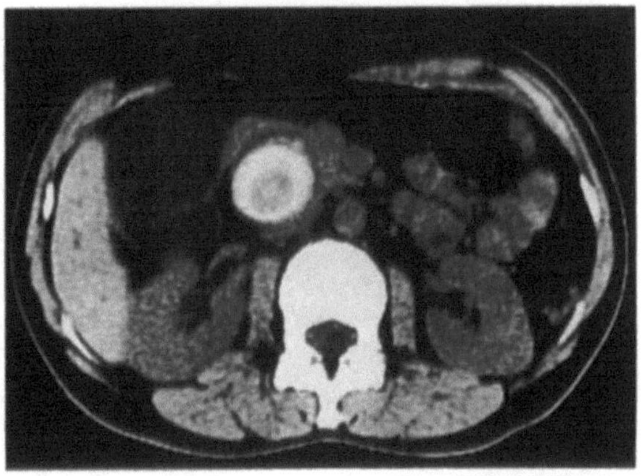

Fig. 4.31. Choledocholithiasis: calcified stone with a diameter of 3 cm in the dilated common bile duct

If scanning sections are made at 1-cm intervals or less, the dilated bile duct can be seen as a variable number of ringlike low-density structures depending on the level of the obstruction and therefore can be used to determine the level of a lesion by the number of these ring images [55] (Fig. 4.34).

The presence of stones, the level of obstruction, the relative size of the ringlike structures, and the shape of the distally visualized ringlike structures are important for determining the cause of the obstruction [56].

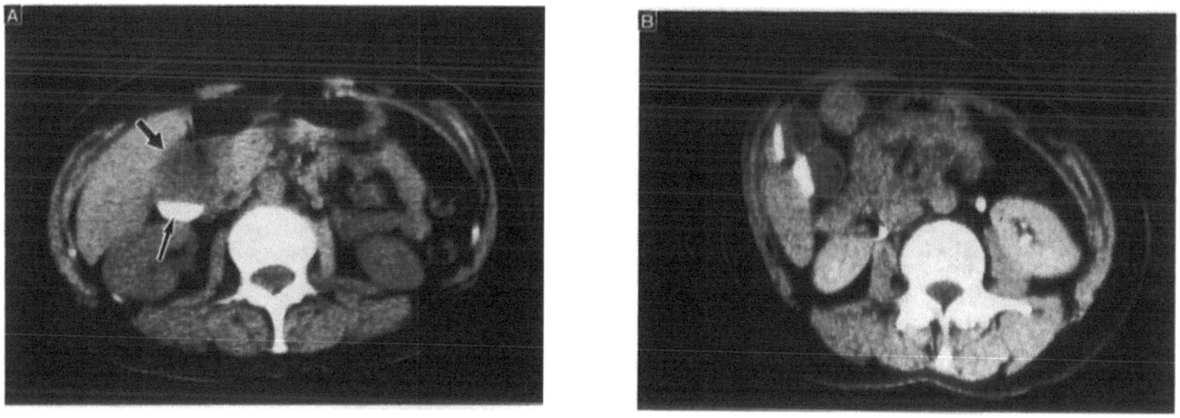

Fig. 4.32 A, B. Milk of calcium bile. **A** supine position: milk of calcium bile (→) observed posteriorly in the gallbladder (→); **B** right lateral decubitus position: milk of calcium bile is shifted in the gravity direction, and the gallbladder is visualized as guitar-shaped. Same case as shown in Figs. 1.14 and 2.27

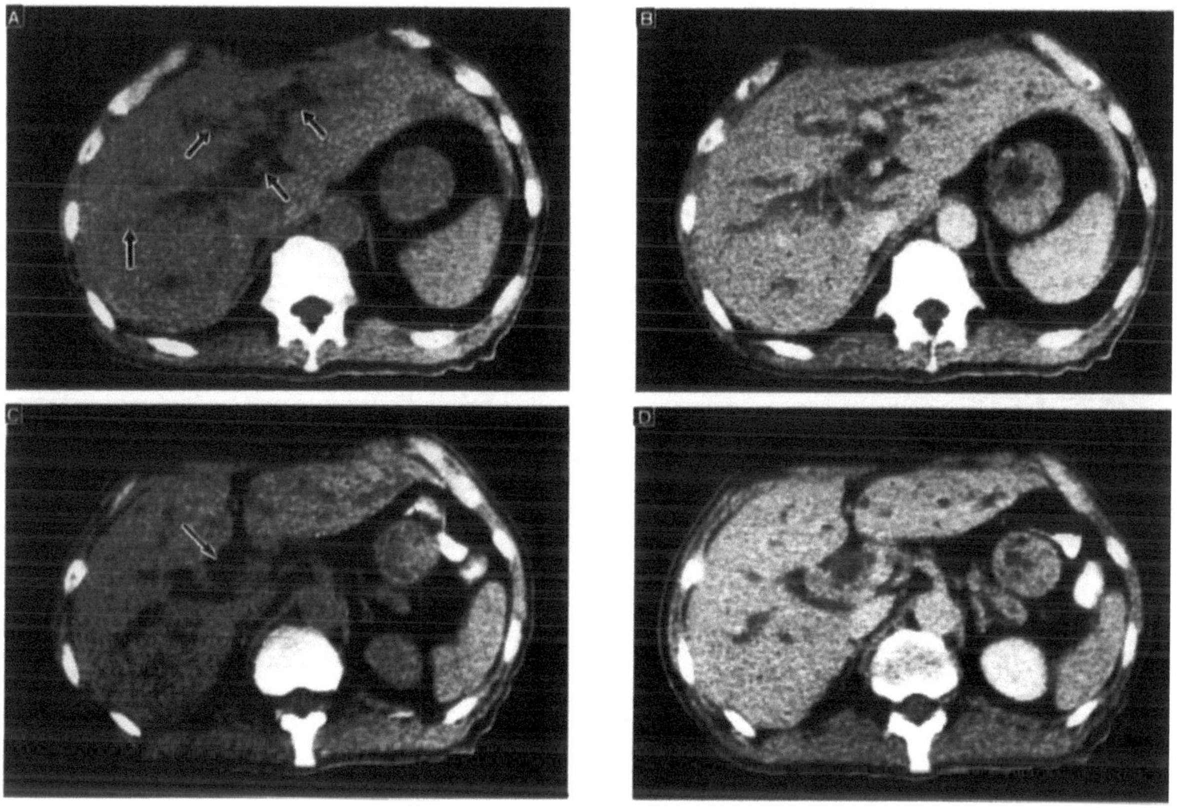

Fig. 4.33 A–D. Dilatation of the biliary tract due to carcinoma of the head of the pancreas. **A, C** before contrast enhancement; **B, D** after contrast enhancement. Dilatation of the intrahepatic bile duct (→) and the common hepatic duct (→) are more clearly visualized by contrast enhancement (**B, D**)

Smooth tapering of a dilated duct indicates benign diseases, and abrupt termination of a dilated duct is characteristic of a malignant tumor [3, 56].

An irregular distal ringlike structure with a protruding nipple or a dilated ringlike structure above it and abrupt change to a nonvisualized duct was present in 100% of the malignant cases in the report of Pedrosa et al. [56]. Intrahepatic ductal dilatation may be more frequent with a malignant lesion than with benign disease [3, 56].

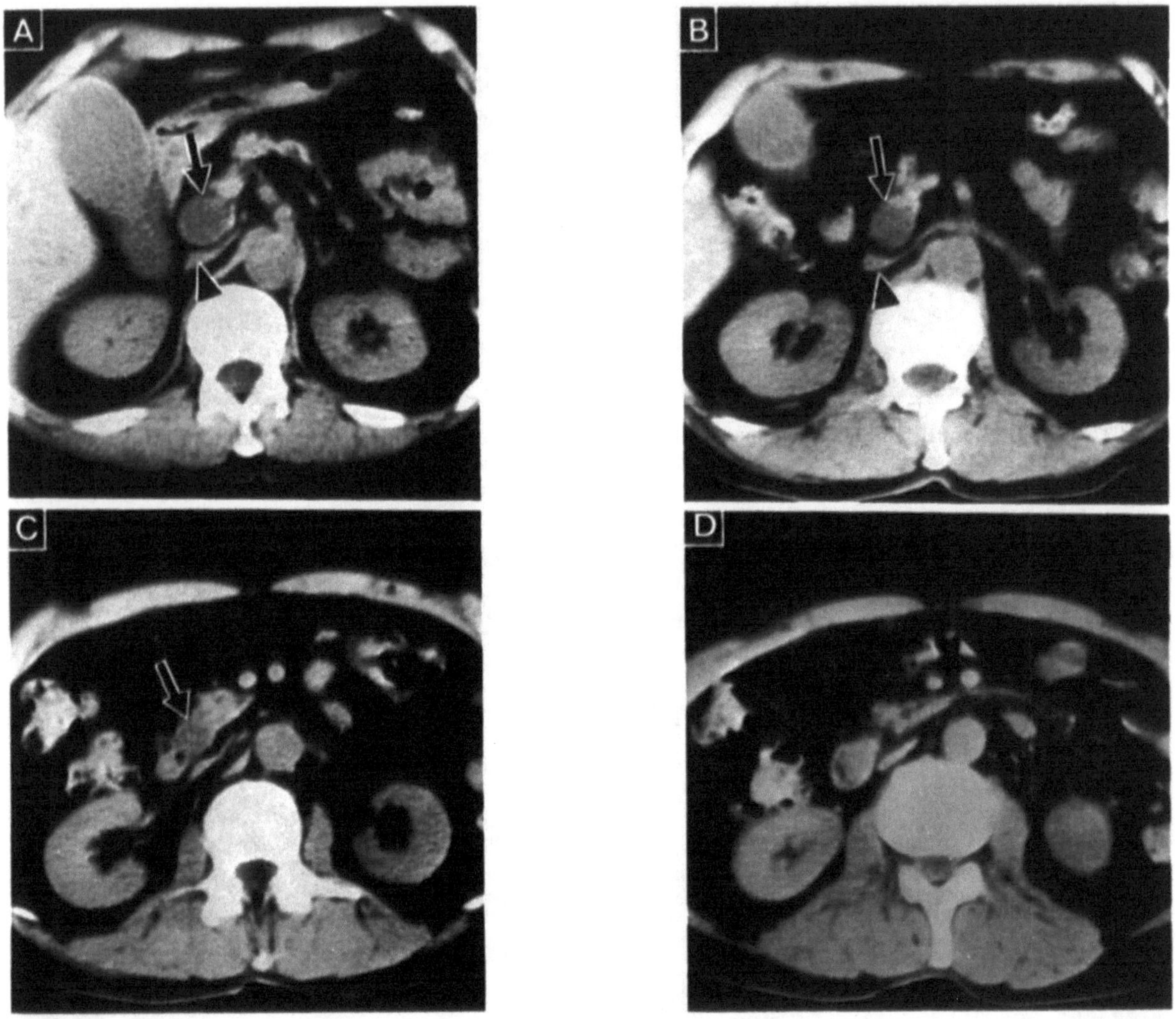

Fig. 4.34 A–D. Dilatation of the extrahepatic bile duct due to carcinoma of the papilla of Vater. The dilated duct is seen as a ringlike shadow (**A, B, C** →) and disappears at the level of the papilla of Vater (**D**). The inferior vena cava is compressed by the dilated bile duct (▶)

Calcium bilirubinate stones of the common bile duct can be readily diagnosed by CT (Fig. 4.31). However, primary cholesterol stones of the common bile duct are difficult to diagnose because their attenuation value is similar to that of the bile juice. A CT finding suggestive of cholesterol stones of the common bile duct is a faint rim of increased density along the periphery of the calculus or punctate areas of increased density within the central part of the stone [37]. In Caroli's disease, the intrahepatic bile duct exhibits localized cystic dilatation [39].

In gallbladder carcinoma at the stage where it has not been filled by tumor, irregular thickening of the wall and an intraluminal mass may be observed [34] (Figs. 4.35 and 4.36). When the gallbladder is filled with a tumor, it is visualized as a structure with the same or somewhat lower density than the liver parenchyma. With invasion of the tumor into the bile duct, intrahepatic bile duct dilatation is observed [27].

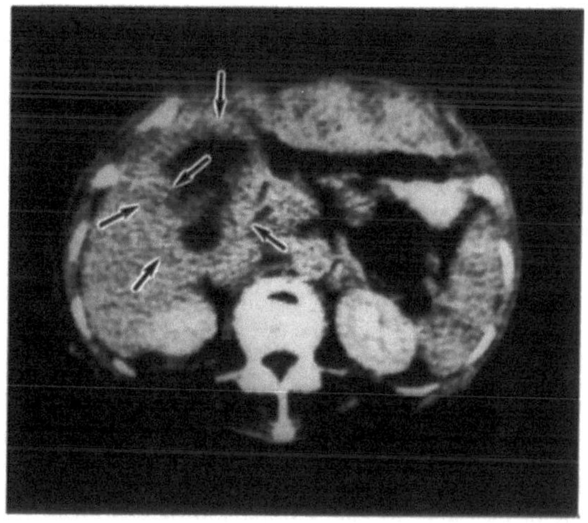

Fig. 4.35. Gallbladder carcinoma: after administration of the contrast medium, an irregular thickened wall (→) and the lumen of the gallbladder almost filled with tumor can be observed

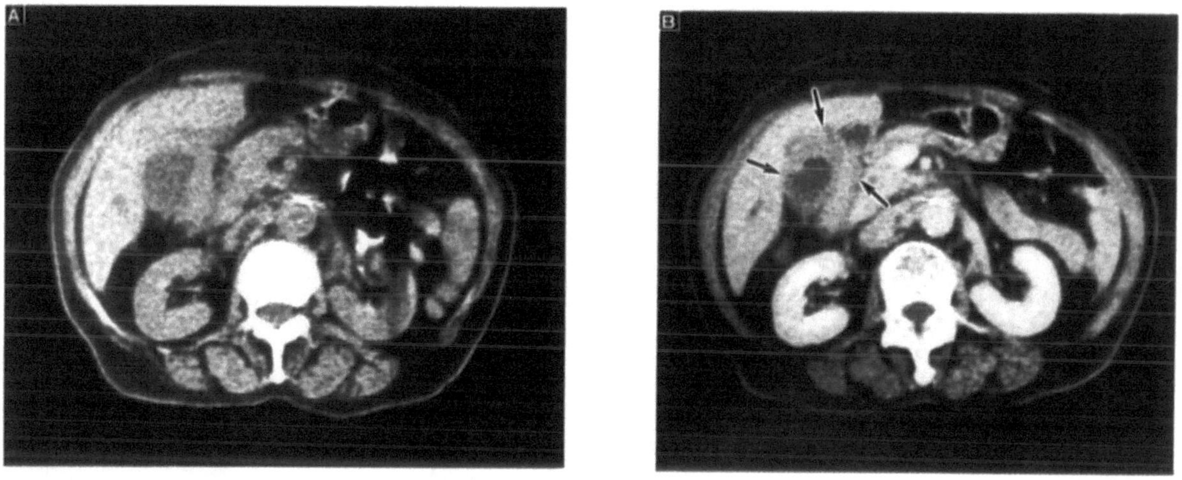

Fig. 4.36 A, B. Gallbladder carcinoma. A before contrast enhancement; B after contrast enhancement. Tumor invades the entire wall of the gallbladder (→). Same case as shown in Figs. 2.32 and 5.22

4.9 CT Images of Diseases of the Pancreas

In acute pancreatitis, a swollen pancreas is observed (Figs. 4.37 and 4.38). The swelling often extends over the entire pancreas, but sometimes it is observed in a localized region. In pancreatitis, the CT number decreases due to the edema, and the peripancreatic fascial plane also disappears.

During the acute phase, diagnosis of the hemorrhage into or around the pancreas is regarded to be possible with CT [31]. In this case, hemorrhage regions are observed as high attenuation images (more than + 60 HU), although in the presence of a hematoma the CT number will progressively decrease within a week.

The extrapancreatic extension of the inflammatory process, abscess, and pseudocyst which occur with acute pancreatitis are also distinctly observed with CT [7, 40]. The extrapancreatic extension of the inflammatory process extends to the lesser sac, anterior pararenal space (Fig. 4.39), and pelvis [10, 47,67].

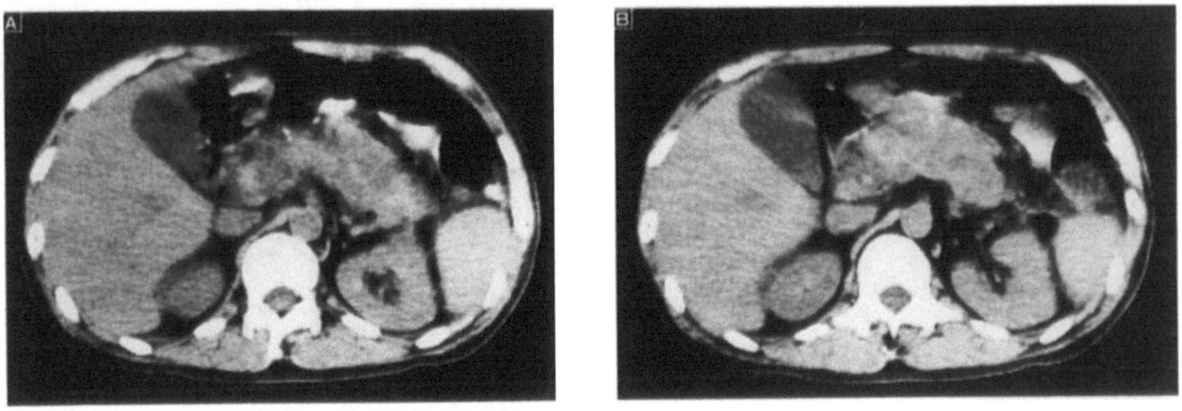

Fig. 4.37 A, B. Acute pancreatitis with complete swelling of the pancreas and multiple low-density areas with a CT number of 33 HU (liver: 50 HU, spleen: 41 HU)

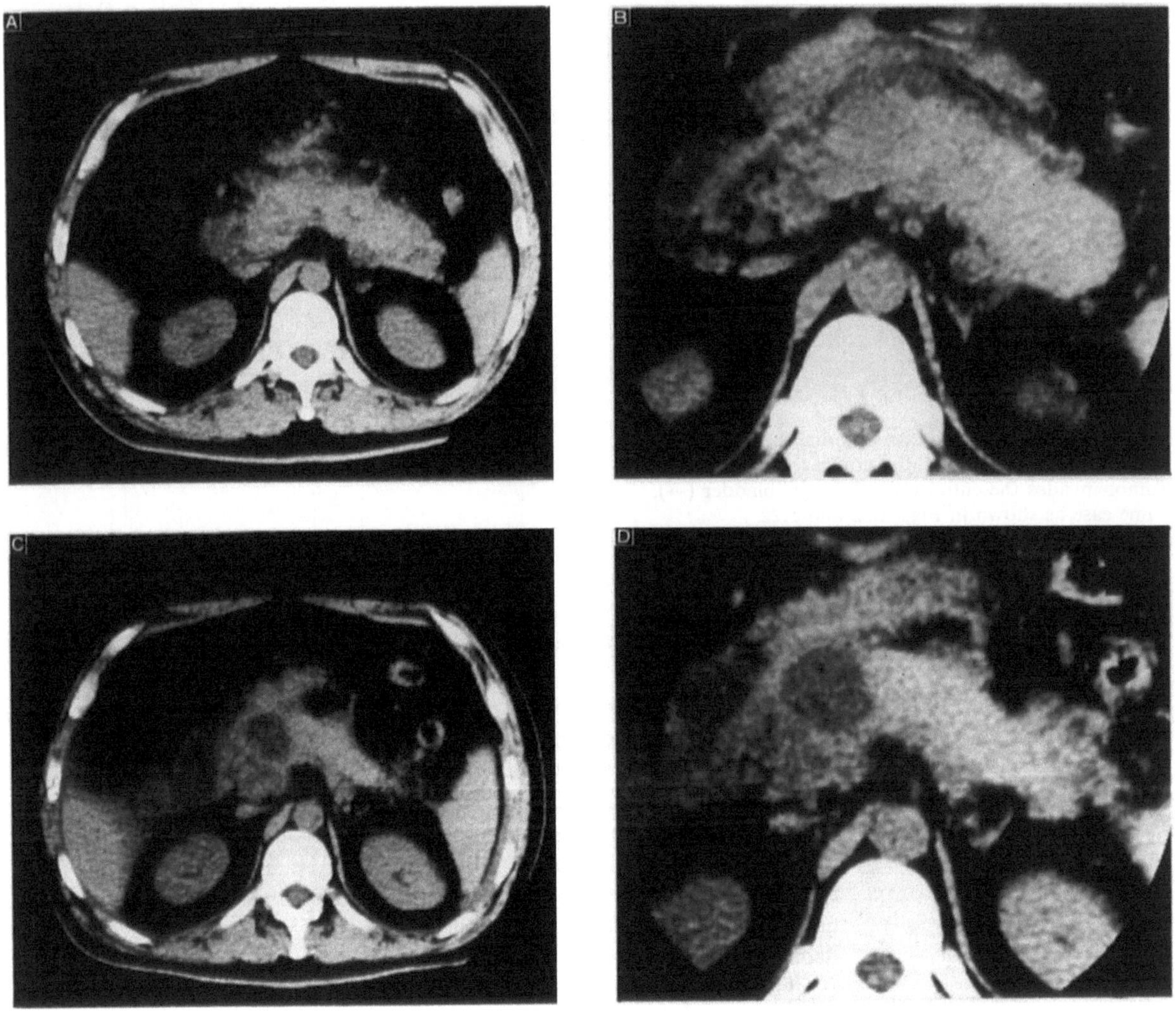

Fig. 4.38 A–D. Acute pancreatitis and chronic relapsing pancreatits. **A, B** an attack of acute pancreatitis with obscure contour of the pancreas and marked swelling of the pancreas with a CT number of 35 HU; **C, D** relapse 1 year after the original attack: pseudocyst in the head and unclear swelling of the body with CT numbers of 15 HU in the cyst and 50 HU in the body

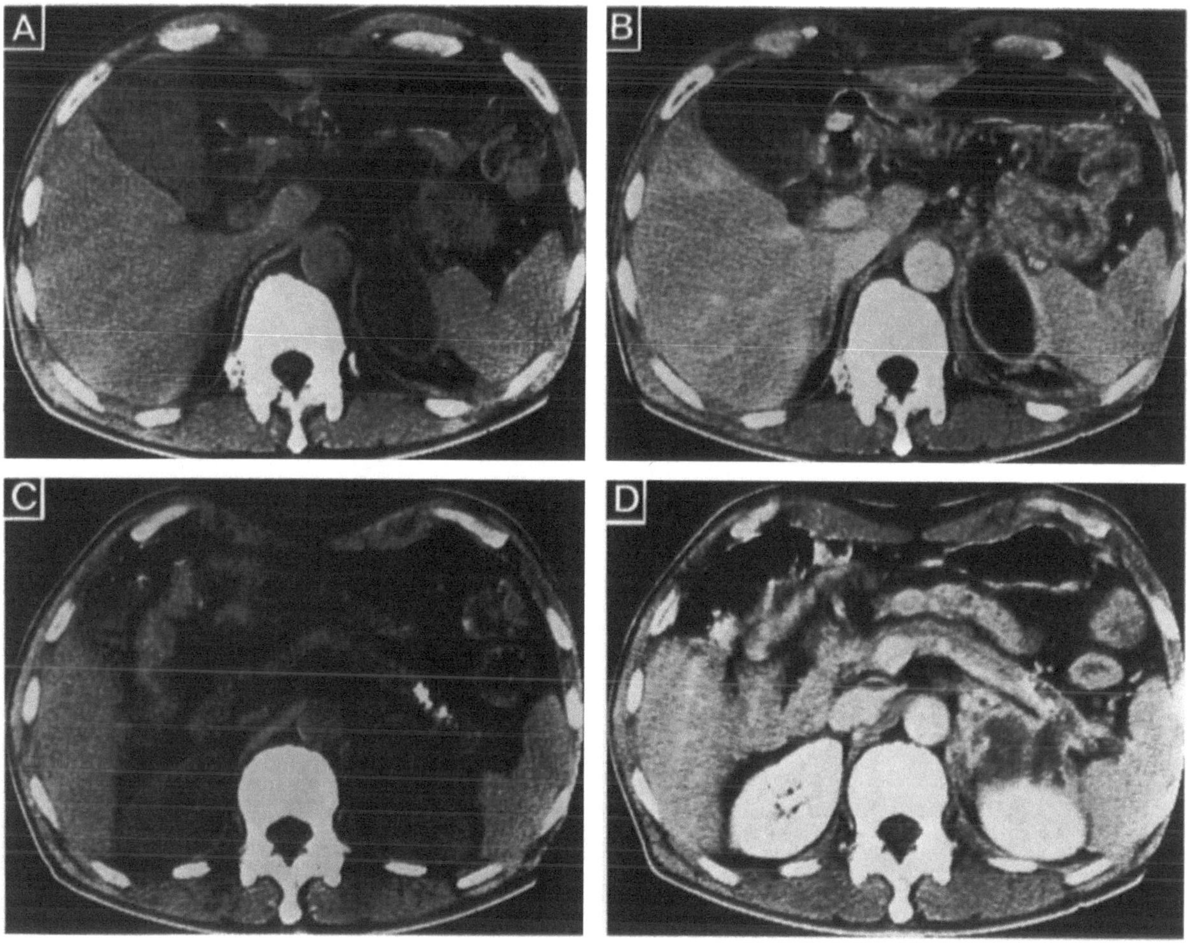

Fig. 4.39 A–D. Pseudocyst and pancreatolithiasis: calcifications are seen in the tail of the pancreas. A main pancreatic duct is dilated. A pseudocyst extending from the tail of the pancreas to the anterior pararenal space is shown. **A, C** before administration of the contrast medium; **B, D** after administration of the contrast medium

In chronic pancreatitis, findings of enlargement, calcification, and pseudocyst can be obtained in 30%–36% of cases [15] (Fig. 4.39). Atrophy of the pancreatic parenchyma and dilatation of the pancreatic duct may sometimes be observed [16]. However, with CT, dilatation of the pancreatic duct cannot be demonstrated without a certain degree of dilatation.

A pseudocyst accompanying pancreatitis is observed as a round or oval low-density image (− 6 ~ + 14 HU) (Fig. 4.38). In this case, with infection, the wall of the pseudocyst becomes thickened, and with abscess, the pancreas attenuation value becomes higher than in the pseudocyst (+ 5 ~ + 22 HU).

With contrast enhancement, the wall of the abscess may be stained so that a high-density image is sometimes observed. Intrapancreatic gases may be visualized in some cases of abscess [46]. Calcification is frequently observed in the case of pancreatic atrophy in chronic pancreatitis. (Fig. 4.40).

In general, pancreatic calculi and calcification can be accurately diagnosed with CT, and pseudocysts and true cysts not caused by pancreatitis can also be diagnosed as above (Fig. 4.41).

In the case of cystadenoma and cystadenocarcinoma of the pancreas, findings of both a solid mass and a cystic image, sometimes accompanied

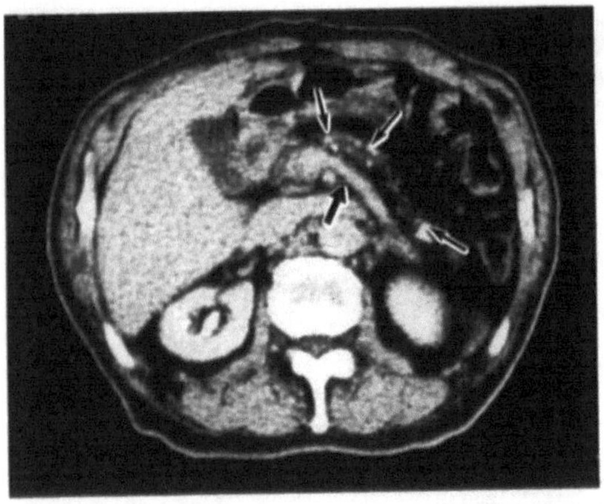

Fig. 4.40. Chronic pancreatitis with calcification. After contrast enhancement; atrophied pancreas in front of the splenic vein (→) accompanied by multiple calcifications (→) can be seen

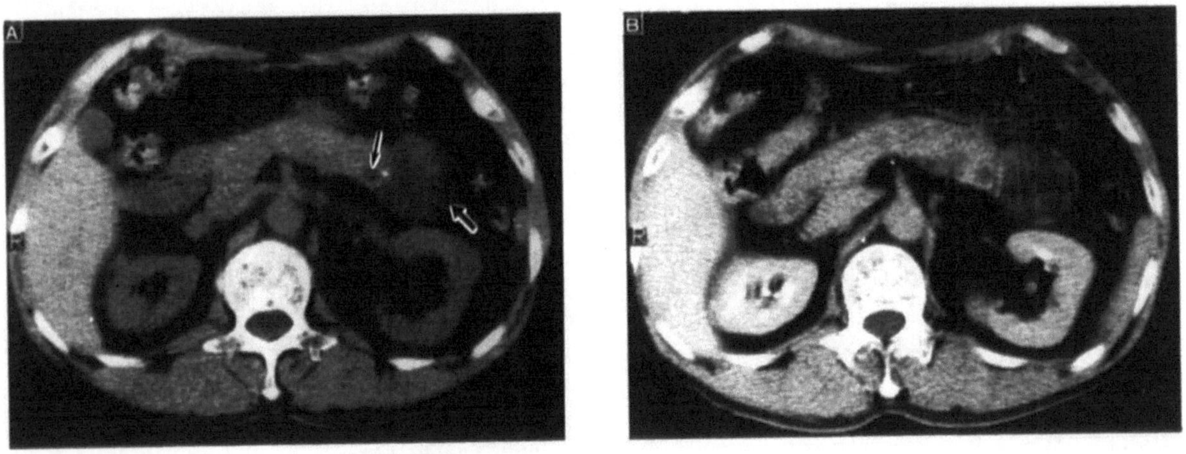

Fig. 4.41 A, B. Cysts of the pancreas with a diameter of 4 cm (→) in the tail and 1 cm (→) on the inner side. There is no change in the CT number of 16.0 HU between before (A) and after (B) administration of the contrast medium

by calcification, can sometimes be visualized; therefore, these characteristic signs are very useful in diagnosis [35, 54].

On the other hand, CT is not effective in conventional techniques for the diagnosis of pancreatic islet cell tumors represented by insulinoma, as the diagnostic accuracy is low at 32%–40% [11, 12]. Dynamic CT should be performed in diagnosing these tumors [26].

In the case of pancreatic carcinoma, CT diagnosis is extremely useful due to the high rate of accuracy of 90%. The direct CT finding of pancreatic carcinoma is a demonstrable tumor with a solid mass image; indirect findings are enlargement of the pancreas due to tumor deformation of the pancreatic contour, and the disappearance of surrounding perivascular and peripancreatic fatty tissues [21, 66] (Figs. 4.42 and 4.43).

Other findings are also obtainable, such as dilatation of the pancareatic duct and secondary enlargement or atrophy of the noninvaded part, pseudocyst, cyst in the tumor, and necrosis in the mass. Secondary findings of carcinoma, observed are dilatation of the biliary tract such as the common or intrahepatic bile duct and cancer metastasis to the lymph node or the liver.

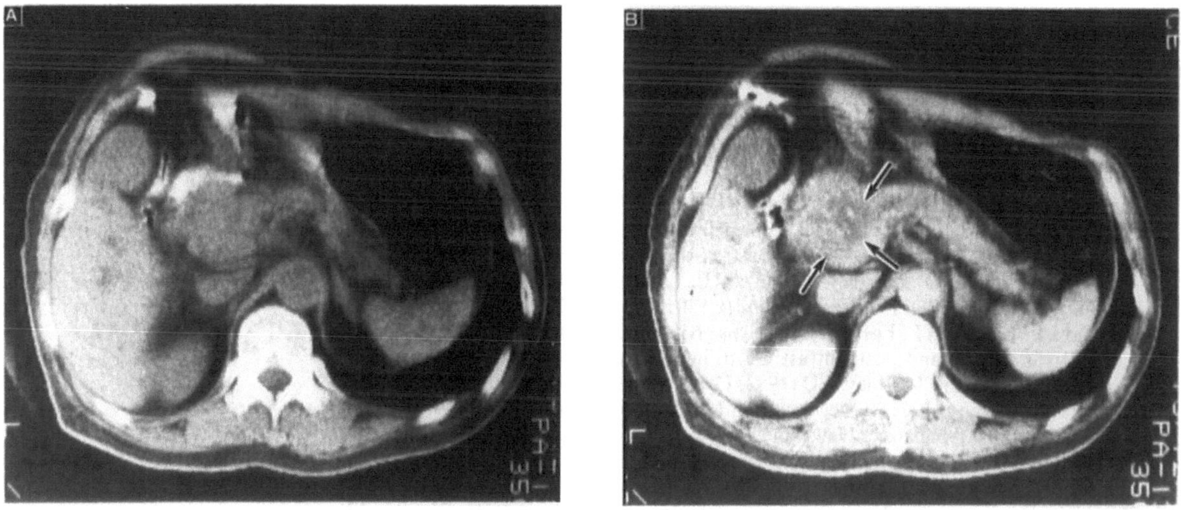

Fig. 4.42 A, B. Carcinoma of the head of the pancreas in the right lateral decubitus position. **A** before contrast medium injection: a swollen head of the pancreas appeared by transoral opacification of the duodenum with the Gastrografin. **B** after administration of the contrast medium: the splenic vein is posterior to the pancreas, the density of the tumor is less than of the body and tail of the pancreas, and there are apparent borders (→) between the tumor and the normal pancreas. Same case as shown in Fig. 2.46

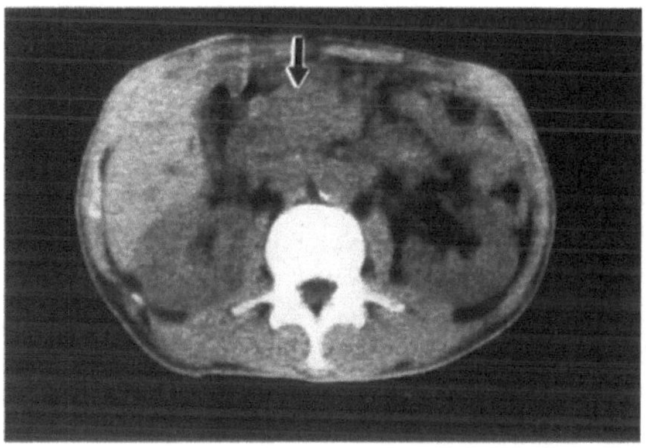

Fig. 4.43. Carcinoma of the head of the pancreas (→)

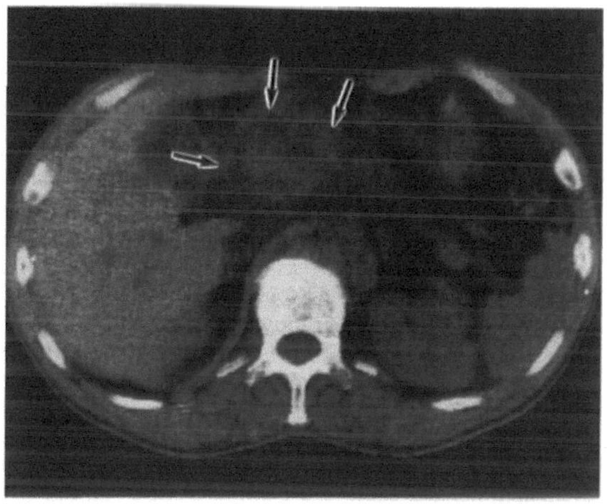

Fig. 4.44. Metastasis of small cell carcinoma of the lung to the pancreas. Swelling of the pancreatic head with a tumor (→) and low-density area inside can be seen

In the case of small pancreatic carcinoma, it is difficult to obtain direct diagnostic signs with conventional CT, and deformation and enlargement of the pancreas due to carcinoma are also not visible; therefore, the diagnostic value of CT is still low in its present state. Useful diagnostic information can be obtained with dynamic CT [5, 26]. In dynamic scanning with bolus injection, carcinoma of the pancreas, due to its hypovascularity, appears to be an area of lower density than the normally enhanced non-tumorous part of the pancreas [26] (Fig. 4.5).

Carcinoma of the pancreatic tail may infiltrate superiorly and inferiorly and sometimes may be found posterior to the splenic vein. This finding may be misdiagnosed for a tumor of the left adrenal gland [8]. Metastatic tumors to the pancreas are also difficult to differentiate from primary pancreatic tumors (Fig. 4.44).

References

Computed Tomography

1. Araki T, Itai Y, Furui S, Tasaka A (1980) Dynamic CT densitometry of hepatic tumors. AJR 135:1037–1043
2. Barnett PH, Zerhouni EA, White RI Jr, Siegelman SS (1980) Computed tomography in the diagnosis of cavernous hemangioma of the liver. AJR 134:439–447
3. Baron RL, Stanley RJ, Lee JKT, Koehler RE, Levitt RG (1983) Computed tomographic features of biliary obstruction. AJR 140:1173–1178
4. Berland LL, Lawson TL, Foley WD, Melrose BL, Chintapalli KN, Taylor AJ (1982) Comparison of pre- and postcontrast CT in hepatic masses. AJR 138:853–858
5. Berland LL, Lawson TL, Foley WD (1983) Dynamic pancreatic scanning. Computed tomography of the pancreas. Siegelman SS (ed) Computed tomography of the pancreas. Churchill Livingstone, New York
6. Bernardino ME (1979) Computed tomography of calcified liver metastases. J Comput Assist Tomogr 3:32–35
7. Braganza JM, Fawcitt RA, Forbes WSC, Isherwood I, Russell JGB, Prescott M, Testa HJ, Torrance HB, Howat HT (1978) A clinical evaluation of isotope scanning, ultrasonography and computed tomography in pancreatic disease. Clin Radiol 29:639–646
8. Callen PW, Breiman RS, Korobkin M, Martini WJD, Mani JR (1979) Carcinoma of the tail of the pancreas: an unusual CT appearance. AJR 133:135–137
9. Callen PW, London SS, Moss, AA (1980) Computed tomographic evaluation of the dilated pancreatic duct. The value of thin-section collimation. Radiology 134:253–255
10. Dember AG, Jaffe CC, Simeone J, Walsh J (1979) A new computed tomographic sign of pancreatitis. AJR 133:477–479
11. Dunnick NR, Doppman JL, Mills SR, McCarthy DM (1980) Computed tomographic detection of nonbeta pancreatic islet cell tumors. Radiology 135:117–120
12. Dunnick, NR, Long JA Jr, Krudy A, Shawker TH, Doppman JL (1980) Localizing insulinomas with combined radiographic methods. AJR 135:747–752
13. Fawcitt RA, Forbes WSC, Isherwood I, Morris AI, Marsh MN, Turnberg LA (1978) Computed tomographic scanning in liver disease. Clin Radiol 29:251–254
14. Federle MP, Filly RA, Moss AA (1981) Cystic hepatic neoplasms: complementary roles of CT and sonography. AJR 136:345–348
15. Ferrucci JT Jr, Wittenberg J, Black EB, Kirkpatrick RH, Hall DA (1979) Computed body tomography in chronic pancreatitis. Radiology 130:175–182
16. Fishman A, Isikoff MB, Barkin JS, Friedland JT (1979) Significance of a dilated pancreatic duct on CT examination. AJR 133:225–227
17. Fishman EK, Farmlett E, Kadir S, Siegelman SS (1982) Computed tomography of benign hepatic tumors. J Comput Assist Tomogr 6:472–481
18. Foley WD, Wilson CR, Quiroz FA, Lawson TL (1980) Demonstation of the normal extrahepatic biliary tract with computed tomography. J Comput Assist Tomogr 4:48–52
19. Freeny PC, Vimont TR, Barnett DC (1979) Cavernous hemangioma of the liver: ultrasonography, arteriography, and computed tomography. Radiology 132:143–148
20. Goldberg HI, Filly RA, Korobkin M, Moss AA, Kressel, HY, Callen PW (1978) Capability of CT body scanning and ultrasonography to demonstrate the status of the biliary ductal system in patients with jaundice. Radiology 129:731–737
21. Haaga JR, Alfidi RJ, Havrilla TR, Tubbs R, Gonzalez L, Meaney TF, Corsi MA (1977) Definitive role of CT scanning of the pancreas. The second year's experience. Radiology 124:723–730
22. Harbin WP, Robert NJ, Ferrucci JT Jr (1980) Diagnosis of cirrhosis based on regional changes in hepatic morphology. A radiological and pathological analysis. Radiology 135:273–283
23. Havrilla TR, Haaga JR, Alfidi RJ, Reich NE (1977) Computed tomography and obstructive biliary disease. AJR 128:765–768
24. Havrilla TR, Reich NE, Haaga JR, Seidelmann FE, Cooperman AM, Alfidi RJ (1978) Computed tomography of the gallbladder. AJR 130:1059–1067
25. Hosoki T, Chatani M, Mori S (1982) Dynamic computed tomography of hepatocellular carcinoma. AJR 139:1099–1106
26. Hosoki, T (1983) Dynamic CT of pancreatic tumors. AJR 140:959–965

27. Hsu-Chong Yeh (1979) Ultrasonography and computed tomography of carcinoma of the gallbladder. Radiology 133:167–173
28. Inamoto K, Sugiki K, Yamasaki H, Miura T (1981) CT of hepatoma: effects of portal vein obstruction. AJR 136:349–353
29. Inamoto K, Tanaka S, Yamazaki H, Okamoto E (1983) Computed tomography in the detection of small hepatocellular carcinomas. Gastrointest Radiol 8:321–326
30. Ishiguchi T, Sakuma S (1983) Dynamic computed tomography with TCT-80A. Toshiba Med Rev 10:49–54
31. Ishikoff MB, Hill MC, Silverstein W, Barkin J (1981) The clinical significance of acute pancreatic hemorrhage. AJR 136:679–684
32. Itai Y, Nishikawa J, Tasaka A (1979) Computed tomography in the evaluation of hepatocellular carcinoma. Radiology 131:165–170
33. Itai Y, Furui S, Araki T, Yashiro N, Tasaka A (1980) Computed tomography of cavernous hemangioma of the liver. Radiology 137:149–155
34. Itai Y, Araki T, Yoshikawa K, Furui S, Yashiro N, Tasaka A (1980) Computed tomography of gallbladder carcinoma. Radiology 137:713–718
35. Itai Y, Moss, AA, Ohtomo K (1982) Computed tomography of cystadenoma and cystadenocarinoma of the pancreas. Radiology 145:419–425
36. Itai Y, Araki T, Furui S, Yashiro N, Ohtomo K, Iio M (1983) Computed tomography of primary intrahepatic biliary malignancy. Radiology 147:485–490
37. Jeffrey, RB, Federie MP, Laing FC, Wall S, Rego J, Moss AA (1983) Computed tomography of choledocholithiasis. AJR 140:1179–1183
38. Johnson CM, Sheedy PF II, Stanson AW, Stephens DH, Hattery RR, Adson MA (1981) Computed tomography and angiography of cavernous hemangiomas of the liver. Radiology 138:115–121
39. Kaiser JA, Mall JC, Salmen BJ, Parker JJ (1979) Diagnosis of Caroli disease by computed tomography: report of two cases. Radiology 132:661–664
40. Kolmannskog F, Kolbenstvedt A, Aakhus T (1981) Computed tomography in inflammatory mass lesions following acute pancreatitis. J Comput Assist Tomogr 5:169–172
41. Korobkin M, Kressel HY, Moss AA, Koehler RE (1978) Computed tomographic angiography of the body. Radiology 126:807–811
42. Kreel L, Haertel M, Katz D (1977) Commputed tomography of the normal pancreas. J Comput Assist Tomogr 1:290–299
43. Levitt RG, Sagel SS, Stanley RJ, Jost RG (1977) Accuracy of computed tomography of the liver and biliary tract. Radiology 124:123–128
44. Marchal GJ, Baert AL, Wilms GE (1980) CT of noncystic liver lesions: bolus enhancement. AJR 135:57–65
45. Mategrano VC, Petasnick J, Clark J, Bin AC, Weinstein R (1977) Attenuation values in computed tomography of the abdomen. Radiology 125:135–140
46. Medenz G Jr, Isikoff MB (1979) Significance of intrapancreatic gas demonstrated by CT: a review of nine cases. AJR 132:59–62
47. Mendez G Jr, Isikoff MA, Hill MC (1980) CT of acute pancreatitis. Interim assessement. AJR 135:463–469
48. Moss AA, Kressel HY, Korobkin M, Goldberg HI, Rohlfing BM, Brasch RC (1978) The effect of gastrografin and glucagon on CT scanning of the pancreas: a blind clinical trial. Radiology 126:711–714
49. Moss AA, Schrumpf J, Schnyder P, Korobkin M, Shimshak RR (1979) Computed tomography of focal hepatic lesions: a blind clinical evaluation of the effect of contrast enhancement. Radiology 131:427–430
50. Moss, AA, Filly RA, Way LW (1980) In vitro investigation of gallstones with computed tomography. J Comput Assist Tomogr 4:827–831
51. Moss, AA, Dean PB, Axel, L, Goldberg HI, Glazer GM, Friedman MA (1982) Dynamic CT of hepatic masses with intravenous and intraarterial contrast material. AJR 138:847–852
52. Mulhern CB, Arger PH, Coleman BG, Stein GN (1979) Nonuniform attenuation in computed tomography study of the cirrhotic liver. Radiology 132:399–402
53. Neumann CH, Hessel SJ (1980) CT of the pancreatic tail. AJR 135:741–745
54. Paricnty RA, Ducellier R, Lubrano JM, Picard JD, Pradel J, Smolarski N (1980) Cystadenomas of the pancreas: diagnosis by computed tomography. J Comput Assist Tomogr 4:364–367
55. Pedrosa CS, Casanova R, Rodriguez R (1981) Computed tomography in obstructive jaundice. Part I: The level of obstruction. Radiology 139:627–634
56. Pedrosa, CS, Casanova R, Lezana AH, Fernandez MC (1981) Computed tomography in obstructive jaundice. Part II: The cause of obstruction. Radiology 139:635–645

57. Piekarski J, Goldberg HI, Royal SA, Axel L, Moss AA (1980) Difference between liver and spleen CT numbers in the normal adult: its usefulness in predicting the presence of diffuse liver disease. Radiology 137:727–729
58. Poleynard GD, Harris RD (1979) Diagnosis of emphysematous cholecystitis by computerized tomography. Gastrointest Radiol 4:153–155
59. Prando A, Wallace S, Bernardino ME, Lindell MM (1979) Computed tomographic arteriography of the liver. Radiology 130:697–701
60. Scatarige JC, Fishman EK, Saksouk FA, Siegelman SS (1983) Computed tomography of calcified liver masses. J Comput Assist Tomogr 7:83–89
61. Scherer U, Rothe R, Eisenburg J, Schidberg, FW, Meister P, Lissner J (1978) Diagnostic accuracy of CT in circumscript liver disease. AJR 130:711–714
62. Scherer U, Santos M, Lissner J (1979) CT studies of the liver in vitro: a report on 82 cases with pathological correlation. J Comput Assist Tomogr 3:589–595
63. Scott WW Jr, Sanders RC, Siegelman SS (1980) Irregular fatty infiltration of the liver: diagnosis dilemmas. AJR 135:67–71
64. Seidelmann FE, Cohen WN, Bryan PJ, Brown J (1977) CT demonstation of the splenic vein – pancreatic relationship: the pseudodilated duct. AJR 129:17–21
65. Shanser JD, Korobkin M, Goldberg HI, Rohlfing BM (1978) Computed tomographic diagnosis of obstructive jaundice in the absence of intrahepatic ductal dilatation. AJR 131:389–392
66. Sheedy PF II, Stephens DH, Hattery RR, MacCarty RL (1977) Computed tomography in the evaluation of patients with suspected carcinoma of the pancreas. Radiology 124:731–737
67. Siegelman SS, Copeland BE, Saba GP, Cameron JL, Sanders RC, Zerhouni EA (1980) CT of fluid collections associated with pancreatitis. AJR 134:1121–1132
68. Simone JF, Simonds BD (1979) Normal anatomy of the pancreas by computed tomography and diagnostic ultrasound: In: Taylor KSW (ed) Diagnostic ultrasound in gastrointestinal disease. Churchill Livingstone, New York, pp 73–84
69. Snow JH Jr, Goldstein HM, Wallace S (1979) Comparison of scintigraphy, sonography and computed tomography in the evaluation of hepatic neoplasms. AJR 132:915–918
70. Stanley RJ, Sagel SS, Levitt RG (1977) Computed tomographic evalution of the pancreas. Radiology 124:715–722
71. Stephens, DH, Sheedy PF II, Hattery RR, MacCarty RL (1977) Computed tomography of the liver. AJR 128:579–590
72. Tada S, Fukuda K, Aoyagi Y, Harada J (1980) CT of abdominal malignancies: dynamic approach. AJR 135:455–461
73. Wooten WB, Bernardino ME, Goldstein HM (1978) Computed tomography of necrotic metastases. AJR 131:839–842
74. Young SW, Turner RJ, Castellino RA (1980) A strategy for the contrast enhancement of malignant tumors using dynamic computed tomography and intravascular pharmacokinetics. Radiology 137:137–147

5 Angiography

The anatomy of the vasculature system is important in the investigation of the morphology and function of organs. The vasculature in the interstitial tissue shows a characteristic distribution particular to the organ. Although they may sometimes provide a primary indication of a lesion, morphological changes of vessels or abnormality of the organs are mostly secondary indicators caused by a disease of the organ.

According to Viamonte [76], angiograms cannot be specific for a disease. Findings of morphological changes of the vascular system caused by tumor are encasement, narrowing, obstruction, dilatation, irregularity, tortuosity, hyper- and hypovascularity, and neovascularity [24]. From these findings, the nature and extension of the tumor can be assumed so that angiography can frequently be utilized as the final morphological diagnostic method [22].

Portography is also useful in the diagnosis of portal hypertension and collateral circulation. Recently, angiography techniques have beeen applied not only to morphological diagnosis but also to treatment for bleeding and tumor.

5.1 Examination Procedures

With stereoangiography [35], the structure of the vascular system is visualized superiorly as an overlapped image due to the three-dimensional location of linear constructions. In angiography, it sometimes may be necessary to observe capillary vessels about 10 μm in diameter, magnification angiography with a small focus X-ray tube may be required [74], and serial radiography with a short exposure time is necessary to follow the quick movement of contrast medium in the vascular blood stream and to observe the change of phase.

5.1.1 Arterial Examination. Arterial examination of the liver, biliary tract, and pancreas can be performed by selective injection of contrast medium into the celiac or superior mesenteric artery or their branches by Seldinger's method.

For puncturing, a catheter needle with a Teflon or polyethylene sleeve is utilized. Using a J-shaped guide wire, injury of the vascular wall can be minimized. The curvature of the tip of the catheter must be selected according to the shape of the particular branch of the aorta. For custom-made catheters, the tip must be carefully shaped according to the curvature of the particular branch of the aorta. Recently, preshaped ready-made catheters have become available.

Although appearing smooth, the surface of the catheter and guide wire is markedly uneven (distinctly observed with an electron microscope); therefore, once it sticks to the surface, blood is hard to remove due to the formation of small clots. Furthermore, disposable catheters and guide wires should be selected because the hepatitis virus may be resistant to heat and sterilizing agents.

Before examination, the patient's history must be referred to, and the present status of hypersensitivity, cardiopulmonary disease, liver dysfunction, renal disease, disease of the thyroid gland, and the degree, if existent, must all be determined. Also, the necessity of angiographic examination must be explained to the patient and the patient's consent obtained.

Thereafter, sensitivity to iodine and anesthetics may be tested. Nausea and vomiting may often occur as side effects so that it is necessary that the patient fast for several hours prior to the examination. An enema is also required to avoid obstruction with stool and bowel gas while reading the angiogram, not to mention complete urination and evacuation of the bowels. Administration of atropine and an antihistaminic is needed 30 min prior to the examination to decrease the patient's anxiety, tension, and pain.

Catheter manipulation must be practiced carefully and the catheter projected correctly into the intended vessel. The catheter operation not only requires training, but the most important factor is that curve in the distal part of the catheter be adapted to the branches of the vasculature.

In angiography, large amounts of contrast medium tend to be used because the medium is immediately carried away after injection due to the speed of the bloodstream. Because of this rapid movement, it is necessary to take a number of films sequentially to obtain fine images. The quantity of contrast medium, intervals of X-ray exposure, and amount of film should be carefully planned. This is also important to protect the patient from unnecessary radiation exposure. After the examination, the patient must be kept quiet and checked for bleeding in the puncture portion and embolism.

In children, angiography of the liver, biliary tract, and pancreas is most often performed with celiac arteriography or superior mesenteric arteriography, less frequently with hepatic venography and percutaneous splenoportography. Superselective angiography, frequently performed in adults, is usually unnecessary in children.

Conventional selective angiography can be easily accomplished using the catheter with the tip bent in a semicircle with a diameter 1.5 times that of the aorta. As a contrast medium, meglumine diatrizoate 65% (Angiografin) is used according to the patient's weight with a standard of 1 ml/kg.

5.1.2 Venous Examination. Venography can be performed following arterial injection or by direct objective intravenous injection. To opacify the portal vein by injection into the superior mesenteric artery, vasodilating agents should be used. For finer opacification of the portal system, in the case of hepatic venography, the contrast medium should be injected through the catheter at the site of the hepatic vein.

Portal venography can be achieved by splenic puncture or by percutaneous transhepatic puncturing using a guide wire with a catheter into the main branch of the portal vein under ultrasonic observation. With percutaneous transhepatic portography, selective catheterization of the intended vein is possible.

5.2 Hepatic Vasculature and Its Findings

The hepatic vasculature [42, 69] is composed of the vasa privata and vasa publica, the vasa privata being the hepatic artery and vasa publica being the portal vein.

5.2.1 Hepatic Artery. The common hepatic artery is made up of branches of the celiac artery. After originating from the celiac trunk, the common hepatic artey forms the proper hepatic artery at the porta hepatis and runs into the right and left hepatic lobe. In the liver, the left and right hepatic arteries generally run along the portal vein. The perfused area of the right and left hepatic arteries does not coincide with the anatomical segment of the liver, but this segment is divided by Cantlie's line, which connects the inferior vena cava and gallbladder fossa.

There is no anastomosis between the right and left hepatic arteries, and collateral circulation is composed of branches from other organs. Branching of the hepatic artery has many variations [42, 69] (Figs. 5.1 and 5.2). The

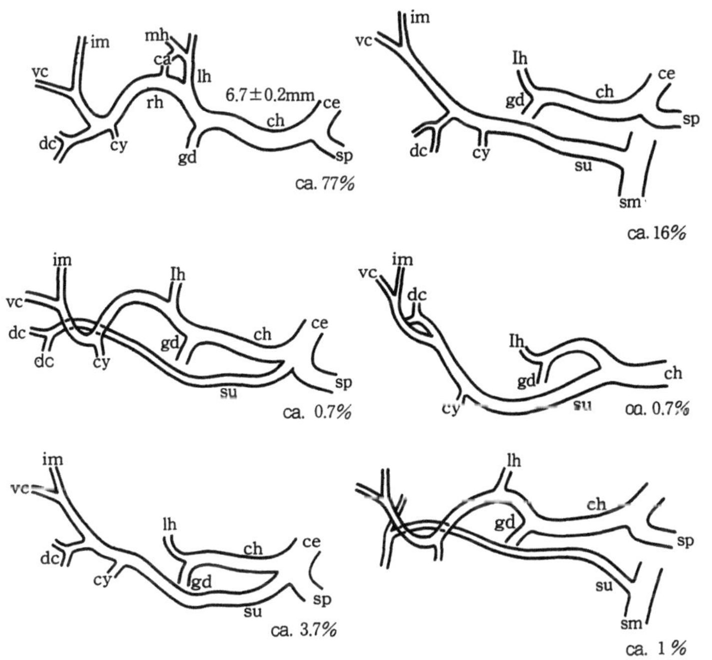

Fig. 5.1. Arterial distribution to the right lobe. The frequency of each type is shown in the right lower corner of each type

ce: Celiac artery
sp: Splenic artery
ch: Common hepatic artery
gd: Gastroduodenal artery
lh: Left hepatic artery
rh: Right hepatic artery
cy: Cystic artery
dc: Dorsocaudal segment artery
vc: Ventrocranial segment artery
im: Intermediate segment artery
sm: Superior mesenteric artery
su: Supplementary artery
ca: Artery supplying cudate lobe
mh: Middle hepatic artery

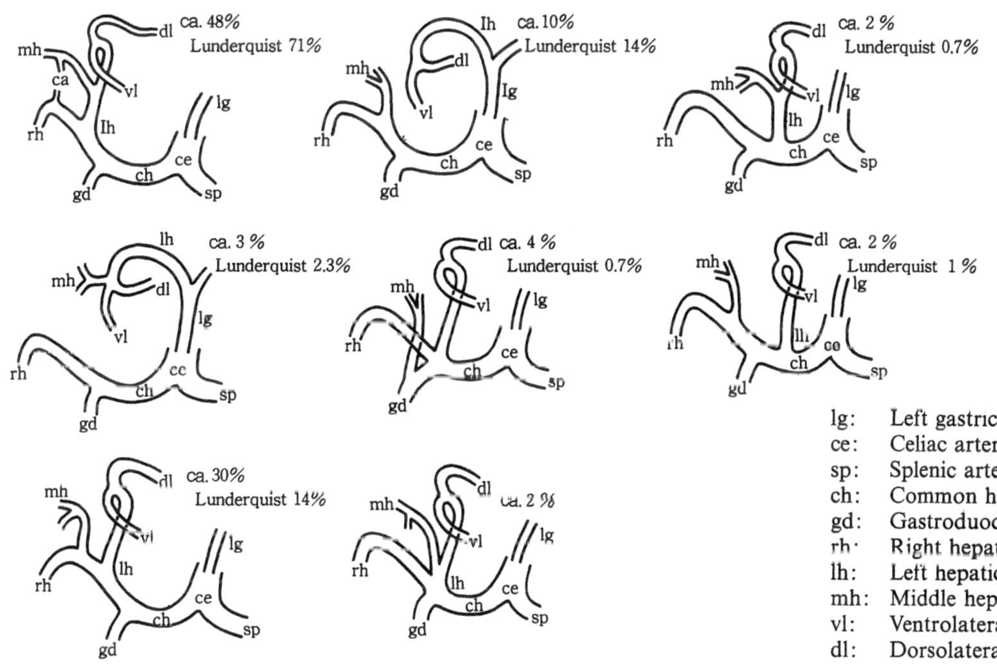

lg: Left gastric artery
ce: Celiac artery
sp: Splenic artery
ch: Common hepatic artery
gd: Gastroduodenal artery
rh: Right hepatic artery
lh: Left hepatic artery
mh: Middle hepatic artery
vl: Ventrolateral segment artery
dl: Dorsolateral segment artery
ca: Artery supplying caudate lobe

Fig. 5.2. Arterial distribution to the left lobe. The frequency of each type is shown in the right upper corner of each type; upper row by the authors [69], lower row by Lunderquist [41]

A.

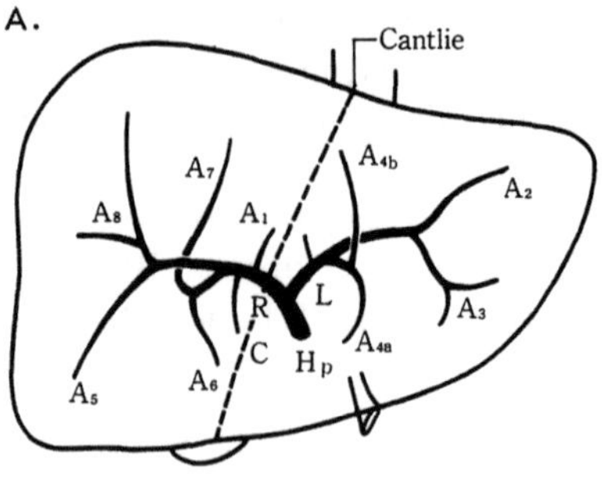

H_p: Proper hepatic artery
R: Right hepatic artery
L: Left hepatic artery
A1: Artery supplying cudate lobe
A2: Dorsolateral segment artery
A3: Ventrolateral segment artery
A4a: Medial segment artery (superficial branch)
A4b: Medial segment artery (profundus branch)
A5: Ventrocaudal segment artery
A6: Dorsocaudal segment artery
A7: Dorsocranial segment artery
A8: Ventrocranial segment artery
C: Cystic artery

(Couinaud [16])

B.

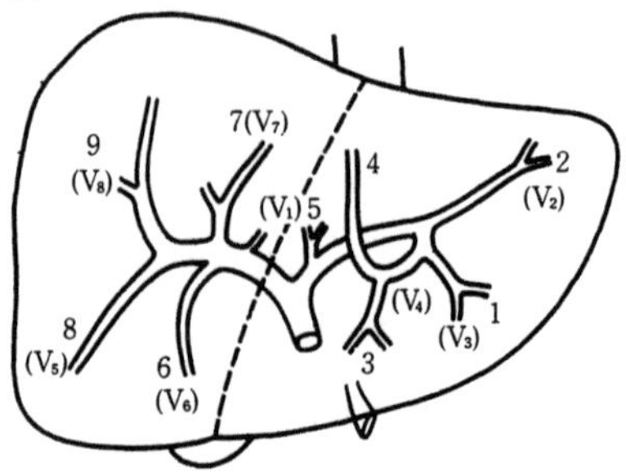

1. Left anterior segment branch (V3)
2. Left posterior segment branch (V2)
3. Median anterior segment branch (V4)
4. Median posterior segment branch (V4)
5. Caudate segment branch (V1)
6. Right median anterior segment branch (V5)
7. Right median posterior segment branch (V8)
8. Right lateral anterior segment branch (V6)
9. Right lateral posterior segment branch (V7)

1–9 by Okudaira's classification [55]
V1–V8 by Couinaud's classification [16]

C.

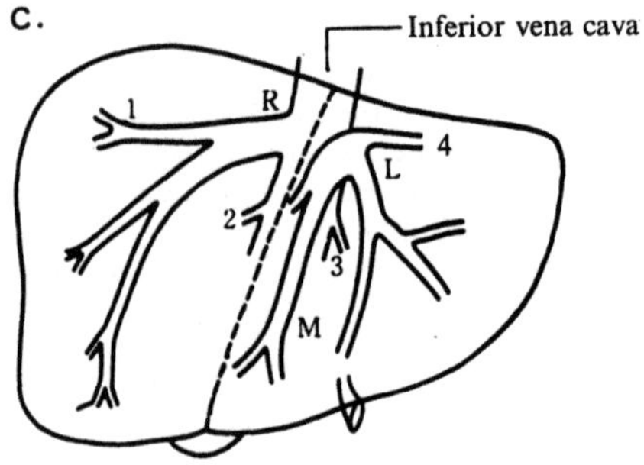

R: Right hepatic vein
1: Right superior hepatic vein
2: Posterior inferior hepatic vein
M: Middle hepatic vein
3: Caudate hepatic vein
L: Left hepatic vein
4: Left superior hepatic vein

Fig. 5.3. A hepatic artery; **B** portal vein; **C** hepatic vein; **D, D′** stereoscopic view of hepatic arteries and portal vein

D

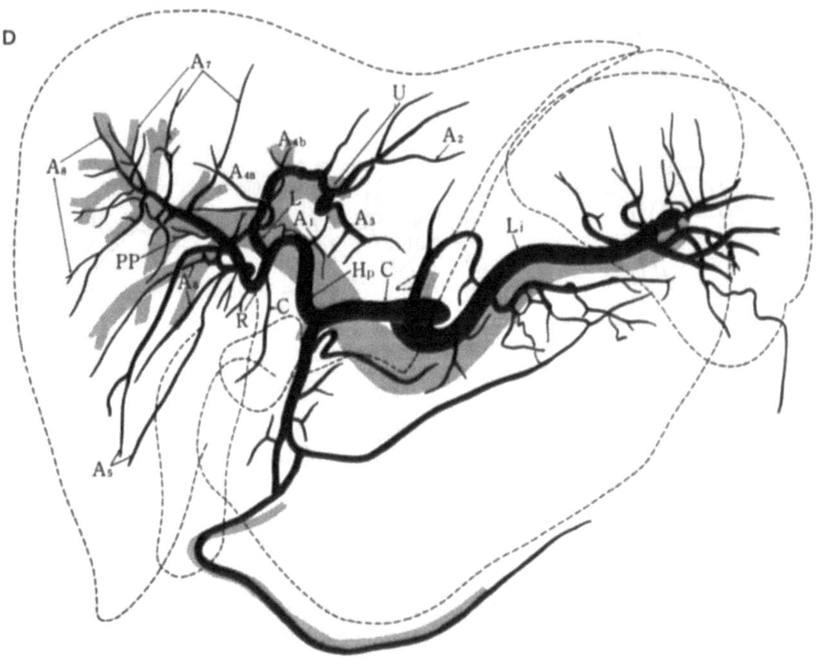

Li: Splenic artery
Hc: Common hepatic artery
G: Gastroduodenal artery
Hp: Proper hepatic artery
L: Left branch
R: Right branch
C: Cystic artery
Lg: Left gastric artery
PP: Periportal arterial plexus
U: Umbilical point

periarterial and periportal plexus are also formed due to anastomosis between the small artery which runs along the hepatic artery [69]. The hepatic artery branches and runs into the liver segment (Fig. 5.3). However, this distribution also has marked variations and is not consistent.

To diagnose the hepatic arteriogram, although Hjortsjo's grouping of hepatic segments [31] is convenient, Couinaud's [16] and Okudaira's groupings [55] are better suited for detailed analyzing. Okudaira's grouping divides the medial segment of Couinaud's grouping into anterior and posterior segments (Fig. 5.4).

Branching again, the segmental arteries become the interlobular artery (Ramus arteriosus interlobularis) and run into the interlobular connective tissues with the interlobular vein and interlobular bile duct. The interlobular artery becomes the capillary vessels which flow into the intralobular capillary vessels. For instance, Elias [19] states the presence of an intralobular arteriole connected from the interlobular artery into the peripheral and radial sinusoid.

D′

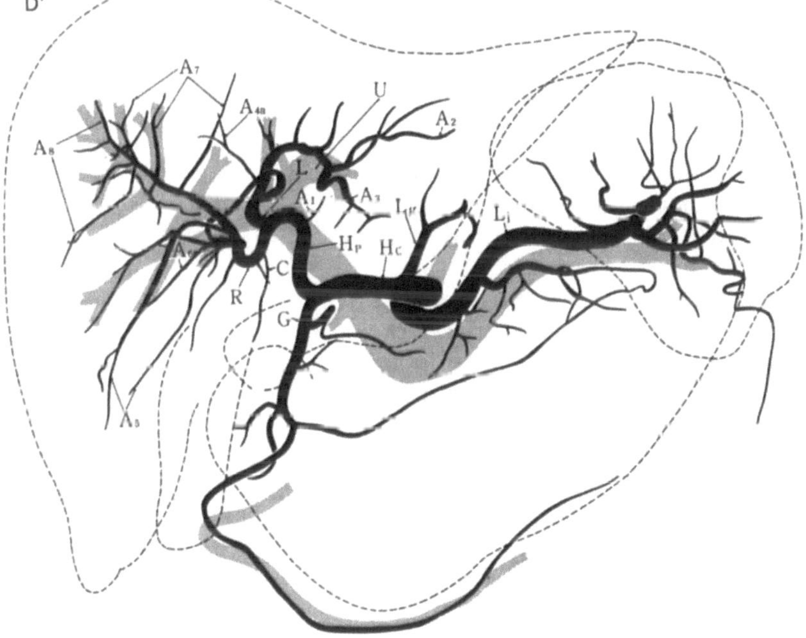

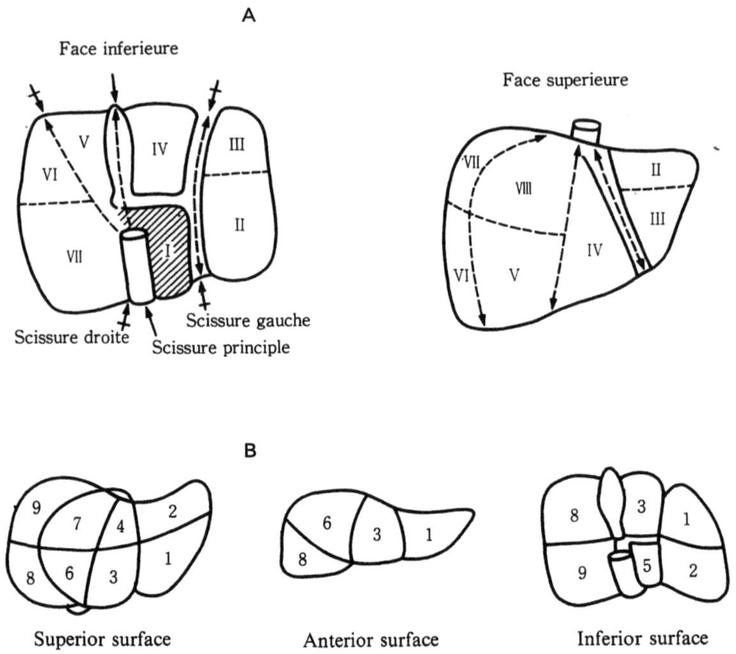

Fig. 5.4 A, B. Hepatic segments

A. Hepatic segment by Couinaud [16]
I: Caudate segment
II: Dorsolateral segment
III: Ventrolateral segment
IV: Medial segment
V: Ventrocaudal segment
VI: Dorsocaudal segment
VII: Dorsocranial segment
VIII: Ventrocranial segment

B. Hepatic segment by Okudaira [55]
1: Left anterior segment
2: Left posterior segment
3: Median anterior segment
4: Median posterior segment
5: Caudate segment
6: Right median anterior segment
7: Right median posterior segment
8: Right lateral anterior segment
9: Right lateral posterior segment

With conventional hepatic arteriography, at most the second branch of the segmental artery can be observed. This is not only because of the limits of resolution, but also because of scattered radiation from the soft tissue of liver parenchyma and hepatic parenchyma stained by contrast medium. All these are undesirable conditions. However, with magnification angiography [69], images of the periportal artery which accompanied the hepatic artery (Fig. 5.11) and the meshy small artery with faint density (the interlobular artery) can be observed (Fig. 5.7).

5.2.2. Portal Vein. The portal vein, the functional vessel of the liver (vasa publica), flows into the liver gathering blood from the stomach, duodenum, small intestine, large intestine, spleen, and pancreas. The wall structure of the portal vein is the same as in the systemic vein, but a valve structure in the systemic vein does not exist.

In the porta hepatis, the portal vein bifurcates into the right and left main trunks at a right angle of about 60°–95° and supplies both sides of the liver with blood. As with the hepatic artery, the right branch of the portal vein supplies blood not to the anatomical right lobe of the liver, but to the right side of Cantlie's line.

In the liver, the portal vein runs along the hepatic artery, but the system of the portal vein is simple and not as complex as the hepatic artery. The portal vein distributes ramifying fan-shaped patterns from the porta hepatis. The portal vein runs through the interlobular connective tissue as the interlobular vein (V. interlobularis) and forms the intralobular capillary network running among cords of hepatic cells in the lobules of the liver. Naturally, the hepatic cells are fed from the portal vein.

The image of the interlobular vein can be observed only by means of portography with an adaptable manner of opacification, such as umbilical venography, splenoportography and percutaneous transhepatic portography.

5.2.3 Hepatic Vein. The intralobular capillary vessels gather at the central vein which runs through the center of the lobule. The length of the central vein is about 1 mm; it joins into the intercalated vein adjacent to the lobule and then unites into the sublobular vein, the so-called collecting vein.

The collecting veins gather and form the hepatic vein. The hepatic vein is a blood vessel with a well-grown tunica media, particularly in the portion opening into the inferior vena cava and the advanced smooth muscle forming the sphincter. The hepatic veins opening into the inferior vena cava are mainly the left, middle, and right hepatic veins. In addition, several small branches of the hepatic vein from the caudate lobe and posterior-inferior part of the right lobe open below the above-mentioned three major hepatic veins.

Like the hepatic artery, there is much variation in the branching form of the hepatic vein. According to Okudaira [55], in 62.5% of cases an independent right hepatic vein and common trunk are formed with the middle and left vein, in 20.9% the right, middle, and left hepatic veins are all independent, in 8.3% a portion of the right vein flows into the middle, and in 4.2% three each of right, middle and left hepatic veins divide into superior and inferior branches. In contrast to the systemic vein, the hepatic vein, which does not have valve structures runs straight to the liver.

Hepatic venography is a fine indicator when measuring the hepatic venous pressure in presinusoidal and postsinusoidal portal hypertension and also examines the morphology of the sinusoid in the case of liver cirrhosis. Magnification venography may be required in this case (Fig. 5.5). Hepatic venography may also be performed as preoperative examination of space-occupying lesions, such as hepatocellular carcinoma, and opacification of all branches of the hepatic vein are necessary.

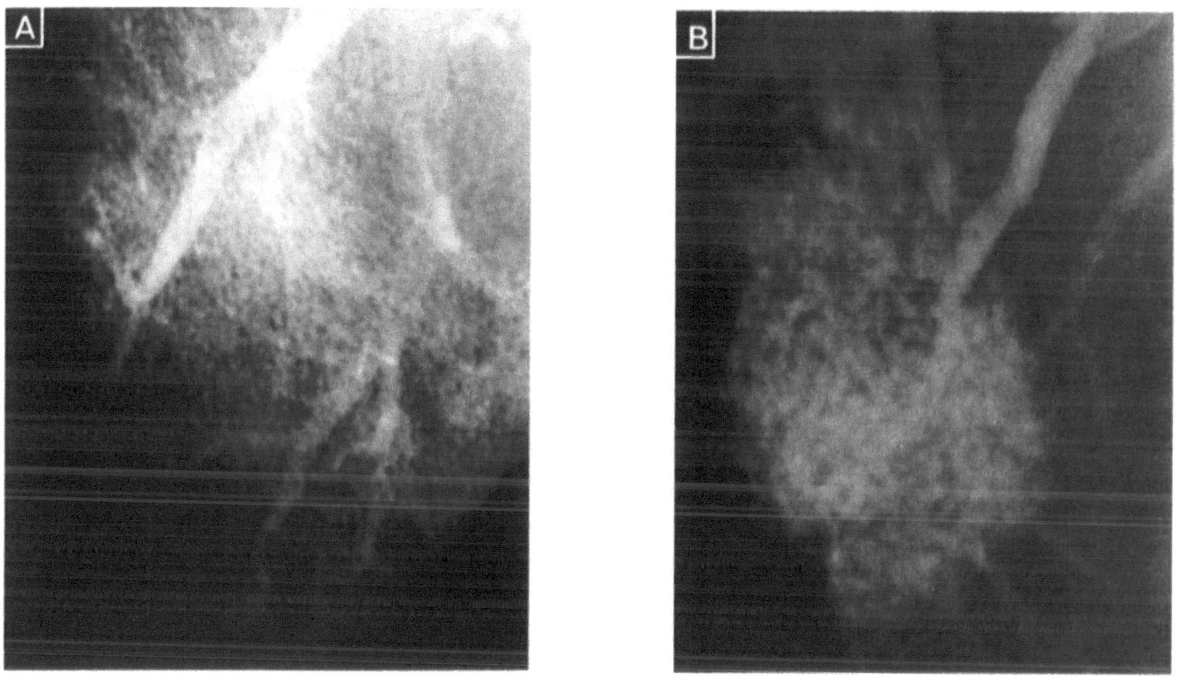

Fig. 5.5 A, B. Fourfold magnifiction venography. **A** Normal liver: sublobular vein, central vein, and homogeneous granular sinusoidal shadows are clearly observed; **B** liver cirrhosis: displacement and distortion of sublobular veins, stenosis of central vein, and inhomogeneous sinusoids with various sizes are visualized. (Courtesy of Kaneko, M., MD. Hamamastsu University Medical School, Hamamatsu)

Selective hepatic venography may be performed with a wedged catheter. Hepatic sublobular veins can be opacified by means of a catheter with a tip of 1.5 mm in diameter, and more detailed information can be obtained using magnification wedged venography simultaneously [12].

After injection of 3 ml of contrast medium, at first the right angular bifurcation at the sublobular vein, and then in succession the central vein and ill-defined granular branching patterns corresponding to a group of sinusoids 0.05–0.2 cm in diameter become opacified (Fig. 5.5).

The opacification images of the group of sinusoids develop rapidly to a homogeneous parenchymal stain, and sometimes branches of the portal vein can be clearly demonstrated exhibiting a characteristic dichotomous pattern. By inserting the tip of the catheter into the main hepatic venous trunk, it is possible to opacify the entire area of the sublobular vein. Sinusoidal opacification by hepatic venography will provide pathological information helpful for the diagnosis of hepatitis, liver cirrhosis, and portal hypertension.

5.3 Angiographic Findings in Diseases of the Liver

Angiography is very useful in examining liver disease in which space-occupying lesions are suspected. In addition, angiography is useful in the diagnosis of trauma, abscess, liver cirrhosis, and portal hypertension.

The method of choice for diagnosing suspected tumors is hepatic angiography. Space-occupying lesions of the liver are classified into localized or diffuse solid tumor, vascular tumor, cystic lesions, and others.

5.3.1 Hepatocellular Carcinoma. In most cases of hepatocellular carcinoma, the tumor vessels are clearly observed [5, 7, 77] (Figs. 5.6 and 5.7). The image of hypervascularity and tumor stain in the angiogram corresponds histologically to the well-differentiated type [36]. Conversely, the finding of hypovascularity without stain may indicate a poorly differentiated type.

With advanced tumor, dilated hepatic arteries are observed due to the increasing blood stream which feeds vessels to the tumor. Furthermore, findings of stretching, displacement, tortuosity, dilatation, obstruction, and encasement of feeding arteries are visualized. Dilatation of the periportal artery can also be noticed as well.

The tumor vessels can be observed in an encased form or of various thicknesses. This finding can be more clearly visualized by magnification angiography. The image of the tumor stain is visible from the capillary phase to the venous phase.

With an arteriovenous shunt, the portal vein and rarely the hepatic vein are visualized in the early phase of opacification [54]. Occlusion of the portal vein caused by the direct invasion of the tumor or thrombus in the portal vein may be observed [53].

Angiography can also be used to treat hepatocellular carcinoma as a transcatheter arterial embolization technique, which involves injecting anticancerous drugs and/or embolization materials into the proximal side of the feeding artery in the tumor via a catheter [15] (Fig. 5.8).

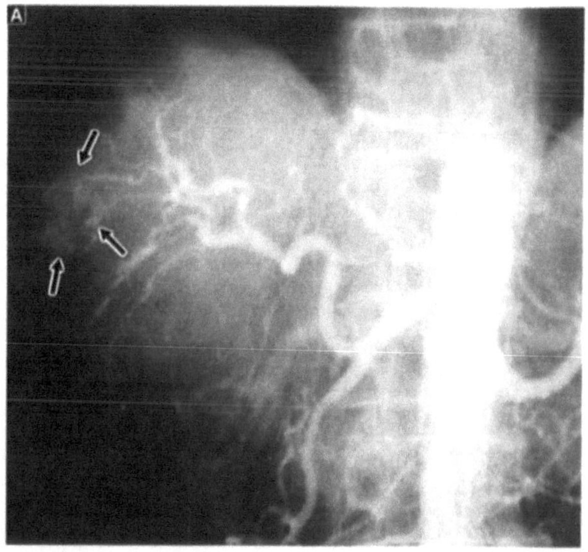

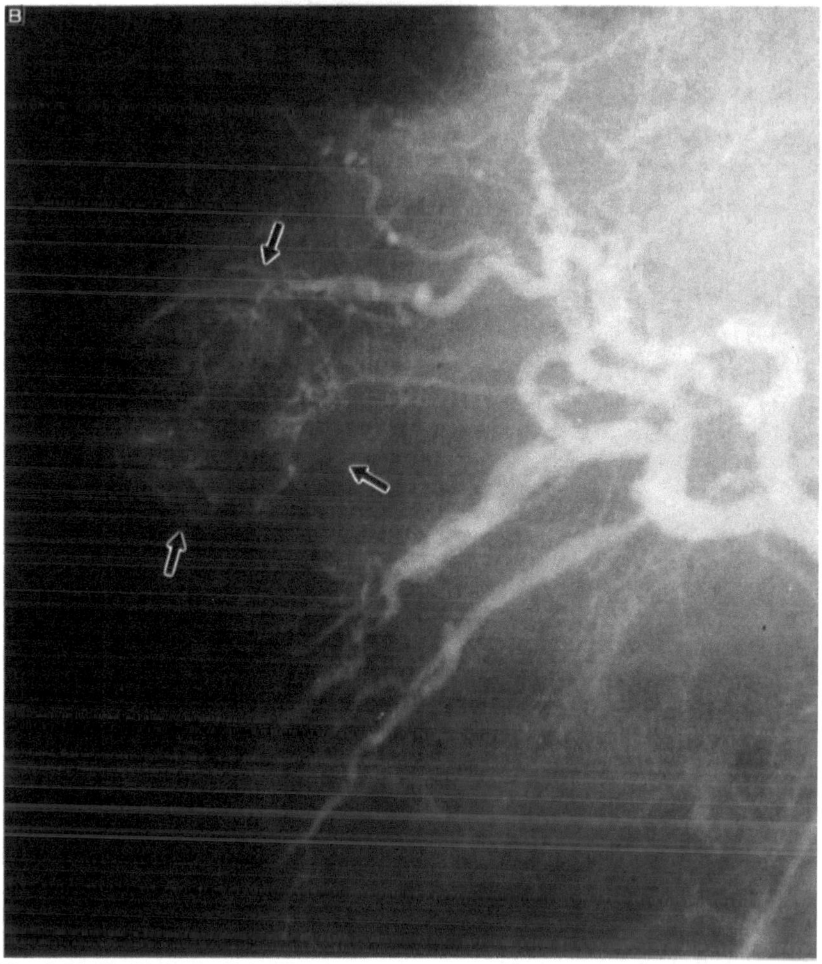

Fig. 5.6 A, B. Hepatocellular carcinoma: tumor (→) with hypervascularity in the right lobe, which is fed by the branches of the right hepatic artery; encasement of the branches of the right hepatic artery and tumor vessels. **A** celiac angiography (arterial phase); **B** threefold magnification angiography (arterial phase)

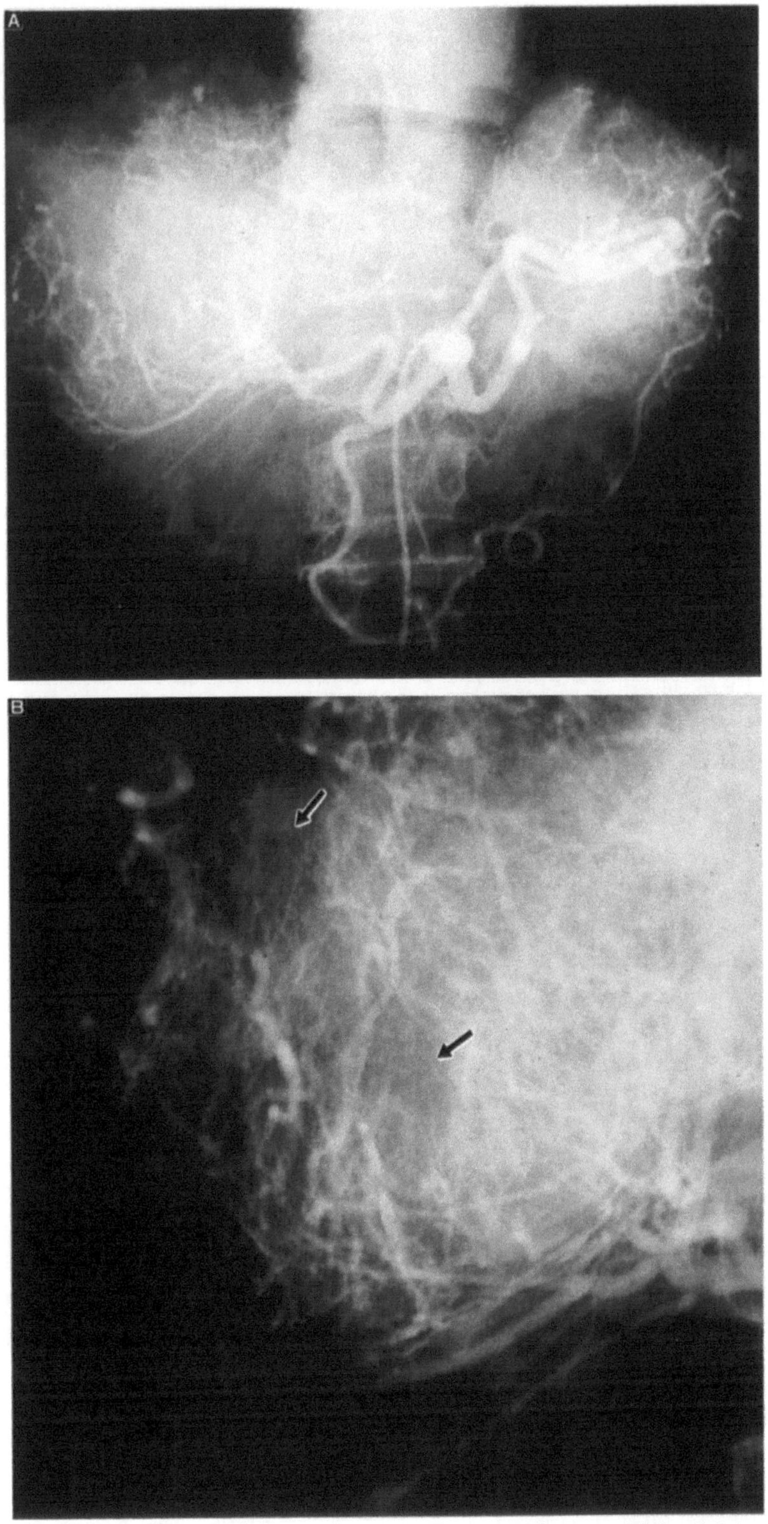

Fig. 5.7 A, B. Hepatocellular carcinoma: tumor occupying two-thirds of right hepatic lobe, which is fed by branches of the right hepatic artery; irregularity of interlobular artery and tumor vessels can be visualized on the threefold magnification angiogram (**B** →) **A** celiac angiography (arterial phase); **B** threefold magnification angiography (arterial phase)

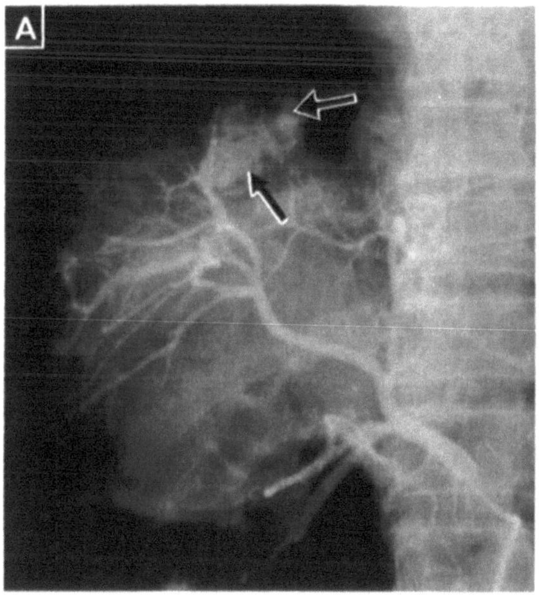

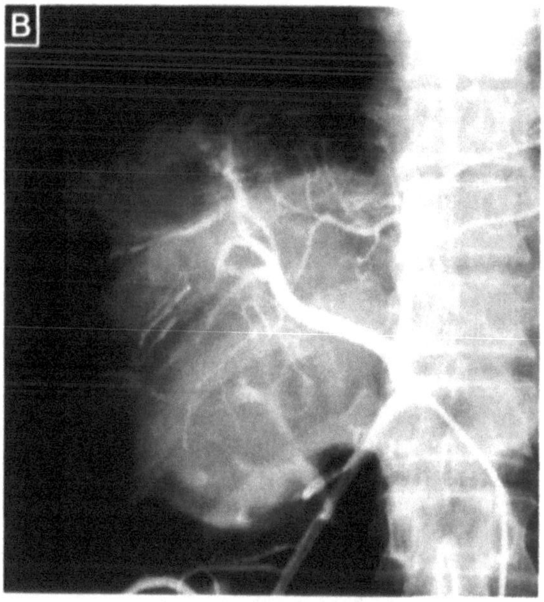

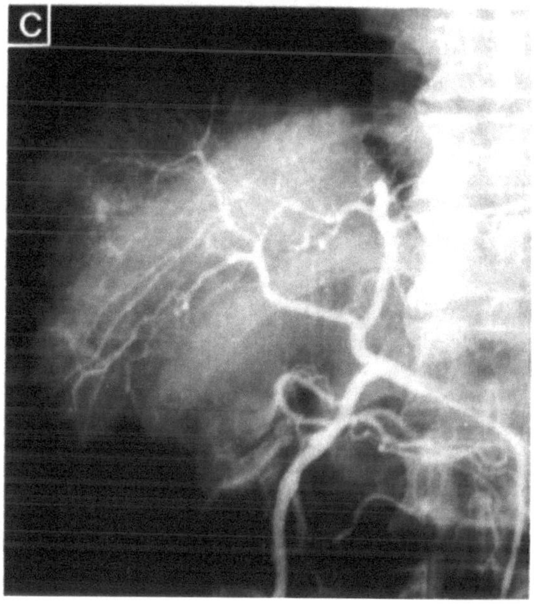

Fig. 5.8 A–C. Hepatocellular carcinoma of the right lobe. **A** pre-embolization angiography: hypervascular tumor (→); alpha fetoprotein: 825 m µg/ml; **B** angiography just after the embolization with Gelfoam; **C** angiography 1 month after the embolization; alpha fetoprotein: 10.5 m µg/ml

5.3.2 Cholangiocarcinoma. Cholangiocarcinoma (Fig. 5.9) occurs in the intrahepatic bile duct and grows infiltratively. Generally, images of rich neovascularity and sinusoidal dilatation cannot be observed as in cases of hepatocellular carcinoma. Thus, a marked tumor stain cannot be seen.

The major findings of angiography are displacement, occlusion, and encasement of the feeding vessels. Tumor vessels, if any, are recognized faintly and are more clearly observed by magnification angiography. In addition, stenosis and obstruction of the portal vein are also noticed, but arteriovenous shunt is scarcely observed.

These angiographic findings occasionally make if difficult to differentiate cholangiocarcinoma from hypovascular hepatocellular carcinoma or metastatic liver carcinoma [63].

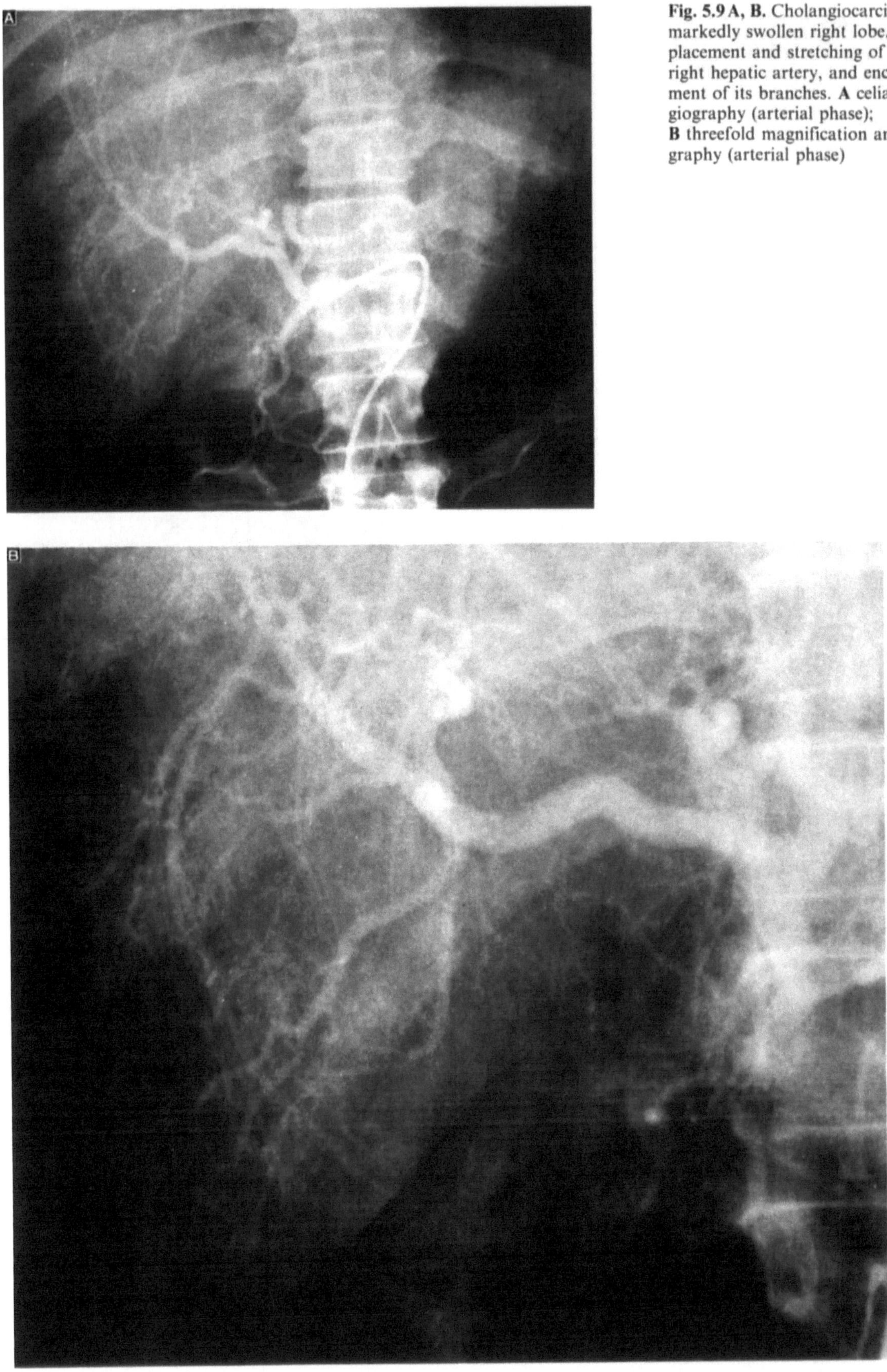

Fig. 5.9 A, B. Cholangiocarcinoma: markedly swollen right lobe, displacement and stretching of the right hepatic artery, and encasement of its branches. **A** celiac angiography (arterial phase); **B** threefold magnification angiography (arterial phase)

5.3.3 Hepatoblastoma. In angiographic findings of hepatoblastoma (Fig. 5.10), the feeding artery of the tumor is observed as dilated. The main branches of the hepatic artery are elongated and stretched to surround the tumor, and hypervascular and often many tumor vessels may also be observed [44, 51]. The image of the tumor stain is observed as a slightly obscure contour, with inhomogeneous density and mottled appearance.

In the early phases of arterial opacification, several long dilated vessels or looped patterns of tumor vessels may be recognized. However, pooling of contrast medium or arteriovenous shunt are generally observed in a few cases. Frequently, it is difficult to differentiate hepatoblastoma from hepatocellular carcinoma solely with angiography.

5.3.4 Liver Metastasis. The angiographic findings of liver metastasis are classified into hyper- and hypovascular patterns (Figs. 5.11 and 5.12). Metastatic hepatic carcinoma with hypervascularity is observed in cases of metastasis from renal cell carcinoma, choriocarcinoma, carcinoid, and islet cell carcinoma of the pancreas. A, hypovascular finding is frequently obtained in cases of metastasis from adenocarcinoma of the gastrointestinal tract, pancreas, and gallbladder. General angiographic findings of metastatic liver carcinoma are indirect findings of displacement and stretching of the feeding vessels; even if the tumor vessels are visualized, they are rarely observed.

In the case of hypervascular lesions, the tumors show round and dense staining images stronger than the hepatic parenchyma in the capillary phase. Necrosis in the center of the tumor is visualized as radiolucent areas. In this case, it is possible to diagnose a tumor the size of 0.5–1 cm. Conversely, a hypovascular tumor is observed only as a finding of a filling defect in the phase of obtaining a hepatogram. Therefore, only tumors larger than 2–3 cm can be diagnosed. In multiple metastatic liver carcinoma, the hepatogram is observed forming a so-called Swiss cheese pattern. In the case of metastatic liver carcinoma, invasion to the portal vein rarely occurs.

Using infusion hepatic angiography [67], metastatic tumors are diagnosed with dense staining images. It is possible to visualize a tumour the size of 0.5–1 cm [34]. This method is also useful in detecting small primary hepatocellular carcinoma, which cannot be identified by conventional hepatic angiography due to its hypovascularity [75]. Differentiating between primary and metastatic carcinoma is supposed to be possible to some extent with this method [43]. A ringlike stain with clear outer and unclear inner margins is thought to be specific for metastasis, and a definite nodular stain with an irregular and notched margin is specific for primary hepatocellular carcinoma.

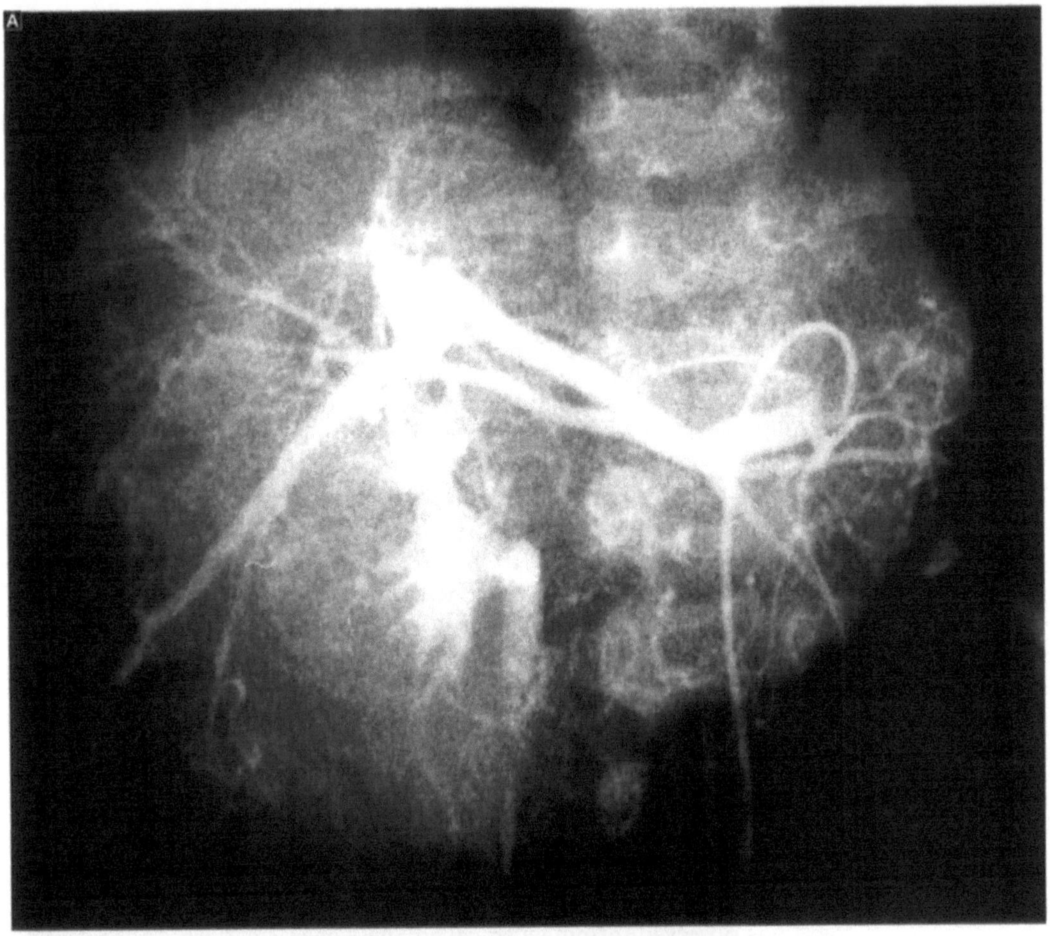

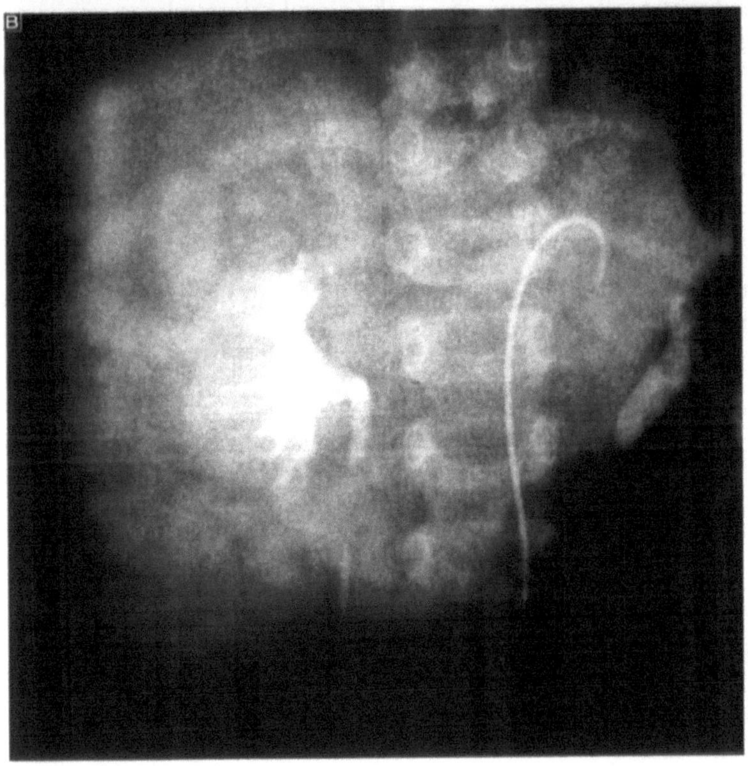

Fig. 5.10 A. B. Hepatoblastoma in a 2-year-old boy: complete swelling of the liver and dilatation of the hepatic artery; stretching and displacement of major branches, which show encasement in the peripheral portion (**A**). In the venous phase, mottled staining appearance is observed (**B**). **A** celiac angiography (arterial phase); **B** celiac angiography (venous phase)

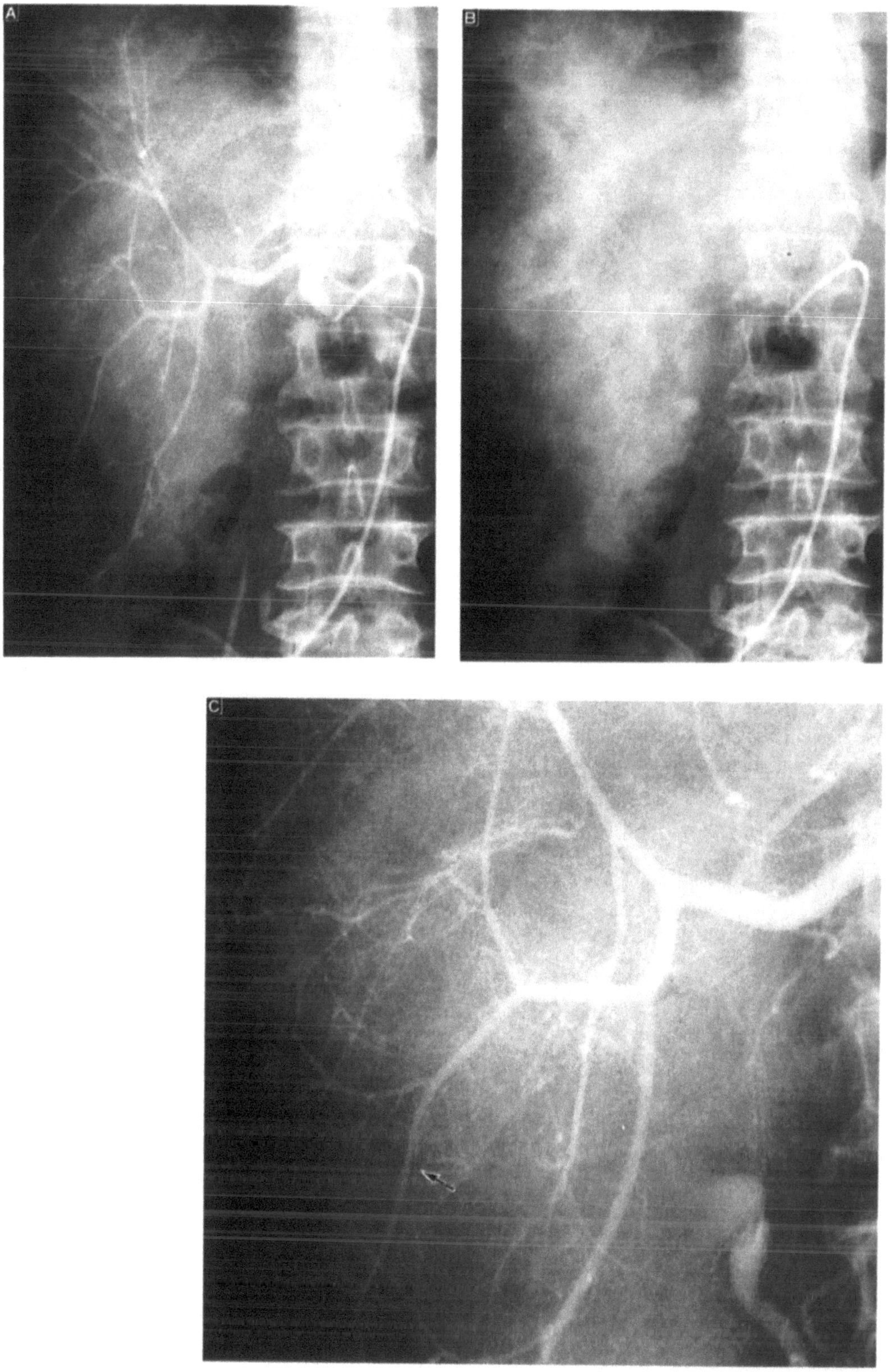

Fig. 5.11 A–C. Metastasis of rectum carcinoma to the liver. **A** common hepatic angiography (arterial phase): notably swollen right lobe of the liver and stretching and displacement of the right hepatic artery; **B** common hepatic angiography (venous phase): radiolucent image on hepatogram; **C** threefold magnification angiography (arterial phase): encasement of the artery, tumor vessels, and periportal artery (→) with hepatic artery

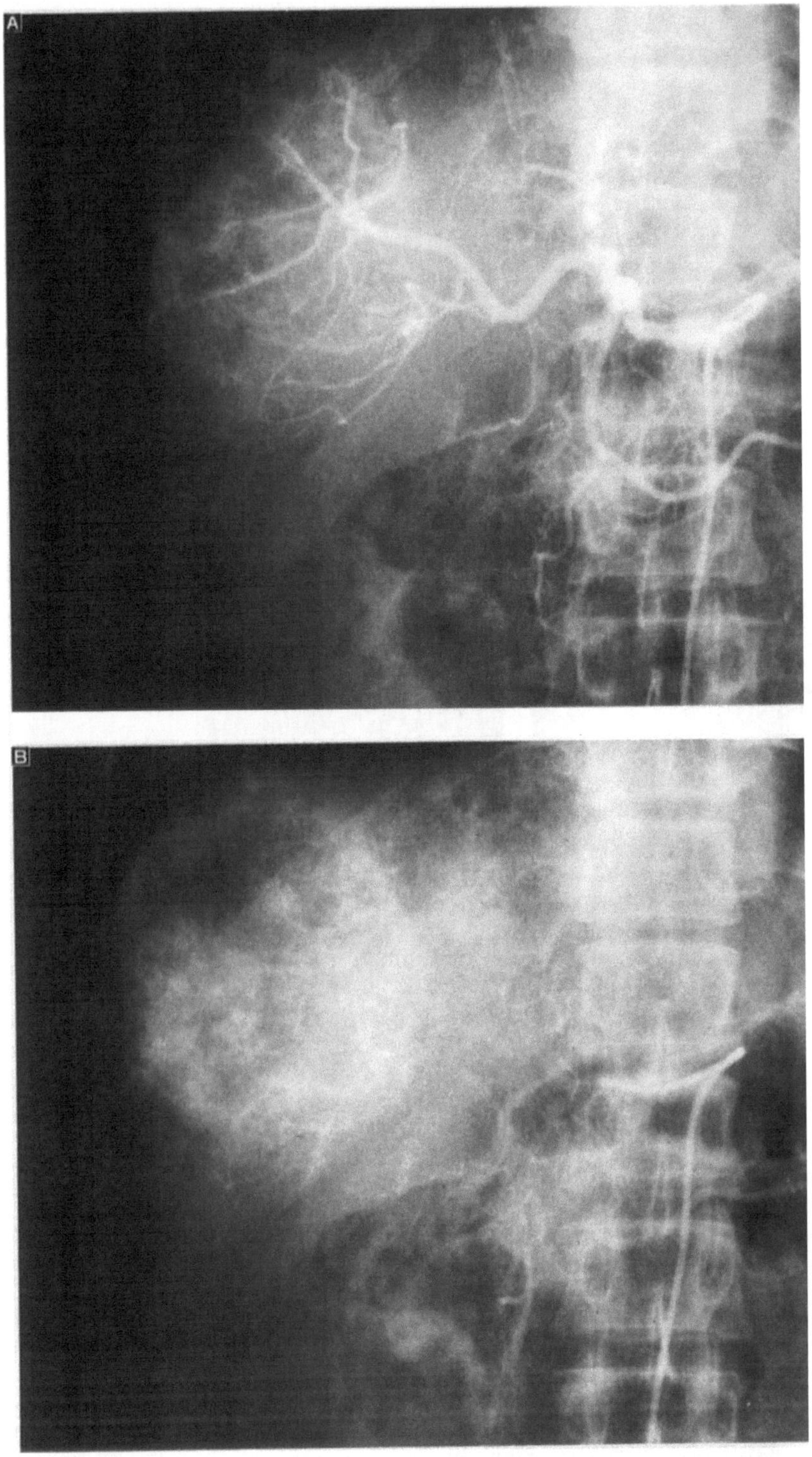

Fig. 5.12 A, B. Metastasis of sigmoid colon carcinoma to the liver. **A** common hepatic angiography (arterial phase): right hepatic artery displaced and stretched surrounding the tumor; **B** common hepatic angiography (capillary phase): dense staining of the tumor and avascular area due to necrosis

5.3.5 Benign Hepatic Tumors. Frequently, benign hepatic tumors are hepatic hemangiomas (Fig. 5.13). In the case of cavernous hemangioma of the liver [2, 56, 67, 68], pooling contrast images in the vascular areas formed with the bloodstream from peripheral branches of the hepatic artery can be observed expanding from the early phase of arterial opacification to the late venous phase. According to McLoughlin [45], "configurations of the hemangioma are ring or C-shaped due to fibrous obliteration in the cener of the lesions." The hepatic artery and its major branches are generally not dilated, and arteriovenous shunt is also rarely observed.

In the case of hemangioendothelioma of the liver [49, 68], the diameter of the hepatic artery dilates, and early opacification of the hepatic veins is frequently visualized due to arteriovenous shunting. Mortensson states [47] that "intrahepatic arteries are wide and stretched but not displaced by the tumours and do not taper towards the periphery. In the early arterial phase clusters of vessel-rich lesions appear along the arteries."

Because of frequent coexistence of a cavernous hemangioma and hemangioendothelioma of the liver, it is often impossible to differentiate between these two findings.

In hepatic adenoma and focal nodular hyperplasia [14, 21, 46], a tumor stain with a sharp outline can be visualized, but arteriovenous shunt is rarely observed. A malignant vascular pattern is generally not observed, although abnormal vessels may be seen. Differentiation between hepatic adenoma and focal nodular hyperplasia may be possible based on vascular patterns [25]. With angiography, they may be difficult to differentiate from hepatocellular carcinoma.

5.3.6 Hepatic Cysts. In nonparasitic hepatic cysts (Fig. 5.14) and polycystic liver disease (Fig. 5.15), displacement and stretching of the hepatic artery are observed, and in the parenchymal phase round filling defects in the hepatogram can be seen. The rims of the cysts may be hypervascular due to displacement of the surrounding hepatic parenchyma.

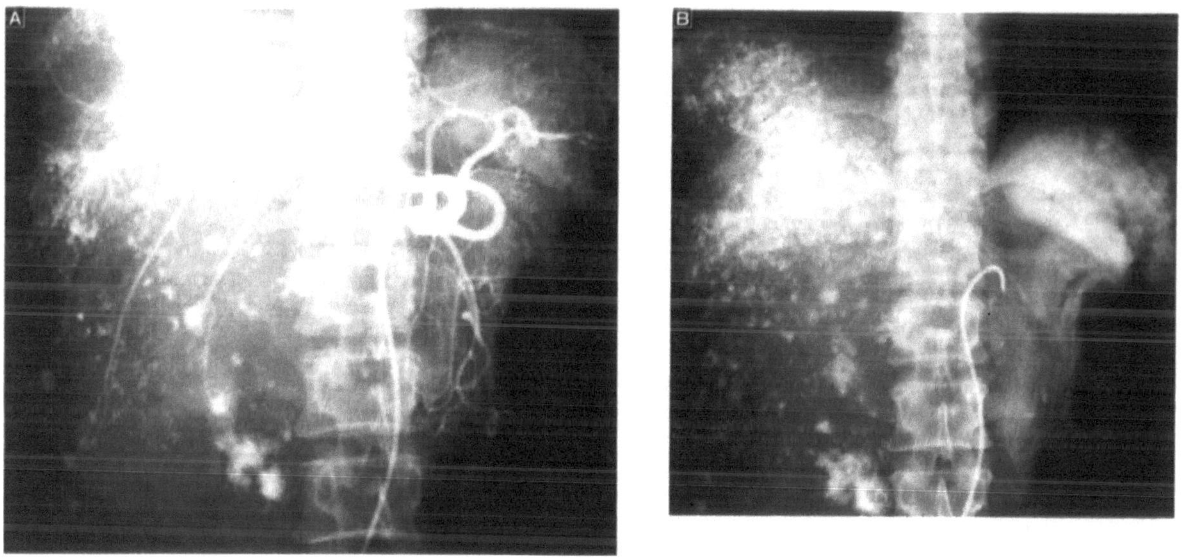

Fig. 5.13 A, B. Hemangioma of the liver. **A** celiac angiography (arterial phase); **B** celiac angiography (venous phase): multiple C-shaped or ring formation of the contrast medium from early arterial to the later venous phase

In an advanced cyst, displacement and stretching of the portal branch are observable. Figure 5.16 is an example of a hepatic echinococcic cyst; the findings on the angiogram are the same as for a hepatic cyst.

5.3.7 Liver Abscesses. In the case of a liver abscess, the branches of the hepatic arteries are observed in an arc shape caused by stretching and displacement of the lesion. In the parenchymal phase of the liver [52], avascular lesions with ill-defined contours, rim signs, and in addition abnormality of the diaphragm may be recognized. A liver abscess may require differentiation from solitary hepatic cysts and polycystic liver disease. A charcteristic sign of cysts is a clear contour in the parenchymal phase of opacification. However, as this differentiation is not always possible, it is necessary to refer to the clinical findings. Liver abscesses may also occasionally be difficult to differentiate from hepatic tumors.

5.3.8 Liver Cirrhosis. In the case of liver cirrhosis (Fig. 5.17), a stretched, angulated, tortuous, and corkscrew appearance of the intrahepatic artery can be observed depending on the stage. These findings, however, are not specific but appear corresponding to the enlargement or shrinkage of the liver [59]. Therefore, it is impossible to diagnose liver cirrhosis with only a hepatic arteriogram.

The diagnostic value of hepatic arteriography lies in the diagnosis of hepatocellular carcinoma, which is frequently accompanied by liver cirrhosis. In the capillary phase, liver cirrhosis may be misdiagnosed for a pathological lesion due to the mottled hepatogram.

With a regenerating nodule exhibiting images of hypervascularity and sometimes arteriovenous shunt [20], differentiation from hepatocellular carcinoma my be necessary [61].

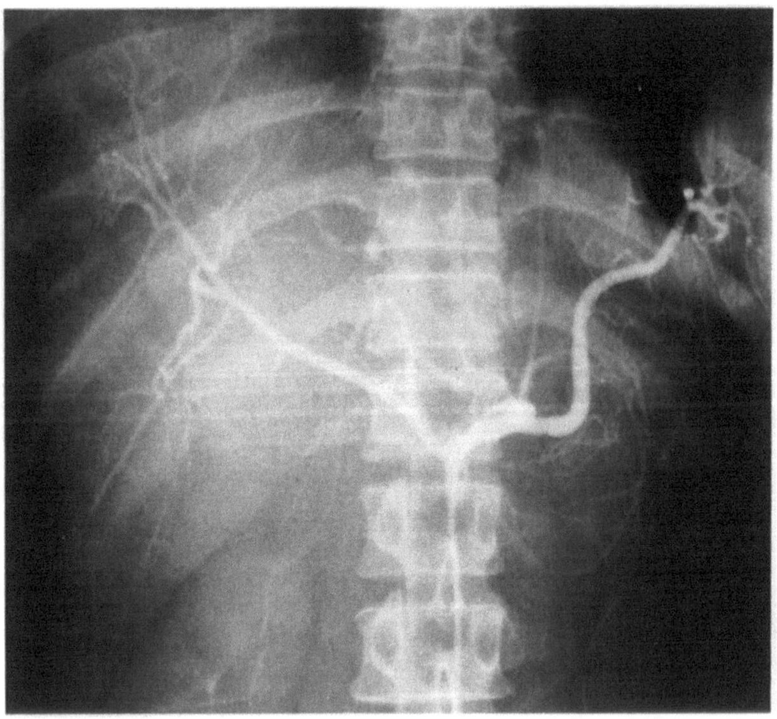

Fig. 5.14. Hepatic cyst: notable displacement and stretching of intrahepatic arterial branches and nonobservable malignant vessels. Same case as shown in Figs. 2.12 and 4.11

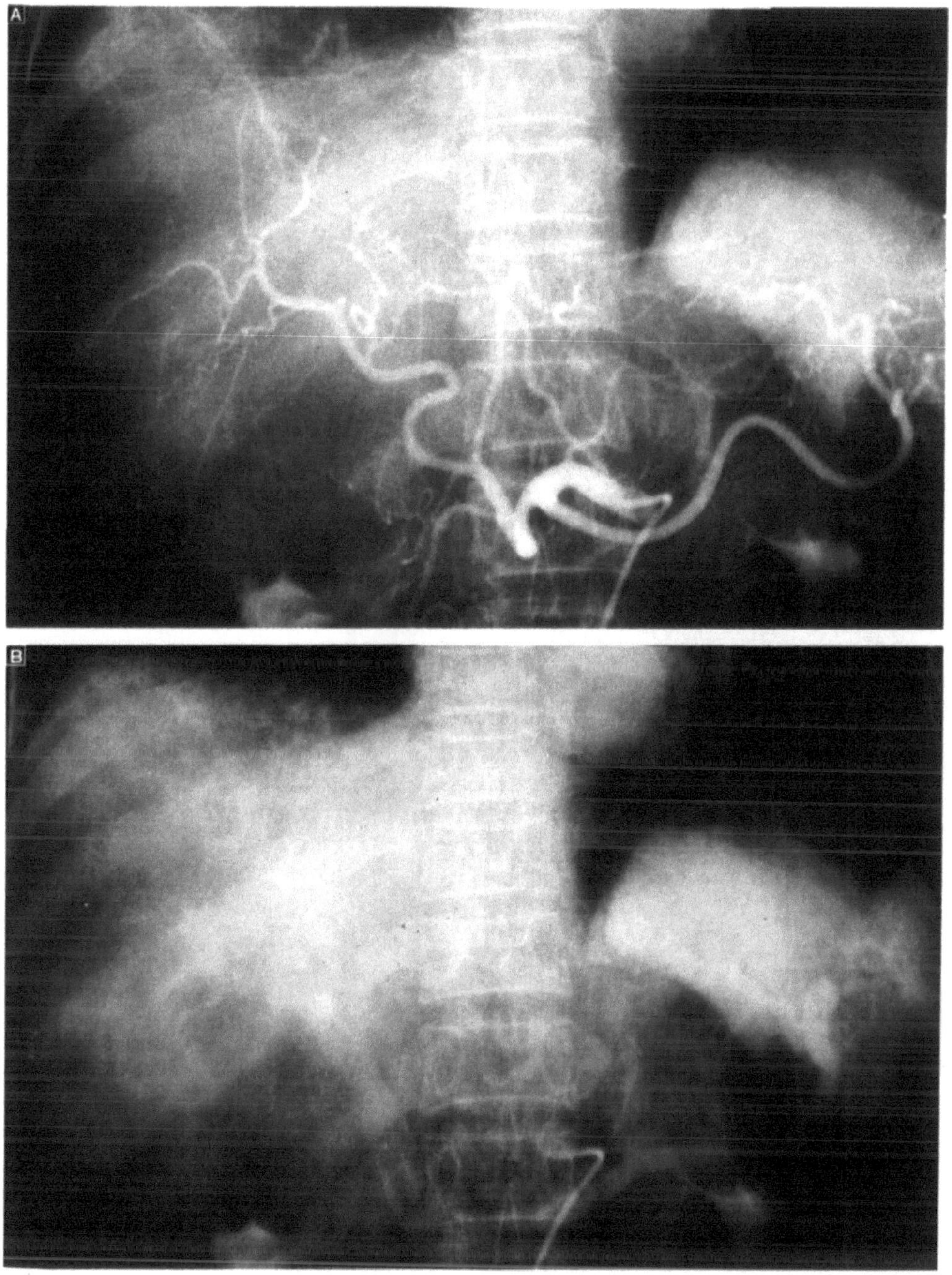

Fig. 5.15 A, B. Polycystic disease of the liver. **A** celiac angiography (arterial phase); **B** celiac angiography (venous phase). Displacement and expansion of the hepatic artery and multiple round radiolucent shadows with slight staining of the wall in the venous phase can be observed

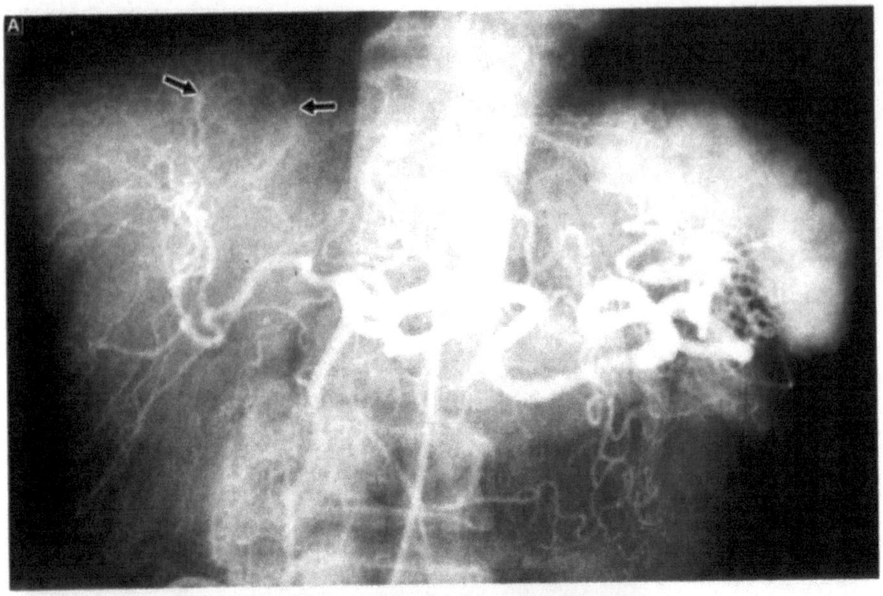

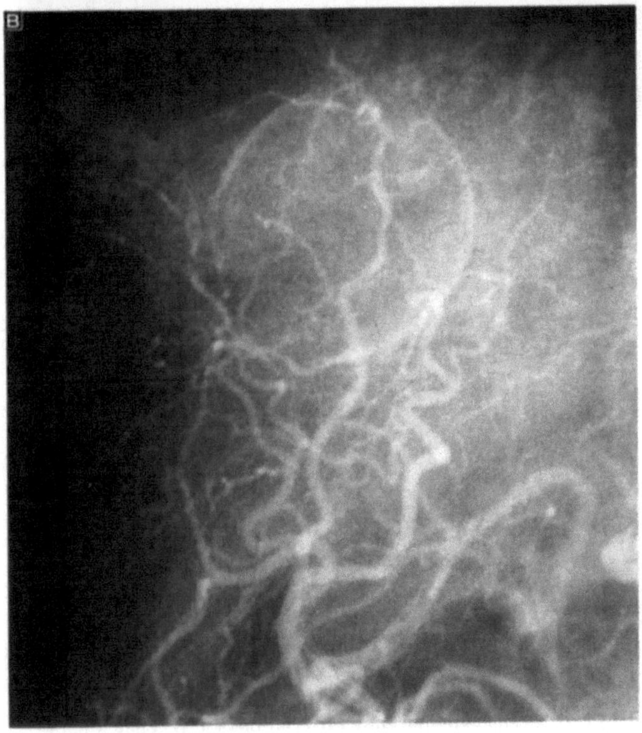

Fig. 5.16 A, B. Hydatid disease of the liver: vasculature surrounding the calcified wall (→) and non-observable vasculature in the tumor. **A** celiac angiography (arterial phase); **B** threefold magnification angiography (arterial phase). Same case as shown in Fig. 1.8

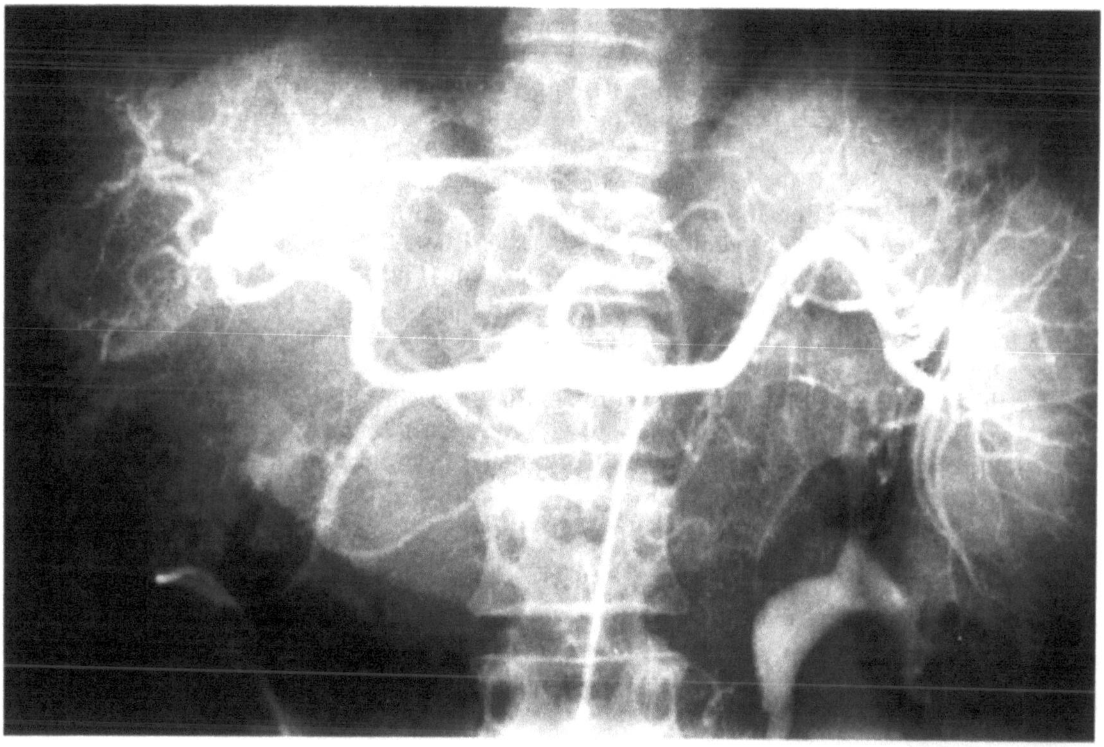

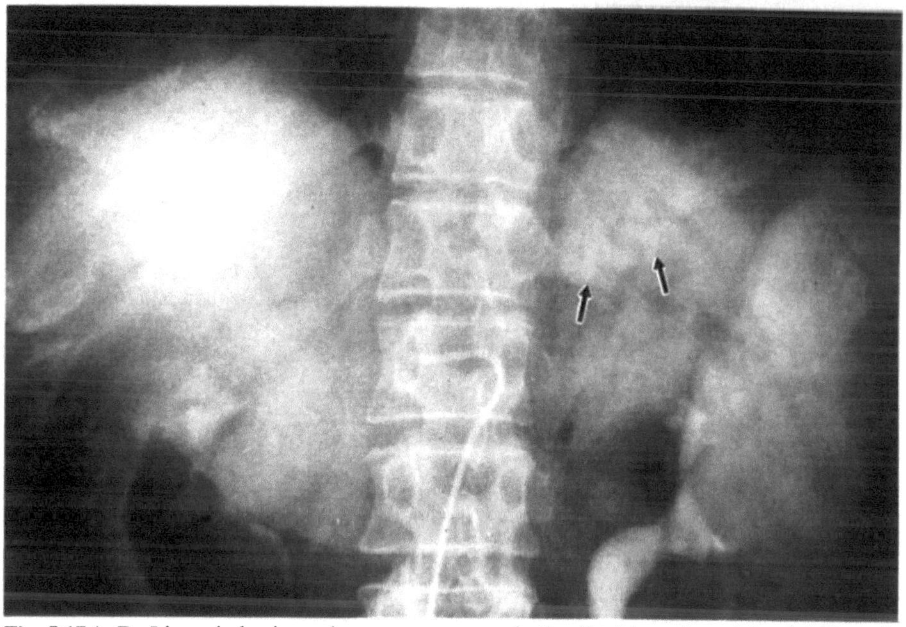

Fig. 5.17 A, B. Liver cirrhosis: corkscrew appearance in the distal branches of the right hepatic artery, stretching of the left branch in the swelling of the left lobe, swelling of the spleen, poor opacification of the splenic vein, and dilatation (→) of the short gastric vein as a collateral channel can be seen. **A** celiac angiography (arterial phase); **B** celiac angiography (venous phase)

5.3.9 Portal Hypertension. In most cases of portal hypertension, portography is required in the presence of portal thrombosis, developmental or acquired portal obstruction, hepatic fibrosis, Banti's syndrome, liver cirrhosis, and schistosomiasis japonica for the main purpose of examining portal obstruction and analyzing collateral circulation [32]. In these diseases, not only hepatic but also splenic arteriography is necessary due to the significance of spleen examination.

Collateral circulation is generally formed between the left portal to umbilical vein (Fig. 5.18), left gastric to esophageal vein (Fig. 5.19), and inferior mesenteric to hemorrhoidal vein; moreover, it may be formed between the splenic to left renal vein and splenic to unidentified retroperitoneal vein.

For the diagnosis of Budd-Chiari syndrome, due to occlusion in the inferior vena cava at the hepatic level, it is necessary to perform cavography above and below the occlusion by inserting the catheter from the antecubital and femoral veins.

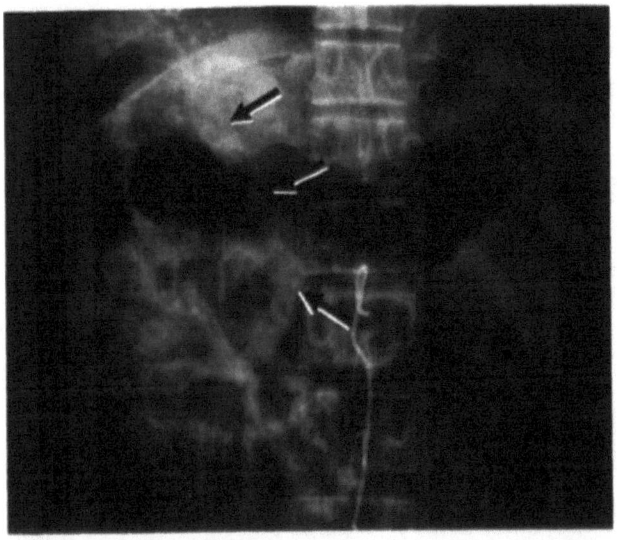

Fig. 5.18. Portal hypertension due to liver cirrhosis: collateral circulation between the left portal vein and the umbilical vein (→) as seen in superior mesenteric arteriography (venous phase)

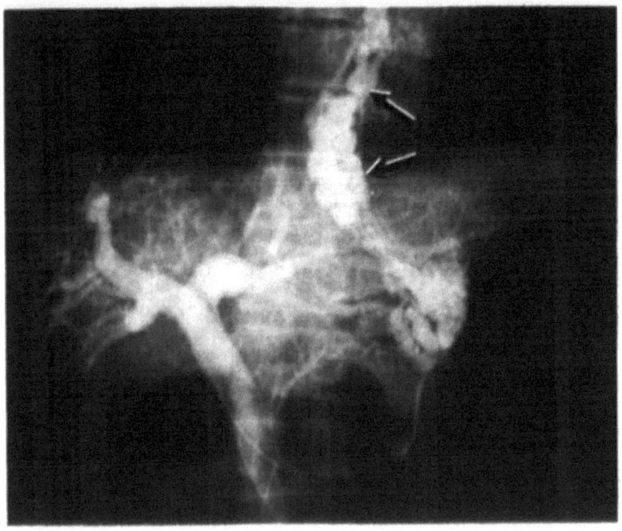

Fig. 5.19. Esophageal varices due to portal hypertenstion (→) as viewed in percutaneous transhepatic portography under ultrasonic guidance

5.4 Vessels of the Biliary Tract and Gallbladder and Their Angiograms

The vessels of the bile duct originate at the point where the posterior superior pancreaticoduodenal artery crosses the common bile duct, and two to five vessels are branched. They anastomose together forming the epicholedochal arterial plexus, which ascends, surrounding the extrahepatic duct (Fig. 5.20).

Among these vessels, the artery which ascends along the right anterolateral side of the common bile duct anastomoses with the cystic artery, forming the so-called marginal anastomotic artery [58]. These arteries also anastomose with the right hepatic artery and cystic artery.

Branching vessels at this epicholedochal arterial plexus pass through the duct wall into the mucosa obliquely and form the first intramural plexus at the outer side of the lamina propria mucosa and the second intramural plexus at the submucosa [58].

The gallbladder is mainly fed by the cystic artery and sometimes directly fed by branches of the hepatic artery. Of the cystic arteries, 75.5% branch from the right hepatic artery, 13.1% from the proper hepatic artery, 6.2% from the left hepatic artery, 2.6% from the gastroduodenal artery, and 2.1% from the region of origin of the proper hepatic artery; 0.5% may branch together with the right hepatic artery.

With conventional selective angiography, the above-mentioned vessels of the biliary tract and gallbladder are not always opacified. Fine vessels can be observed to a certain extent by performing magnification angiography with a high resolution. In our experience, the arteries of the extrahepatic bile duct were observed in 85% of the cases by using magnification techniques.

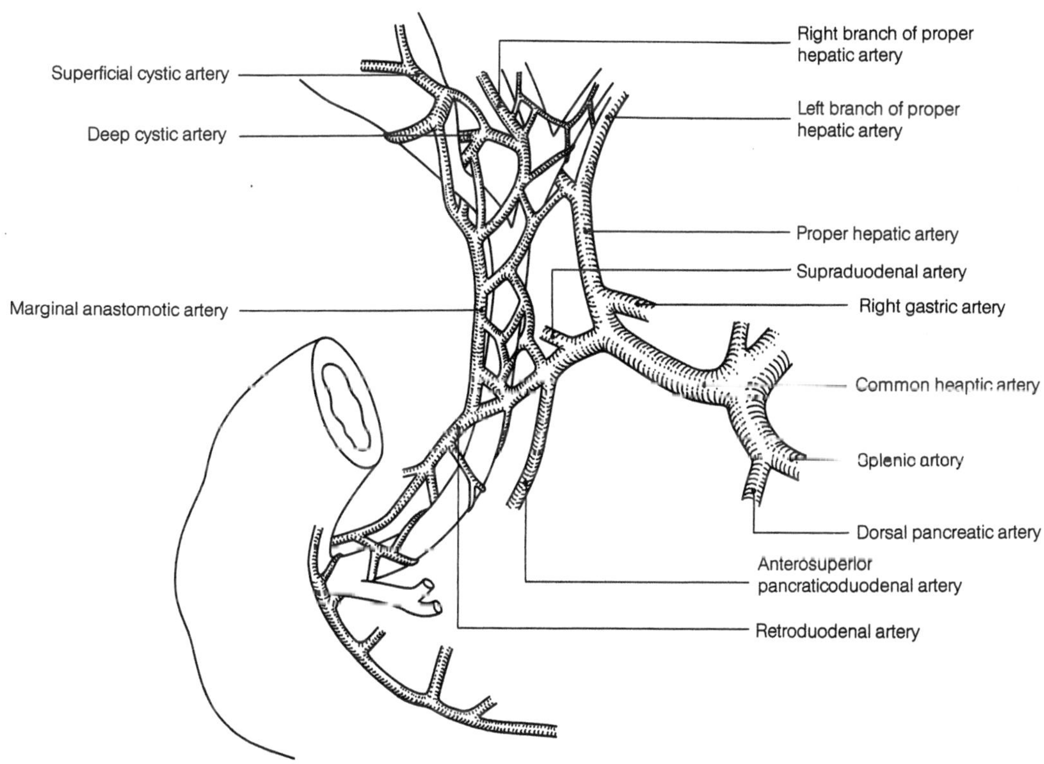

Fig. 5.20. Blood supply of the bile duct. (Modified from Parke et al. [58] by the author [69])

Table 5.1. Angiogram of epicholedochal arterial plexus. Number of apparent vessels corresponds to the number of circle marks

Original artery \ Case		1	2	3	4	5	6	7	8	9
Cystic artery			•••	• ○	•• ○○	••				
Right hepatic artery		•	•	•	•	•• ○	•	•		•
Right gastric artery							•			
Superior pancreaticoduodenal artery		••• ○	•	• ○	•• ○	•• ○	••• ••• ○○	•	•••	
Gastroduodenal artery				••						
Total	Magnification	4	5	5	5	6	8	2	3	1
	Conventional	1	0	2	3	2	2	0	0	0
Marginal anastomotic artery	Magnification	+	+	+	+	+	+	+	+	–
	Conventional	–	–	–	–	–	–	–	–	–

(• magnification, ○ conventional)

With conventional selective angiograpy, the extrahepatic biliary arteries are observed 44% of the time, even in abnormal cases where opacification is easily achieved [39] because these vessels are narrow and overlapped with other vessels. Therefore, to make a detailed observation of the vascular system in the extrahepatic bile duct, it is necessary to carry out magnification angiography and stereoangiography together (see Table 5.1).

The frequency of observing the eggshell-thin shadow of the wall of the gallbladder is low, about only 25%. The artery of the gallbladder frequently anastomoses to the anterior or posterior superior pancreaticoduodenal artery. The venules of the gallbladder cross together forming a venous plexus, which forms the cystic vein.

The cystic vein runs from the fundus to the corpus and the neck of the gallbladder, and then it may flow directly into the portal vein, or enter into the quadrate lobe of the liver by connecting with the venoplexus of the bile duct, and then it flows into the hepatic veins.

In addition, 2–20 veins flow into the quadrate lobe of the liver through the gallbladder bed. Hence, after cystic arteriography, opacification of the hepatic vein can generally rarely be observed, and it is limited to cases where gallbladder veins flow directly into the portal vein.

5.4.1 Abnormal Findings in Diseases of the Gallbladder. In diseases of the gallbladder, angiography is necessary when gallbladder carcinoma is suspected [17, 37, 66] (Figs. 5.21 and 5.22). Angiographic findings of gallbladder carcinoma are dilatation and encasement of the cystic artery and neovascularity in the tumor region. Also, tumor staining may be observed with a finding of uneven thickness of the gallbladder wall [3]. In the case of a small carcinoma, differentiation from chronic cholecystitis may occasionally be difficult [28] so that magnification angiography can provide useful diagnostic information.

Gallbladder carcinoma frequently invades the liver via the gallbladder fossa. Characteristic findings of this expansion are encasement, stenosis,

Fig. 5.21 A, B. Gallbladder carcinoma. **A** celiac angiography (arterial phase); **B** threefold magnification angiography (arterial phase). Tight encasement of the anterior (→) and posterior (→) branches of the cystic artery and infiltration into the extrahepatic bile duct (▶) can be observed

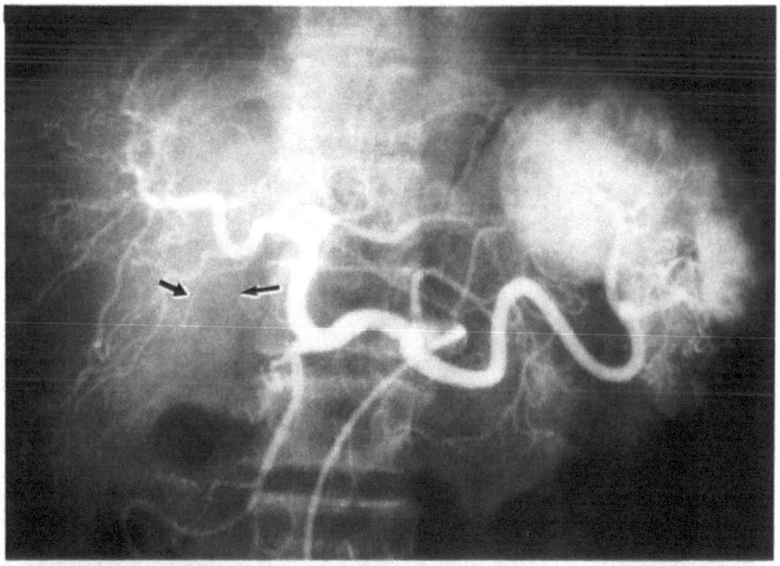

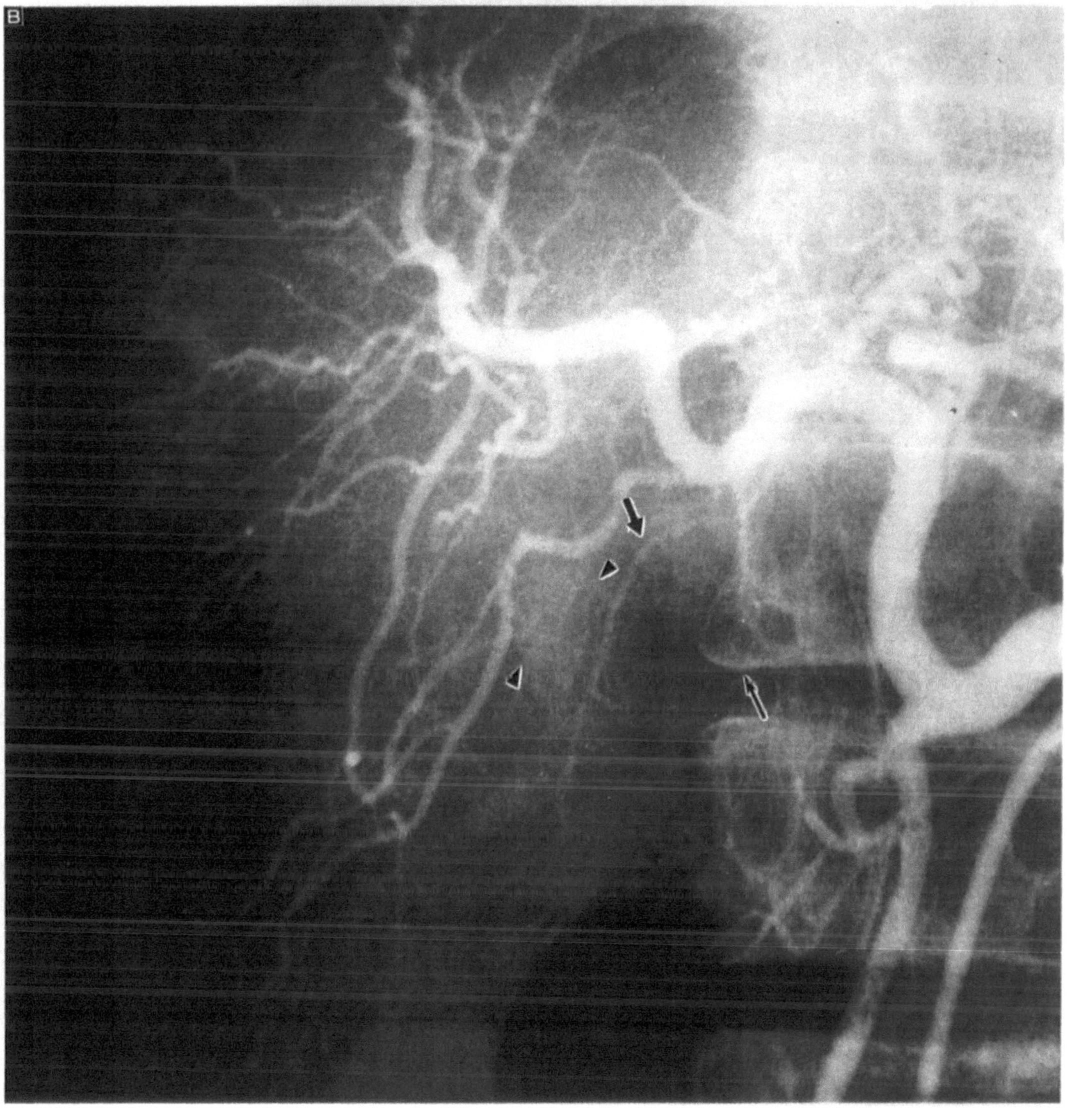

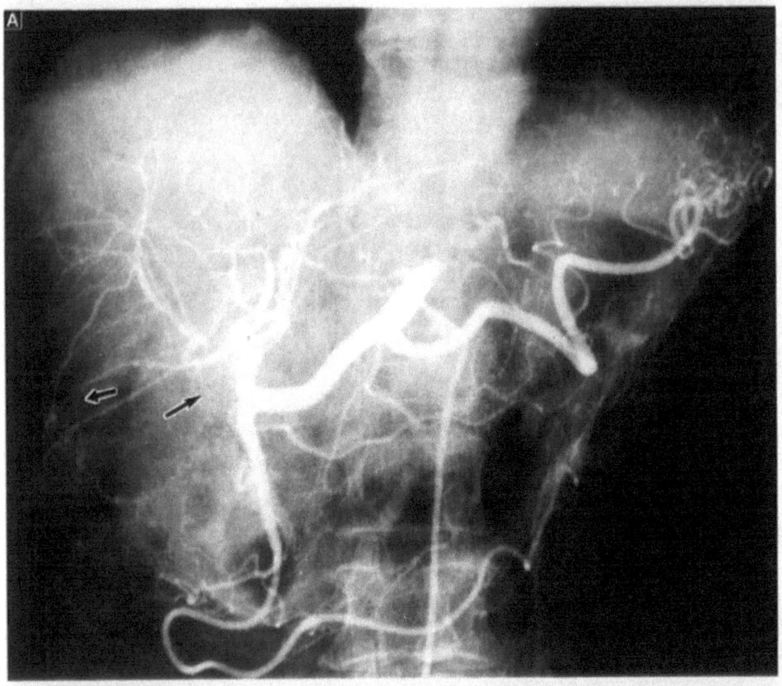

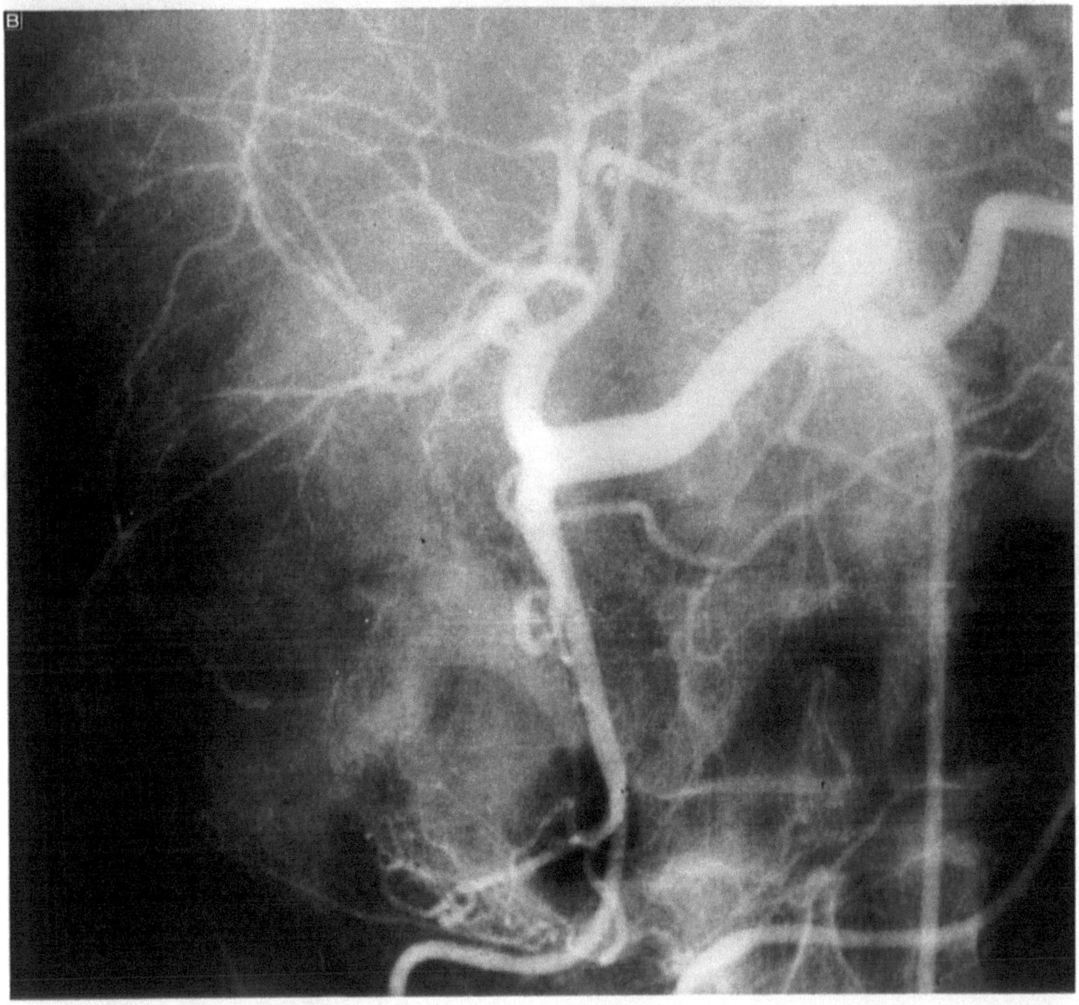

Fig. 5.22 A, B. Gallbladder carcinoma. **A** celiac angiography (arterial phase); **B** threefold magnification angiography (arterial phase). Encasement of the anterior (→) and posterior (→) branches of the cystic artery with fine tumor vessels; a major change in the region of the gallbladder bed and tight encasement of the hepatic artery suggest infiltration of carcinoma into the liver. Same case as shown in Figs. 2.32 and 4.36

Fig. 5.23 A, B. Carcinoma of the extrahepatic bile duct. **A** celiac angiography (arterial phase); **B** threefold magnification angiography (arterial phase). Marked irregularity of the wall of the proper and common hepatic arteries, tight encasement of the epicholedochal arteries, which branch from the posterior superior pancreaticoduodenal artery (→), and a finding of tumor vessels can be observed

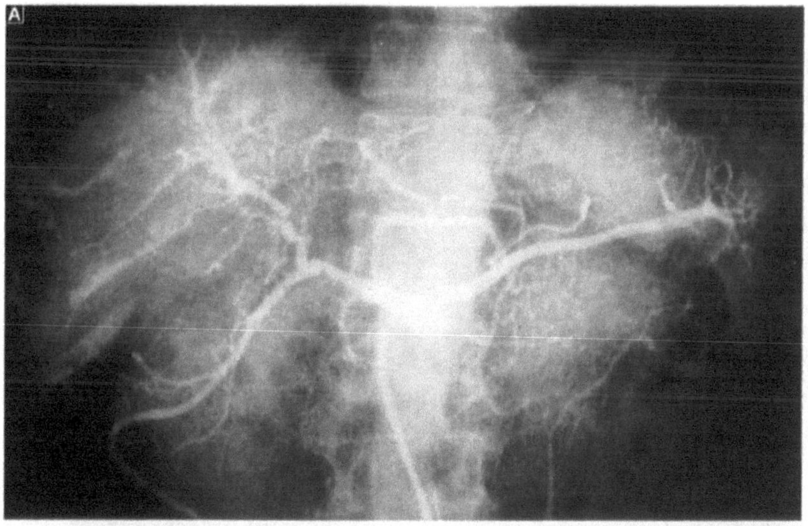

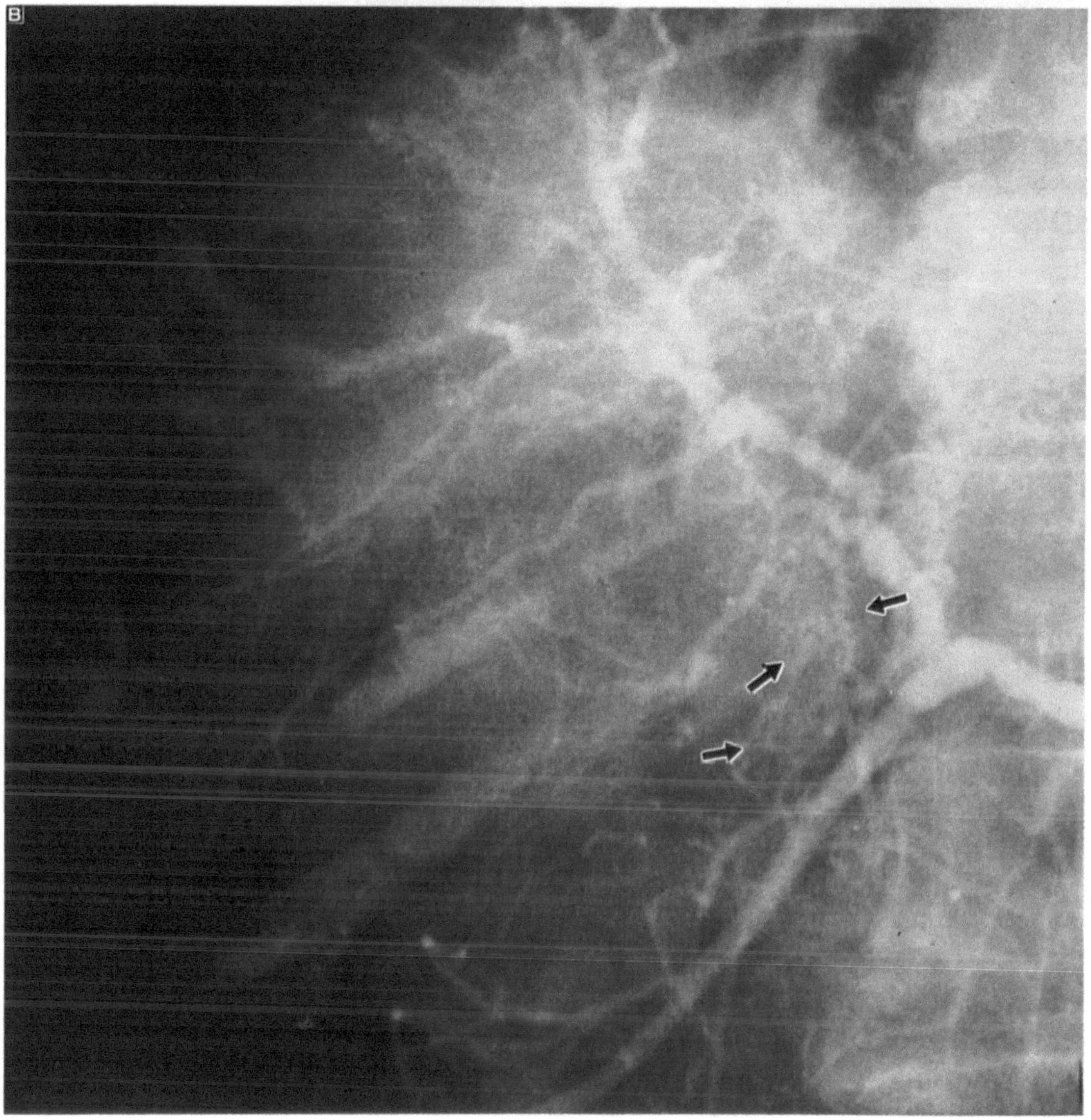

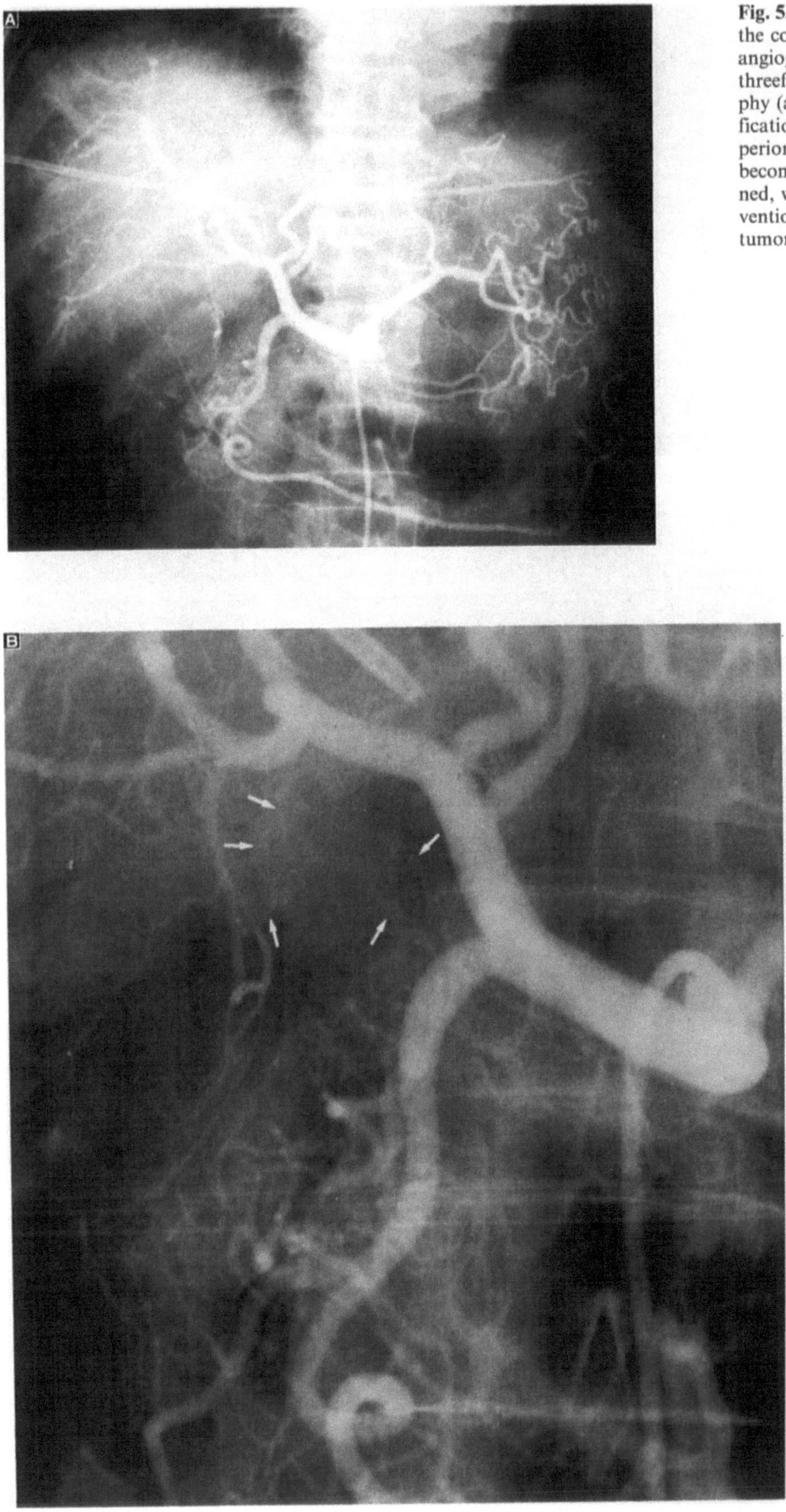

Fig. 5.24 A, B. Small carcinoma of the common bile duct. **A** celiac angiography (arterial phase); **B** threefold magnification angiography (arterial phase). Using magnification angiography (**B**), the superior epicholedochal arteries (→) become irregular and slightly stained, which are not seen with conventional angiography (**A**). The tumor size is 15 × 20 mm

and obstruction of the proper hepatic artery and its right branch. Sometimes, findings of stenosis and obstruction may also be observed in the portal vein.

In the case of a giant massive legion formed by infiltration, differentiation from hepatocellular carcinoma and cholangiocarcinoma is difficult.

In extrahepatic bile duct carcinoma, tumor vessels may only be slightly visualized. The major characteristic findings on the angiogram [39, 64] are encasement and amputation of the epicholedochal arteries, although a case in which encasement of the feeding arteries is visible may be inoperable (Fig. 5.23). In operable cases, abnormal characteristic angiographic findings are generally not observed. Even though magnification angiography can indicate abnormal changes or vessels more clearly (Fig. 5.24), it has not proven to be helpful for diagnosing operable cancer in the early stage.

5.5 Angiographic Findings in the Pancreas

5.5.1 Roentgenographic Anatomy. The pancreas is fed by the branches of the celiac artery and the branch of the superior mesenteric artery, such as the posterior superior and anterior superior pancreaticoduodenal arteries, inferior pancreaticoduodenal artery, dorsal and transverse pancreatic arteries, great pancreatic artery, and caudal pancreatic artery (Fig. 5.25).

The superior and the inferior pancreaticoduodenal arteries form an arcade, and anastomosis between arcades is observed in 60% of cases [41]. The arcades perform the part of anastomosing branches between the celiac and the superior mesenteric arteries.

The dorsal pancreatic artery branches from the splenic artery in 40% of cases; 20% of the cases branch from the celiac artery, 20% from the com-

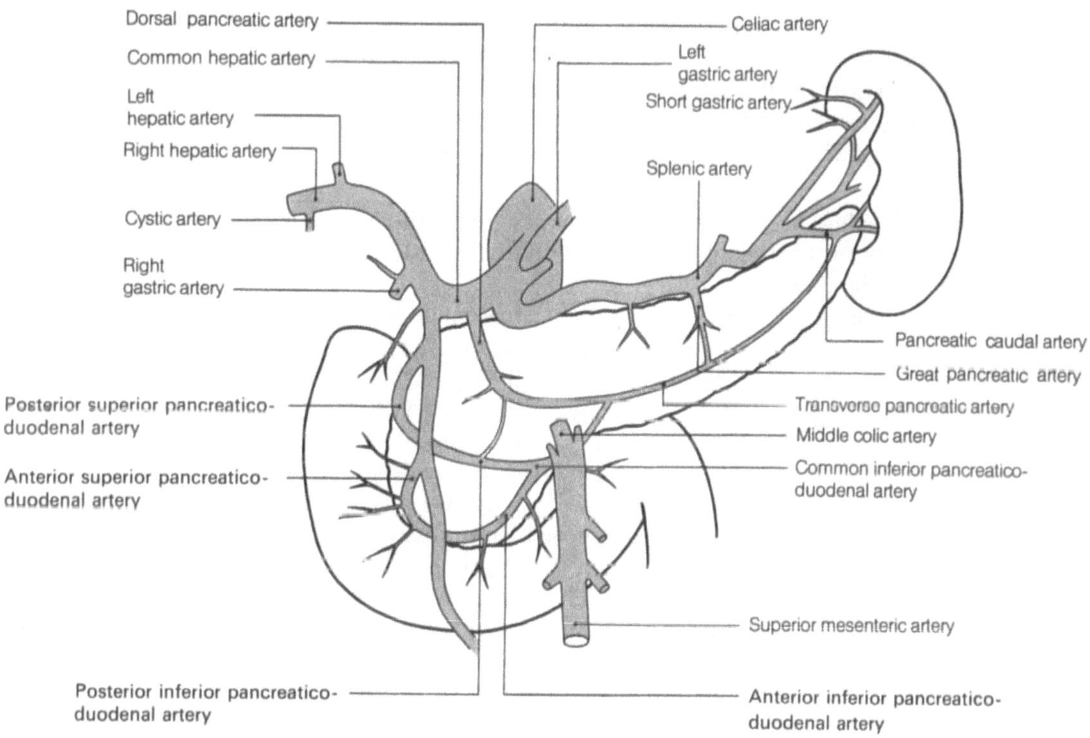

Fig. 5.25. Blood supply of the pancreas. [69]

mon hepatic artery, and 15% from the superior mesenteric artery or sometimes the middle colic artery [41].

The dorsal pancreatic artery takes the part of an anastomosing branch between the splenic and the common arteries, also between superior mesenteric and the middle colic arteries. Ninety percent of the transverse pancreatic arteries are branched from the major left branches of the dorsal pancreatic artery. The great pancreatic and caudal arteries branch from the splenic artery. The head of the pancreas is mainly fed by the superior and the inferior pancreaticoduodenal arteries and sometimes supplementarily by the dorsal pancreatic artery. The body of the pancreas is fed by the dorsal, transverse, and great pancreatic arteries. These vessels are anastomosed together by many different branches. In addition, the distribution of the vessels differs between the uncinate process of the head of the pancreas and the group forming the body and tail of the pancreas, indicating their embryologic background.

With angiography, the posterior superior pancreaticoduodenal artery, which is about 1.5 mm in diameter, is demonstrated in 96% of cases [69]. The anterior superior pancreaticoduodenal artery is about 1.8 mm in diameter and observed 96% of the time. The frequency of anastomosis of these two arteries is 52%–64% and corresponds closely to frequencies reported by anatomists. The visualization of the dorsal pancreatic artery is achieved 100% of the time, and the transverse pancreatic artery is demonstrated in around 74.4% of cases. In contrast, although the pancreatic vein runs in a pattern similar to the artery, it cannot be visualized in the venous phase, which continuously opacifies after the arterial phase.

Göthlin [27] has achieved success in selective pancreatic venography by the mothod of transumbilical or transhepatic catheterization of the portal vein. Fine images of the pancreatic vein can be obtained by direct injection of the contrast medium into the intended vein.

Vessels distributed in the pancreas are branches of the celiac and the superior mesenteric arteries so that angiography of both arteries is requird to obtain an entire image of the pancreatic vessel. Furthermore, to observe the thin peripheral arteries, it is necessary to perform superselective angiography [4] of the intrapancreatic artery or magnification angiography [26, 35]. Occasionally, pharmacoangiography may be valuable [26, 72].

5.5.2 Abnormal Findings in the Pancreas. Of the pancreatic diseases, angiography is necessary for chronic pancreatitis, pseudocyst, islet cell tumor, and carcinoma of the pancreas.

In chronic pancreatitis, findings of stenosis or encasement in large extrapancreatic arteries, such as a celiac artery or splenic artery, may be observed [9, 26, 48], the so-called sleevelike narrowing [62] (Fig. 5.26). A beaded appearance of the intrapancreatic arteries may also be seen [9, 35] and is said to be characteristic of pancreatitis [62]. Compression or occlusion of the marjor portal vein may be observed in pancreatitis due do pseudocyst, abscess, or swelling of the pancreas [9, 26, 35, 65]. However, in some cases, chronic pancreatitis cannot be directly diagnosed from angiography.

In the case of islet cell tumors [8, 10, 18, 23, 29], hypervascularity or hypovascularity occurs at a ratio of 2:1. The characteristic findings of hypervascular types of islet cell tumor are images of hypervascularity in the tumor region and clear contour staining in the capillary phase (Fig. 5.27). Therefore, even a small tumor of less than 1 cm can be diagnosed with angiography; however, false-positive angiographic findings diagnosed only with staining are a source of error in the localization of tumors [38]. Cyst-

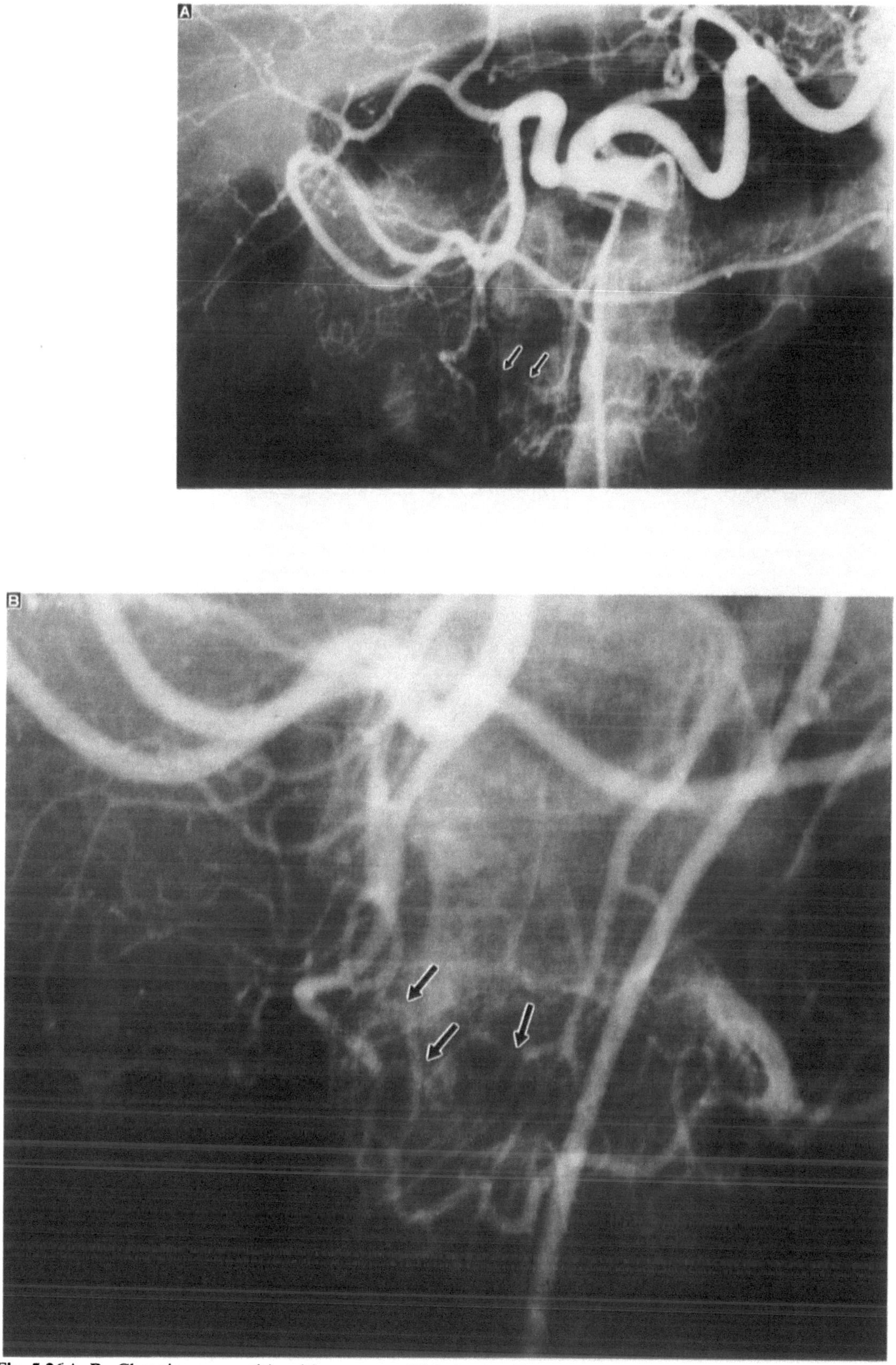

Fig. 5.26 A, B. Chronic pancreatitis with pancreatolithiasis. **A** celiac angiography (arterial phase); **B** threefold magnification angiography (arterial phase). Calcification along the pancreatic ducts and irregular and beaded formation (→) in the vessels of the pancreatic arcade can be seen

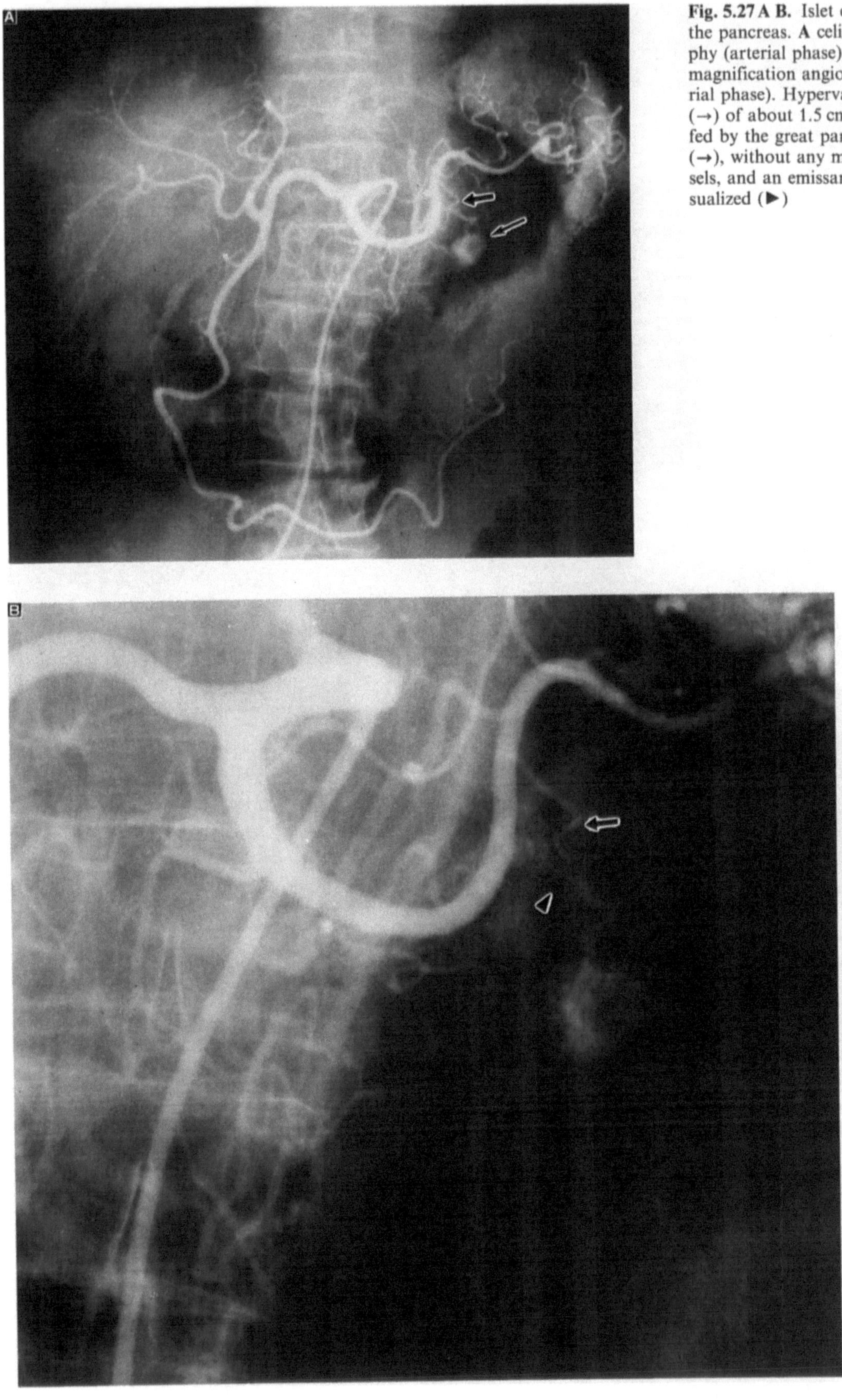

Fig. 5.27 A B. Islet cell tumor of the pancreas. **A** celiac angiography (arterial phase); **B** threefold magnification angiography (arterial phase). Hypervascular tumor (→) of about 1.5 cm in diameter fed by the great pancreatic artery (→), without any malignant vessels, and an emissary vein are visualized (▶)

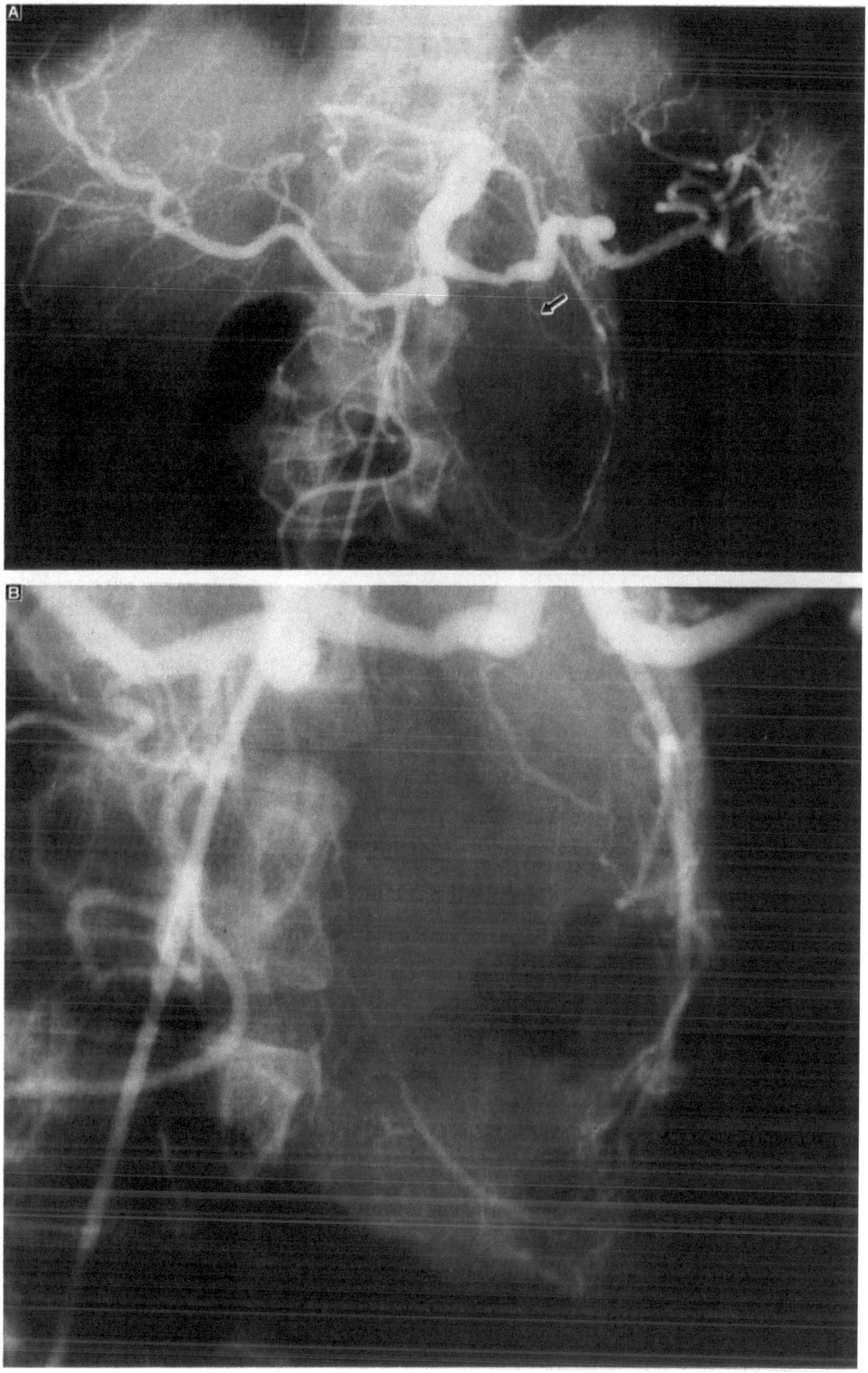

Fig. 5.28 A, B. Pseudocyst of the pancreas. **A** celiac angiography (arterial phase); **B** threefold magnification angiography (arterial phase). Smooth encasement of the splenic artery and great pancreatic artery (→) without malignant appearances can be observed

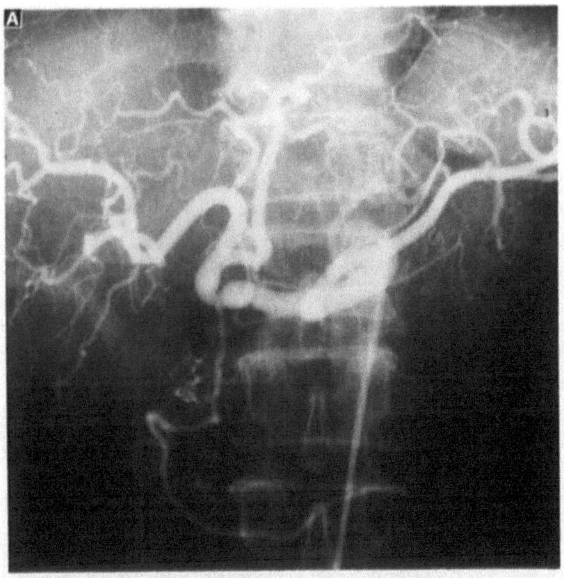

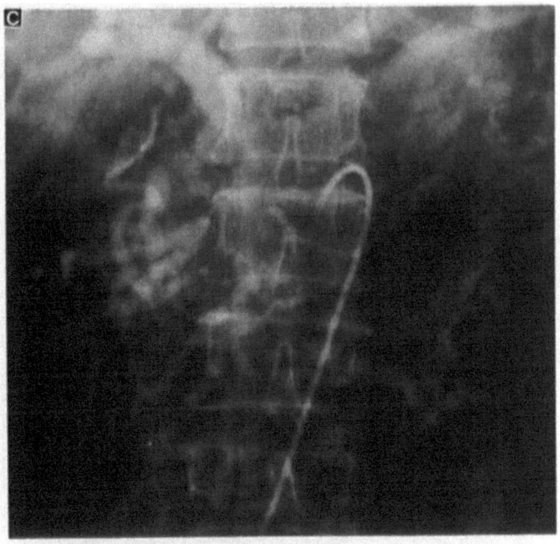

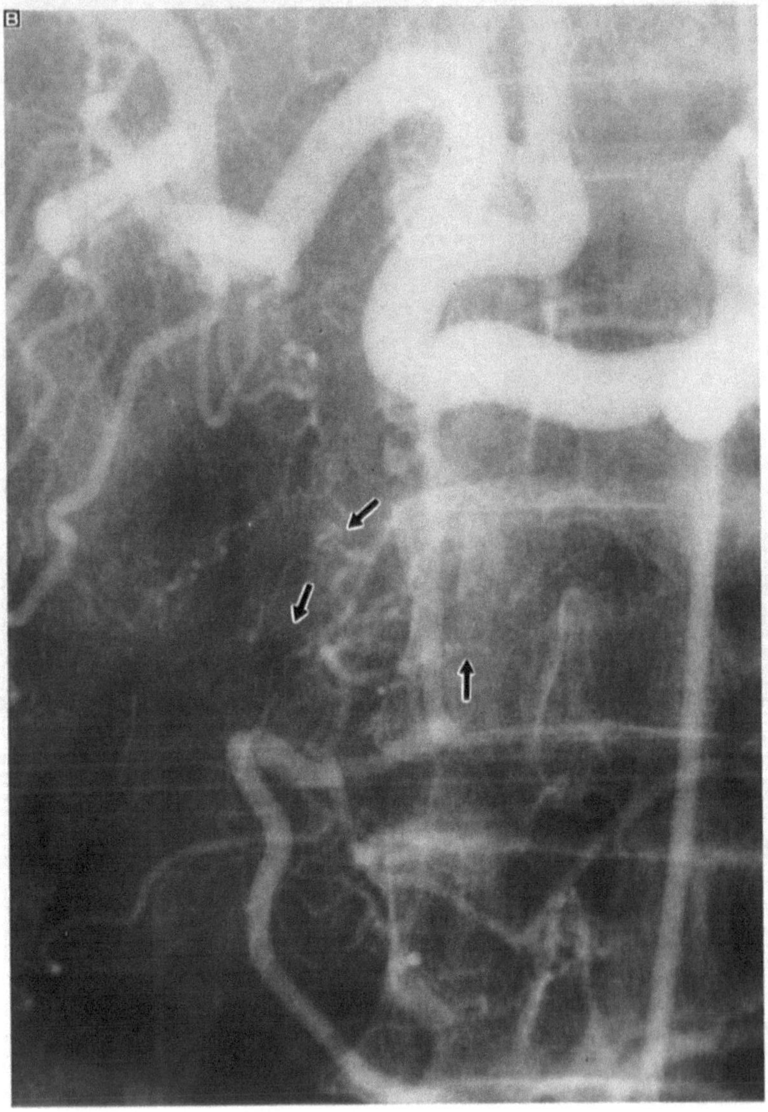

Fig. 5.29 A–C. Carcinoma of the head of the pancreas: gastroduodenal artery with stretching and partial encasement and encasement and obstruction (→) in the arteries of the arcade of the pancreatic head can be seen. Obstruction of the superior mesenteric vein causes the contrast medium to flow into the portal vein via a collateral channel. **A** celiac angiography (arterial phase); **B** threefold magnification angiography (arterial phase); **C** superior mesenteric arteriography (venous phase)

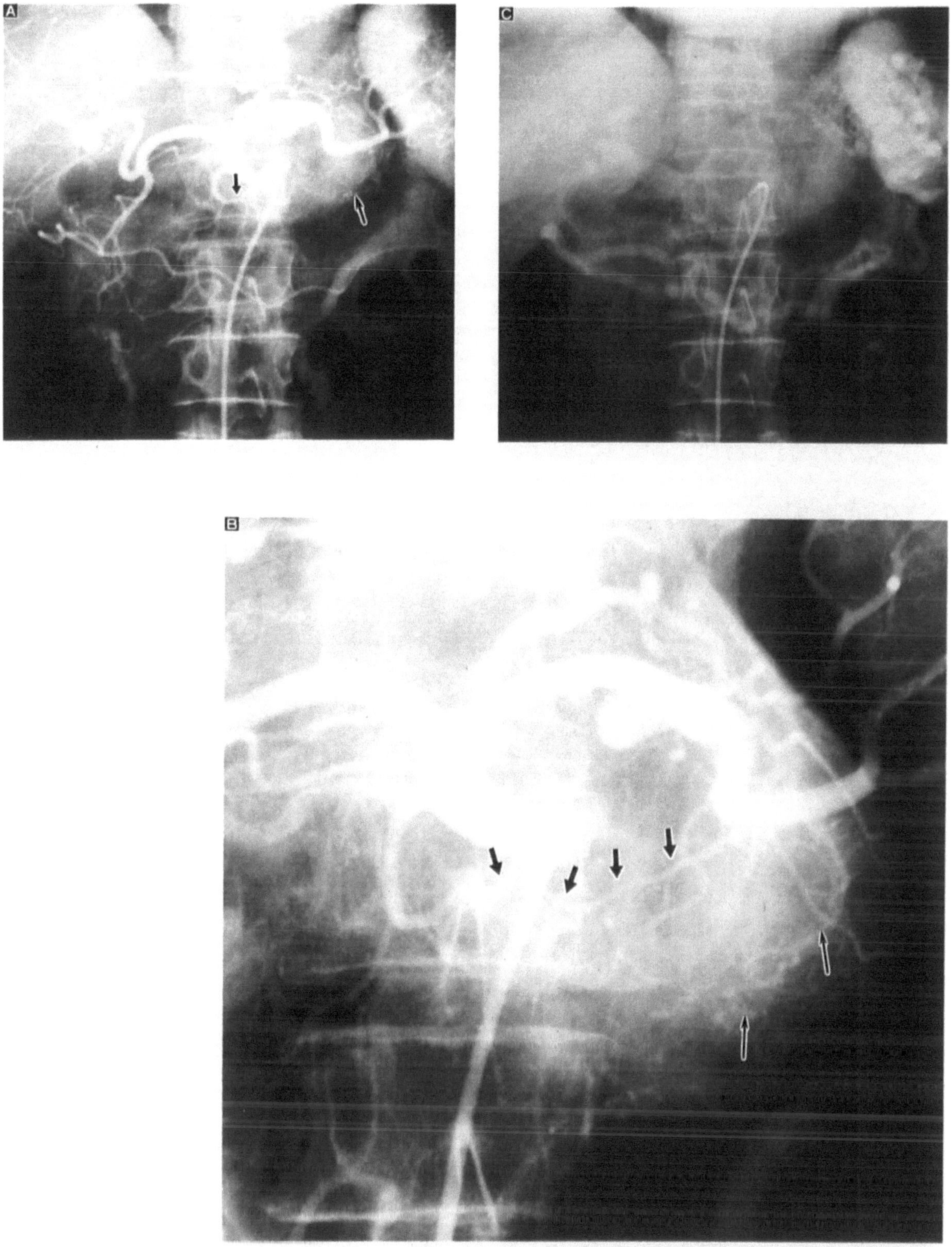

Fig. 5.30 A–C. Pancreatic carcinoma in the body and tail. **A** celiac angiography (arterial phase); **B** threefold magnification angiography (arterial phase); **C** celiac angiography (venous phase). Tight encasement in a junction of the dorsal and great pancreatic artery (→) and hypervascularity (→) in the distal portion of the left gastroepiploic artery surrounding the tumor with partial encasement can be seen. The splenic vein is not opacified, and contrast medium flows into the portal vein via the collateral channel (**C**)

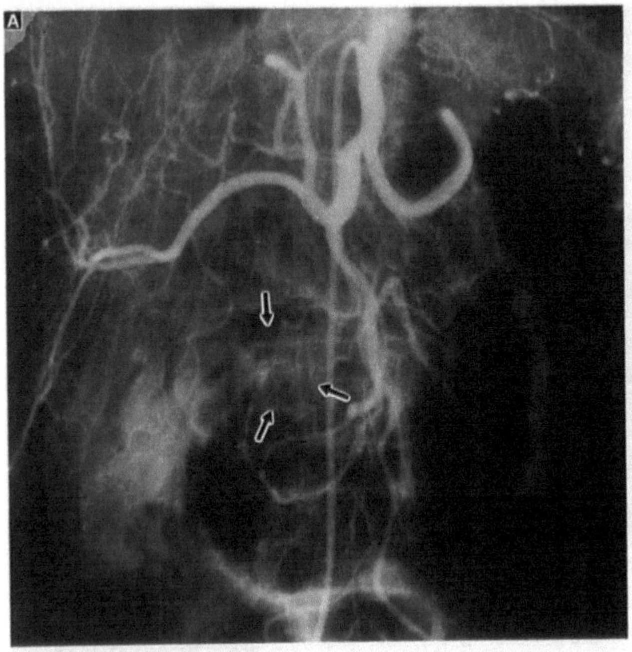

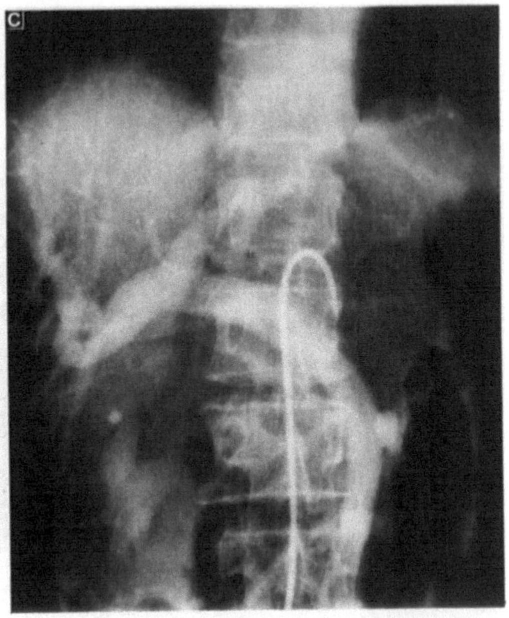

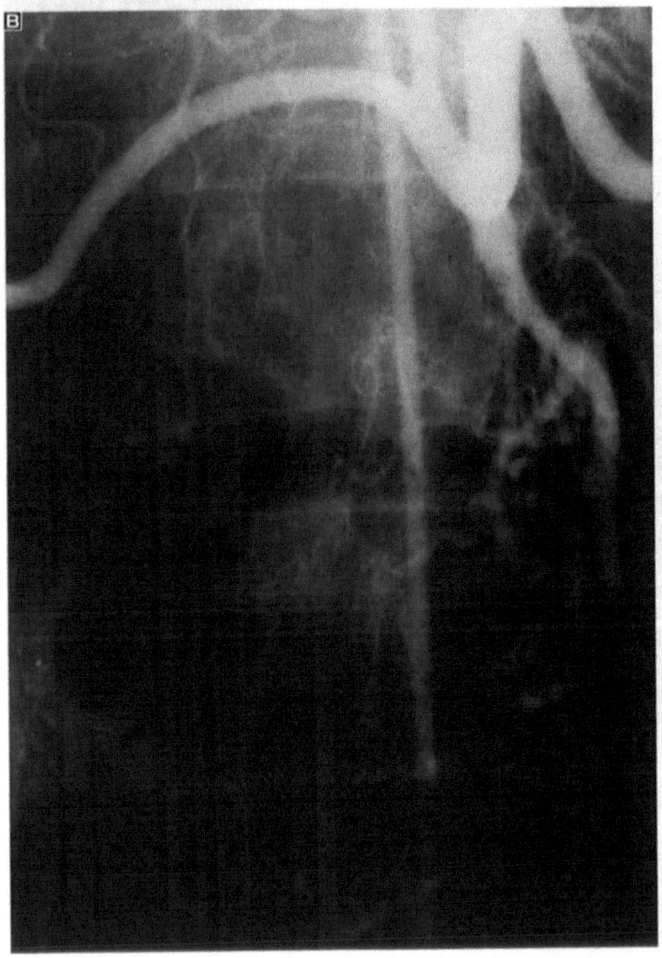

Fig. 5.31 A–C. Carcinoma of the head of the pancreas. **A** celiac angiography (arterial phase); **B** threefold magnification angiography (arterial phase); **C** superior mesenteric arteriography (venous phase). The encasement in the branches of the posterior superior pancreaticoduodenal artery and anterior superior pancreaticoduodenal artery (→) is more clearly observed with magnification angiography (**B**). There were no abnormal findings in the superior mesenteric veins. Pancreaticoduodenectomy was performed, and adenocarcinoma of 17 mm in diameter was found with no infiltration into the superior mesenteric vein and no metastasis to the lymph node. No tumor was found on examination with CT and ultrasonography

adenoma and cystadenocarcinoma may show similar staining images, although they may be uneven due to the cystic portion being unstainable [1, 6, 60].

The major characteristic findings of pancreatic cyst and pseudocyst are displacement and stretching of the vessels [9, 35] (Fig. 5.28), and occasionally it may be difficult to differentiate from hypovascular cystadenoma or cystadenocarcinoma. Hemorrhage from pseudoaneurysm in pseudocyst patients can be diagnosed by angiography [33, 40].

In most cases of pancreatic carcinoma, when symptoms are apparent, it is at the advanced stage. Angiographic findings of irregular stenosis or obstruction in the celiac artery, the common hepatic artery, gastroduodenal artery, and splenic artery (Figs. 5.29 and 5.30) that surround the pancreas can be observed.

Cases with abnormality of peripancreatic arteries are generally inoperable [11]. Even after surgery, the prognosis is poor [73]. Radical operation is only possible in a case which shows a change such as encasement and obstruction only in the intrapancreatic artery [4, 72] (Fig. 5.31). Encasement and obstruction of these intrapancreatic arteris are caused mainly by perivascular fibrosis induced by infiltration of cancer cells [70, 71].

Superselective and magnification angiography [26, 35] are necessary to diagnose operable pancreatic carcinoma because the diagnosis must be based slight changes of the intrapancreatic arteries due to its hypovascularity [30, 50]. In addition, it is also necessary to perform portography by opacifying the superior mesenteric artery since pancreatic carcinoma may cause encasement and obstruction of the superior mesenteric vein and the portal vein [13].

References

Angiography

1. Abrams RM, Beranbaum ER, Beranbaum SL, Ngo NL (1967) Angiographic studies of benign and malignant cystadenoma of the pancreas. Radiology 89:1028–1032
2. Abrams RM, Beranbaum ER, Santos JS, Lipson J (1969) Angiographic features of cavernous hemangioma of liver. Radiology 92:308–312
3. Abrams RM, Meng CH, Firooznia H, Beranbaum ER, Epstein HY (1970) Angiographic demonstration of carcinoma of the gallbladder. Radiology 94:277–282
4. Ariyama J, Shirakabe H, Ikenobu H, Kurosawa A, Owman T (1977) The diagnosis of the small resectable pancreatic carcinoma. Clin Radiol 28:437–444
5. Bartley, O, Edlund, Y, Helander CG (1967) Angiography in primary hepatic carcinoma. Acta Radiol (Diagn) 6:81–90
6. Bieber, WP, Albo RJ (1963) Cystadenoma of the pancreas: its arteriographic diagnosis. Radiology 80:776–778
7. Boijsen E, Abrams HL (1965) Roentgenologic diagnosis of primary carcinoma of the liver. Acta Radiol (Diagn) 3:257–277
8. Boijsen E, Samuelsson L (1970) Angiographic diagnosis of tumours arising from the pancreatic islets. Acta Radiol (Diagn) 10:161–176
9. Boijsen E, Tylén U (1972) Vascular changes in chronic pancreatitis. Acta Radiol (Diagn) 12:34–48
10. Bookstein JJ, Oberman HA (1966) Appraisal of selective angiography localizing islet-cell tumours of the pancreas. Radiology 86:682–685
11. Bookstein JJ, Reuter SR, Martel W (1969) Angiographic evaluation of pancreatic carcinoma. Radiology 93:757–764
12. Bookstein JJ, Appelman HD, Walter JF, Foley WD, Turcotte JG, Lambert M (1975) Histological-venographic correlates in portal hypertension. Radiology 116:565–573
13. Buranasiri S, Baum S (1972) The significance of the venous phase of celiac and superior mesenteric arteriography in evaulating pancreatic carcinoma. Radiology 102:11–20

14. Casarella WJ, Knowles DM, Wolff M, Johnson PM (1978) Focal nodular hyperplasia and liver cell adenoma: Radiologic and pathologic differentiation. AJR 131:393–402
15. Chuang VP, Wallace S (1981) Hepatic artery embolization in the treatment of hepatic neoplasms. Radiology 140:51–58
16. Couinaud C (1954) Lobes et segments hépatiques. Notes sur l'architecture anatomique et chirurgicale du foie. Presse Med 62:709–712
17. Deutsch V (1967) Cholecysto-angiography. Visualization of the gallbladder by selective celiac and mesenteric angiography. AJR 101:608–616
18. Deutsch V, Adar R, Jacob ET, Bank H, Mozes M (1973) Angiographic diagnosis and differential diagnosis of islet-cell tumors. AJR 119:121–132
19. Elias H (1949) A re-examination of the structure of the mammalian liver. II. The hepatic lobule and its relation to the vascular and biliary systems. Am J Anat 85:379–456
20. Farrell R, Steinman A, Green WH (1972) Arteriovenous shunting in a regenerating liver simulating hepatoma. Report of a case. Radiology 102:279–280
21. Fechner RE, Roehm JO (1977) Angiographic and pathologic correlation of hepatic focal nodular hyperplasia. Am J Surg Pathol 1:217–224
22. Fredens M, Egeblad M, Holst-Nielsen F (1967) The value of selective angiography in the diagnosis of tumors in pancreas and liver. Radiology 93:765–769
23. Fujii K, Yamagata S, Sasaki R, Ohneda A, Shoji T, Suzuki J (1974) Arteriography in insulinoma. AJR 120:634–647
24. Gammill SL, Shipkey, FH, Himmelfarb EH, Parvey LS, Rabinowitz JG (1976) Roentgenology-pathology correlative study of neovascularity. AJR 126:376–385
25. Goldstein HM, Neiman HL, Mena E, Bookstein JJ, Appelman HD (1974) Angiographic findings in benign liver cell tumors. Radiology 110:339–343
26. Goldstein HM, Neiman HL, Bookstein JJ (1974) Angiographic evaluation of pancreatic disease. A further appraisal. Radiology 112:275–282
27. Göthlin J, Lunderquist A, Tylén U (1974) Selective phlebography of the pancreas. Acta Radiol (Diagn) 15:474–480
28. Göthlin J, Pettersson H (1976) Angiography in malignant and chronic inflammatory lesions of the gallbladder. Acta Radiol (Diagn) 17:343–352
29. Gray, RK, Rosch J, Grollman JH Jr (1970) Arteriography in the diagnosis of islet-cell tumors. Radiology 97:39–44
30. Herlinger H, Finlay DBL (1978) Evaluation and follow-up of pancreatic arteriograms. A new role for angiography in the diagnosis of carcinoma of the pancreas. Clin Radiol 29:277–284
31. Hjortsjo CH (1951) The topography of the intrahepatic duct systems. Acta Anat 11:599–615
32. Itzchak Y, Adar R, Bogokowski H, Mozes M, Deutsch V (1974) Intrahepatic arterial portal communications: angiographic study. AJR 121:384–387
33. Kadell BM, Riley JM (1967) Major arterial involvement by pancreatic pseudocysts. AJR 99:632–636
34. Kaude J, Jensen R, Wirtanen GW (1973) Slow injection hepatic angiography. A comparison with a high injection rate. Acta Radiol (Diagn) 14:700–712
35. Khademi M, Lazaro JE, Rickert RR (1973) Selective arteriography in the diagnosis of chronic inflammatory pancreatic disease. AJR 119:141–150
36. Kido C, Sasaki T (1971) Angiography of primary liver cancer. AJR 113:70–81
37. Kido C, Hibino, K, Kaneko M, Sasaki T (1974) Angiography of gallbladder cancer. Nippon Acta Radiol 34:1–11
38. Korobkin MT, Palubinskas AJ, Glickman MG (1971) Pitfalls in arteriography of islet-cell tumors of the pancreas. Radiology 100:319–328
39. Kuroda C, Uchida H, Nakamura H, Sato T, Yshioka H, Tokunaga K (1979) Diagnostic value in angiography on malignancies of the extrahepatic bile ducts, with special reference to the epicholedochal arterial plexus (in Japanese). Nippon Acta Radiol 39:1332–1343
40. Levin DC, Eisenberg H, Wilson R (1977) Arteriography in the evaluation of pancreatic pseudocysts. AJR 129:234–248
41. Lunderquist A (1965) Angiography in carcinoma of the pancreas. Acta Radiol [Suppl] 235:
42. Lunderquist A (1967) Arterial segment supply of the liver. An angiographic study Acta Radiol [Suppl] 272:
43. Matsui O (1979) Clinical usefulness of infusion hepatic angiography for the diagnosis of space occupying lesions of the liver (in Japanese). Nippon Acta Radiol 39:1–16

44. Matsuyama K, Sakuma S (1980) Angiographic appearance of diseases of the liver, biliary tract and pancreas in infants and children (in Japanese). Jpn J Pediatr 33:1223–1230
45. McLoughlin MJ (1971) Angiography in cavernous hemangioma of the liver. AJR 113:50–55
46. McMullen CT, Montgomery JL (1973) Ateriographic findings of focal nodular hyperplasia of the liver and review of the literature. AJR 117:380–387
47. Mortensson W, Pettersson H (1979) Infantile hepatic hemangioendothelioma. Angiographic considerations. Acta Radiol (Diagn) 20:161–169
48. Moskowitz H, Chait A, Mellins H (1968) Tumor encasement of the celiac axis due to chronic pancreatitis. AJR 104:641–645
49. Moss, AA, Clark RE, Palubinskas AJ, DeLorimier AA (1971) Angiographic appearance of benign and malignant hepatic tumors in infants and children. AJR 113:61–69
50. Nebesar RA, Pollard JJ (1967) A critical evaluation of selective celiac and superior mesenteric angiography in the diagnosis of pancreatic disease, particularly malignant tumor: facts and artefacts. Radiology 89:1017–1027
51. Novy S, Wallace, S, Medellin H, McBride C (1974) Angiographic evaluation of primary malignant hepatocellular tumors in children. AJR 120:353–360
52. Novy SB, Wallace S, Goldman AM, Ben-Menachem Y (1974) Pyogenic liver abscess. Angiographic diagnosis and treatment by closed aspiration. AJR 121:388–395
53. Okuda K, Musha H, Yoshida T, Kanda Y, Tamazaki T, Jinnouchi S, Moriyama M, Kawaguchi S, Kubo, Y, Shimokawa Y, Kojiro M, Kuratomi S, Sakamoto K, Nakashima T (1975) Demonstration of growing casts of hepatocellular carcinoma in the portal vein by celiac angiography: the thread and streaks sign. Radiology 117:303–309
54. Okuda K, Musha H, Yamazaki T, Jinnouchi S, Nagasaki Y, Kubo Y, Shimokawa Y, Nakayama T, Kojiro M, Sakamoto K, Nakashima T (1977) Angiographic demonstration of intrahepatic arterioportal anastomoses in hepatocellular carcinoma. Radiology 122:53 58
55. Okudaira M (1969) Hepatic lobes with reference to vascular structures (in Japanese). Acta Hepatoloiga Japonica 10:98–101
56. Olmsted WW, Stocker JT (1975) Cavernous hemangioma of the liver. Radiology 117:59–62
57. Pantoja E (1968) Angiography in liver hemangioma. AJR 104:874–879
58. Parke WW, Michels NA, Ghosh GM (1963) Blood supply of the common bile duct. Surg Gynecol Obstet 117:47–55
59. Pollard JJ, Nebesar RA, Mattoso LF (1966) Angiographic diagnosis of benign diseases of the liver. Radiology 86:276–283
60. Pressman BD, Asch T, Casarella WJ (1973) Cystadenoma of the pancreas. A reappraisal of angiographic findings. Radiology 119:115–120
61. Rabinowitz, JG, Kinkabwala M, Ulreich S (1974) Macro-regenerating nodule in the cirrhotic liver. Radiologic features and differential diagnosis. AJR 121:401–411
62. Reuter SR, Redman HC, Joseph RR (1969) Angiographic findings in pancreatitis. AJR 107:56–64
63. Reuter SR, Redman HC, Siders DB (1970) The spectrum of angiographic findings in hepatoma. Radiology 94:89–94
64. Reuter SR, Redman HC, Bookstein JJ (1971) Angiography in carcinoma of the biliary tract. Br J Radiol 44:636–641
65. Reuter SR, Redman HC (1977) Gastrointestinal angiography. Saunders, Philadelphia
66. Rösch, J, Grollman JH, Steckel RJ (1969) Arteriography in the diagnosis of gallbladder disease. Radiology 92:1485–1491
67. Rösch J, Freeny P, Antonovic R, Gutierrez OH (1976) Infusion hepatic angiography in diagnosis of liver metastases. Cancer 38.2278–2286
68. Stanley P, Gates GF, Eto, RT, Miller SW (1977) Hepatic cavernous hemangiomas and hemangioendotheliomas in infancy. AJR 129.317–321
69. Sakuma S (1977) Roentgenographic anatomy in abdomen (in Japanese). Kanehara Shuppan, Tokyo
70. Sumida M, Takagi T, Fukuda, Y, Ariyama J, Ikenobe H, Kurosawa A, Ohashi K, Kawai S, Shirata I, Shimaguchi H, Shirakabe H (1978) Histopathological study of arterial encasement in pancreatic carcinoma. Comparison of in vivo and specimen angiography, and reconstruction of histological serial section of arterial encasement (in Japanese). Jpn J Clin Radiol 23:445–451

71. Sumida M, Ariyama J, Shimaguchi S, Shirata I, Ikenobe H, Shirakabe H, Takagi T, Fukuda Y, Hashimoto K (1980) Histopathological study of arterial occlusion in pancreatic carcinoma (in Japanese). Jpn J Clin Radiol 25:71–78
72. Suzuki T, Kawabe K, Nakayasu A, Takeda H, Kobayashi K, Kubota N, Honjo I (1971) Selective arteriography in cancer of the pancreas at a resectable stage. Am J Surg 122:402–407
73. Suzuki T, Kawabe K, Imamura M, Honjo I (1972) Survival of patients with cancer of the pancreas in relation to findings on arteriography. Ann Surg 176:37–41
74. Takahashi S, Sakuma S (1975) Magnification radiology. Springer, Berlin Heidelberg New York
75. Takashima T, Matsui O (1980) Infusion hepatic angiography in the detection of small hepatocellular carcinomas. Radiology 136:321–325
76. Viamonte M Jr, Roen, S, LePage J (1973) Nonspecificity of abnormal vascularity in the angiographic diagnosis of malignant neoplasms. Radiology 106:59–63
77. Yü C (1967) Primary carcinoma of the liver (Hepatoma): its diagnosis by selective celiac arteriography. AJR 99:142–149

B: Other Imaging Modalities

6 Hypotonic Duodenography

Hypotonic duodenography is the roentgenographic examination performed under hypotonic conditions by administering an antispasmodic agent. There are two methods of hypotonic duodenography. One is the tube-assisted method [4], which is achieved by inserting a tube into the duodenum, and the other is a tubeless method [2].

The tube-assisted method is suitable for precise examination, because selective duodenography can be achieved by controlling the amount of barium and air.

The tubeless method is performed by administering barium orally and filling the stomach with air using a gastric tube or effervescent agent, then introducing the desirable ratio of air and barium into the duodenum by changing the patient's position. This method is beneficial as a routine examination owing to less invasion to the patient just after examining the esophagus and stomach.

6.1. Application

6.1.1 Tube-Assisted Method

1. Intubation Technique. First, the guide wire is inserted through the duodenography tube; the application of Xylocaine jelly facilitates easy sliding of the guide wire through the duodenography tube. Then, the patient assumes a supine position, and the tube is inserted transorally or transnasally under fluoroscopic control. When the tip of the tube reaches the pylorus ring, the guide wire is removed 2–4 cm, then manually pushed up the greater curvature between the angular incisure and antrum; then, the inserted tube can pass through easily. When the tip of the tube reaches near to the interior duodenal flexure, the guide wire is pulled out completely, and the edge of the manipulation side of the tube is fixed to the cheek of the patient with tape.

2. Administration of Anticholinergic Drug. The anticholinergic drug is administered intramuscularly or intravenously. The intramuscular injection can extend the effective time, although it differs depending is on the individual. The intravenous injection, with minor individual differences, is quickly effective, provides enough effective time for routine examination, and is more desirable than an intramuscular injection. As an anticholinergic drug, 40 mg of Buscopan (Scopolamine butylbromide) is suitable. This injection is given just before the instillation of barium.

3. Examination Technique. Normally, the patient is in the supine position, the barium is injected slowly (50–100 ml) through the tube, and then the barium-filled image is photographed. Thereafter, a double-contrast image is photographed in the supine frontal position by suction of 20–50 ml of barium and supplying air with a 100 ml syringe. Next, the patient is turned to the left decubitus and then to the prone position. While sending air in the prone frontal, prone left posterior oblique, and prone right posterior oblique positions, the double-contrast images are photographed.

Subsequently, the patient is turned to the left decubitus and then to the supine position, and a mucosal image is photographed. After sending air, double-contrast images in the supine frontal, supine right anterior oblique, and supine left anterior oblique positions are photographed.

Only in the case of a projecting lesion in the duodenum must compression photography be performed by adding barium. During examination, if overlapping images of the duodenum and the stomach are observed due to a backflow of barium, it is necessary to separate them using a cotton pad.

6.1.2 Tubeless Method

1. Administration of Anticholinergic Drug. The same amount of anticholinergic drug as used in the tube-assisted method is injected transmuscularly 5–10 min prior to examination. However, a reliable method is to give another intravenously injection shortly before the opacification. With this method, 20 mg of Buscopan are injected, transmuscularly, then another 20 ~ 40 mg are injected intravenously just before opacification.

2. Opacification Technique. After 150–200 ml of barium have been administered transorally, the stomach is filled with over 300 ml of air supplied through a gastric tube or by transoral administration of effervescent agents.

The contrast medium in the stomach is transported to the duodenum by moving the patient into the right decubitus position. Then, the anticholinergic drug is injected. The air in the stomach is moved to the duodenum by shifting the patient into the left decubitus position. The patient is then changed to the prone position holding a cotton pad on the right upper abdomen. After repeating the process of turning the patient from the left decubitus to the prone projection, double-contrast images in the prone frontal, prone right anterior oblique, and left anterior oblique projections are photographed. Subsequently, double-contrast images in the supine frontal and supine right anterior oblique projections and then mucosal relief images are photographed.

6.2 Roentgenographic Anatomy of the Duodenal Loop

The duodenum is 25–30 cm in length and forms a C shape (Fig. 6.1). The duodenal loop is divided into four portions; the first portion contains the duodenal bulb and the horizontal part (the duodenal bulb constitutes approximately one-half or two-thirds of the first portion).

The junction zone of the first and second portions is called the superior duodenal flexure and that of the second and third portions the inferior duodenal flexure.

The second portion contains the major and the minor duodenal papillae.

Fig. 6.1. **A** normal case (supine position); **B** normal case (prone position)

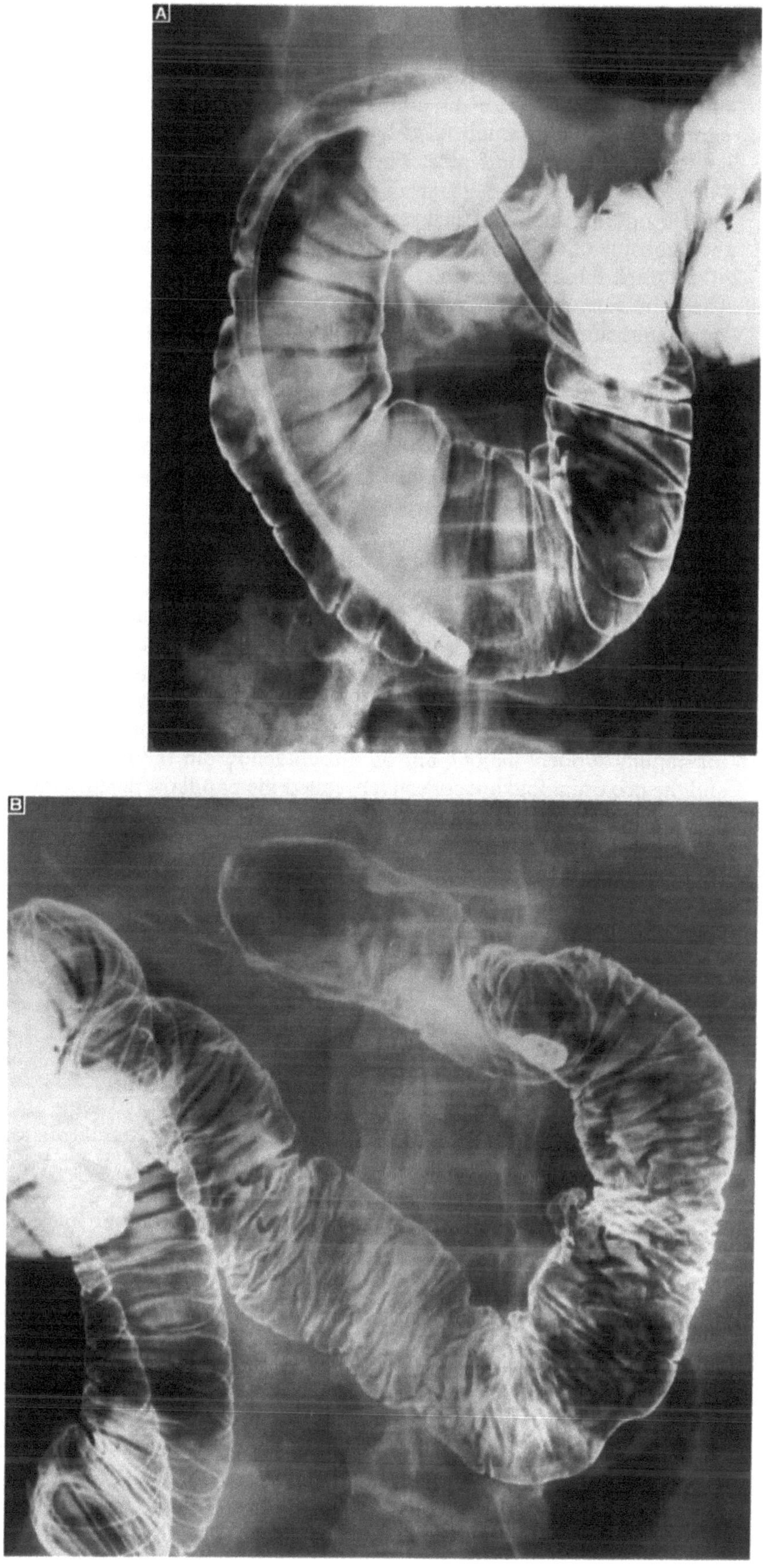

1. The first portion is 4–5 cm in length, extending from the pylorus ring of the stomach to the superior duodenal flexure, and runs to the right direction transversely at the level of the first lumbar vertebra or runs in the right posterosuperior direction. The duodenal bulb is covered with peritoneum, and although fixed by the hepatoduodenal and duodeno-colic ligaments, it is movable. Furthermore, it lacks Kerckring's fold.
2. The second portion is 6 – 8 cm in length, located between the superior and the inferior duodenal flexures. It descends almost perpendicularly at the right side of the lumbar spine, and its distal end is almost at the level of the third lumbar vertebra.
3. The third portion, the so-called inferior horizontal portion, is 4–7 cm in length and runs horizontally from the inferior duodenal flexure in a left direction.
4. The fourth portion is 5–7 cm in length and runs in a left superior direction to the duodenojejunal junction. The distal end is on the left side of the lumbar spine at the level of the second lumbar vertebra. The junction zone of the jejunum and duodenum, the so-called duodenoje-junal junction, is tightly fixed with the ligament of Treitz so that is almost immovable.
5. The papillary portion can be observed on the posterior wall close to the inner border near the middle of the second portion. The common bile duct and main pancreatic duct open at this portion, and at the oral side of the duodenal papilla, a ridge is formed by these ducts which run on the duodenal wall. It is called the plica longitudinalis duodeni. At the anal side, there are one to several longitudinal folds called the frenulum. Anatomically, the duodenal papillary portion means the papilla of Vater (or papilla duodeni major), but on a roentgenogram the major papilla and the proximal fold are collectively called the papillary portion due to the difficulty of differentiation.
6. The minor papilla is a protrusion of 3 cm and is located proximal to the major papilla at the site of the opening of the accessory pancreatic duct. However, the accessory pancreatic duct dose not always open; histologi-cally, there may be only a residue of the pancreatic duct.

6.3 Hypotonic Duodenography in Diseases of the Biliary Tract and Pancreas

Abnormal duodenographic findings [1] of the entire duodenal loop are a widened loop, an inverted "3" sign, stenosis, dilatation, triangular distor-tion of the descending segment, and a round shape of the superior or inferior duodenal flexure.

The characteristic finding of a widened duodenal loop is the image of superior, inferior, and lateral displacement of the duodenum (Fig. 6.2) and of the inverted "3" sign the image of concave superior and inferior portions of the inner wall protrusion of the descending portion. Both are regarded as characteristic findings in carcinoma of the head of the pancreas; how-ever, these findings cannot always be observed.

According to Ito [3], the widened loop and inverted "3" sign can be observed in 10.8% and 4.1%, resepectively, of all cases of disease of the pancreas and biliary tract, and in 17.6% and 5.9% of cases of carcinoma of the head of the pancreas. Findings helpful for the diagnosis of disease of the pancreas and biliary tract are localized abnormal findings rather than a widened duodenal loop or the inverted "3" sign [3].

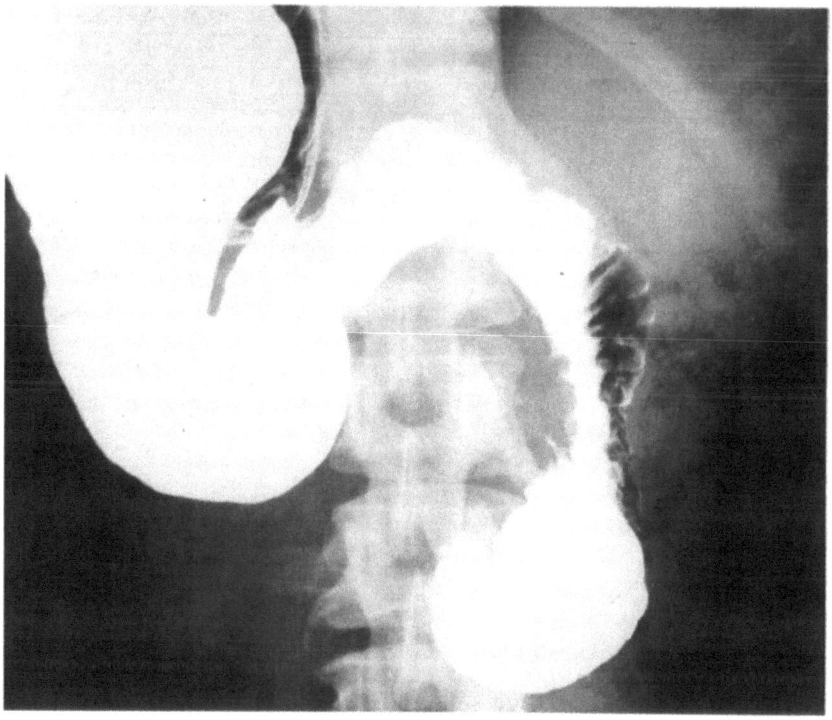

Fig. 6.2. Enlargement of the duodenal loop duo to the pancreatic cyst. A pancreatic stone is also observable

Localized abnormal findings are images of flattening, irregularity, spiculation, compression, filling defects, and double contour in the margin of the duodenal wall. Further abnormal images in the duodenal lumen are fold thickening, irregular course of the fold, amputation of the fold, niche, and pseudodiverticulum of the mucosa and skeletal images composed of string shapes in the mucosa.

Of the above-mentioned characteristic findings, abnormal images of the inner and outer margins are important because an irregular infiltrated pattern and displacement are observed in 50% – 60% of cases of diseases of the pancreas and biliary tract [3].

In cholelithiasis, an abnormal finding in the lateral margin of the duodenum between the duodenal bulb and upper part of the second portion may be a major diagnostic sign. An abnormal finding is an image of a smooth indentation caused by dilatation of the gallbladder and extrahepatic bile duct, or an irregularly contoured image of the lateral margin of the duodenum resulting from an inflammatory process of chole- and/or pericholecystitis.

The above findings are more often observed in choledocholithiasis or cholecysto-choledocholithiasis than in cholecystolithiasis alone.

In the case of cholelithiasis, an image of a swollen duodenal papilla can also be an indicative finding. Additionally, when a gallstone is in the common bile duct, an image of smooth swelling over 15 mm may often be visualized.

In cases of carcinoma of the gallbladder and the biliary tract, images of an irregular infiltration or abnormal displacement of the lateral margin between the duodenal bulb and the upper part of the second portion (especially in the center of the horizontal part) are frequently observable. Abnormal findings in the inner margin of the duodenum are rarer than in the

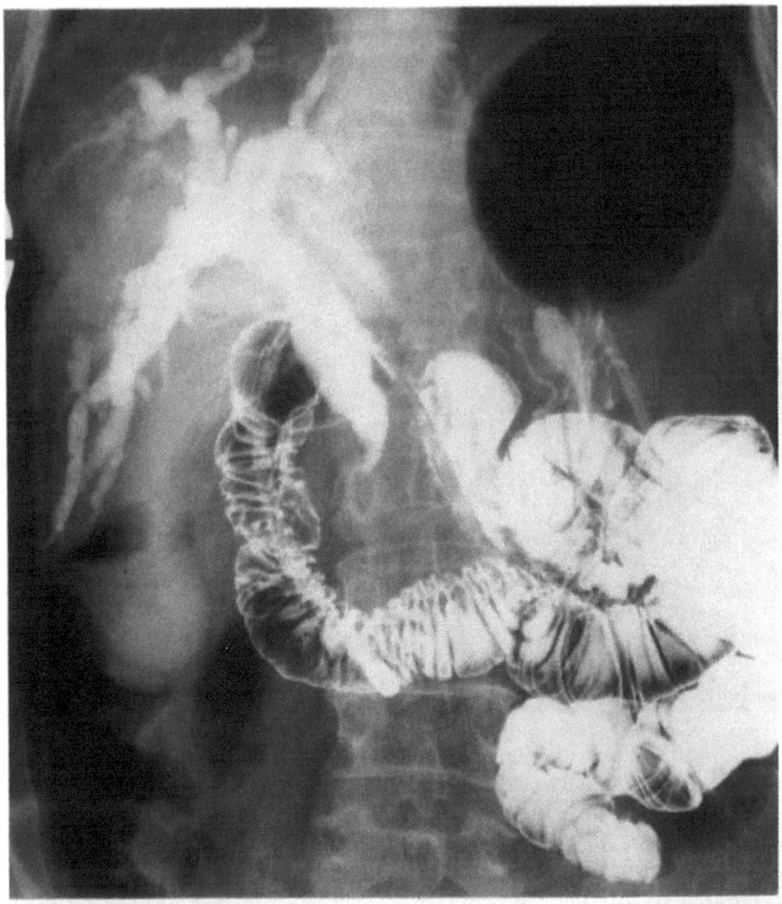

Fig. 6.3. Carcinoma of the head of the pancreas causing irregularity and infiltration in the inner descending portion of the duodenum. With PTC, a V-shaped obstruction in the common bile duct corresponding to the head of the pancreas is seen

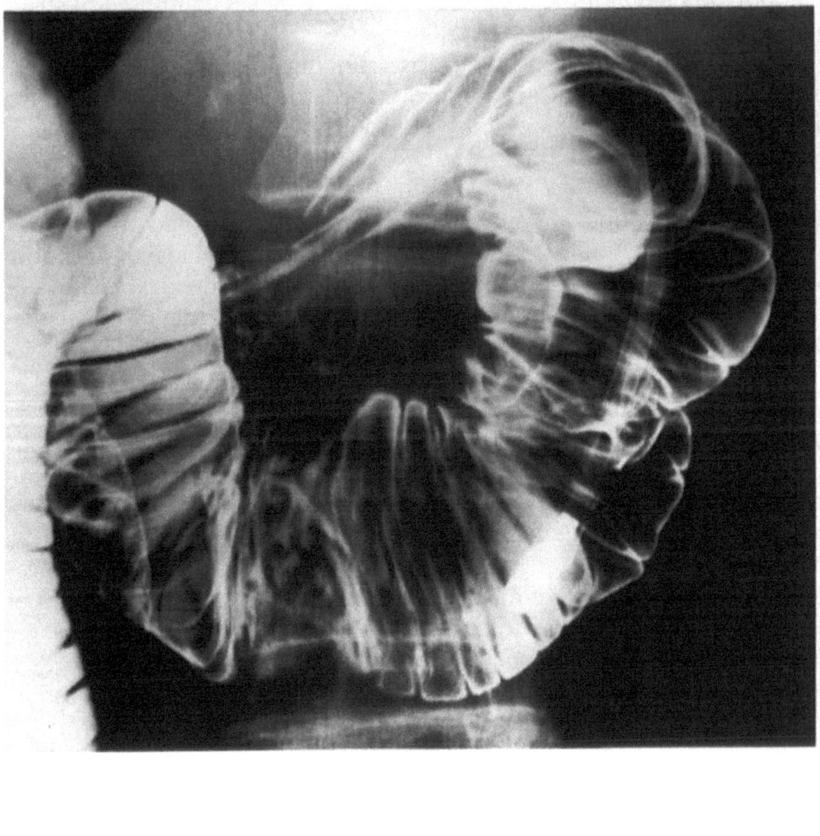

Fig. 6.4. Small carcinoma of the head of the pancreas

lateral margin because pathological changes of the inner margin extend from the outer margin.

Conversely, in carcinoma of the head of the pancreas, symptomatic findings are mainly observed in the inner margin of the duodenum. Various findings, such as irregular infiltration, spiculation, and a double contour of the inner margin, can be observed in the inner margin of the second portion (Figs. 6.3 and 6.4). In carcinoma of the head of the pancreas accompanied by dilatation of the gallbladder and biliary tract, an image of smooth displacement may sometimes be visible in the lateral margin between the duodenal bulb and the upper part of the second portion.

References

Hypotonic Duodenography

1. Eaton SB, Ferrucci JT Jr (1973) Radiology of the pancreas and duodenoum. Saunders, Philadelphia
2. Goldstein HM, Zboralske FF (1969) Tubeless hypotonic duodenography. JAMA 210:2086–2088
3. Ito M (1976) Clinical studies on diagnosis of diseases in pancreas and biliary system. – Diagnosis by combined methods of percutaneous transhepatic cholangiography, hypotonic duodenography and cytology (in Japanese). J Nagoya City University Med Assoc 27:54–93
4. Liotta D (1955) Pour le diagnostic des tumeurs du pancréas: la duodénographie hypotonique. Lyon Chir 50:455–460

7 Excretory Cholecystocholangiography

The first generation of excretory cholecystocholangiography was cholecystography, which was originally performed by Graham and Cole [4] using tetrabromophenolphthalein sodium. Since then, contrast media have been improved, and with various new techniques and X-ray photographing techniques, today's excretory cholecystocholangiography has been refined.

There are two methods of excretory cholecystocholangiography; oral administration and intravenous injection. A combined method can also be employed. Compared with the direct method, which is performed by injecting contrast medium directly into the gallbladder and bile duct, the excretory method is easier to perform and has fewer side effects. Thus, it is a useful method for routine examinations. The excretory method can be a basic examination for diagnosing diseases of the biliary tract because entirely opacified images can be obtained.

7.1 Oral Cholecystography

Iopanoic acid (Telepaque), copodate sodium (Biloptin), and iobenzamic acid are usually used as contrast media. These are triiodophenyls and contain 60% of iodate. Opacification can be achieved to essentially the same degree.

Orally administered contrast medium is absorbed in the small intestine, bound to the serum protein, transported to the liver via the portal vein, and then excreted 2.5–3 h later metabolically.

The liver excretes the contrast medium into the bile juice, which then enters into the gallbladder by way of the common hepatic duct and the cystic duct, and the contrast medium is concentrated 8–10 times. The contrast medium excreted into the small intestine with the bile juice is also reabsorbed into the blood; then one part is fed back to the liver (called enterohepatic circulation) and is utilized to reopacify the gallbladder.

The contrast medium concentrated in the gallbladder produces an X-ray image of the gallbladder. To obtain an image of the bile duct [11], 0.3%–0.5% contrast medium in iodine is required. However, the contrast medium excreted from the liver into the biliary tract is far lower in density; it is therefore necessary to send the concentrated contrast medium to the biliary tract by contracting the gallbladder to opacify the extrahepatic bile duct. Orally administered contrast medium is excreted 60%–80% into the urine and only 20%–40% into the stool.

Special premedication is unnecessary for the examination. It is necessary to exclude intestinal gas as it hinders assessment of the X-ray image. For this purpose, the patient must avoid indigestible food and eat low-fat food for supper prior to the day of examination. It is also effective to give absorbents and carminatives and for severe constipation purgatives 1–2 days before administration of the contrast medium.

Generally, 3 g of contrast medium must be administered in doses of 0.5 g with a little water every 5 min between 9 and 10 p.m. After administration of the contrast medium, the patient must fast until the examination is completed.

The density of concentration in the gallbladder is highest about 12 h after administering the contrast medium. Therefore, it is preferable to take roentgenograms between 9 and 10 a.m. the next day.

To produce positive images of a bilirubinic stone, oral contrast medium is given after every meal dividing the amount for a day (3 g) into three doses. This is continued for 3–4 days. With this method, as the contrast medium acts upon the bilirubin, it deposits on the surface of the bilirubinic stone [9], and a rim sign can be visualized. This method is helpful for diagnosing not only a stone in the gallbladder but also in the biliary tract, and its diagnostic accuracy is 68% when performed together with tomography. However, one must be cautious of side effects due to the large amount of contrast medium administered.

To opacify the bile duct including the gallbladder, twice the volume divided into two fractions is used [1]. This is achieved by giving 3 g of contrast medium in the evening before the examination and another 3 g at 6 a.m. the next morning. Roentgenography is performed 3–4 h after the last administration. The image of the bile duct obtained with the oral method is inferior in quality to that obtained with an intravenous injection.

7.2 Intravenous Cholangiography

With an intravenous injection of contrast medium, the gallbladder and bile duct can be opacified simultaneously and opacification is high, thus efficiently improving diagnostic ability. Even if the absorption of contrast medium is not influenced by the digestive organs, the frequency rate of side effects is higher than with the oral method.

As a contrast medium, 20 ml of 30% or 50% iodipamide meglumine (Biligrafin) is used. Generally, 30% Biligrafin is utilized; 50% Biligrafin is used for obese patients, cases of poor opacification and postoperative cholangiography. Meglumine sodium of iodoxamic acid (40.3% Endobil 20 ml) is also excellent.

Injected contrast medium binds to the serum protein, is taken into the hepatic cells, excreted into the bile juice, and then enters into the gallbladder via the bile duct. With this procedure, the biliary tract including the gallbaldder and bile duct is entirely opacified because the iodine content of the bile juice exceeds the opacification threshold.

About 90% of Biligrafin is excreted into the intestine without feedback to the liver due to lack of enterohepatic circulation; 10% is excreted in the urine. In the case of hypoproteinemia, the amount excreted in the urine increases.

With rapid injection, the rate of nonbinding Biligrafin increases, thus decreasing the efficiency of opacification. A pyelogram can then be obtained due to increased excretion in the urine. The same situation is observed in cases of liver dysfunction and renal failure.

In preparation for the procedure, bowel gas should be removed and hypersensitivity testing must be performed.

The contrast medium must be injected slowly in 5–10 min. Generally, the image of the bile duct is clearly visualized 30–70 min and of the gallbladder 60 min after the injection. With diseases of the biliary tract, opacification may be delayed because of accompanying liver dysfunction. Therefore, it is necessary to make exposures 30, 60, 90, and 120 min after injection.

With drip infusion cholangiography (DIC), enhancement of opacification by the cholagogue effect and a decrease in side effects can be accomplished by slowing the infusion speed [2]. As it is possible with this method to increase the dose of contrast medium injected, the accuracy of opacification of the biliary tract increases more than with the method of intravenous injection. However, Biligrafin is limited to being excreted into the bile juice. Therefore, the accuracy of opacification does not always increase with more contrast medium; additionally, the frequency of side effects will increase.

A specially designed injection medium to balance side effects and opacification efficiency is commercially available; for instance, using the 250 ml injection medium for 4.8% Biligrafin DIC, opacification efficiency is elevated and side effects can be decreased.

Dripping time influences opacification ability, and one of 30–60 min is adequate. Roentgenography is performed 30, 60, 90, and 120 min after drip infusion. To increase opacification capacity, cholagogues, anti-inflammatory agents (steroids, etc.) and relaxants for Oddi's sphincter (morphine, anticholinergic agents) may occasionally be used simultaneously.

In any case, with DIC, suitable emergency treatment can be provided in a case with side effects via the needle inserted into the vein.

There are various other methods available for effective contrast medium injection. A combined method of oral and intravenous administration is applied to efficiently opacify the gallbladder and bile duct simultaneously. With this method, six tablets of Telepaque are administered at 9 p.m. the day prior to examination, and roentgenography is performed at 9 a.m. the next day. At 9:30 a.m., 20 ml of 30% Biligrafin is injected intavenously in

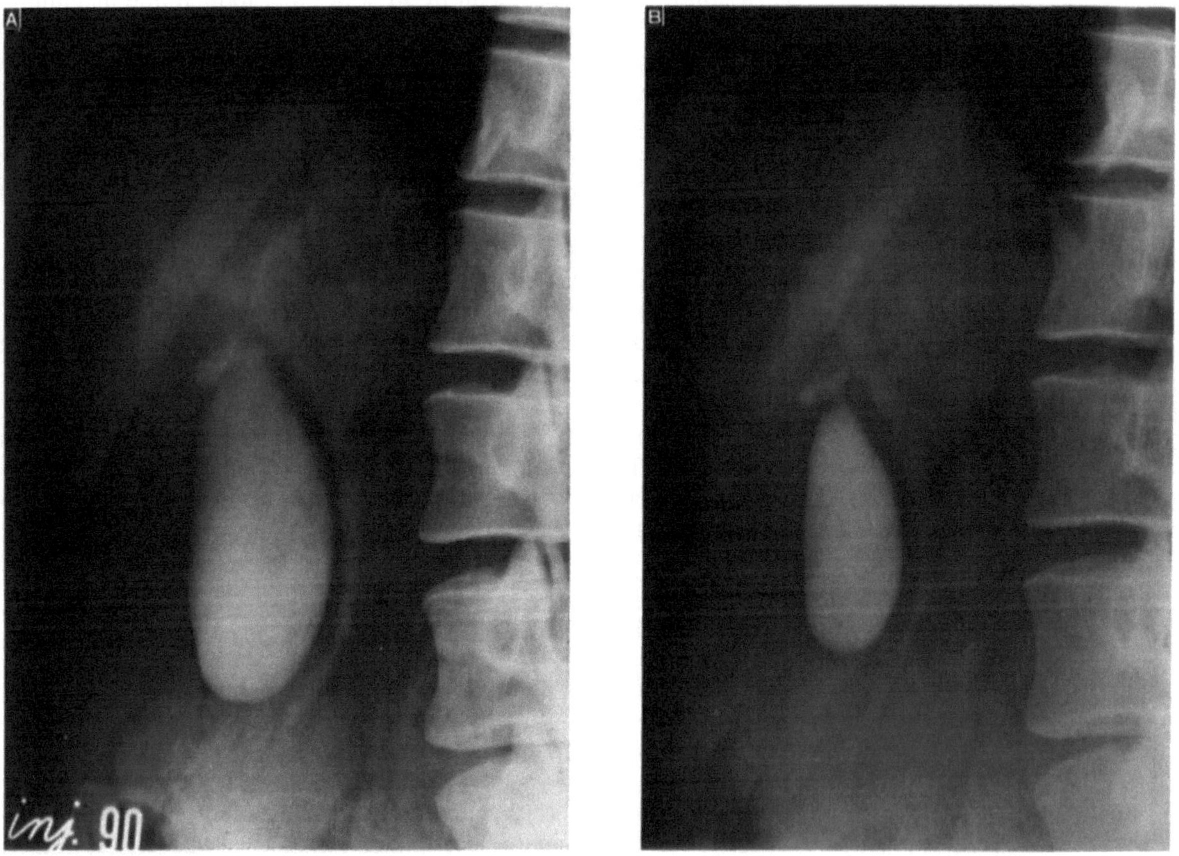

Fig. 7.1 A, B. Normal gallbladder and bile duct (combination of transoral and intravenous administration). **A** 90 min after the intravenous injection; **B** 30 min after administrating a cholecystokinetic agent

5–10 min and exposures are made 30, 60 and 90 min after the injection. Then, the cholecystokinetic agent is given and additional exposures are made 30 and 60 min later (Fig. 7.1).

A combined method of oral administration and DIC is also employed [12]. Examination of the contractility of the gallbladder can be achieved by administering various cholecystokinetic agents after the above – mentioned roentgenography. The yolks of one or two eggs or Caerulein (ceruletide diethylamine) are used as cholecystokinetic agents. Although physiologic, egg yolk has a poor rate of absorption and is allergenic. Caerulein, which rarely elicits an allergic reaction, can be injected intramuscularly and produces faster contraction of the gallbladder [13]. In this examination, 0.2 μg/kg body weight are administered, and roentgenography is performed 15, 30 and 60 min after intramuscular injection.

In most cases of without biliary tract disease, contraction of the gallbladder of more than half size can generally be observed; around 30 min later, maximum contraction occurs, and redilatation is frequently observed 60 min later. A decisive criterion for normal contractility of the gallbladder is a change in size by more than half after 30 and 60 min of yolk administration.

7.3 Examination Procedures

Generally, the prone position is used for the left anterior oblique projection to avoid overlapping of the biliary tract and spine. Roentgenography is also performed in the supine, erect, and lateral decubitus positions when the best cholecystogram can be obtained (normally about 90 min after intravenous injection). With an intravenous injection, right anterior oblique projections in the supine position are also effective for observing the bile duct. The lateral projection is useful for examining the location and running pattern of the bile duct.

Tomography is helpful for further examination of diseases of the biliary tract, such as stones of the common bile duct or cystic duct, and for clearer observation in the region of the distal end of the common bile duct [7].

The tomographic scanning level is at 1 cm intervals and 4–9 cm (5–10 cm in obese patients) above the tomographic table in the slight left anterior oblique projection in the prone position. The gallbladder is finely photographed at a level of 4–6 cm and the bile duct 7–9 cm above the table.

To diagnose polypoid lesions, diverticulum and small calculi, a compression method in the erect and supine positions is useful. It is even more useful for differentiation between bowel gas and stones.

7.4 Side Effects

Side effects may occur with both oral and intravenous methods, although they are less frequent and less severe with the oral method. With intravenous administration, side effects are fewer with the drip infusion method than with a single injection. Side effects caused by contrast medium given orally [5] are eruption, diarrhea nausea, and vomiting and may be severer with hepatic dysfunction.

Using Telepaque, the mortality rate is regarded to be 0.00003%. With an intravenous injection, it is necessary to check for side effects such as local reddening, edema, eruption, itching, sneezing, epiphora and dyspnea by injecting 1 ml of contrast medium prior to examination.

With Biligrafin, slight side effects occur in 10%–30% of cases, and severe symptoms such as drop in blood pressure, sweating and breathlessness occur in about 0.5% of cases. However, cases of mortality are rare, and the rate is 0.00035% according to Frommhold's report [3]. At any rate, it is necessary to be very cautious of side effects during performance of excretory cholecystocholangiography, and a different examination should be performed in patients with a history of drug eruption or allergic disease.

7.5 Roentgenographic Findings

With excretory cholecystocholangiography, lower density images are obtained than with direct cholecystocholangiography. Therefore, roentgenogram must be carefully interpreted. By carefully observing the contours of the opacified gallbladder, the Rokitansky-Aschoff sinus (Fig. 7.2) and septated gallbladder can be easily identified. Also, disease of the extrabiliary tract can be recognized from the image of extrinsic displacement.

7.5.1 Morphological Abnormality. The location and size of the gallbladder differs depending on body habitus, photographing position and opacification technique. For instance, the image of the gallbladder obtained with an intravenous injection is observed to be 1.2–1.5 times larger than in the oral method.

The diameter of the common bile duct is normally 4–8 mm and abnormally over 10 mm, which is mostly caused by common bile duct stones (Fig. 7.3). However, as the diameter of the common bile duct may also dilate due to a malignant tumor, examination of the cause is necessary.

Morphological abnormalities of the gallbladder are exhibited in the following patterns: agenesis of the gallbladder, multiple gallbladder, intrahepatic and floating gallbladder, phrygian cap (Fig. 7.4), and hourglass-type gallbladder; also, multiseptate gallbladder and diverticulum of the gallbladder are present.

A congenital abnormality of the bile duct is congenital dilatation of the common bile duct, in which case opacification is hardly achieved, and the entire biliary tracts are rarely opacified. A dilated common bile duct may sometimes be misdiagnosed as a gallbladder if the true gallbladder cannot be opacified.

On the other hand, findings of stenosis of the common hepatic duct are observed in the case of a gallstone protruding to the neck of the gallbladder and cystic duct (Mirizzi's syndrome). Similiar findings are also obtained in carcinoma of the gallbladder so that careful diagnosis is necessary.

7.5.2 Gallbladder Stones. While a calcified stone is observed in about 15% of gallbladder stones, gallstones are generally visualized as images of radiolucency (Fig. 7.5). If the radiolucency adjoining the contour of the gallbladder is visible, a mass lesion and localized adenomyomatosis are suspected.

Images of stones in the biliary tract can be diagnosed by careful observation when excretion of the bile juice is normal and no liver dysfunction is present (Fig. 7.6). However, in the case of gallstones with high-density opacification of the gallbladder, the image of the stone cannot be observed

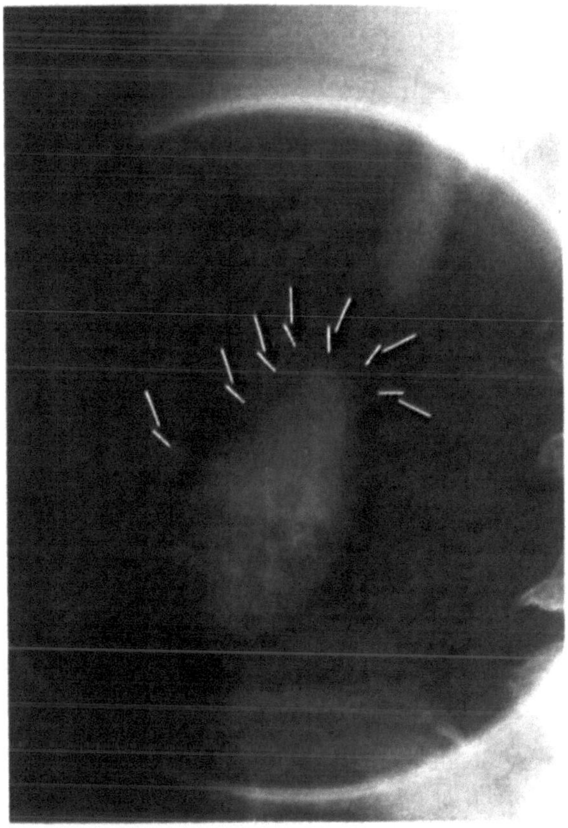

Fig. 7.2. Rokitansky-Aschoff sinus with gallstones, observed from body to fundus of the gallbladder (→)

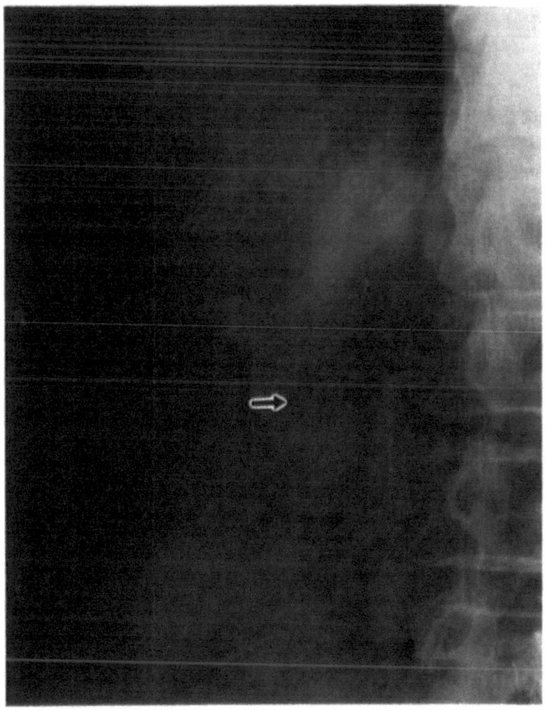

Fig. 7.3. Common hepatic duct stone (→)

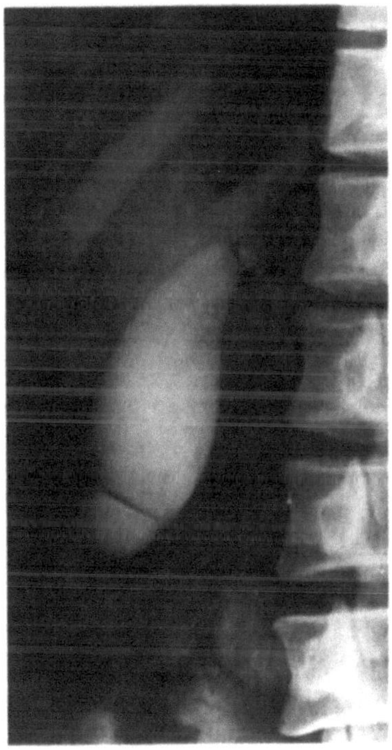

Fig. 7.4. Phrygian cap

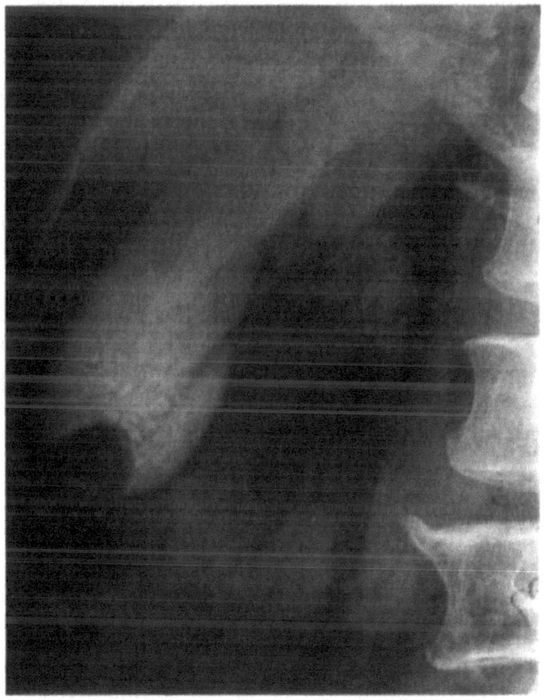

Fig. 7.5. Gallbladder stone

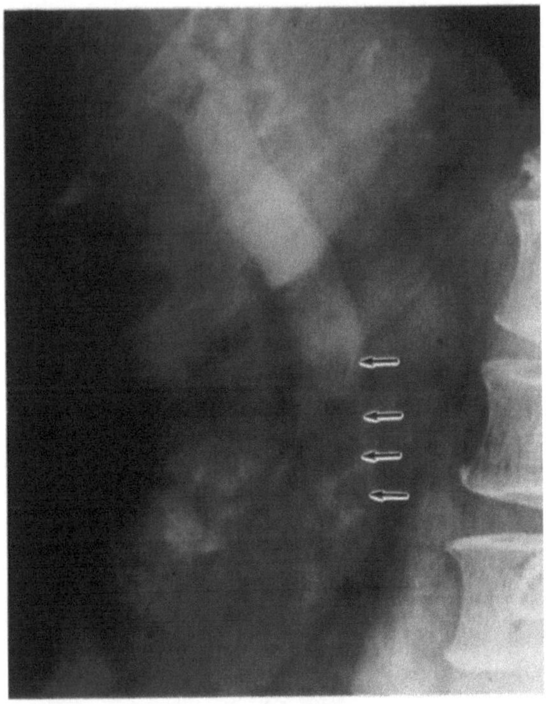

Fig. 7.6. Common bile duct stone (→)

because of a masking effect. Floating gallstones are easily diagnosed by filming in the erect position.

A radiolucent image in the gallbladder is required to differentiate from bowel gases. In the case of gallstones, the radiolucent image of the stone is observed in the gallbladder, and it never protudes from the contour of the gallbladder. In the intravenous injection method, an inhomogeneous shadow of the gallbladder may sometimes be visualized because contrast medium flowing into the gallbladder does not mix with the bile juice, the Hornykiewytsch-Stender sign [6], and because of stratification [10]. Although this image disappears in 1–2 h, in a quick examination it may be misdiagnosed for a giant solitary gallstone or floating gallstone.

7.5.3 Dyskinesia of the Bile Duct. Dyskinesia of the bile duct is a general term for choledocal dysfunction of the sphincter and can be diagnosed by examinations of duodenal juice and assessment of gallbladder kinetics. Dyskinesia can be classified into hyperkinetic dyskinesia, hypertonic dyskinesia and hypotonic dyskinesia.

In hyperkinetic dyskinesia, the image of contraction is quickly observed after administration of a cholecystokinetic agent, and sometimes abnormal marked contraction or disappearance of the gallbladder image may be caused.

Hypertonic dyskinesia is divided into the Oddi's sphincter type and neck-cystic duct type. In a typical case of the Oddi's sphincter type, the cystic duct can be opacified even with the oral method, and by giving an agent that relaxes Oddi's sphincter, excretion of contrast medium can be easily observed. In the neck-cystic duct type, the gallbladder exhibits a round pattern and contraction starts later, is slower and prolonged.

In hypotonic dyskinesia, the gallbladder relaxes and is generally observed with poor density and a large size. Also, contractility is poor, and prolonged opacification of the gallbladder can be observed.

Chronic inflammation can be determined based on opacification density, contraction function, size, shape, hardening of the gallbladder contour and visualization of the Rokitansky-Aschoff sinus.

7.5.4 Poor Opacification

1. Dysfunction of the Gastrointestinal Tract, Pancreas, and Liver. With the oral method, poor opacification is caused by low absorption of contrast medium due to disturbances of absorption or passage of the gastrointestinal tract. Even liver dysfunction causes insufficient excretion of contrast medium into the biliary tract resulting in poor opacification or nonvisualization in severe cases. Generally, nonvisualization is apparent when data from clinical examinations do not reach the following standards:

20% – 30% in BSP clearance test
2 – 3 mg/dl in total serum bilirubin
30 King-Armstrong units in serum alkaline phosphatase

According to Nanbu [8], with 2.0 mg/dl in total serum bilirubin, 50% of cases are not opacified; when values detected were over 30% in the BSP clearance test, or over 30% or under 0.05 of the numerical value of K, in the ICG (indocyanine green) clearance test, opacification was not achieved in all cases.

In liver dysfunction, the opacification effect differs between the primary liver diseases and primary biliary diseases or extrinsic obstruction of the bile duct. Generally, clearer opacification can be obtained in liver diseases than in biliary diseases. Many cases of biliary diseases are poorly opacified because of functional or organic insufficiency of the distal end of the bile duct even with slight liver dysfunction.

2. Negative Findings of the Gallbladder Caused by Diseases of the Biliary Tract. In excretory cholangiography, negative opacification of the gallbladder is the most serious case. In acute biliary inflammation, negative opacification occurs due to transitional liver dysfunction and obstruction of the cystic duct. Also, in the case of stasis of bile juice in the gallbladder and cholecystitis, opacification of the gallbladder is poor because of the decreased concentrating ability of bile juice and hyperabsorption of contrast medium in the mucosa of the gallbladder wall.

Furthermore, poor or nonopacification is produced by gallstone filling in the gallbladder, atrophy of the gallbladder, impaction of a gallstone in the neck of the gallbladder, cicatricial obstruction of the cystic duct, obstruction due to inflammation, and carcinoma of the gallbladder. In addition, obstruction of the common bile duct caused by carcinoma of the common bile duct, the papilla of Vater and the head of the pancreas will result in nonopacification. Conversely, rapid excretion of contrast medium due to duodenal-biliary fistula or hyperkinetic dyskinesia also results in poor opacification (Table 7.1).

3. Other Causes of Poor Opacification. Poor opacification is caused by overly rapid injection and faulty administration of the contrast medium and also by inadequate decisions regarding photographing time, condition and position. Hypoproteinemia, thyroid gland disease and anemia may also result in poor opacification.

Table 7.1 shows itemized examples of negative opacification of the gallbladder without the presence of liver and gastrointestinal tract diseases

Table 7.1. Causes and frequency of nonopacified gallbladder

Cholecystolithiasis	68 (57.6%)
Cholecystocholedocholithiasis	13 (11.0%)
Noncalculus cholecystitis	10 (8.5%)
Gallbladder carcinoma	10 (8.5%)
Carcinoma of the bile duct	4 (3.4%)
Hepatocellular carcinoma	3 (2.5%)
Carcinoma of the pancreas	3 (2.5%)
Liver cirrhosis	2 (1.7%)
Metastatic liver carcinoma	1
Cholecystolithiasis with liver cirrhosis	1
Dialtation of the bile duct	1
Hemangioma of the liver	1
Agenesis of the gallbladder	1

using the combined method of intravenous injection and oral administration. These cases were determined by direct cholangiography and surgery.

In most cases of nonvisualization of the gallbladder in excretory cholangiography, organic lesions of the biliary tract can be suspected if liver disease has been ruled out. It is necessary to perform further examinations, such as direct cholangiography, to obtain detailed diagnostic information.

References

Excretory Cholecysto-cholangiography

1. Bogatzki M (1959) Perorale, fraktionierte Cholezysto- und Cholangiographie. Fortschr Röntgenstr 91:729–734
2. Feldman MI, Keohane M (1966) Slow injection intravenous cholangiography. Radiology 87:355–356
3. Frommhold W, Braband H (1960) Zwischenfälle bei Gallenblasenuntersuchungen mit Biligrafin und ihre Behandlung. Fortschr Röntgenstr 92:47–59
4. Graham EA, Cole WH (1924) Roentgenologic examination of the gallbladder; preliminary report of a new method utilizing the intravenous injection of tetrabromphenolphthalein. JAMA, 82:613–614
5. Hashimoto E, Matsuno K, Maeda J, et al (1980) Side effects of contrast agents for oral cholecystography. (in Japanese). Biliary Tract Pancreas 1:1043–1049
6. Hornykiewytsch T, Stender HS (1953) Intravönese Cholangiographie. Fortschr Röntenstr 79:292–309
7. Melnick GS, Lo Curcio SB (1973) The nonvisualized gallbladder. A tomographic re-evaluation. Radiology 108:513–515
8. Nanbu K, Kurosawa A, Yamaguchi T, Namihisa AT, Shirakabe H (1971) Cholecysto-cholangiography (in Japanese). Jpn J Clin Radiol 16:922–929
9. Salzman E, Watkins DH (1958) Opacification of radiolucent biliary calculi. JAMA 167:1741–1743
10. Shaffer HA Jr, Harrison RB (1978) Stratification in the gallbladder during intravenous cholangiography. Gastrointest Radiol 3:33–37
11. Taenzer V (1964) Das negative Cholezystogramm und seine klinische Bedeutung. Dtsch Med Wochenschr 89:827–832
12. Takeuchi T, Goto K, Miyaji M, Katagiri K, Takahata M (1975) Studies on the cholelithiasis in the aged (in Japanese). The Saishin-Igaku 30:995–1001
13. Wetner SM, Vincent ME, Robbins AH (1979) Ceruletide-assisted cholecystography: a clinical assessment. Radiology 131:23–26

8 Endoscopic Retrograde Cholangiopancreatography (ERCP)

Endoscopic retrograde cholangiopancreatography (ERCP) is carried out to obtain opacified images of the pancreatic and common bile ducts by inserting a catheter into the duodenal papilla. The examination is performed by inserting a duodenoscope into the descending portion of the duodenum.

This examination has evolved from technical developments in the field of endoscopic diagnosis [1, 5, 8, 10]. However, it belongs to the category of X-ray diagnosis. With this procedure, not only the pancreatic duct and the common bile duct can be opacified, but also the image of the duodenal papilla is easily observed by endoscopy.

8.1 Examination Procedures

Premedication is the same as in duodenoscopy, although testing of hypersensitivity to iodine is indispensable because water-soluble contrast media such as 60% Urografin and 64% Angiografin are used. Additional administration of sedatives may occasionally be required.

The endoscopic manipulation is also the same as for fiber gastroscopy. Generally, the fiberscope can be quickly inserted into the descending portion of the duodenum. This manipulation is aimed at the duodenal papilla, which is situated in the descending portion of the duodenum and is seen along the longitudinal axis which intersects with the circular fold. The duodenal papilla is usually located 7–9 cm from the pylorus.

Figure 8.1 shows the regional anatomy around the duodenal papilla [11]. With an endoscope, however, images cannot always be observed in the same form because they are seen differently depending on functional movements and the conditions of observation.

According to endoscopic classification, the morphology of the duodenal papilla is divided into hemispheric, oval and flat types [11]. The hemispheric type is the most frequent, followed by the oval type.

The morphology of the orifice of the duodenal papilla can be classified into five types: villous, granular, lacerate, split and hard hole [11]. Needless to say, to insert a cannula through the orifice of the duodenal papilla, it

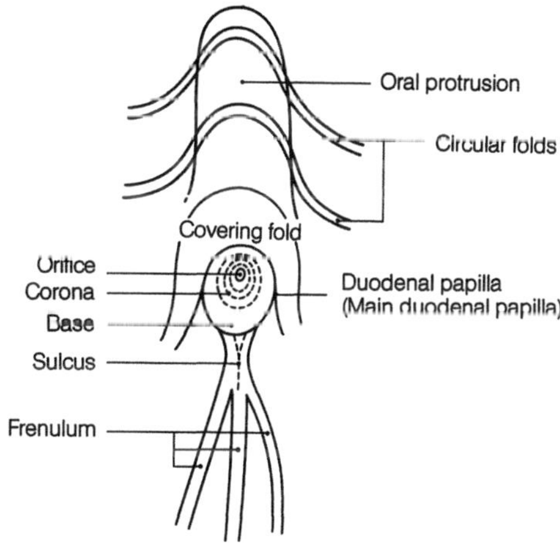

Fig. 8.1. Anatomy of the duodenal papilla. [11]

must first be found, and skillful handling is required [9]. For detailed technical questions, the reader is referred to specialized literature [4, 8, 11, 12].

To opacify the pancreatic duct, 3–5 ml of contrast medium is injected and 20–30 ml are required to enhance the image of the common bile duct.

It is desirable to control the injection of the contrast agent by use of a manometer to measure the pressure [2]. Roentgenography must be performed quickly because the contrast agent is excreted from the pancreas soon after removing the cannula. To opacify the fine branches of the pancreatic duct, it is necessary to keep the cannula inserted during roentgenography, and careful operation is required to avoid X-ray hazard to the physician.

The opacification procedure should be done with care to avoid complications of acute pancreatitis and infection.

Colangitis (0.39%) and acute pancreatitis (0.24%) occur occasionally, and their mortality rates in Japan are, respectively, 0.08% and 0.01% [3]. To avoid these complications, sterile examinations, giving a mixed injection of antibiotics and contrast medium and intensive care after the operation are standard procedures.

8.2 Findings from Opacification of the Pancreas

8.2.1 Normal Pancreatogram. On a normal pancreatogram, an image of the main pancreatic duct can be observed running from the orifice of the papilla of Vater, through the center of the pancreas, to the pancreatic tail gradually tapering off (Figs. 8.2 and 8.3). An accessory pancreatic duct branches upward from the main pancreatic duct in the head of the pancreas forming a triangle with the duodenal wall.

Branching from the main pancreatic duct, fine ducts forming a brush pattern can be seen, and usually can be observed up to a second or third branch. Observation of these brush patterns, however, is limited to the head or the tail; they cannot be clearly seen in the body of the pancreas because the contrast medium is flushed out by the massive secretion from the body of the pancreas.

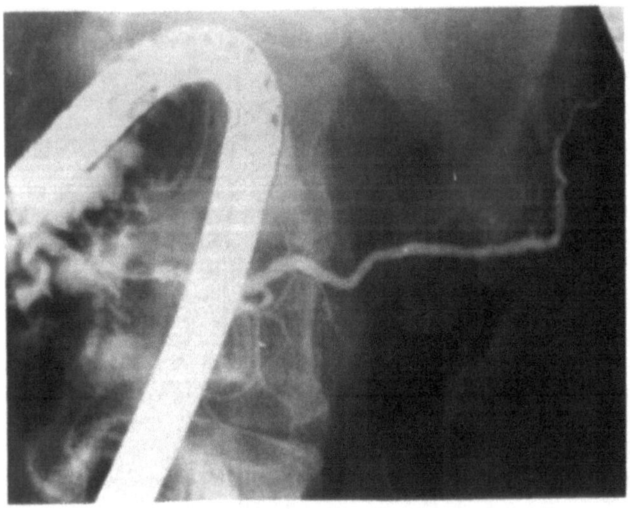

Fig. 8.2. Normal pancreatic duct

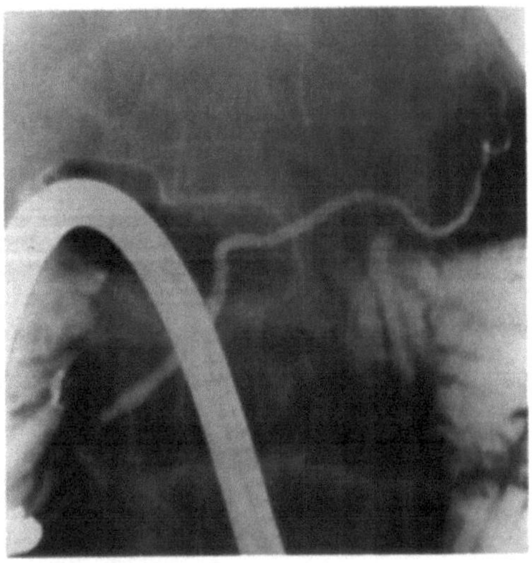

Fig. 8.3. Normal pancreatic duct

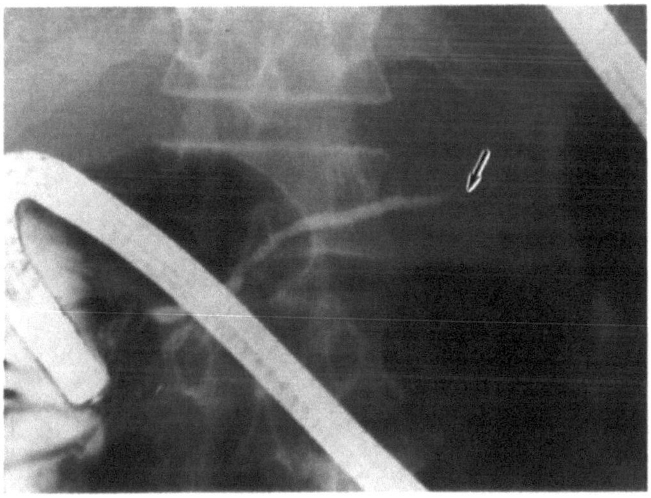

Fig. 8.4. Carcinoma of the tail of the pancreas with obstruction in the tail of the pancreatic duct (→)

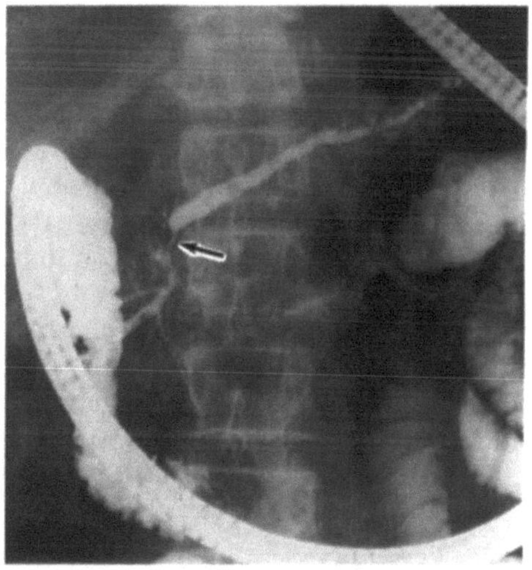

Fig. 8.5. Carcinoma of the head of the pancreas with main pancreatic duct stenosis in the head of the pancreas (→)

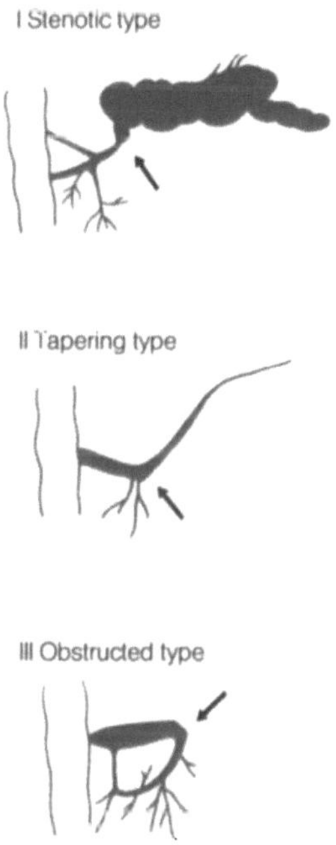

Fig. 8.6. Classification of pancreatic carcinoma based on opacification of the pancreatic duct. [6]

The normal pancreatic duct smoothly tapers off to the pancreatic tail, and sudden constriction does not occur. Even if contriction takes place in normal cases, it affects less than 50% of the maximal diameter of the main pancreatic duct. If an image of the main pancreatic duct thinner than this is observed, it can considered to be a stenosis.

8.2.2 Carcinoma of the Pancreas. Abnormal findings characteristic for pancreatic carcinoma [9, 11] are obstruction (Fig. 8.4), irregularity, stenosis (Fig. 8.5), dilatation, displacement and narrowing. Ogoshi [6] has classified the patterns of the pancreatic duct found in pancreatic carcinoma into four types (Fig. 8.6).

Type I is the stenotic type, which causes localized stenosis. The distal portion of the stenosis shows poststenotic dilatation depending on the grade of stenosis.

Type II is the tapering type, which shows a hardening pattern in the course of the main pancreatic duct due to the wide area of compression caused by the cancer.

Type III is the obstructed type, which shows a sudden disappearance of the main pancreatic duct due to the even greater compression caused by the cancer.

Type IV is the unclassified type, which, although not frequent, shows various patterns without any special characteristics.

These classifications are regarded as closely correlated to prognosis.

With pancreatography, it may be difficult to differentiate between pancreatic carcinoma and inflammatory changes of the pancreas. Oguri [7], however, observing the wall of the pancreatic duct by magnification radiography, reported that chronic pancreatitis shows a concave pattern whereas pancreatic carcinoma exhibits a convex pattern.

8.2.3 Pancreatitis. Pancreatography of acute pancreatitis sometimes provides an image similar to a pseudocyst due to leakage of the contrast medium into the necrotic area or shows coarse opacification of the acini due to increased permeability in the epithelial cells of the pancreatic duct.

However, in acute pancreatitis, pancreatography is regarded to be contraindicated since reverse flow of the pancreatic juice caused by pressure elevation due to injection of the contrast medium into the pancreatic duct results in a worsening of the condition.

Characteristic images of the pancreatic duct in chronic pancreatitis [9, 11] are partial stenosis or obstruction of the pancreatic duct, irregular stenosis or dilatation of the entire pancreatic duct, or a combination of these findings (Fig. 8.7). In addition to these findings, an image of a filling defect due to calculi and protein plug, an image of a pseudocyst and small cyst, or an interrupted image of the pancreatic duct may occasionally be observed.

In the case of pancreatic carcinoma, partial stenosis or obstruction is more common than in chronic pancreatitis. If localized stenosis and obstruction of the pancreatic duct are observed, carcinoma should be suspected.

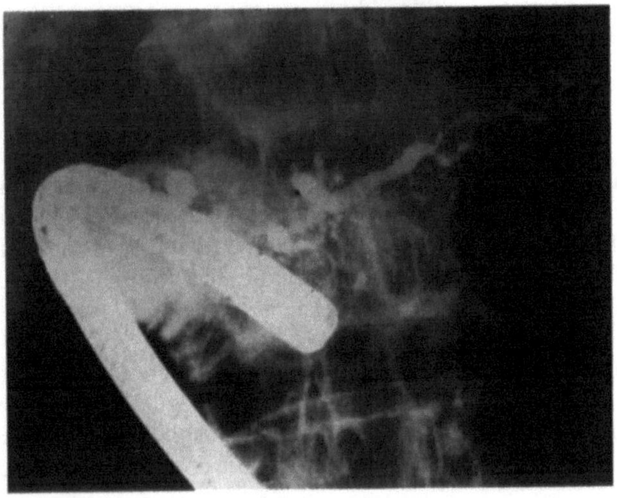

Fig. 8.7. Chronic pancreatitis

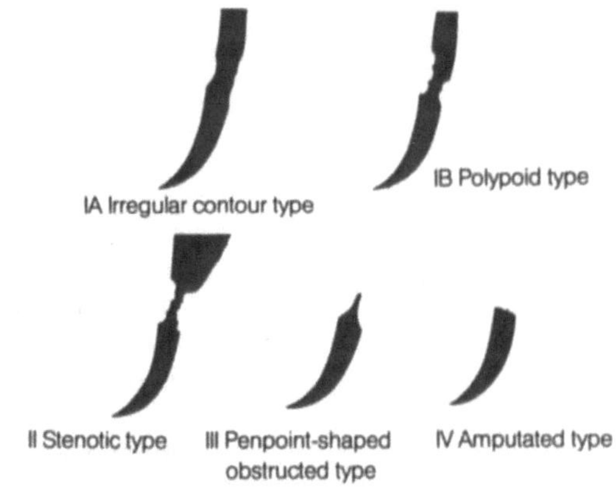

Fig. 8.8. Classification of carcinoma of the bile duct based on endoscopic retrograde cholangiography. [4]

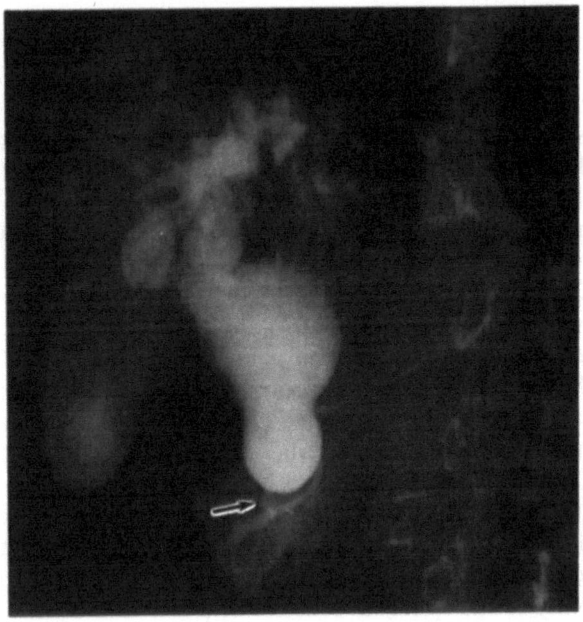

Fig. 8.9. Congenital dilatation of the common bile duct. Anomalous connection between the pancreatic and biliary ducts (→)

8.3 Findings from Opacification of the Bile Duct

8.3.1 Carcinoma of the Bile Duct. The major characteristic findings of bile duct carcinoma are obstruction, stenosis and filling defect. Kishi [4] classified the opacification findings of bile duct carcinoma into four types (Fig. 8.8).

In obstructive jaundice, bile duct opacification using ERCP reveals a condition of obstruction at the distal portion. By also using percutaneous transhepatic cholangiography, it is possible to examine the tumor extent. However, these cases are frequently inoperable, and even if correct diagnosis is achieved, its contribution to treatment is minimal. Opacification of the bile duct has great significance in the diagnosis of the early stage of bile duct carcinoma before the occurrence of jaundice.

8.3.2 Cholelithiasis. ERCP is a useful method for the diagnosis of cholelithiasis when opacification by oral or intravenous administration is inadequate.

Cholelithiasis is frequently accompanied by diseases of the pancreas, and ECRP may provide significant diagnostic signs by opacifying both the bile and pancreatic ducts [4].

When cholecystography does not sufficiently opacify the gallbladder, conditions of the cystic duct and neck of the gallbladder can be easily diagnosed with ERCP. However, it is not always possible to differentiate whether the obstruction is caused by a stone or tumor.

8.3.3 Congenital Dilatation of the Bile Duct. This abnormal condition frequently occurs among the Japanese. Diagnostic ability has been greatly improved by development of the ERCP technique since the biliary tract can be directly opacified (Fig. 8.9).

With ERCP, it is clearly noticeable that in many cases congenital dilatation of the bile duct shows an anomalous connection between the common bile duct and the pancreatic duct [11]. Some believe that the cause of this disease is the anomalous connection between the distal end of the common bile duct and the pancreatic duct.

ERCP has made it possible to diagnose stenosis of the distal end of the bile duct (papillary portion).

References

Endoscopic Retrograde Cholangiopancreatography

1. Cotton PB (1972) Cannulation of the papilla of Vater by endoscopy and retrograde cholangiopancreatography (ERCP). Gut 13:1014–1025
2. Kasugai T, Kuno N, Kizu M (1973) Endoscopic pancreatography – With special reference to manometric method (in Japanese). Stomach and Intestine 8:303–314
3. Kasugai T (1978) E.R.C.P.; Complications and counter measures (in Japanese). J Clin Surg 33:1533–1541
4. Kishi S, Urakami Y, Ito S (1977) Endoscopic retrograde cholangiopancreatography and its application (in Japanese). Nanzando, Tokyo
5. Oi I, Kobayashi S, Kondo T (1970) Endoscopic pancreatocholangiography. Endoscopy 2:103–106

6. Ogoshi K, Hara Y (1972) Retrograde pancreatocholangiography (in Japanese). Jpn J Clin Radiol 17:455–466
7. Oguri T, Kasugai T, Kuno N, Matsuura A, Fujiwara K, Kurimoto K, Kido C (1979) Direct magnification during ERCP. Discrimination between carcinoma of the pancreas and chronic pancreatitis by the use of convex type and concave type in ERCP (in Japanese). Jpn J Gastroenterol 76:2232–2241
8. Okuda K, Someya N, Goto A, Kunisaki T, Emura T, Yasumoto M, Shimokawa Y (1973) Endoscopic pancreato-cholangiography: a preliminary report of technique and diagnostic significance. AJR 117:437–445
9. Rohrmann CA, Silvis SE, Vennes JA (1974) Evaluation of the endoscopic pancreatogram. Radiology 113:297–304
10. Takagi K, Ikeda S, Nakagawa Y, Sakaguchi N, Takahashi T, Kumakura K, Maruyama M, Someya N, Nakano H, Takada T, Kin T (1970) Retrograde pancreatography and cholangiography by fiberduodenoscope. Gastroenterology 59:445–452
11. Takemoto T, Kasugai T (1979) Endoscopic retrograde cholangiopancreatography. Igaku-Shoin, Tokyo
12. Takemoto T, Oi I (1975) Endoscopy of the duodenum (in Japanese). Nagai Shoten, Osaka

9 Percutaneous Transhepatic Cholangiography (PTC)

Percutaneous transhepatic cholangiography (PTC) is carried out by various methods according to puncture sites. With the right lateral approach [4, 6, 7], the puncture site is selected in the intercostal space on the right lateral chest wall; the anterior approach [1] is situated below the right costal arch. These two methods are frequently utilized. Another method is via the retroperitoneum. The right lateral approach is advantageous to obtain cholangiograms [7] because the liver can be punctured adequately, leakage of bile juice and hemorrage from the liver are prevented due to the long distance from the punctured bile duct, and the risk of puncturing the gallbladder remains minor. Although it is also valuable for the technique of internal bile drainage, the anterior approach is more useful not only to drain the internal bile but to excrete the bile juice to the duodenum in inoperable cases of bile duct carcinoma by introduction of the catheter through the tumor [2]. The inserted catheter in the anterior approach is holded more stably than in the lateral method because the catheter is less moved by respiration.

9.1 Opacification Procedure

After performing the puncture into the biliary tract, intrahepatic bile juice is withdrawn prior to injection of the contrast medium to decrease the internal pressure of the bile duct and to increase the level of opacification. The withdrawn bile juice can also be utilized for cytologic examination [3].

The injection of contrast medium must be performed slowly. Roentgenography is carried out properly while the injection is taking place and finally when the bile duct is fully filled with contrast medium. However, in cases of bile duct obstruction, the injection of contrast medium is halted once for several minutes while the bile duct is only half filled.

In cases of bile duct stones, after a while the contrast medium flows into the space between the walls of the bile duct and the stone, and an image of the contour of the stone is then gradually visualized.

As far as obstruction of the bile ducts due to tumor is concerned, the distal end of the obstruction and the image of the gallbladder in cases with obstruction in the lower part of the common bile duct can be clearly seen. Better opacification can be achieved in the semierect position by making use of gravitational force.

The amount of contrast medium needed to fill the biliary tract is indicated by the quantity of bile juice priorly withdrawn. However, the injection of contrast medium must be done carefully so as not to increase the pressure in the bile duct due to overinjection. After completion of roentgenography, it is necessary to withdraw the contrast medium as soon as possible, remove the needle slowly, and stop bleeding by pressure with a gauze bandage.

9.2 Roentgenographic Anatomy of the Biliary Tract

The biliary tracts, conduits for bile juice, start from the bile canaliculi at the interhepatic cells, then become the interlobular bile ducts, which finally gather to form the right and left hepatic ducts. They become the common hepatic duct after passing through the porta hepatis, then join with the cystic duct to form the common bile duct; it curves slightly posterior to the duodenum, and passing through the parenchyma of the head of the pancreas, it finally opens to the duodenal papilla. Figure 9.1 shows an image of normal biliary tracts.

The right hepatic duct divides into anterior and posterior branches, and the left hepatic duct bifurcates into medial and lateral branches. In the absence of any mechanical obstruction in the bile duct, PTC can only opacify up to second branch of the intrahepatic bile duct. However, further peripheral branches can be opacified in the case of mechanical obstruction.

On an X-ray image of a normal biliary tract, the diameter of the hepatic duct is on average 4.9 mm on the right and 4.6 mm on the left. In our experience, the largest diameter never exceeds 5.2 mm.

According to Yamaguchi's anatomical measurement of the Japanese [8], the length of the extrahepatic bile duct is 2.8 cm in the common hepatic duct and 6.7 cm in the common bile duct. By X-ray measurement, the common hepatic duct is 3.3 cm in length and 0.6 cm in diameter, and the common bile duct is 7.4 cm in length and 0.7 cm in diameter on average.

In most cases, the cystic duct opens at a portion one-third from the top of the extrahepatic bile duct, but in some cases it may join at the proximal or distal portion of the orifice point above. The average diameter of the cystic duct measured from an X-ray image is 3.4 mm. The length cannot be exactly measured from an X-ray image, and anatomically it is 2.8 cm on average.

The distal end of the common bile duct is located close to the main pancreatic duct.

Millbourn's classification indicates three types of orifices [5]. The case of the main pancreatic duct and the common bile duct forming a common duct together is most frequently observed. A part of the main pancreatic duct may be observed during opacification of the biliary tract by PTC.

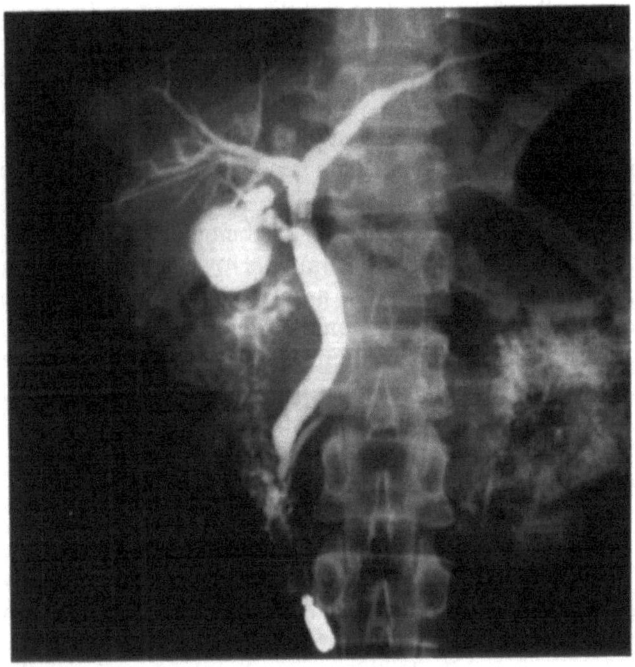

Fig. 9.1 Normal findings of the biliary tract

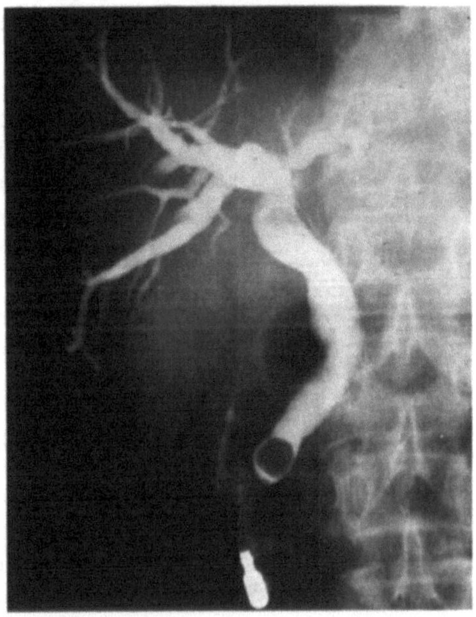

Fig. 9.2 Bile duct stone

The gallbladder is seen as pear-shaped, with a volume of 30–50 ml. Its average anatomical size in the Japanese is 8.6 cm in the long axis and 3.8 cm in the short axis.

9.3 PTC Images of Diseases of the Pancreas and Biliary Tract

9.3.1 Diameter of the Bile Duct. The extrahepatic bile duct may dilate in the case of cholelithiasis. As regards our measurement [3], the diameter of the extrahepatic bile duct is 10.9 ± 3.9 mm due to dilatation in the case of cholelithiasis, 23.3 ± 9.2 mm in choledocholithiasis, and 18.4 ± 5.4 mm in cholecystocholedocholithiasis. Conversely, it is 16.4 ± 5.9 mm in gallbladder carcinoma, 24.1 ± 8.1 mm in bile duct carcinoma, and 21.6 ± 6.2 mm in pancreatic head carcinoma. Even though these are seen as marked dilatations, no clear differentiation can be made between a stone and carcinoma.

On the other hand, the diameter of the intrahepatic bile duct is 6.0 ± 2.6 mm in gallbladder stones, 12.4 ± 7.4 mm in stones of the common bile duct, and 11.5 ± 4.0 mm in cholecystocholedocholithiasis. In comparison, diameters of 17.6 ± 6.7 mm in gallbladder carcinoma, 18.5 ± 6.1 mm in bile duct carcinoma, and 15.1 ± 4.3 mm in pancreatic head carcinoma can be found.

Thus, so dilatation of the intrahepatic bile duct caused by carcinoma is much greater than that due to stones. This difference can be more clearly noticed by comparing the diameter of the first branch of the intrahepatic bile duct, which is 5 ~ 6 mm in cholelithiasis and 9 ~ 10 mm in carcinoma.

Generally, in cholelithiasis, dilatation of the intrahepatic bile duct is less than that found in cancer even with a markedly dilated extrahepatic bile duct. This is because of incomplete obstruction of the extrahepatic bile duct in most cases of cholelithiasis, while obstruction advances irreversibly with cancer.

9.3.2 Image of Obstruction of the Bile Duct. In cholelithiasis, obstruction of the extrahepatic bile duct is caused at a rate of about 7%, and it can be observed with a stone impacted to the papillary portion. Other portions may be seen as fully obstructed, but a radiolucent image due to the passing of the contrast medium will be observed as time passes.

Most cases of carcinoma, however, show images of complete obstruction, although incomplete obstruction may sometimes be caused by invasion from the lateral wall of the bile duct in cases of gallbladder and pancreatic carcinoma.

Obstruction tends to occur in the papilla or the common bile duct in the case of cholelithiasis (Fig. 9.2). In gallbladder carcinoma, obstruction tends to be observed in the porta hepatis or common hepatic duct, and in carcinoma of the bile duct frequently in the common hepatic duct (Fig. 9.3), as it is dependent on the site of origin of the cancer. In carcinoma of the head of the pancreas (Fig. 9.4), obstruction is mainly observed distal to the junction of the cystic duct and common bile duct; therefore, gallbladder opacification can frequently be seen with PTC (Table 9.1).

Table 9.2 shows a classification of the obstruction images of the bile duct into five patterns: U, V, inverted L, inverted U, and unclassified type. The outline of the contour of the obstruction is divided into smooth and irregular types [3].

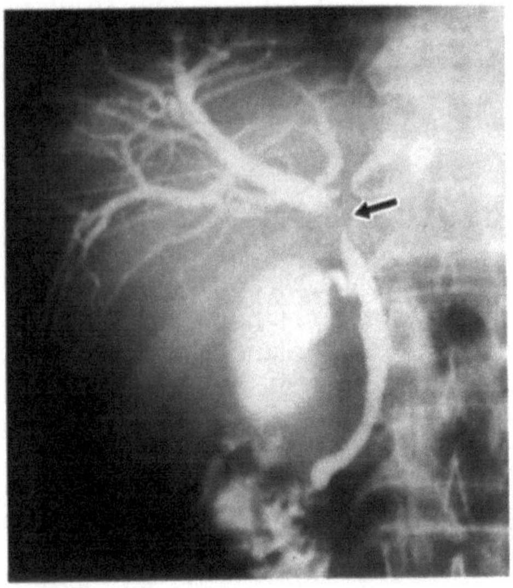

Fig. 9.3 Stenosis due to bile duct carcinoma (→)

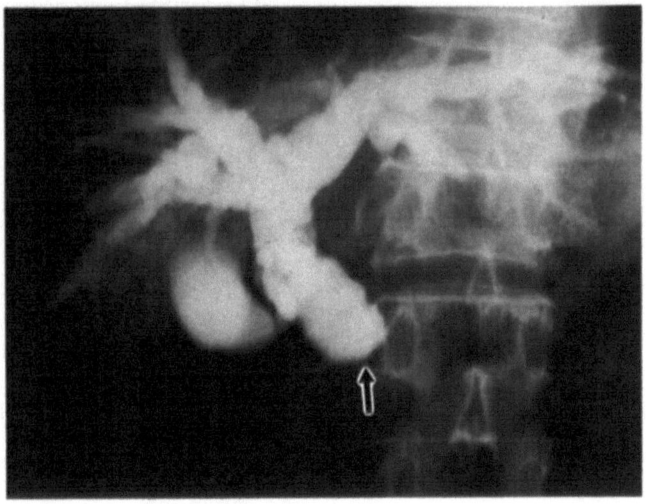

Fig. 9.4 Obstruction due to carcinoma of the pancreatic head (→)

Table 9.1. Obstructed portion of the bile duct related to its causes [3]

Disease / Obstructed portion	Malignancy				Cholelithiasis		
	Gallbladder carcinoma	Carcinoma of the bile duct	Carcinoma of the papilla of Vater	Carcinoma of the pancreas head	Cholecysto-lithiasis	Choledocho-lithiasis	Cholecysto-choledocho-lithiasis
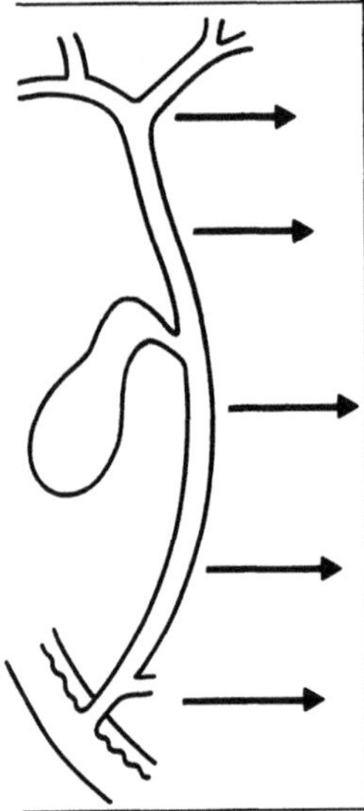 →	●●●●● ●●●●● ●	●●●●● ●●●●● ●●●●● ●●		●			
→	●●●	●●●●● ●●●●● ●●●		●●			
→	●●	●●●●● ●		●●●●● ●●●●● ●●●●●			●
→	●	●●●●●		●●●●● ●●●●● ●●●●● ●		●	
→		●	●●●●● ●●●●● ●●●●● ●●	●●●●●		●	●●
Nonobstruction	●●●●●				●●●●●●●● ●●●●●●●● ●●●●●●●● ●●●●●●●● ●●●●●●●● ●●●●●●●	●●●●●●●● ●●●●●●●● ●●●●●	●●●●●●●● ●●●●●●●● ●●●●●●●● ●●●●●●●● ●●●●●●●● ●
Total	22	42	17	39	47	23	44

Table 9.2. Obstructed pattern in the bile duct [3]

	Disease \ Obstructed pattern	Irregular contour		Smooth contour				Unclassified	Non-obstruction	total
Malignancy	Gallbladder carcinoma	●● ●	●●●	●●●●●	●●●●●●	●	●●	●●	●●●	22
	Carcinoma of the bile duct	●●●●●● ●●	●●●●●●● ●●●●●●● ●●●●●●●	●	●●●●●● ●		●	●●●●		42
	Carcinoma of the papilla of Vater	●●	●●●●●● ●●●●●●		●●	●				17
	Carcinoma of the pancreas head	●	●●●●●●	●●●●●● ●●●●●● ●●●●●	●●●●●● ●●●●●		●●	●●		39
Cholelithiasis	Cholecystolithiasis								●●●●●● ●●●...47	47
	Choledocholithiasis						●	●	●●●●●● ●●...21	23
	Cholecystocholedocholithiasis						●●●		●●●●●● ●●...41	44

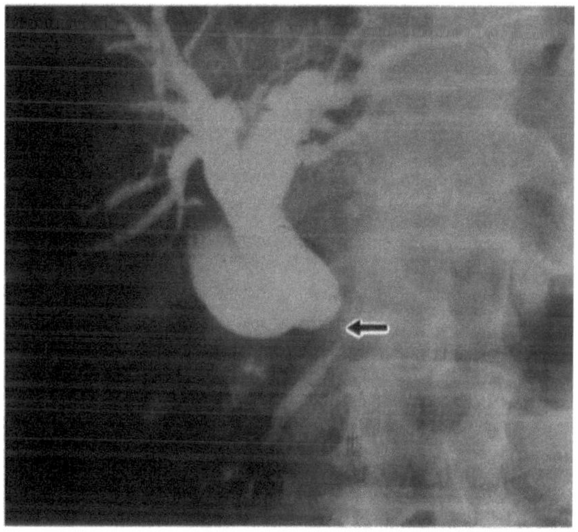

Fig. 9.5 Stenosis of the bile duct due to carcinoma of the pancreatic head (→)

Most cases of cholelithiasis show an inverted U pattern (Fig. 9.2). Gallbladder carcinoma and carcinoma of the head of the pancreas exhibit a smooth outline with U and V patterns due do infiltration from outside into the wall of the bile duct (Fig. 9.5). However, when marked infiltration reaches into the lumen of the bile duct, irregular contours with V pattern or occasionally U pattern will be observed. In bile duct carcinoma, an irregular contour with V pattern is exhibited because the cancer grows in the lumen of the bile duct.

References

Percutaneous Transhepatic Cholangiography

1. Carter FR, Saypol GM (1952) Transabdominal cholangiography. JAMA 148:253–255
2. Hoevels J, Lunderquist A, Ihse I (1978) Percutaneous transhepatic intubation of bile ducts for combined internal-external drainage in preoperative and palliative treatment of obstructive jaundice. Gastrointest Radiol 3:23–31
3. Ito M (1976) Clinical studies on diagnosis of diseases in pancreas and biliary system. Diagnosis by combined methods of percutaneous transhepatic cholangiography, hypotonic duodenography and cytology (in Japanese). J Nagoya City University Med Assoc 27:54–93
4. Lang EK (1974) Percutaneous transhepatic cholangiography. Radiology 112:283–290
5. Millbourn E (1950) On excretory ducts of pancreas in man with special reference to their relations to each other, to common bile duct and to duodenum. Radiological and anatomical study. Acta Anat 9:1–34
6. Tsuchiya Y (1969) A new safer method of percutaneous transhepatic cholangiography (in Japanese). J Gastroenterol 66:438–455
7. Wiechel KL (1963) Percutaneous transhepatic cholangiography. Acta Clin Scand [Suppl] 309:1
8. Yamaguchi H (1930) Anatomy of the biliary tract (in Japanese). Acta Anat Nipponica 3:191–229

Part II
Clinical Presentation

Introductory Remarks

Flow chart (Sequence of diagnostic imaging)

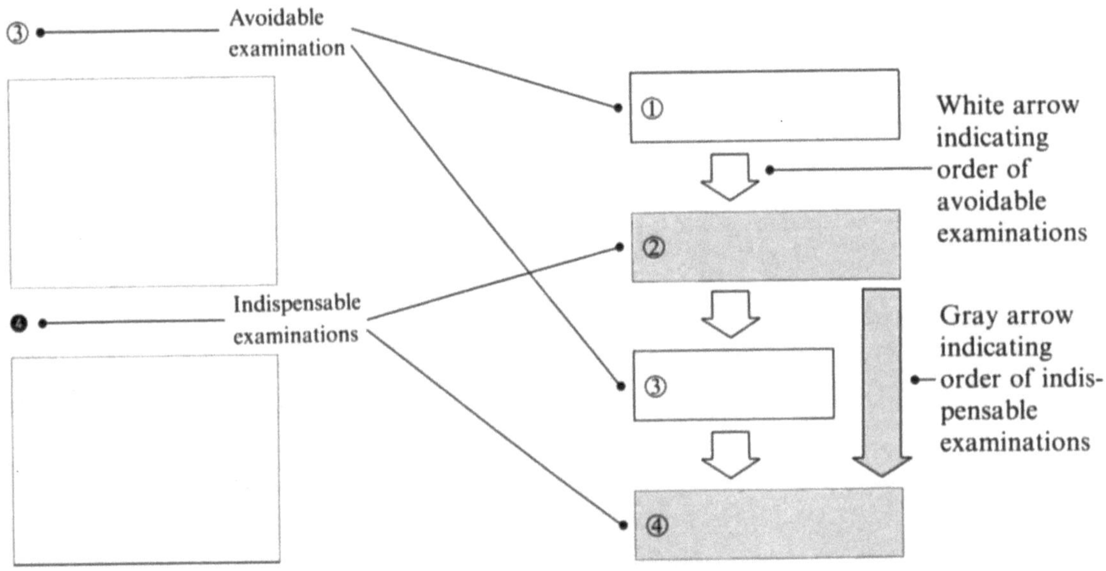

Indispensable examinations are indicated by gray-colored backgrounds on the flow chart and by a white Arabic numeral in a black background (❹ etc.)

Sequence of diagnostic imaging are indicated by gray-colored arrows, which indicate the order of indispensable examinations, and white arrows, which indicate avoidable examinations, i.e., gray arrows (🡇) connect indispensable examinations

A pair of angiograms, e.g., A, A′, B, B′, are shown in the case of stereo-angiography.

A: Diagnostic Imaging of Diseases of the Liver

1 Procedure

In diagnosing diseases of the liver, especially space-occupying lesions, diagnostic imaging can provide valuable information. While selecting a suitable examination method, it is necessary to carefully consider the accuracy, sensitivity, specificity, and invasiveness to the patient of each method.

Table 1 shows the detection rates of space-occupying lesions with liver scintigraphy, ultrasonography, and X-ray CT examined in 67 cases [27]. In liver scintigrams, although highly sensitive, the ability to detect a pathological lesion may often result in false-positive diagnosis; therefore, specificity is inferior to ultrasonography and CT. Although the sensitivity of ultrasonic diagnosis and of CT examination is inferior to that of a hepatic colloid scintigram, it can be increased and accuracy improved by combined usage of both methods. However, this data was obtained around 1980, and recently the sensitivity of ultrasonic diagnosis and CT examination has been improved.

Ultrasonic diagnosis and CT examination are almost equal in diagnostic ability, but considering the hazards involved, an ultrasonic examination should be chosen at the first diagnostic method. Table 2 shows the relationship between each diagnostic imaging approach and patient discomfort [28]. There is no discomfort in ultrasonic, nuclear, and X-ray CT examination, but angiography causes a great deal of discomfort.

Figure 1 shows a procedure of diagnosis which is performed in cases in which the level of alpha-fetoprotein (AFP) is under 400 ng/ml and hepatic tumor is suspected. If a mass in the liver is palpable, diagnosis is begun with an ultrasonic examination. Without a palpable mass, in cases with or without hepatomegaly, hepatic scintigraphy is suitable as a first examination due to its simplicity and high sensitivity. However, with hepatic scintigraphy, it is difficult to find a mass smaller than 2 cm so that in cases in which

Table 1. Detection rates of space-occupying lesions according to method

		RN		US		CT	
		+	−	+	−	+	−
Final diagnosis	+	16	1	21	4	20	5
	−	5	32	1	41	2	40

	RN	US	CT	CT + US
Sensitivity	87.5 ± 4.4	78.4 ± 11.4	78.9 ± 9.4	88.9 ± 7.2
Specificity	78.9 ± 9.9	86.0 ± 15.5	87.5 ± 9.0	87.8 ± 5.3
Accuracy	82.2 ± 5.7	82.3 ± 11.4	83.4 ± 5.8	88.3 ± 4.2

RN = radionuclide study; US = ultrasonography; CT = computed tomography

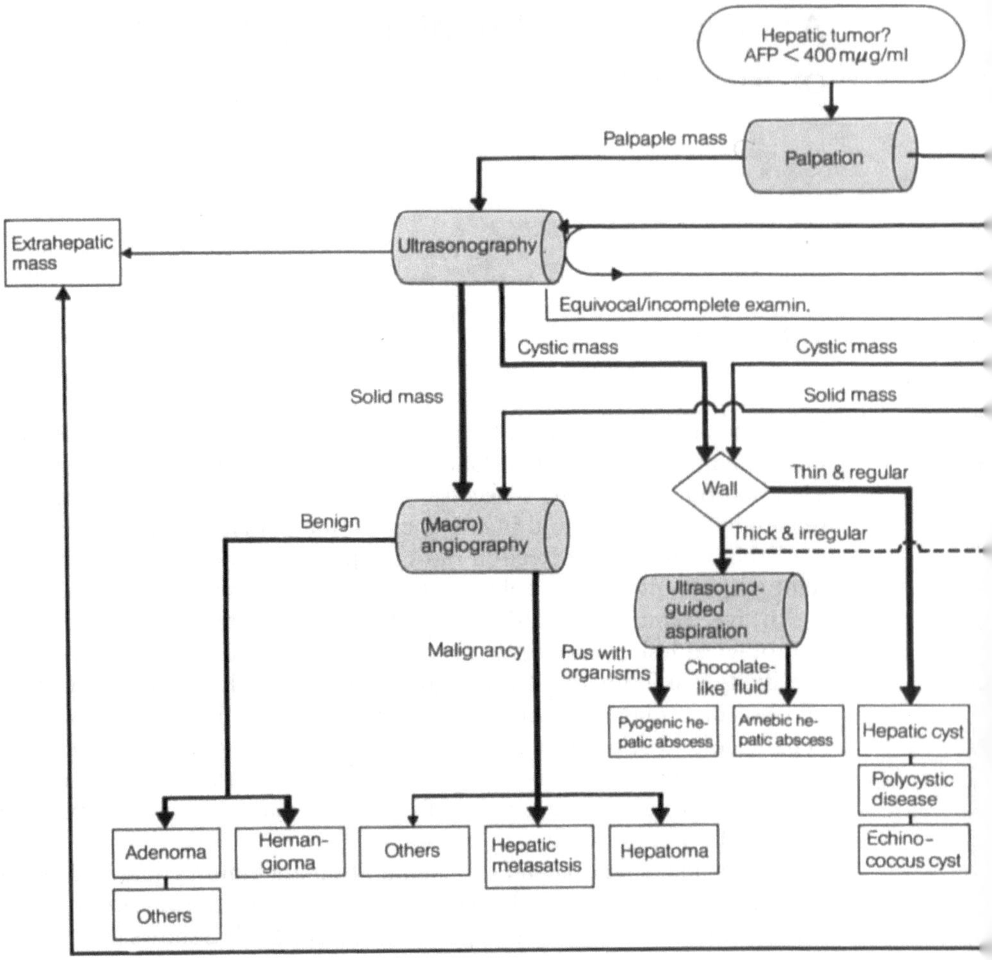

Fig. 1. Procedure of diagnostic imaging in suspected hepatic tumor.

Table 2. Evaluation of patient discomfort (Wittenberg et al. [27])

	No. Patients	Rating (%)				
		Comfortable	Some Discomfort	Uncomfortable	Very uncomfortable	Extremely uncomfortable
Body CT	100	61	28	4	5	2
Ultrasonography	53	83	17	0	0	0
Radionuclide study	9	55	45	0	0	0
Angiography	13	15	8	8	23	46
Lymphangiography	10	30	40	10	10	10
Endoscopic retrograde cholangiopancreatography	10	0	0	50	50	0

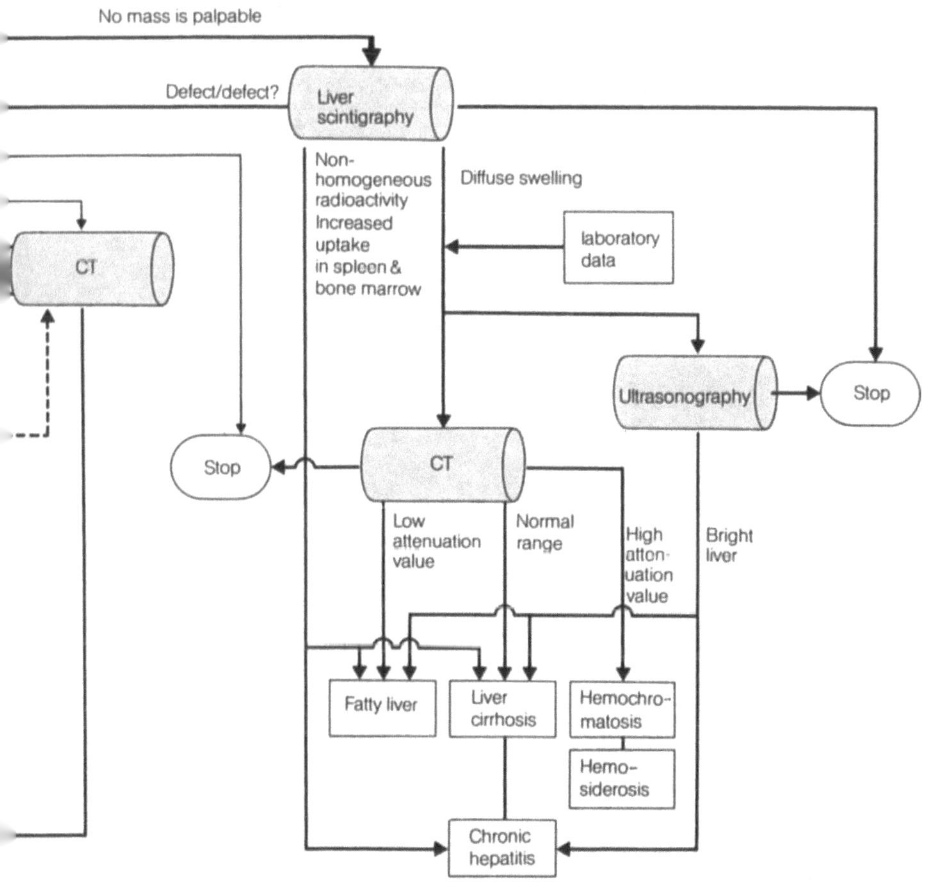

a tiny hepatic tumor is suspected, ultrasonic examination is advisable. If a hepatic tumor is still suspected, angiography is necessary for conclusive diagnosis. Hepatocellular carcinoma is often suspected in cases in which the level of AFP exceeds 400 ng/ml. Therefore, it is necessary to perform angiography even if lesions cannot be found by other noninvasive diagnostic imaging methods.

Figure 2 shows the diagnostic procedure in a case of swelling of the liver accompanied by fever. The procedure is simple when there are definite symptoms of fever. It is of great value to design diagnostic procedures that sufficiently consider clinical conditions to avoid an unnecessary series of examinations.

Among the diffuse hepatocellular diseases of the liver, definite diagnosis is possible with diagnostic imaging in cases of fatty liver, hemochromatosis, and hemosiderosis, while conclusive diagnostic information is difficult to obtain in cases of chronic hepatitis and liver cirrhosis, especially in the early stage. The possibility of hepatic carcinoma accompanying chronic hepatitis and liver cirrhosis exists so that diagnostic imaging must be performed with this taken into consideration.

In Southeast Asia, there is a large incidence of hepatic carcinoma. Mortality rates have also been increasing greatly in Japan. According to

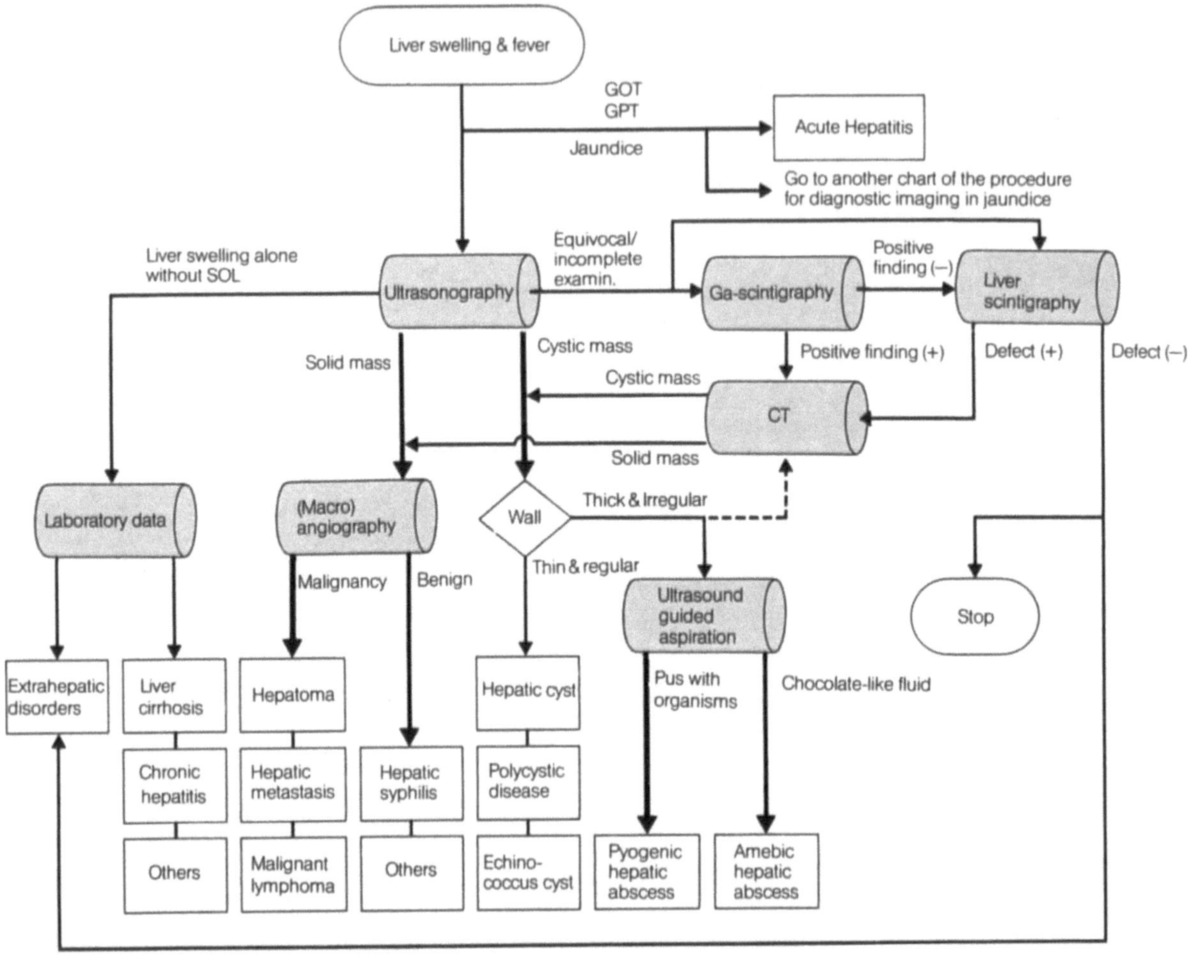

Fig. 2. Procedure of diagnostic imaging in liver swelling with fever

1978 statistics, 8143 males (15.5 males in 100 000) and 4308 females (7.4 females in 100 000) had hepatic carcinoma [15].

Hepatocellular carcinoma is frequently associated with liver cirrhosis: 25% of liver cirrhosis is accompanied by hepatocellular carcinoma, and 85% of hepatocellular carcinoma is coupled with liver cirrhosis.

Viral hepatitis, alcohol abuse, drug, toxicity, congestive liver, metabolic disorders, and parasites are also responsible for liver cirrhosis. In Japan, liver cirrhosis is not usually caused by alcohol consumption, but quite often advances from hepatitis virus B. Twenty percent of patients with chronic hepatitis, especially those with chronic active hepatitis, develop liver cirrhosis, and some reports also suggest that hepatocellular carcinoma advances from chronic pancreatitis. Conversely, in Western societies, alcohol abuse is quite often responsible for liver cirrhosis. For the above-mentioned reasons, a IRD classification (Index of Roentgen Diagnosis, from the American College of Radiology) cannot be regarded as adaptable for actual conditions in Japan.

2 Cases

2.1 Liver Cyst

Sequence of Diagnostic Imaging.

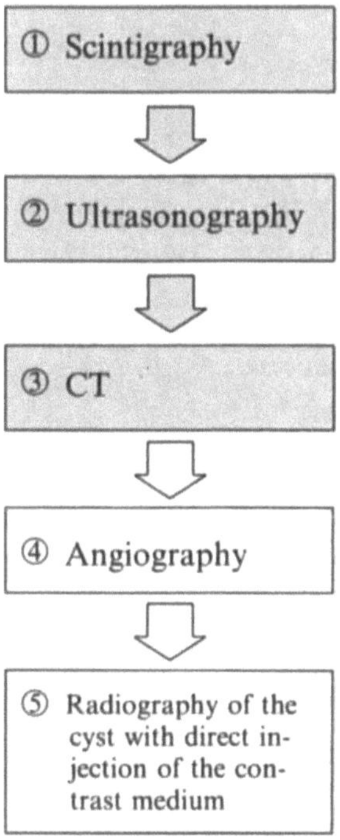

Patient. A 56-year-old woman.

Main Complaint. Epigastralgia.

History. Operation for uterine myoma had been performed 3 year previously.

Present History. Back pain and epigastralgia occasionally occurred in the past 4 years. The patient was admitted to this clinic for a precise examination because a gallstone and an epigastric tumor had been diagnosed at another clinic 3 months before

Present Status. The liver edge is palpable 3 FB (fingerbreadth) below the epigastrium. The liver is elastic and soft with no jaundice.

Laboratory Data.

SGOT	34 mU/ml	Normal
SGPT	24 mU/ml	Normal
ALP	188 mU/ml	↑
LDH	289 mU/ml	↑
γ-GTP	35 mU/ml	Normal
Cho E	296 U/dl	Normal
HBs Ag	(–)	
ZTT	3.7 U	Normal
TB	0.5 mg/dl	Normal
TP	7.3 g/dl	Normal

Cho E, cholinesterase; HBs Ag, hepatitis B antigen; ZTT, zinc sulfate turbidity test; TB, total bilirubin; TP, total protein.

Purpose of Diagnostic Imaging. Precise examination of the swollen liver.

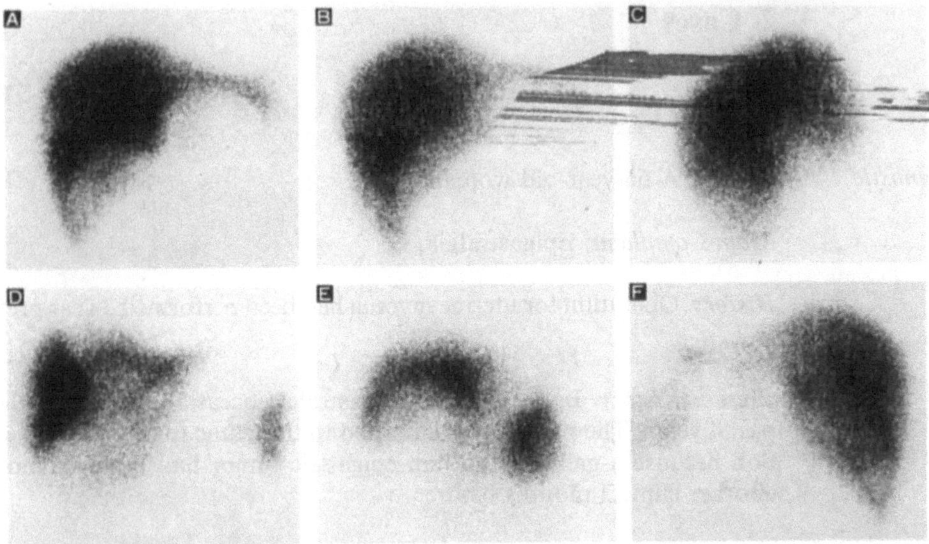

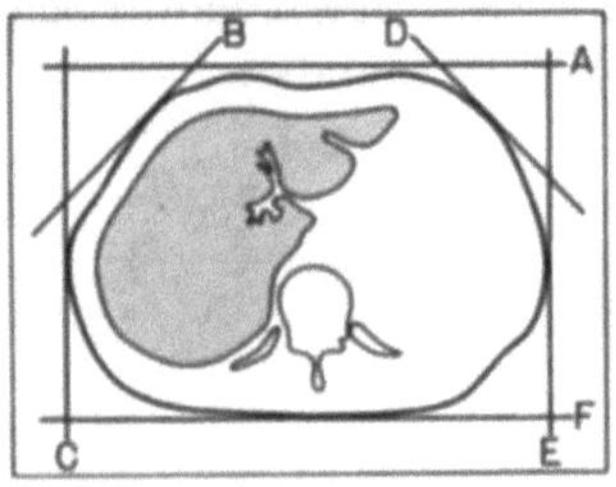

❶ Scintigram

A Frontal view
B Right anterior oblique view
C Right lateral view
D Left anterior oblique view
E Left lateral view
F Posterior view

Liver scintigram. A defective image suggesting an intrahepatic space-occupying lesion is observed in the lateral lobe of the left lobe of the liver.

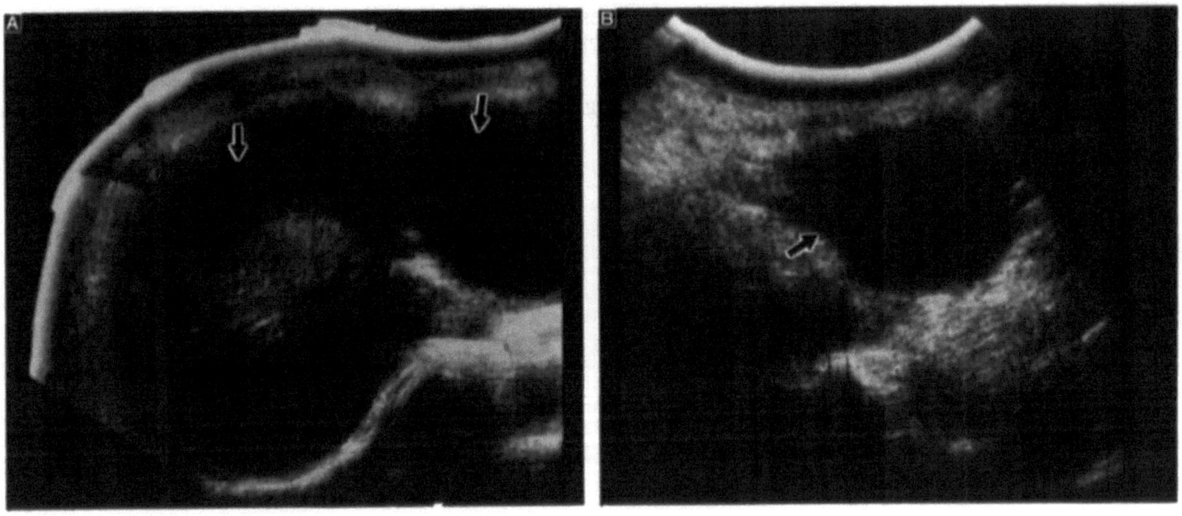

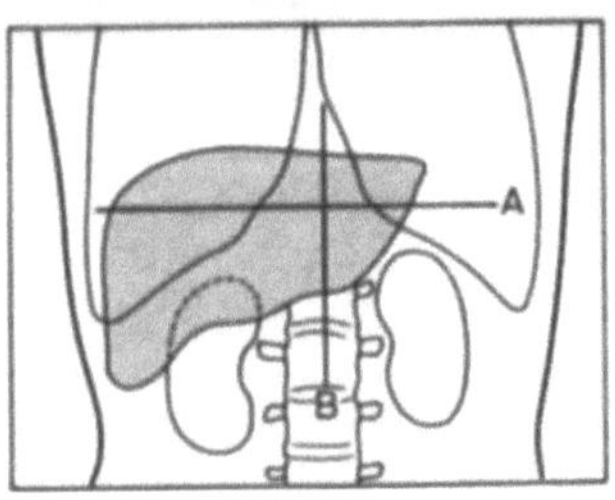

❷ Contact compound ultrasonic scanning image

A, B Unechoic, cystic lesions are observed (→) in the left lobe and right anterior segment of the liver. Regular contour and no internal echo are seen, and posterior enhanced echoes are observed.

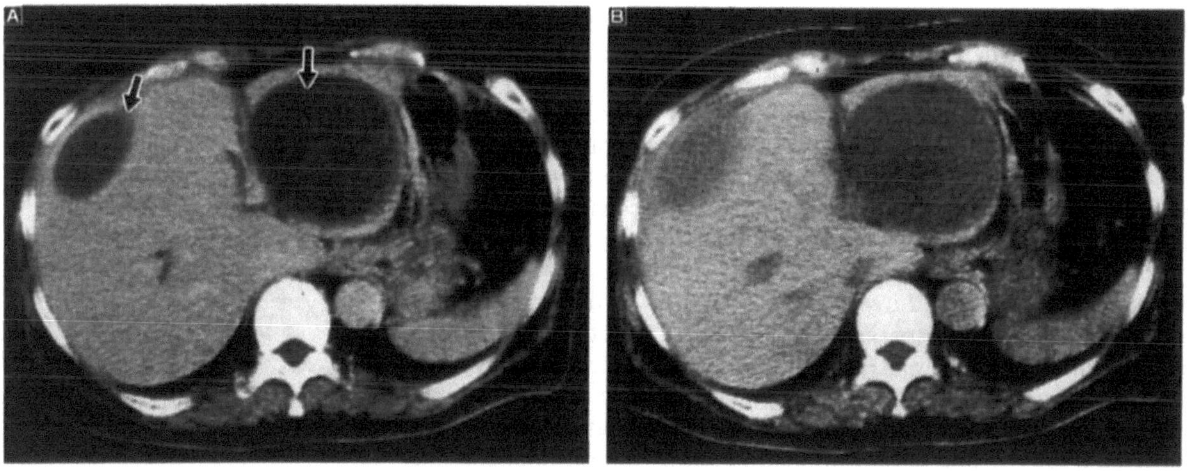

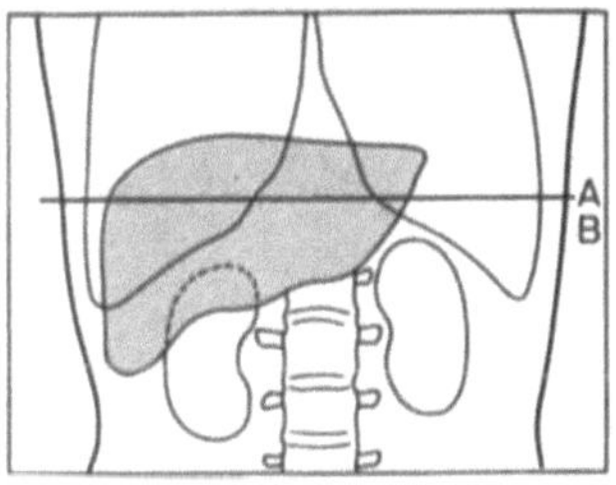

③ CT image
A Before contrast enhancement
B After contrast enhancement

Low attenuation area with regular contour is seen (→) in the lateral segment of the left lobe and anterior segment of the right lobe where the CT number does not increase after the contrast enhancement (CT number is 15.3 HU).

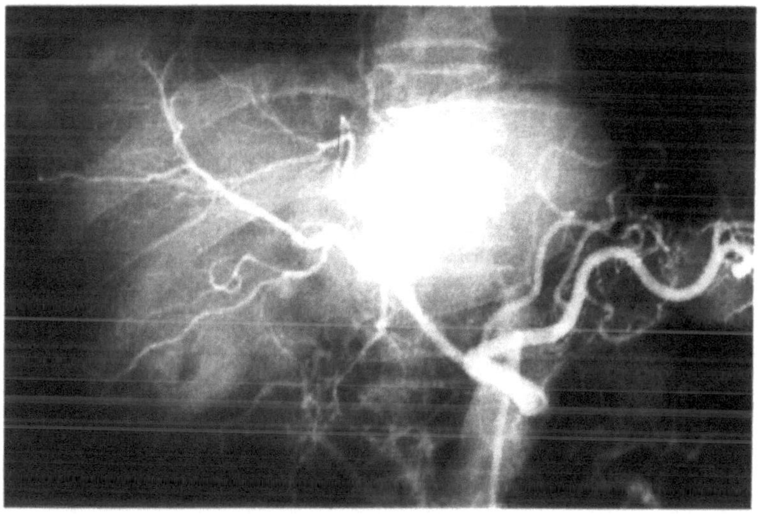

④ Angiogram
Celiac arteriography (arterial phase): The left hepatic artery running along the cyst opacified by cystography is observed without any findings of irregular vessels.

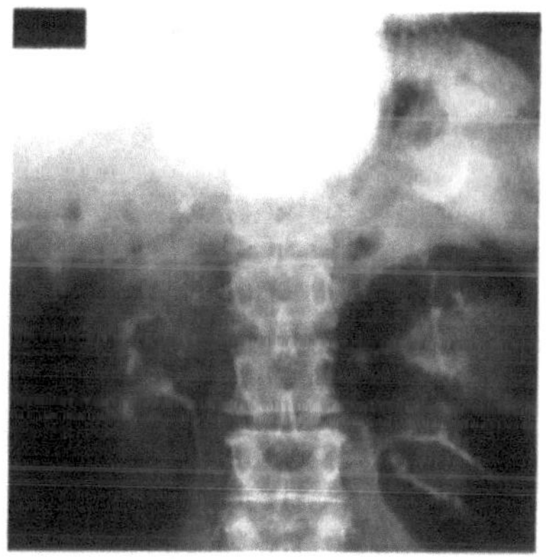

⑤ Radiogram of the cyst
The cyst in the left lobe is isolated without communicating with the bile duct.

Operative Findings. Cystectomy was performed. The liver cyst originated in the bile duct, and no malignancy was found.

Significance of Diagnostic Imaging. Image of a defect of the left hepatic lobe and the "beaksign" were clearly seen on the liver scintigram. Therefore, a liver cyst is suspected and definite diagnosis can be made by ultrasonic examination and CT. Angiography is unnecessary because there were no findings of malignancy in ultrasonography and CT.

General Matters Concerning Liver Cyst [22]. Causes of liver cyst can be divided into parasitic and nonparasitic. Nonparasitic liver cysts are divided into the congenital multiple cysts forming in the liver accompanied by renal cysts and pancreatic cysts and the simple cysts which have acquired (sometimes congenital) solitary or multiple cysts in the liver. A retention cyst may frequently be observed due to partial obstruction of the intrahepatic bile duct.

The ratio of occurrence between males and females is 1:4–5, i.e., overwhelming more frequent in females.

The cyst grows gradually. When advancing, a sense of fullness and abdominal pain may be symptoms; additionally, hemorrhage in the cyst, rupture, and infection may occur. Surgery should be carried out in cases with symptoms due to compression by the cyst.

In general, liver cysts often show no symptoms, but since the use of CT and ultrasonic examination has spread, the frequency of finding a liver cyst without prior symptoms has been greatly increased.

2.2 Parenchymal Hamartoma

Sequence of Diagnostic Imaging.

① IVP

② Scintigraphy

③ CT

④ Angiography

Patient. An 8-month-old baby boy.

Main Complaint. Abdominal mass.

Present History. A distended abdomen was observed 7 months after birth. An abdominal mass was diagnosed during the periodical examination 8 months after birth. The patient was hospitalized for precise examinations.

Present Status. A large, smooth, elastic, and solid tumor extending over the midline and entirely occupying the right abdomen was palpated.

Laboratory Data.

Blood		
WBC	14100/mm^3	Slightly↑
RBC	383 × 10^4/mm^3	↓
Hb	9.7 g/dl	↓
Platelets	33.8 × 10^4/mm^3	Normal
TP	6.5 g/dl	Normal
SGOT	31 mU/ml	Normal
SGPT	9 mU/ml	Normal
LDH	171 mU/ml	Normal
AFP	3200 mμg/dl	↑
CRP	(−)	Normal
Urine		
Protein	(−)	Normal
Gluc.	(−)	Normal
Urobilinogen	(±)	Normal
VMA	(−)	Normal

Purpose of Diagnostic Imaging. To identify the localization and characteristics of the abdominal mass.

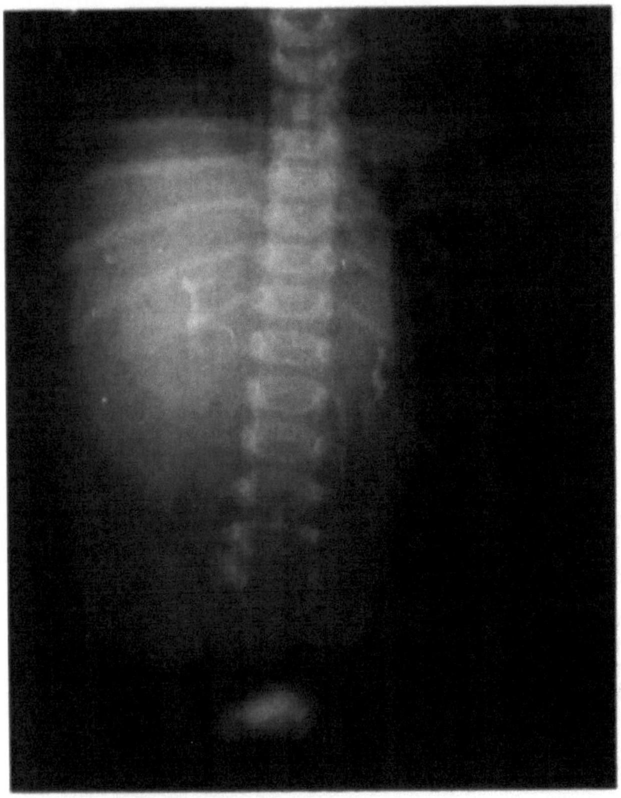

① Excretory intravenous pyelogram
Both sides of the kidney are normally opacified. A large massive image expanding to the pelvic cavity is seen continuously from the soft tissue density of the liver. Calcification is not observed in the tumor.

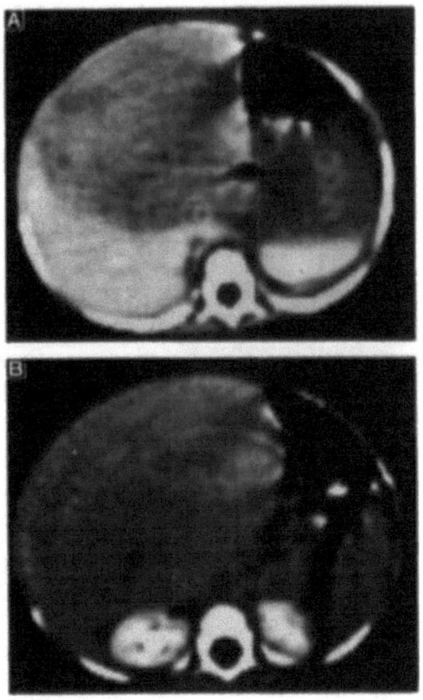

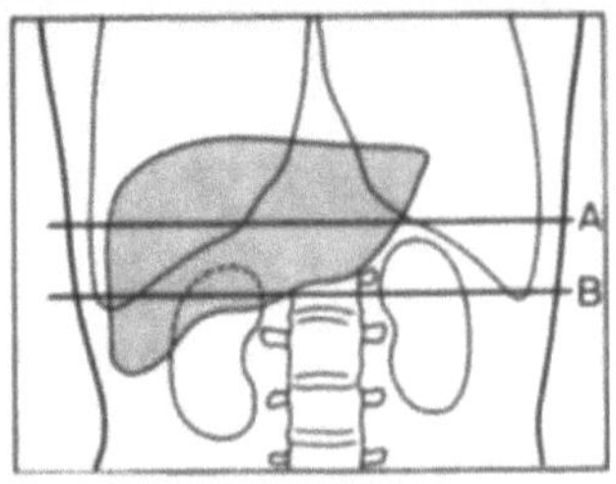

③ CT image (after administration of contrast medium) A nonhomogeneous, low-attenuation region is observed in the liver. The CT number is about one-third that of the normal liver. Contrast enhancement makes a clear differentiation from the nomal liver possible.

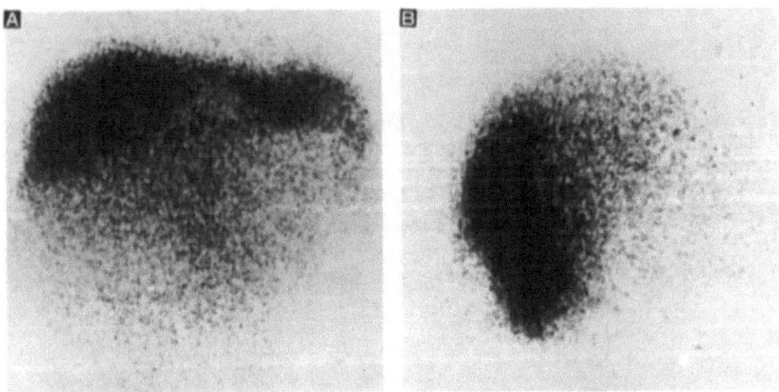

② Scintigram
A Frontal view
B Right lateral view
Liver scintigram (^{99m}Tc-phytate): Image of a large defect is seen in the lower part of the right lobe.

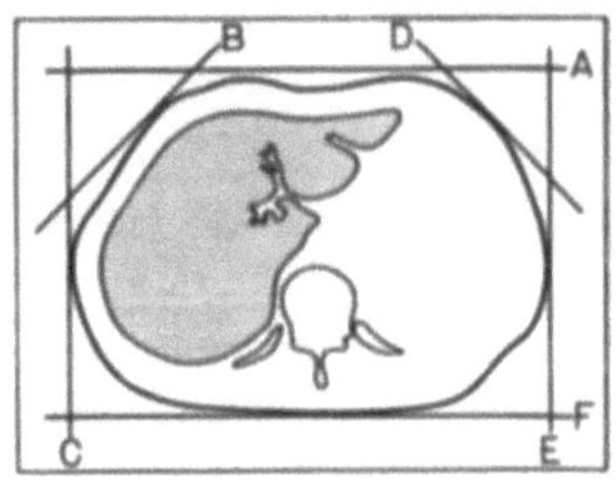

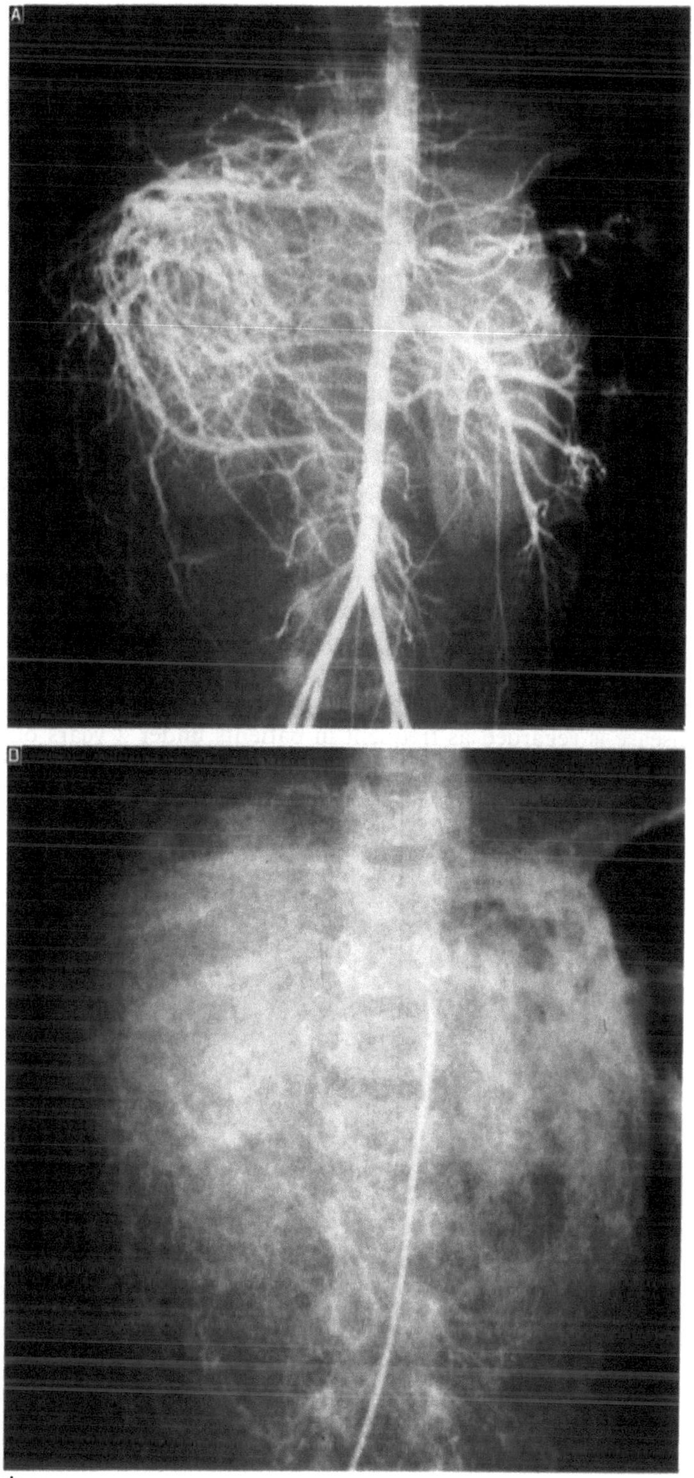

❹ Angiogram

A Abdominal aortography (arterial phase): The right hepatic artery is enlarged in diameter. Many tumor vessels from its branches extend downward forming willow shapes. Encasement, angulation, and tortuosity of tumor vessels are not severe. Obvious arteriovenous shunting is not observed. A few large, sinuslike vessels from unknown origins are seen in the capillary phase.

B Abdominal aortography (venous phase): Tumor stain is not markedly observable.

Operative Findings. A pedunculated massive tumor (16.5 × 14 × 8 cm) with a stalk approximately 4 cm in length was found on the inferior surface of the right lobe of the liver, and a right hemilobectomy was performed. Histologically, it was a parenchymal hamartoma with findings of a bile-duct-like tubular structure and increased fibroblastic cells.

Clinical Progress. The level of AFP lowered to 11 ng/ml after the operation, and there have been no recurrent symptoms for 3 years.

Significance of Diagnostic Imaging. Tumors in the liver can clearly be diagnosed from hepatic scintigrams and CT. An angiogram provides a basis for suspecting hamartoma or hepatoblastoma although it is not definitive in differential diagnosis. From an angiogram of a hamartoma, findings of the tumor region can be either hypovascular or hypervascular depending on the proportion between the cystic and solid components, and hence there is no fixed pattern. If hypervascularity is recognizable, tumor vessels may frequently be observed running directly in a definite direction, forming a willow-branch shape.

Arteriovenous shunt could not be seen. In this case, the diagnosis based on the angiogram led to tumorectomy.

General Matters Concerning Parenchymal Hamartoma [10]. Parenchymal hamartoma is rather rare, and only 20 cases have been reported in Japan. This disease is regarded as frequent in patients under 2 years of age and more often in males. The liver function test is almost normal, and the level of AFP may occasionally rise. After tumorectomy, prognosis is fine.

2.3 Chronic Active Hepatitis (Lupoid Hepatitis)

Sequence of Diagnostic Imaging.

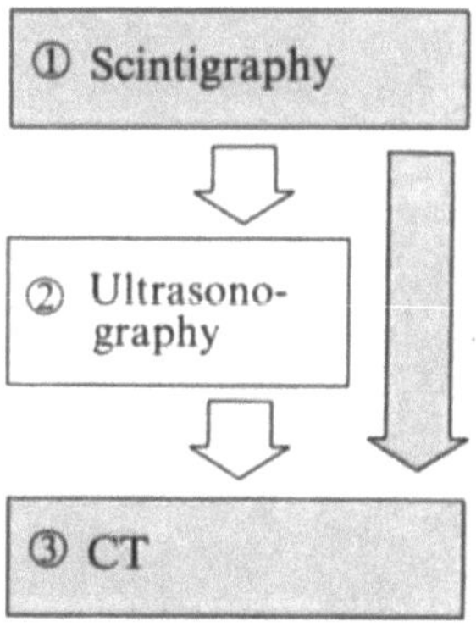

Patient. A 46-year-old woman.

Main Complaint. General fatigue.

History. Not specified.

Present History. The patient had pyrexia half a year before and experienced general fatigue. Liver dysfunction was diagnosed in another clinic where progress had been monitored. As the liver dysfunction turned to the worse 1 month previously the patient was admitted to the internal department; a precise examination was performed by the department of radiology.

Present Status. The sharp-edged liver is palpable 2 FB below the right costal margin.

Laboratory Data.

SGOT	330 m/ml	↑
SGPT	340 mU/ml	↑
ALP	89 mU/ml	↑
LDH	193 mU/ml	Normal
γ-GTP	56 mU/ml	↑
Cho E	279 U/dl	Normal
ZTT	15.1 U	↑
TB	1.1 mg/dl	Normal
TP	6.9 g/dl	Normal
AFP	Under 20 mμg/ml	Normal
HBs Ag	(−)	
R_{15} ICG*	13%	↑
KICG**	0.136	↓
Antinuclear antibody	(+)	
Smooth muscle antibody	(+)	

* R_{15}ICG: indocyanine green (ICG) clearance test at 15 min.
** KICG: plasma disappearance rate of ICG

Purpose of Diagnostic Imaging. To identify the morphological status of the liver and presence of space-occupying lesions.

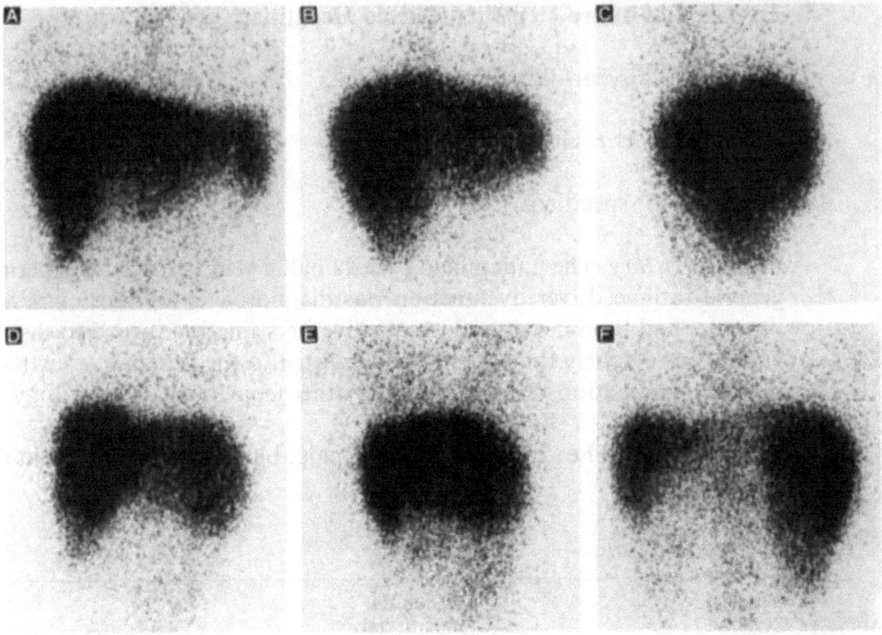

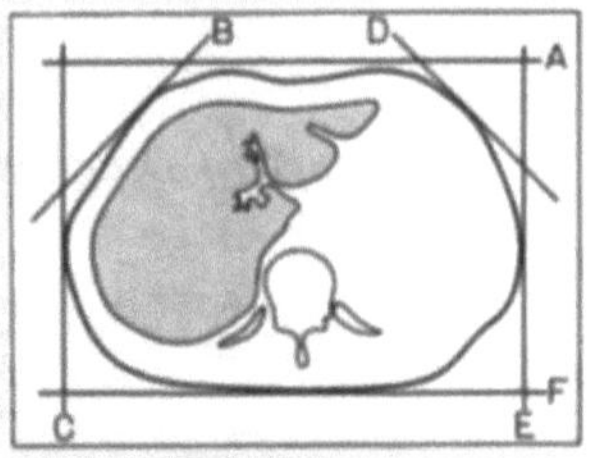

❶ Scintigram
A Frontal view
B Right lateral oblique view
C Right lateral view
D Left anterior oblique view
E Left lateral view
F Posterior view
Liver scintigram: Swelling of the left lobe and slightly swollen spleen are observed with visualization of the bone marrow. There are no findings suggesting space occupying lesions in the liver.

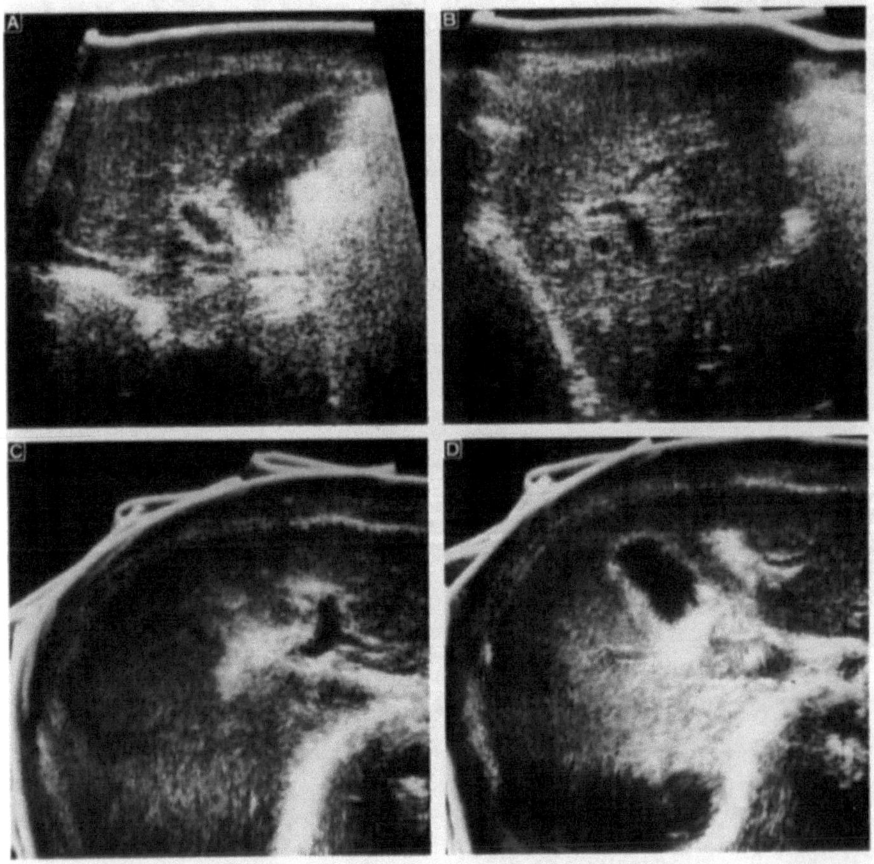

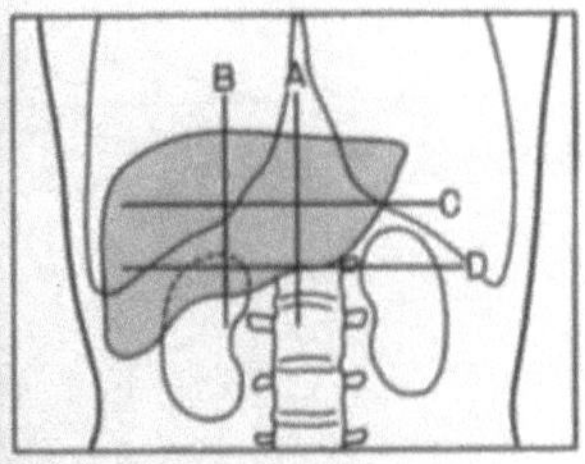

② Ultrasonogram
A–D Contact compound scan: Neither "bright liver" nor any findings showing decreasing of echo are seen. Swelling in the left lobe is observable, but no space-occupying lesions.

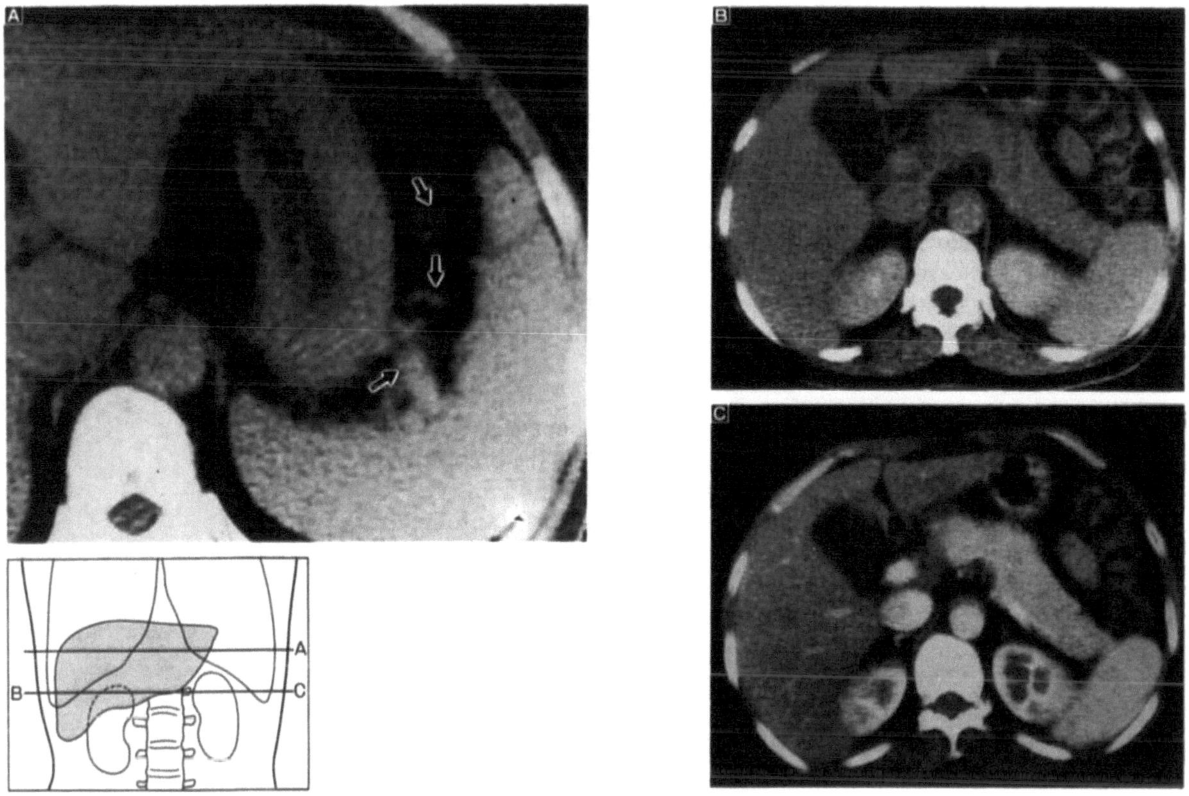

❸ CT image
B Before contrast enhancement
A, C After contrast enhancement
There are no space-occupying lesions in the liver. The lateral segment of the left lobe swells expanding to the anterior of the spleen. The quadrate lobe does not swell but contracts, and the porta hepatis becomes wider. The caudate lobe swells slightly. No changes are observed in the right lobe. The CT number of the liver is normal (55 HU). Findings of slight splenomegaly are recognized. Dilatation and tortuosity of the coronal and short gastric veins are seen, suggesting the existence of varices (→). A slightly swollen pancreas can be observed.

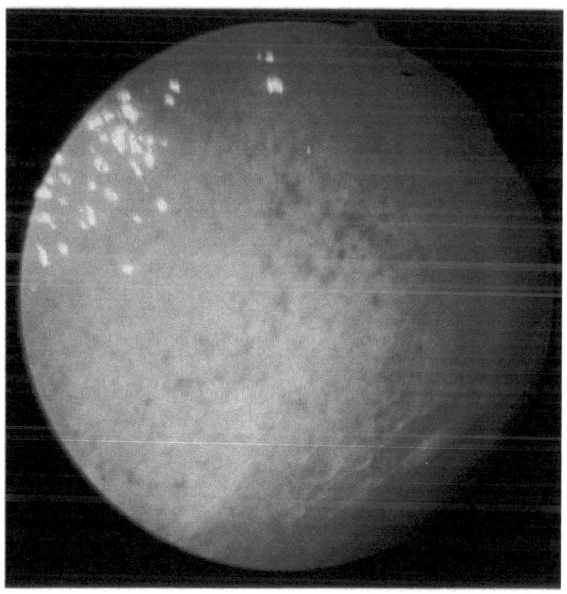

Laparoscopic findings: The surface of the liver is smooth and taut. Dilatation and bleeding of capillary vessels are observable.

Significance of Diagnostic Imaging. This case was already recognized as chronic active hepatitis, after biopsy of the liver, and diagnostic imaging was carried out for insurance. Chronic hepatitis cannot be diagnosed by any diagnostic imaging methods. However, it is possible to perceive morphological changes in ther liver, especially since CT is capable of examining morphological changes caused by process of chronic hepatitis progressing to liver cirrhosis.

An image of the swollen spleen and bone marrow can often be seen on the hepatic scintigram in cases of chronic active hepatitis. Hepatoma may occur in chronic hepatitis with or without going through the condition of liver cirrhosis. The importance of diagnostic imaging lies in detecting space-occupying lesions.

General Matters Concerning Lupoid Hepatitis [21]. Lupoid hepatitis (autoimmune hepatitis) is a chronic active hepatitis characterized by the presence of positive LE cells. The major finding is liver dysfunction although some clinical symptoms similar to systemic lupus erythematosus, SLE (autoimmune disease) appear because of an autoimmunological mechanism.

In Western countries lupoid hepatitis or autoimmune hepatitis, which occurs as a result of autoimmune factors, accounts for approximately half of all chronic active hepatitis cases, while in Japan it is just present in some. It is frequent in girls and women at menarche and during the menopause and rare in boys and men.

In the case of classic lupoid hepatitis, the LE cell phenomenon is present. However, in cases of lupoid chronic active hepatitis or autoimmune hepatitis, the LE cell phenomenon and antinuclear antibodies may not always be present. In such cases, the appearance of autoantibodies, such as antinuclear antibody, antismooth muscle antibody, and antihepatic antibody, SLE-like symptoms, and hypergammaglobulinemia serves as a guide for the diagnosis.

2.4 Liver Cirrhosis

Sequence of Diagnostic Imaging.

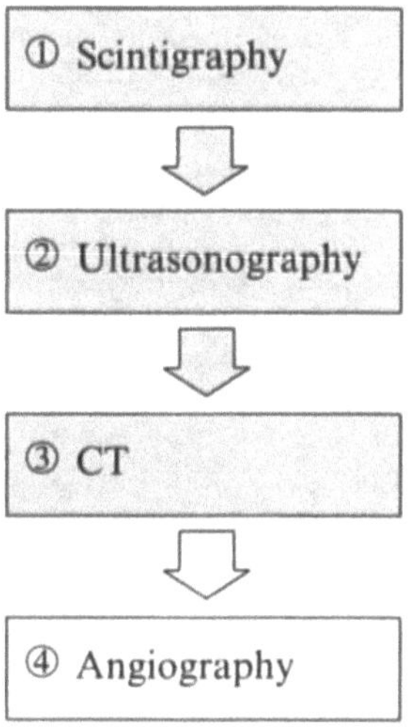

Patient. A 50-year-old man.

Main Complaint. Fatigue in the past 6 months.

Present Status. Vascular spider in the anterior chest wall. Varices in the esophagus were diagnosed from an esophagogram.

Laboratory Data.

SGOT	113 mU/ml	↑
SGPT	84 mU/ml	↑
LDH	277 mU/ml	↑
ALP	122 mU/ml	↑
γ-GTP	51 mU/ml	↑
Cho E	188 U/dl	↓
HBs Ag	(+)	
AFP	1.88 mμg/ml	Normal
Bleeding time	3 min	Normal
Coagulation time	12 min 30 s	Normal

Purpose of Diagnostic Imaging. To identify the presence of a space-occupying lesion associated with liver cirrhosis.

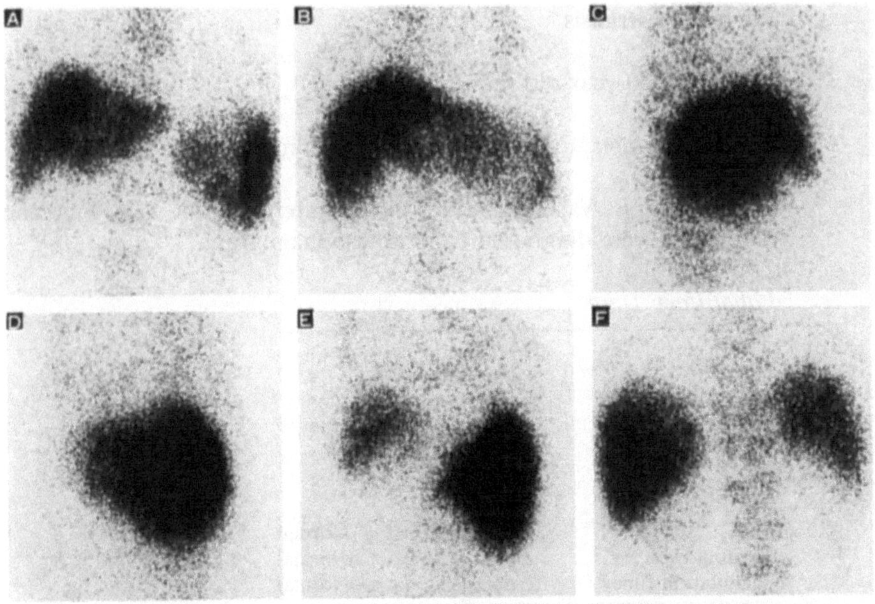

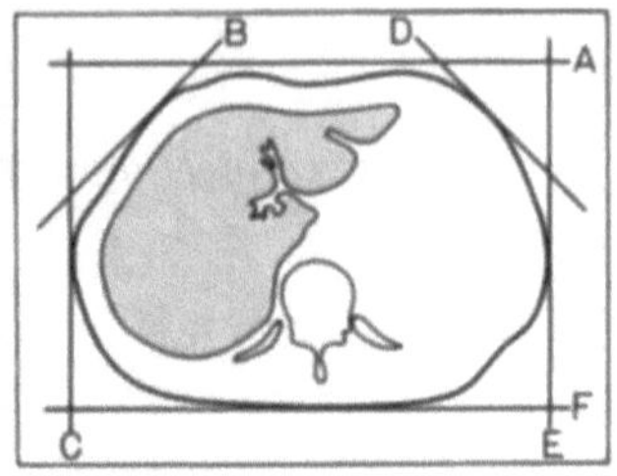

❶ Scintigram
A Frontal view
B Right anterior oblique view
C Right lateral view
D Left lateral view
E Left anterior oblique view
F Posterior view

Liver scintigram (^{99m}Tc-phytate). A marked atrophy of both lobes of the liver is observed with inhomogeneous uptake. Increased uptake of radioisotope (RI) into the spleen and bone marrow can be seen. A finding of splenomegaly is obtained.

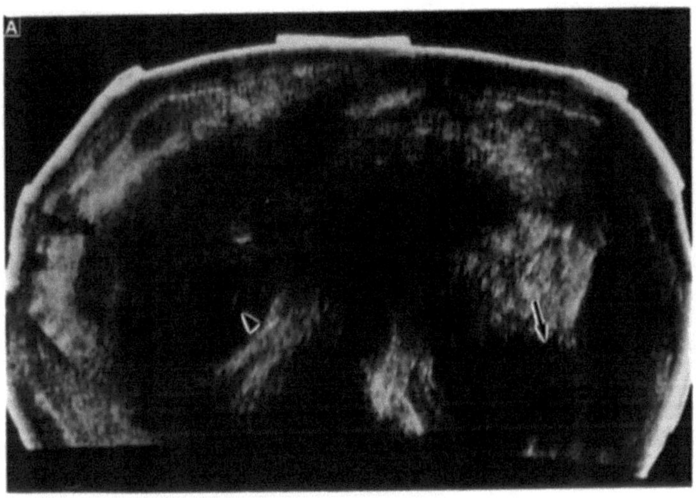

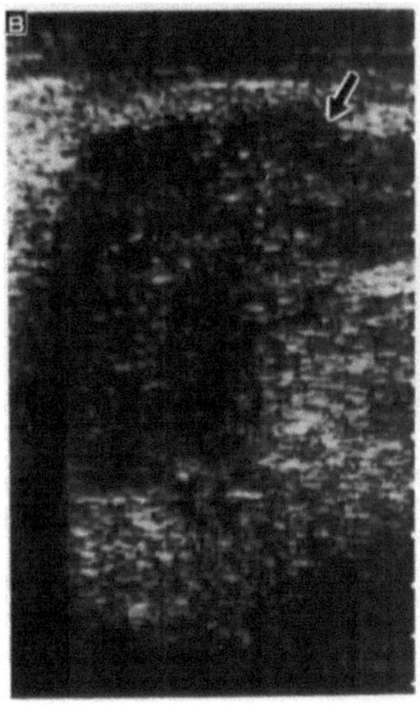

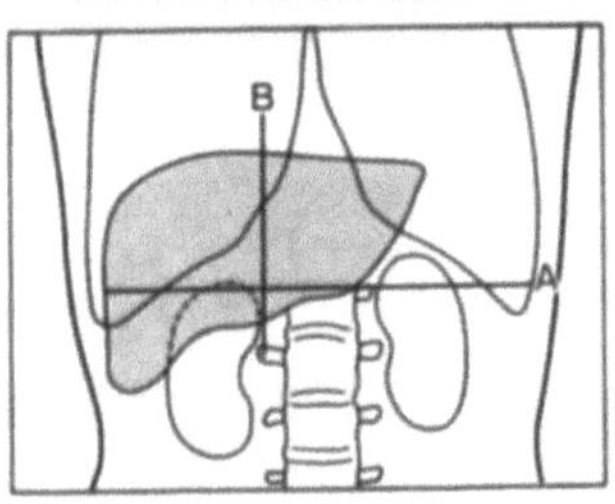

❷ Ultrasonogram
A Contact compound scanning image
B Linear electronic scanning image
The liver echo is coarse and uneven on the surface (→) showing the regenerating nodule. Echogenicity of the liver is markedly higher than the right kidney (▶) suggesting advancement of fibrosis. Splenomegaly is observed (→).

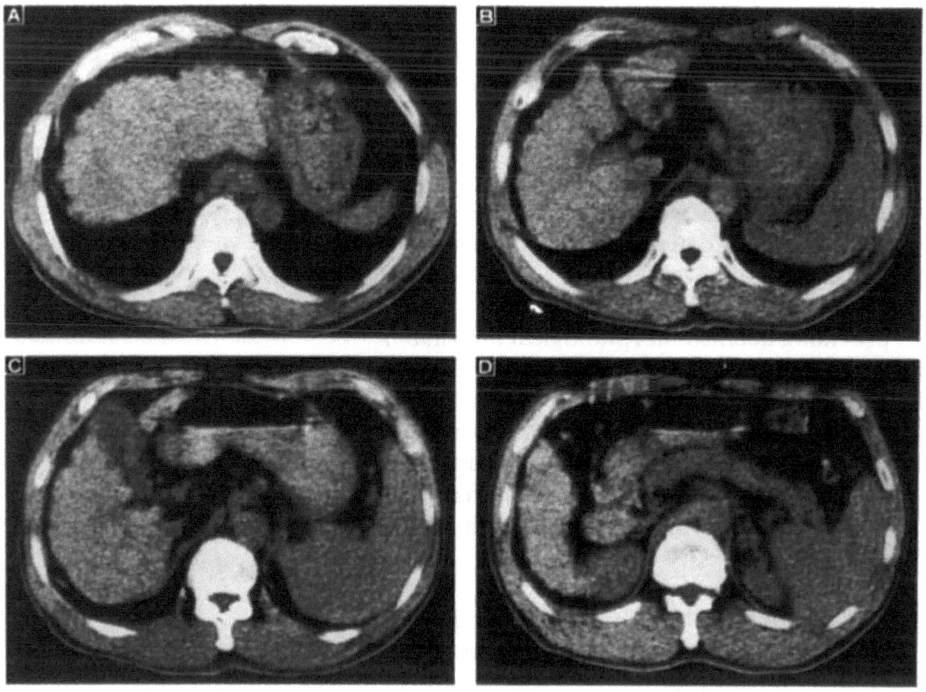

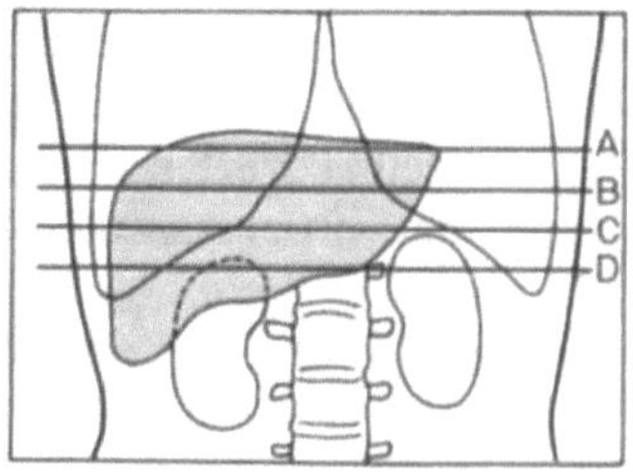

❸ CT image
Both lobes of the liver are shrunken and uneven on the surface. A round shadow showing the regenerating nodule is observed in the liver parenchyma indicating that this is the cause of the uneven surface. Ascites is seen in the lateral border of the liver. Varices from the stomach to the esophagus are recognizable.

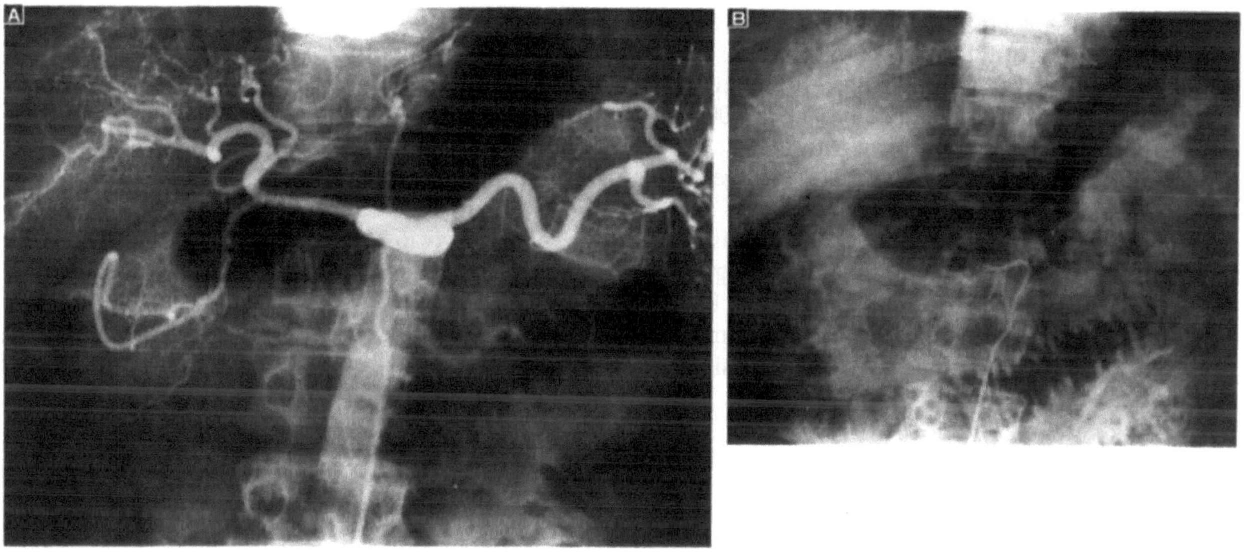

④ Angiogram
A Celiac arteriogram (arterial phase)
B Celiac arteriogram (venous phase)
The liver is entirely shrunken, and angulation and tortuosity of the intrahepatic arteries are observed without any findings of malignant tumors. In the venous phase, the splenic vein is poorly opacified and collateral bypath formation is marked.

Clinical Progress. Outpatient treatment for liver cirrhosis was initiated. The ascites and edema of the legs appeared after 9 months, and when hepatic coma occurred after 1 year and 3 months, the patient was hospitalized. After that, progress was fine and AFP was negative.

Significance of Diagnostic Imaging. With CT, findings of rgenerating nodule and ascites without space-occupying lesions were obtained. The presence of a space-occupying lesion was also not determined from the ultrasonic examination.

In advanced liver cirrhosis causing shrinkage of the liver, ultrasound may frequently be incapable of providing detailed morphological information due to parenchymal fibrosis. Therefore, CT is superior due to its capacity to observe the entire liver.

Liver scintigraphy is useful for examining morphological changes in the liver over a period of time, while its ability to diagnose space-occupying lesions is not high due to too many false-positive results. Hence, in cases in which space-occupying lesions are suspected from CT, determination by angiography is required.

General Matters Concerning Liver Cirrhosis [7, 8, 13, 21, 24]. Liver cirrhosis is an excessive state of liver dysfunction which can never be reversed. Specific morphological findings of liver cirrhosis are:

1. Nodular formation over the entire liver.
2. Degeneration and necrosis of the hepatocyte with regenerating nodule.
3. Increasing connective tissue (mainly interstitial septa formation between Glisson's capsule and the hepatic vein).

Liver cirrhosis is mainly caused by viral hepatitis, alcohol abuse, malnutrition, toxicity, and immunological factors, and in a few cases, congestion, biliary disease, parasitic infestation, syphilis, hemochromatosis, and Wilson's disease may cause liver cirrhosis. In Japan 90% of liver cirrhosis are caused by virus infection, while in Western countries, alcoholic cirrhosis accounts for 70% of all cases.

The mortality rate of liver cirrhosis in Japan has been increasing annually, and today it is considered that 12 per 100000 people die from liver cirrhosis. The frequency of liver cirrhosis in Japan is high in the west and low in the east, and patients with HBs antigen are also found more frequently in the west than in the east.

Generally, the prognosis for liver cirrhosis is poor, and the 50% survival interval is only 3–4 years after the initial diagnosis of liver cirrhosis. The major fatal causes are hepatic coma, intestinal bleeding, and hepatocellular carcinoma. The mortality rate from hepatic coma has been decreasing while that from intestinal bleeding has been increasing.

2.5 Liver Cirrhosis

Sequence of Diagnostic Imaging.

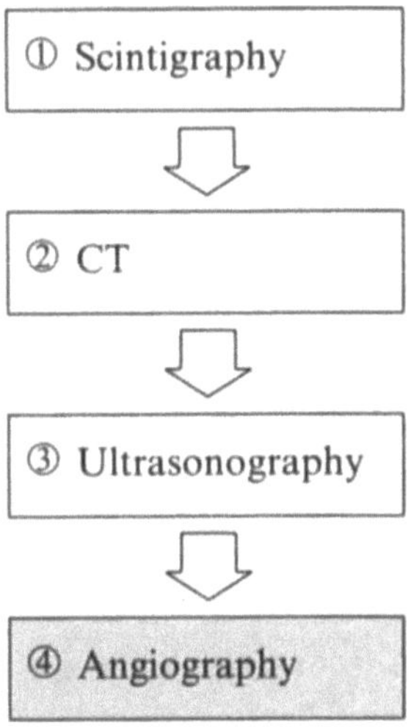

Patient. A 59–year-old man.

Main Complaint. Not specified.

History. In the past 10 years, the patient was medically treated in the internal medicine department for diabetes mellitus and chronic hepatitis. The patient has a low alcohol intake. The patient was admitted to the department of radiology for further examination because liver dysfunction had continued and the level of AFP was elevated with the liver swelling.

Present Status. The liver is palpable 3 FB below the right costal margin. Palmar erythema and vascular spider in the anterior chest wall are recognized without jaundice.

Laboratory Data.

SGOT	166 mU/ml	↑
SGPT	204 mU/ml	↑
ALP	177 mU/ml	↑
LDH	184 mU/ml	Normal
γ-GTP	147 mU/ml	↑
Cho E	181 U/dl	↓
TP	7.1 g/dl	Normal
TB	1.8 mg/dl	↑
Direct bilirubin	0.7 mg/dl	Normal
ZTT	17.0 U	↑
HBs Ag	(−)	
AFP (2 months prior)	318 mμg/ml	↑
(1 month prior)	629 mμg/ml	↑
(at the time of admission)	2628 mμg/ml	↑

Purpose of Diagnostic Imaging. Hepatic carcinoma was suspected from the rapid increase of AFP.

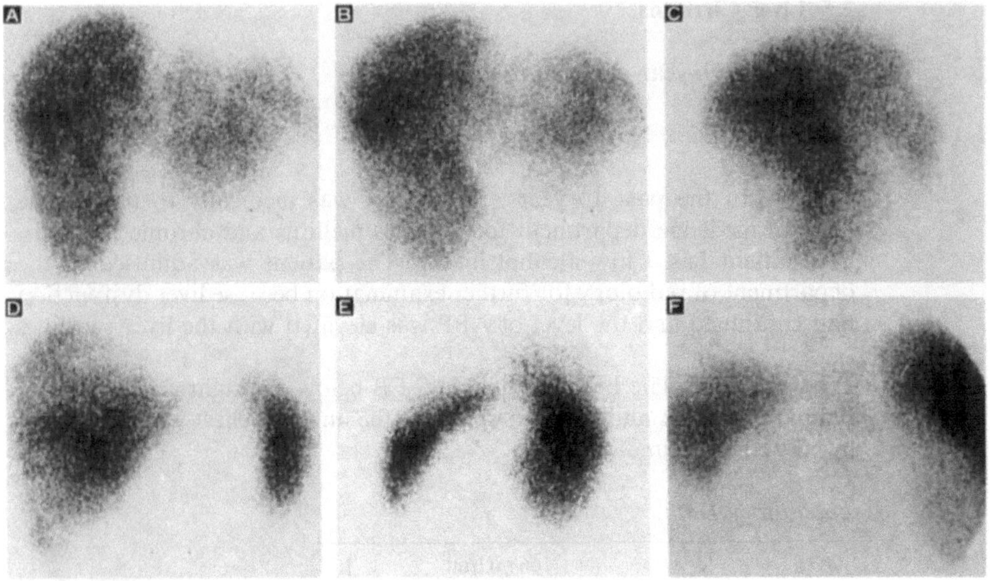

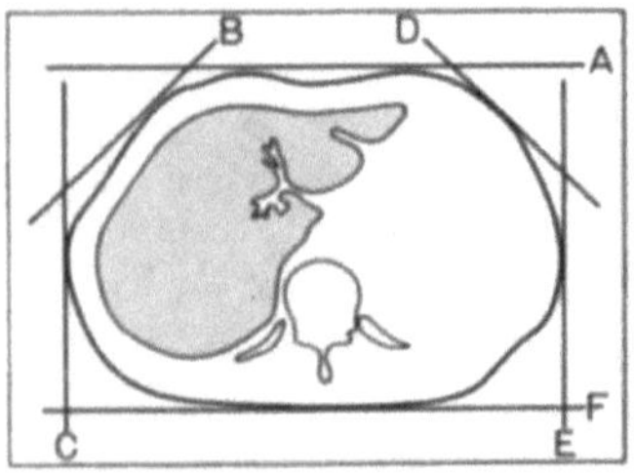

① Scintigram
A Frontal view
B Right anterior oblique view
C Right lateral view
D Left anterior oblique view
E Left lateral view
F Posterior view
Liver scintigram (^{99m}Tc-phytate in sitting position): Swelling of the right lobe and deep incisions of the porta hepatis are observed. Uptake into the liver is inhomogeneous suggesting a regenerating nodule. Hyperfunction of the spleen is noticed and bone marrow is visualized.

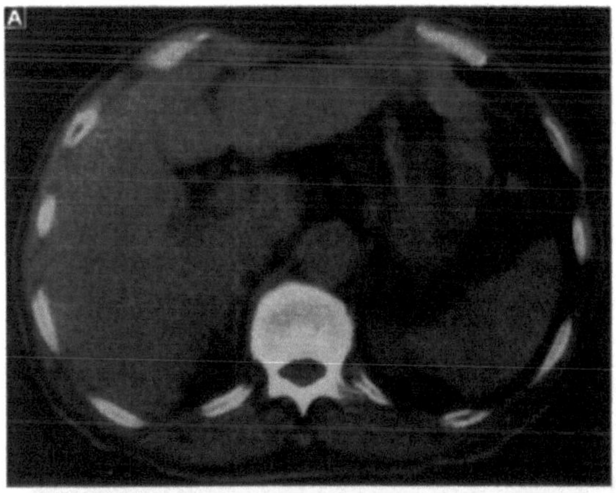

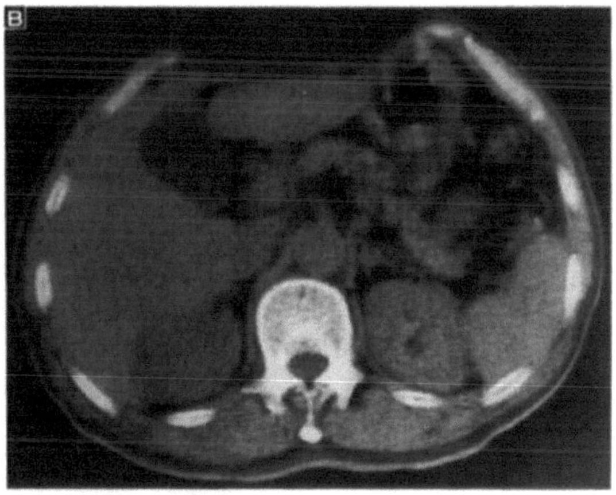

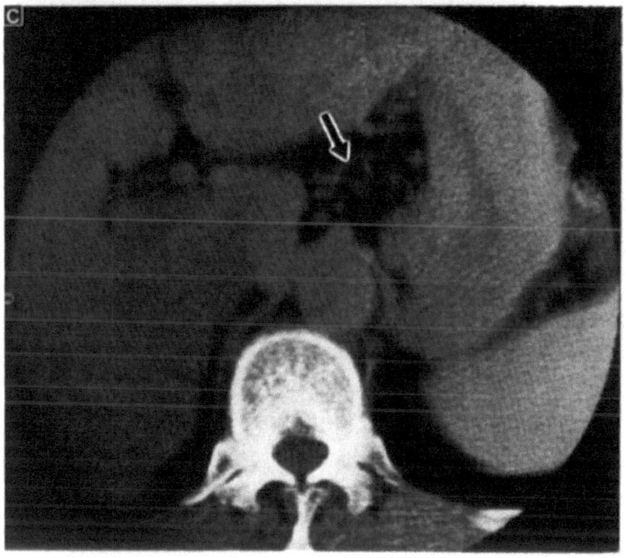

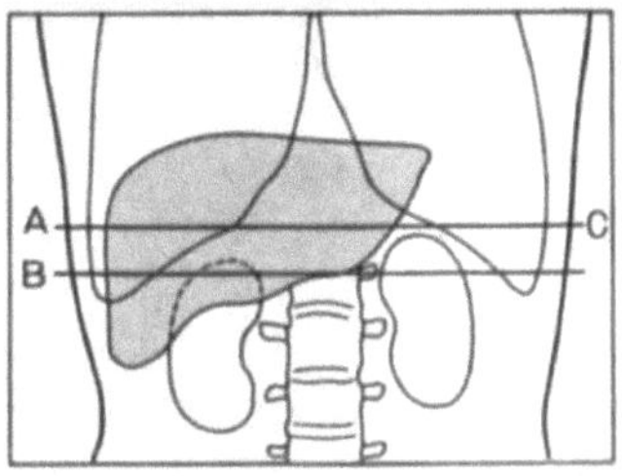

② CT image
Atrophy of the quadrate lobe, swelling of the caudate lobe, nodule formation, deep incision of the porta hepatis of the right lobe and dilatation of the short gastric and coronal veins forming varices are observed (→). An intrahepatic space-occupying lesion is not recognized.

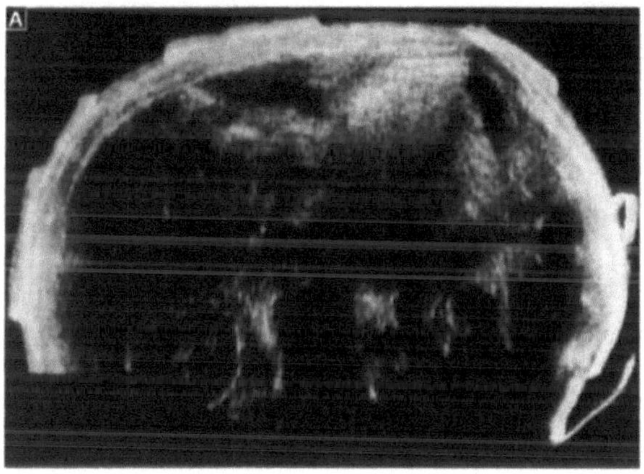

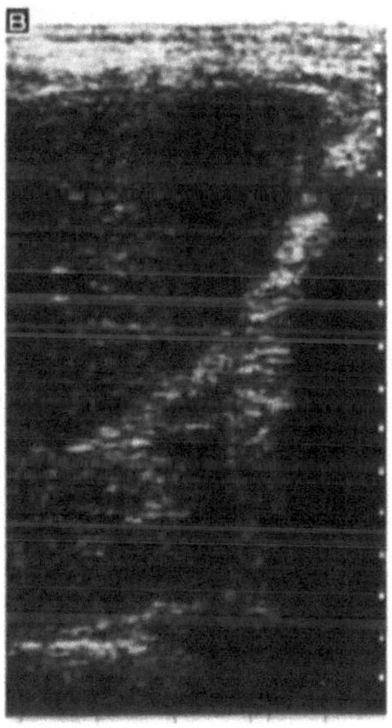

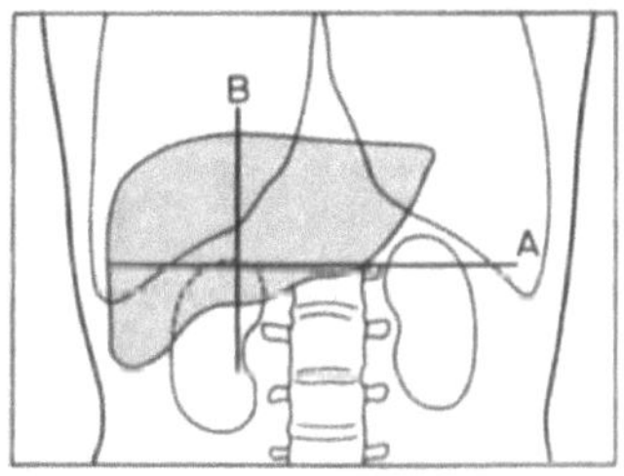

③ Ultrasonogram
A Contact compound scanning image
B Linear electronic scanning image
Intrahepatic echogenicity is not homogeneous, and a space-occupying lesion is not observed.

④ Angiography

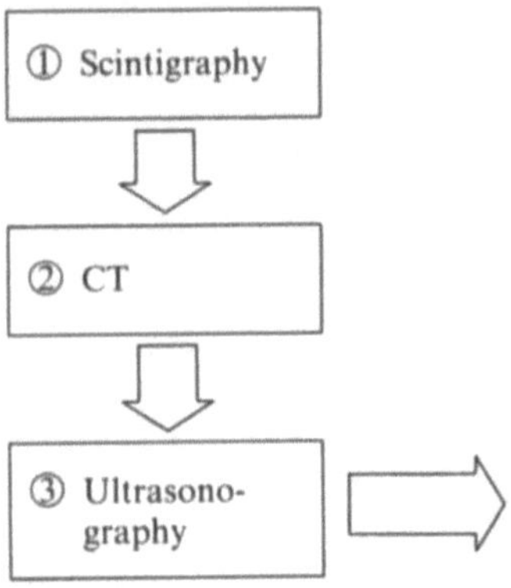

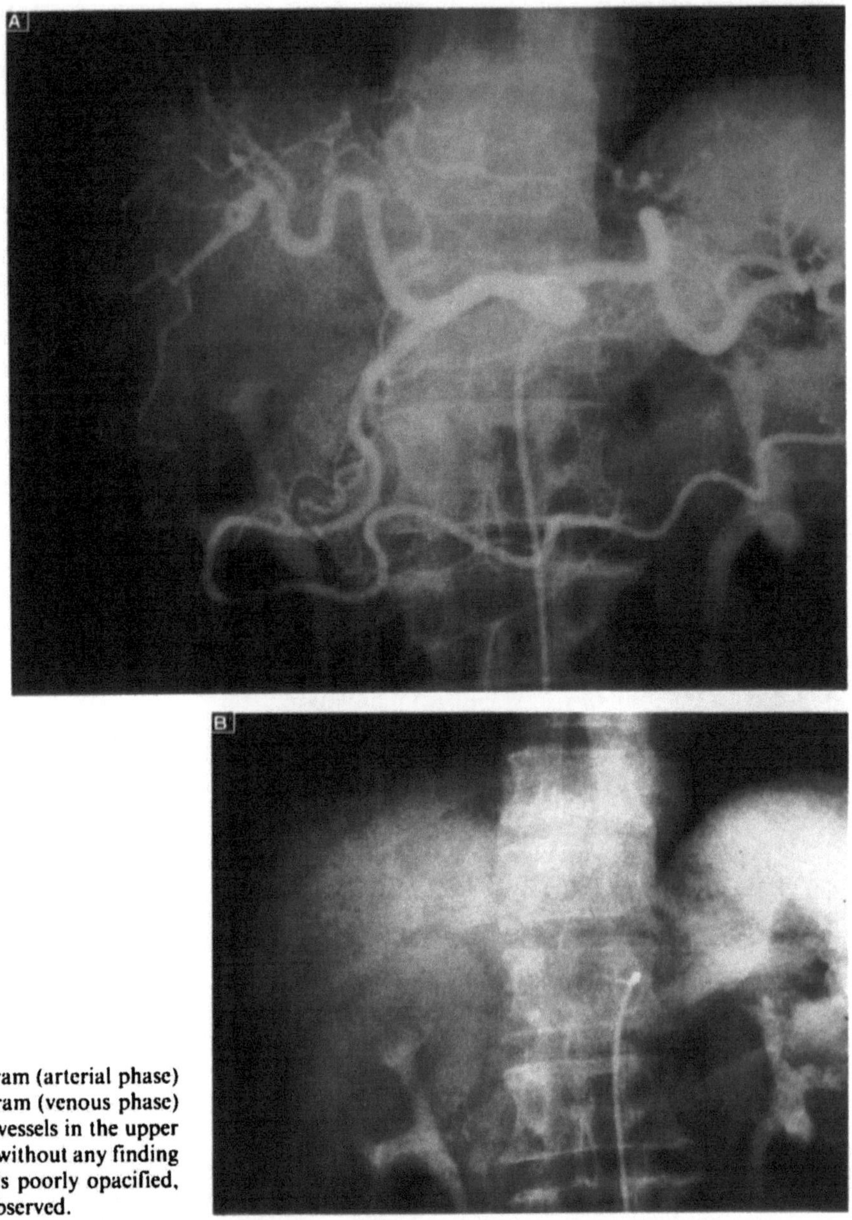

❹ Angiogram
A, A′ Stereoscopic celiac arteriogram (arterial phase)
B, B′ Stereoscopic celiac arteriogram (venous phase)
Angulation and tortuosity of the vessels in the upper segment of the right lobe are seen without any finding of malignancy. The splenic vein is poorly opacified, and varices in the stomach are observed.

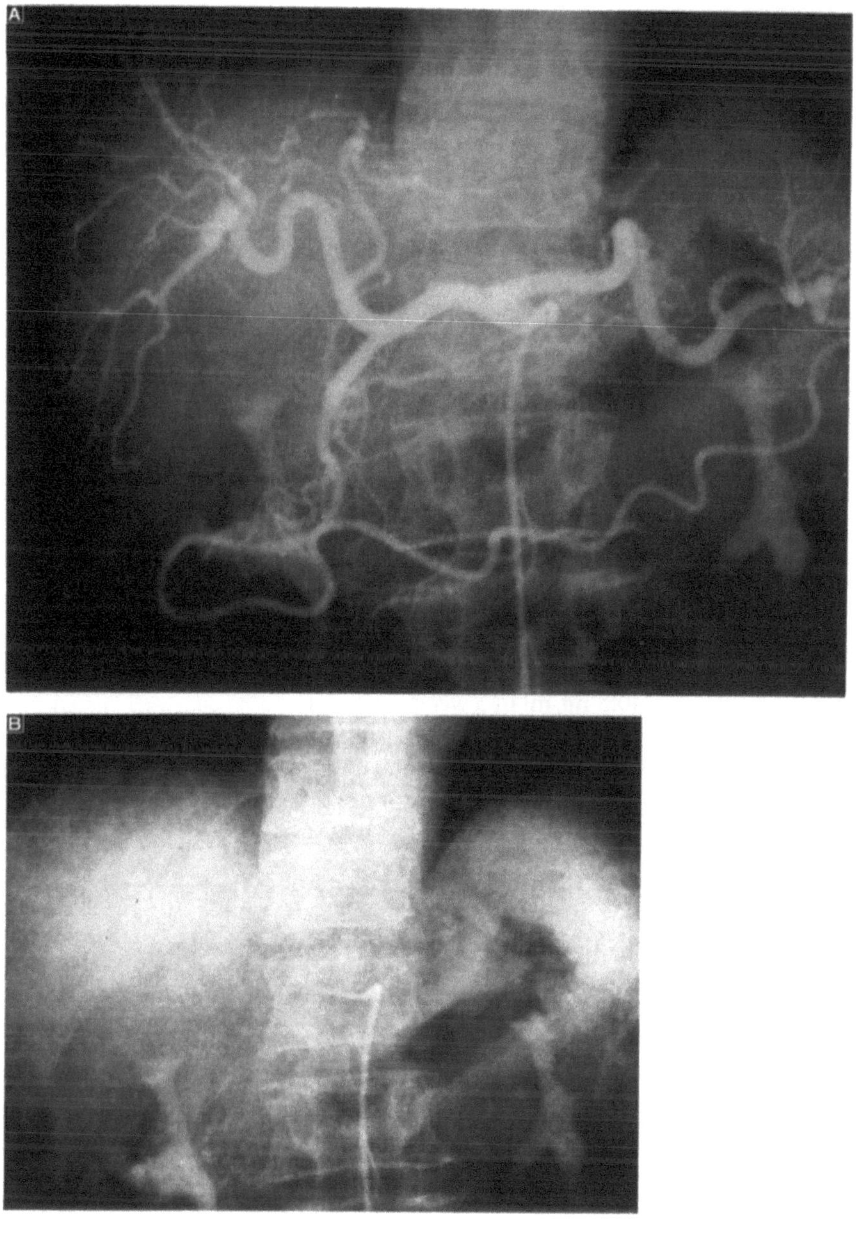
A
B

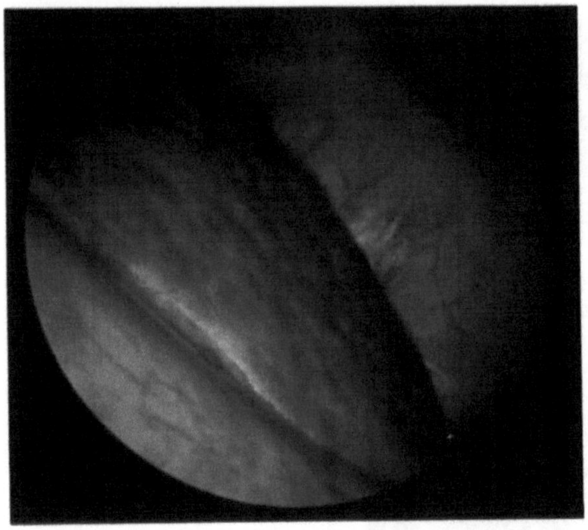

Laparoscopic findings: The liver is reddish-brown. Nodule formations of various sizes are observed with cicatricial indentations in the space between them.

Clinical Diagnosis. With laparoscopy, white liver was observed with abnormal findings of nodule formation and swelling in the right lobe. Liver cirrhosis was determined from the liver biopsy.

Clinical Progress. The level of AFP declined to 240.5 ng/ml in 3 weeks after the first diagnosis in the department of radiology, and it has been hovering around 200 ng/ml in the following year. After a year, liver scintigraphy and ultrasonic examination were performed, and no space-occupying lesions were observed.

Significance of Diagnostic Imaging. In this case, hepatic carcinoma was suspected because of the rapid increase in the level of AFP, and the diagnostic imaging was performed. In such a case, although no lesions are recognized by liver scintigraphy, ultrasonic examination, and CT, examination by angiography is indispensable. Other examinations are unnecessary only if angiography is performed.

General Matters Concerning Liver Cirrhosis. Even in liver cirrhosis with regeneration of hepatic cells, the level of AFP may sometimes exceed 400 ng/ml, and this state may persist for over half a year. Generally, however, an elevated level of AFP exceeding 400 ng/ml due to the regeneration of hepatic cells is transitional. This case shows the remarkable transitional elevation of AFP, but usually the level of AFP seldom rises so high.

2.6 Fatty Liver

Sequence of Diagnostic Imaging.

① Scintigraphy
⇩
② Ultrasonography
⇩
③ CT

Patient. A 21-year-old woman.

Main Complaint. General fatigue and hepatomegaly.

History. The patient had pyrexia a year earlier. Slight liver dysfunction was diagnosed in the internal medicine department, but the cause was not determined. At that time, the department of radiology examined the upper abdomen. Four months prior, Crohn's disease was diagnosed and the patient was hospitalized. Corticosteroid therapy and intravenous hyperalimentation had been carried out resulting in improvement of the Crohn's disease. Recently, the patient has experienced severe general fatigue, and the liver, which was not palpated at the time of hospitalization, is now palpable 2 FB below the right costal margin.

Laboratory Data.

SGOT	102 mU/ml	↑
SGPT	255 mU/ml	↑
ALP	85 mU/ml	Normal
LDH	188 mU/ml	Normal
γ-GTP	50 mU/ml	↑
Cho E	321 U/dl	Normal
HBs Ag	(−)	
AFP	under 1.0 mμg/ml	Normal

Purpose of Diagnostic Imaging. To precisely examine the swelling of the liver associated with liver dysfunction (fatty liver was suspected).

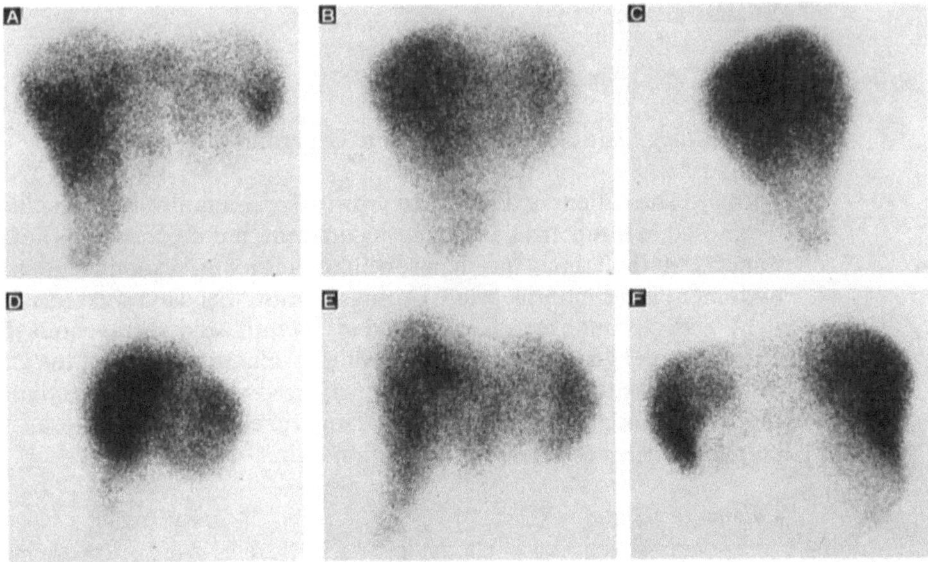

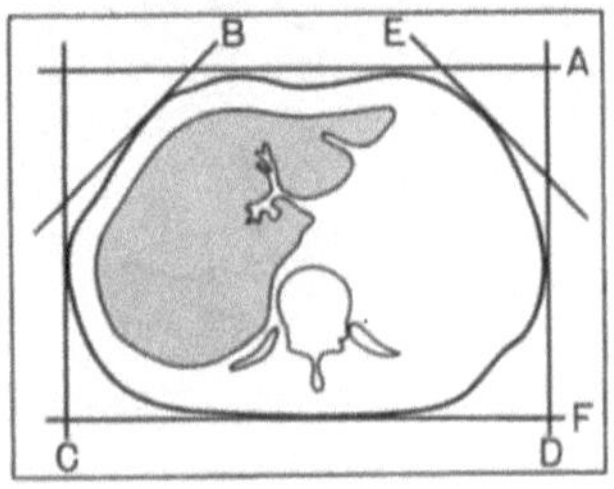

① Scintigram
A Frontal view
B Right anterior oblique view
C Right lateral view
D Left lateral view
E Left anterior oblique view
F Posterior view
Liver scintigram (^{99m}Tc-phytate in sitting position): Swelling of the left lobe and deep incisions of the porta hepatis are observed. Descent of the right lobe in a sitting position indicated that elasticity of the liver was preserved.

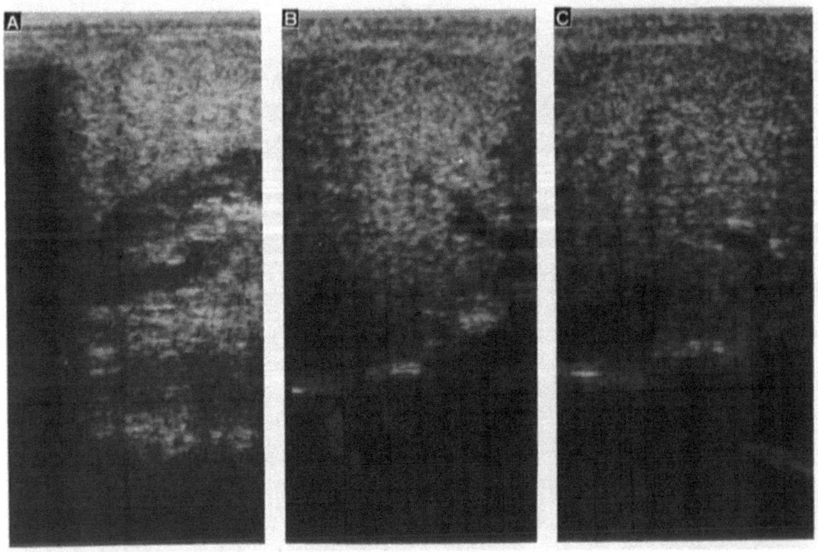

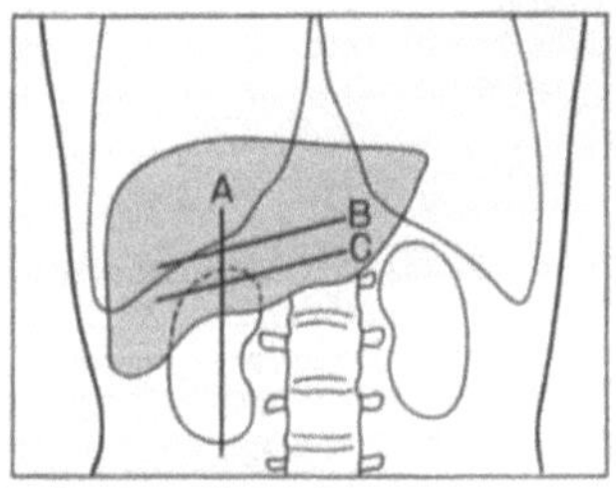

❷ Ultrasonogram
A–C Linear electronic scanning image: A "bright liver" remarkably higher in echo level than the right kidney is observed. Vascularity in the liver is poorly visualized.

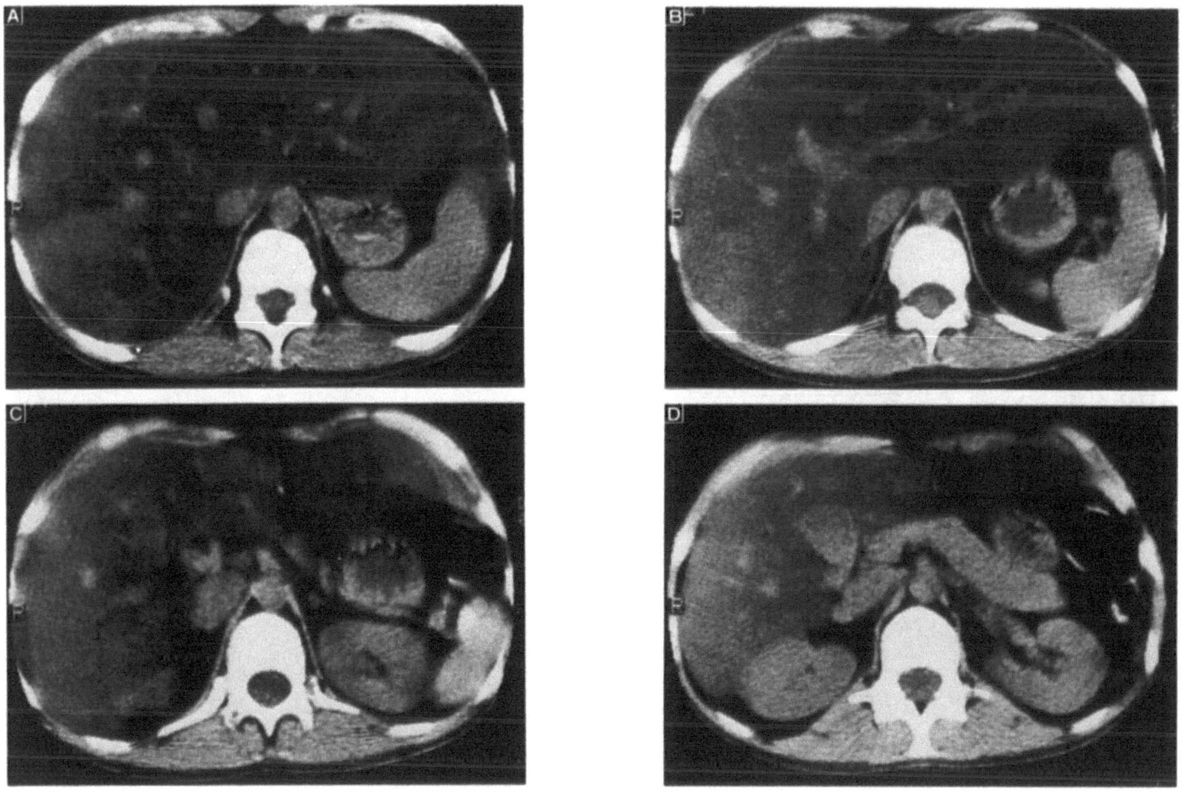

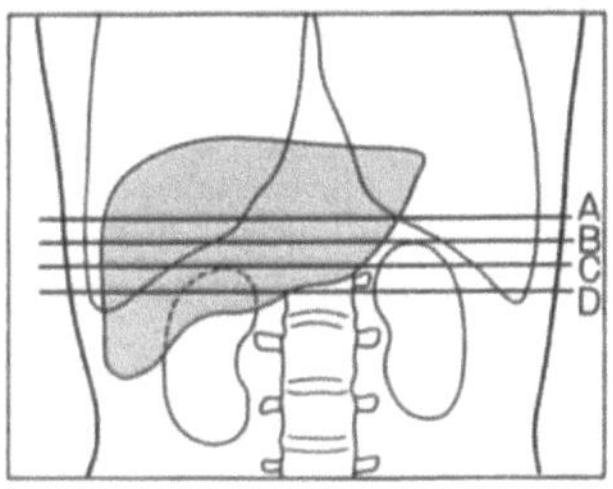

❸ CT image

The X-ray absorption ratio of the liver (the CT number is 5 HU) is lower than the intrahepatic vessels and vastly lower than the pancreas, kidney, spleen, and gallbladder. Morphologically, swelling of the left lobe (beak sign of the lateral segment) and caudate lobe is observed.

12 months prior

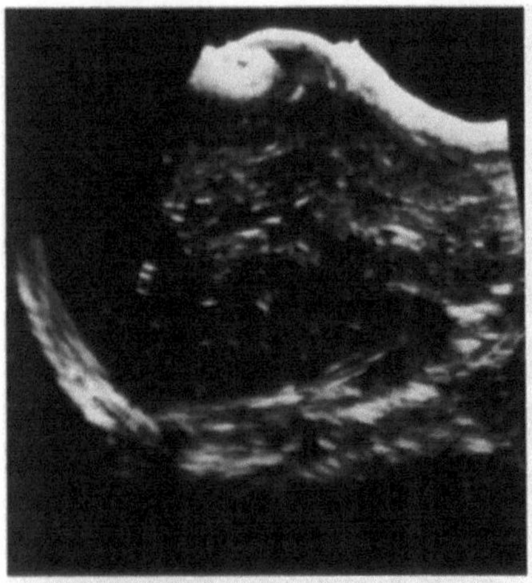

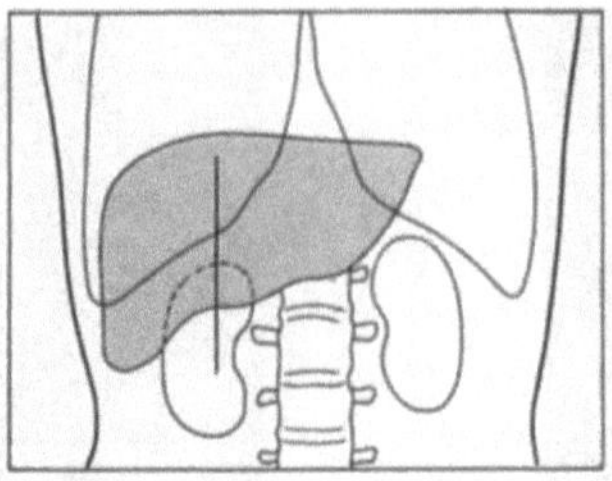

① Ultrasonogram
Contact compound scanning image: The echo pattern of the liver is normal without large differences from the right kidney in echo level. Vascularity in the liver is clearly visualized.

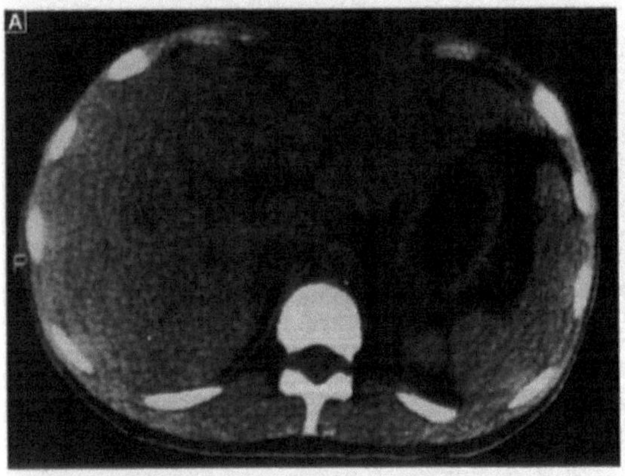

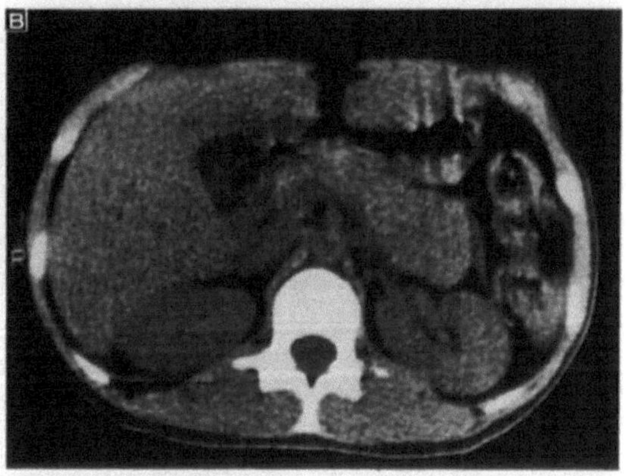

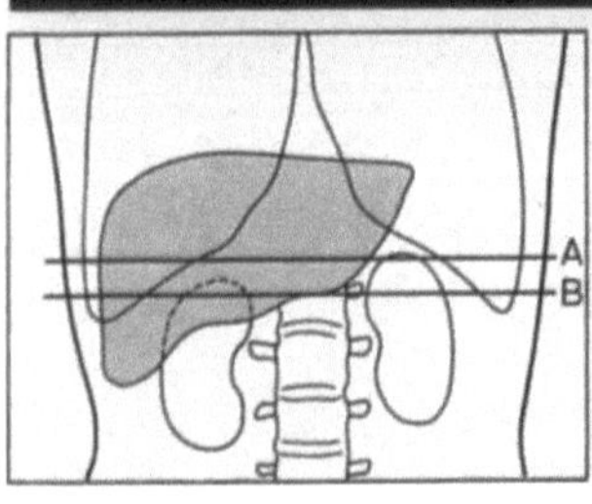

② CT image
The CT number of the liver is 60 HU, remaining in the normal range. Slight swelling of the left lobe of the liver is observed.

After 2 months

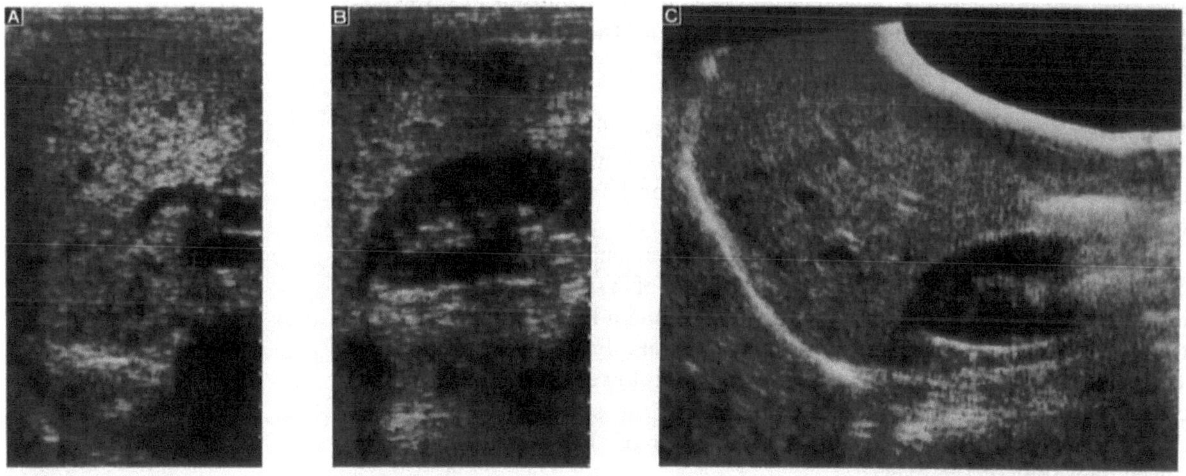

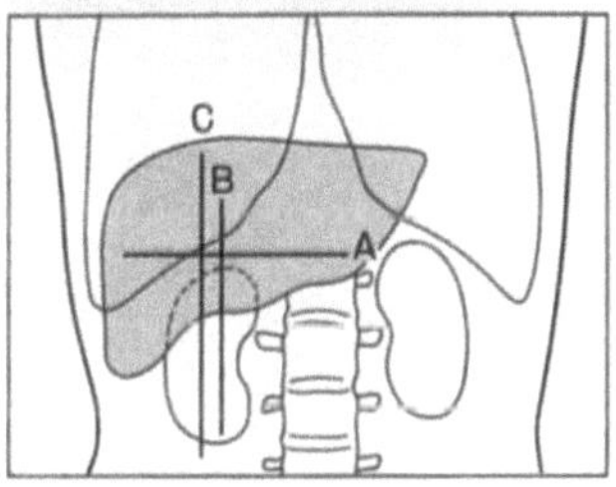

① Ultrasonogram
A, B Linear electronic scanning image
C Contact compound scanning image
The bright liver is still observed showing a higher echo level than the right kidney, but the difference has slightly decreased, and vascularity in the liver can be visualized.

② CT image
The X-ray absorption of the liver is increasing (the CT number is 56 HU) although low attenuation areas are still observed in certain segments. The beak sign of the lateral segment has dissappeared, and the swelling of the left lobe has improved. The CT number of the spleen is 62.5 HU and still higher than the liver.

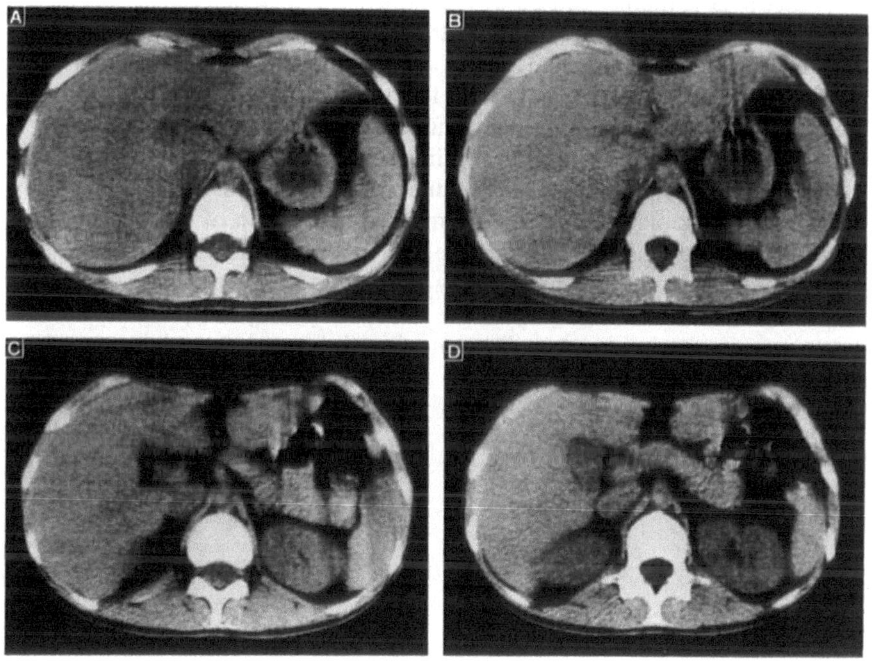

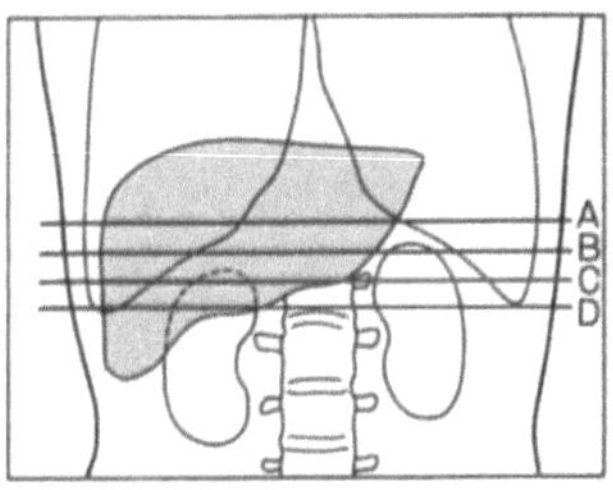

Clinical Progress. After determining severe fatty liver with our diagnostic imaging, the use of steroids was stopped after decreasing administration and then the high-calorie fluid therapy was ceased, resulting in improvement of SGOT down to 29 mU/ml, SGPT to 80 mU/ml, and 2 months later the liver was not palpable at all.

Significance of Diagnostic Imaging. The progress of this case can be well traced because the ultrasonic and CT examinations were performed 12 months before the fatty liver appeared and 2 months after the beginning of medical treatment.

The diagnosis of an advanced fatty liver can easily be obtained from a CT image, which is characterized by a decline of X-ray absorption in the liver parenchyma due to increasing fatty tissue and a high contrast between the liver parenchyma and the intrahepatic vessels. Fatty liver can be fully suspected only when the CT number of the liver is lower than that of normal cases (40 HU–70 HU). The image density of the spleen is indicative in determining fatty liver because the CT number of the spleen is normally lower than that of the liver.

In this case, the CT number of the liver parenchyma improved and was higher than that of the intrahepatic vessels 2 months after the initiation of medical treatment for fatty liver. Compared to the spleen, however, the liver parenchyma was still lower in CT number and nonhomogeneous in density. On the other hand, the sign of the bright liver could still be visualized on the ultrasonic image, and the echo level of the liver parenchyma was also much higher than that of the kidney. Needless to say, the ultrasonic and CT images photographed 12 months before the occurrence of fatty liver were both normal.

General Matters Concerning Fatty Liver [11, 21]. Fatty liver is an abnormal accumulation of triglycerides in the liver. The finding of fat droplets in more than half of the hepatic cells in the microscopic field under normal magnification is called fatty liver and in less than half of the hepatic cells is called the accumulation of fat or fatty deposition.

Fatty liver is mainly caused by alcoholism, drug toxicity, diabetes mellitus, and supernutrition. So far, in the cases in which autopsy was performed, it was most frequent in the age group of 50–60 years, and the distribution ratio between males and females was 2:1.

The macroscopic findings include an increase in the volume and weight of the liver, which corresponds to swelling of the liver. The liver is soft, nonelastic, and fragile, but it may harden due to the fibrotic or cirrhotic change.

The microscopic findings include marked deposition of fat in the cytoplasm of hepatic cells and balloon cells with eccentric nucleus. The progression of fatty liver is accompanied by inflammation of the mesenchymal tissue and fibrotic change around the portal vein. Further progression of fatty liver results in cirrhosis. By removing the cause, fatty liver may be entirely reversed.

2.7 Hemochromatosis

Sequence of Diagnostic Imaging.

① Scintigraphy

⇩

② Ultrasonography

⇩

③ CT

Patient. A 59-year-old woman.

Main Complaint. Pigmentation of the skin.

Present History. A year prior, another clinic diagnosed liver dysfunction and pigmentation of the face and the back of the hand. The patient was admitted to the department of radiology for further examinations.

Present Status. The patient has tenderness on pressure below the right costal margin without palpability of the liver. Pigmentations of the face and the back of the hand are observed and no jaundice is apparent.

Past History. Seven years prior, chronic hepatitis was diagnosed in another clinic. During medical treatment, anemia was determined and iron medication was given for 2 years.

Laboratory Data.

SGOT	153 mU/ml	↑
SGPT	240 mU/ml	↑
LDH	164 mU/ml	↑
ALP	103 mU/ml	↑
Serum iron	267 mg/dl	↑
HBs Ag	(−)	
AFP	298 mμg/ml	↑

Purpose of Diagnostic Imaging. To identify the morphology of the liver and the existence of space-occupying lesions.

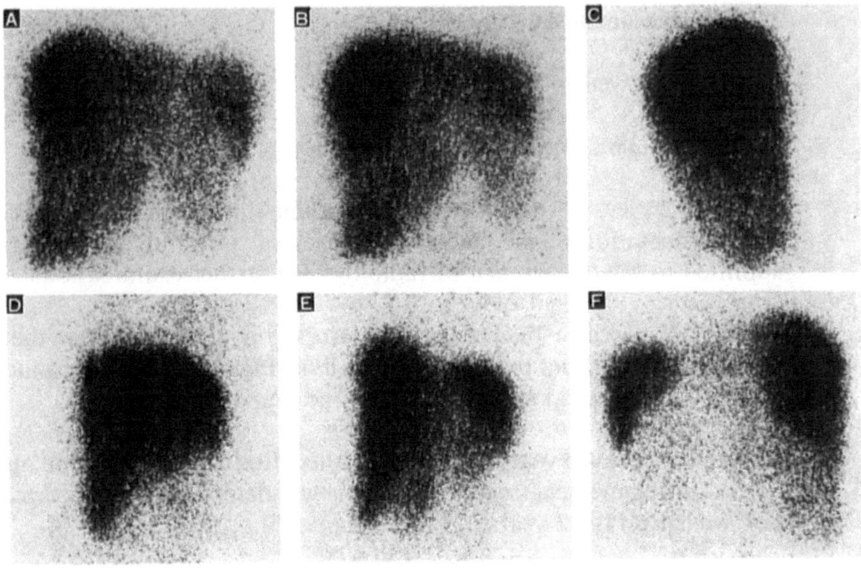

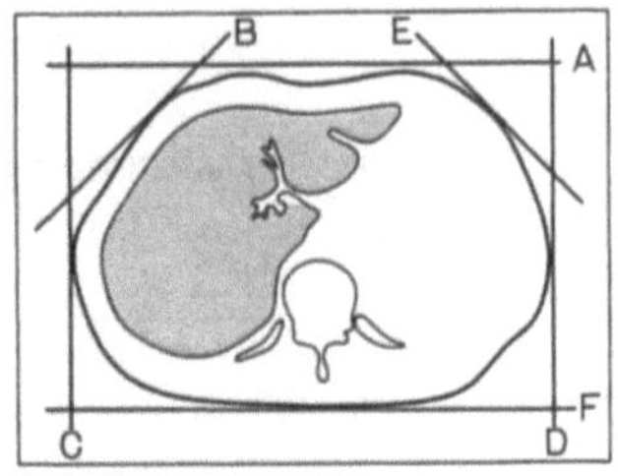

① Scintigram
A Frontal view
B Right anterior oblique view
C Right lateral view
D Left lateral view
E Left anterior oblique view
F Posterior view

Liver scintigram (^{99m}Tc-phytate in sitting position): Swelling of the liver in both hepatic lobes and inhomogeneous uptake of RI without any findings of space-occupying lesions are observed. Uptake of RI into the spleen and bone marrow is increasing.

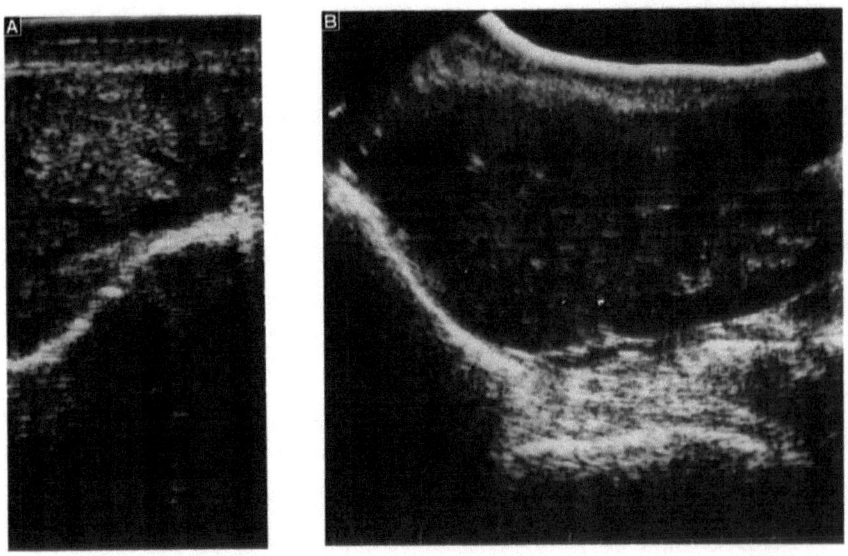

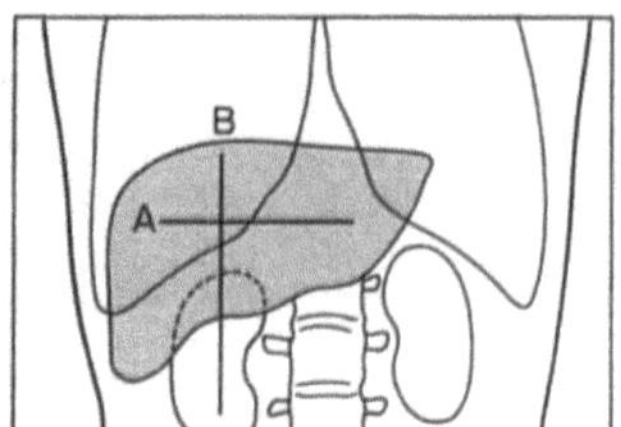

② Ultrasonogram
A Linear electronic scanning image
B Contact compound scanning image
The echogenicity of the liver is not homogeneous and the echo level is slightly higher than the kidney.

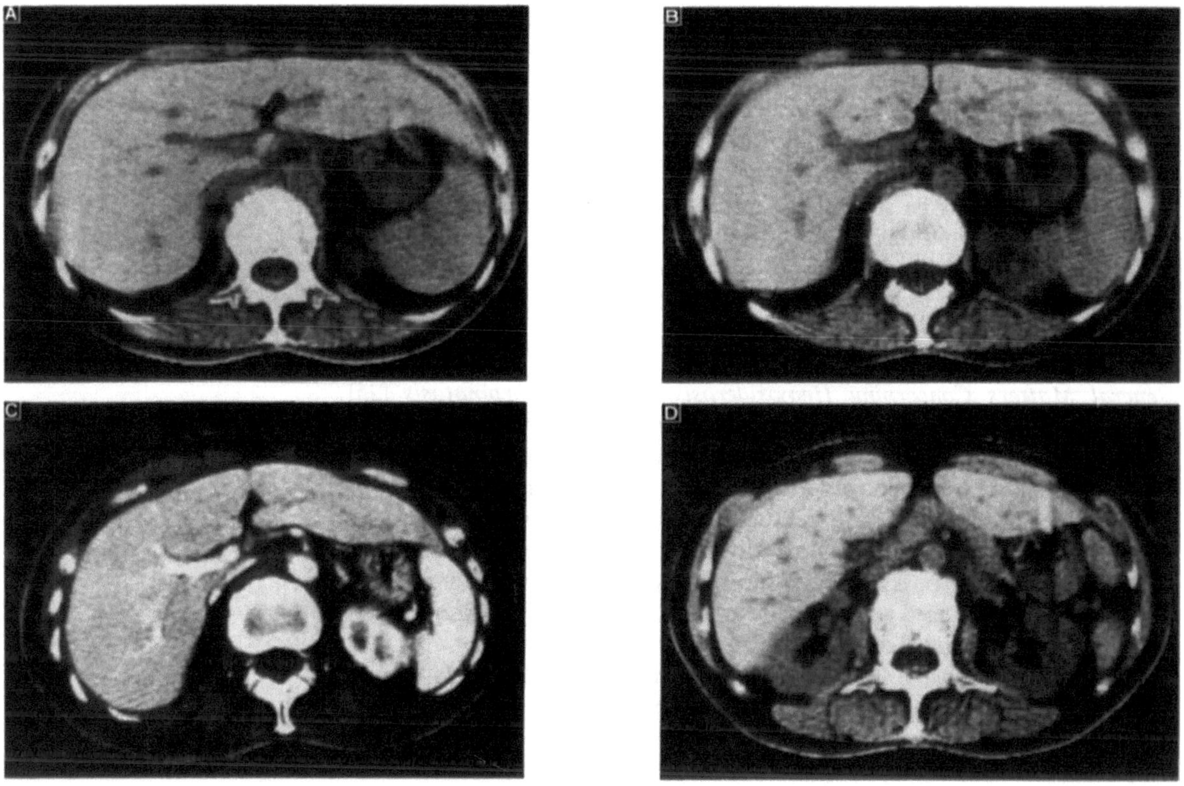

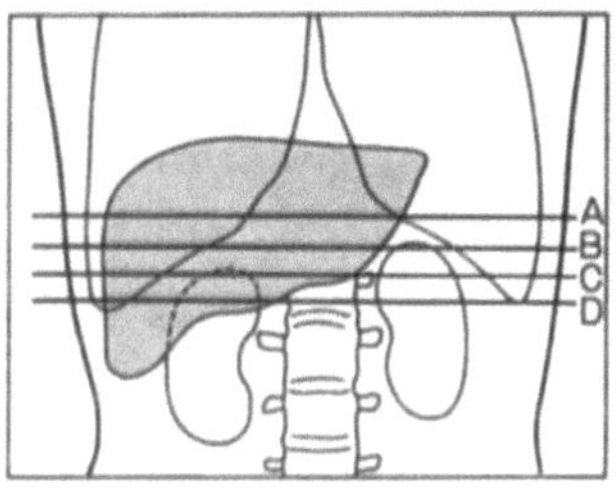

❸ CT image
A, B, D Before contrast enhancement
C After contrast enhancement

High X-ray absorption of the liver and comparatively low attenuation image of the intrahepatic vessels are visualized. The CT number of the liver parenchyma is 87 HU, increasing to 120 HU after contrast enhancement. The morphological findings include extention of the liver to the left with a sharp tip and highly advanced swelling of the left lobe. Atrophy of the quadrate and caudate lobes and rib compression on the lateral surface of the right lobe suggesting progression of fibrosis are also observed.

Clinical Progress. Large amounts of "brown pigment" with a positive iron reaction were detected from skin biopsy, and liver biopsy indicated increasing deposits of hemosiderin.

Significance of Diagnostic Imaging. In hemosiderosis and hemochromatosis, accumulation of iron in the liver causes increasing X-ray absorption by the liver parenchyma so that the intrahepatic vasculature is visualized with less attenuation allowing easy diagnosis with CT.

Although liver scintigraphy and ultrasonography are both excellent means to determine space-occupying lesions, they do not permit diagnosis of hemosiderosis or hemochromatosis.

General Matters Concerning Hemosiderosis and Hemochromatosis [25]. Hemosiderosis and hemochromatosis are characterized by abnormally increasing accumulation of excess iron in the body. Hemosiderosis is defined as an increase of iron deposits in the liver, pancreas, and bone marrow without liver dysfunction, and hemochromatosis is accompanied by dysfunction in those organs. They are divided into primary and secondary types. The primary type is an idiopathic increase of iron absorption, and the secondary type is caused after chronic anemia, multiple blood transfusion, and long-term iron medication.

A histopathological finding of the liver, in the case of hemochromatosis, is diffuse or localized existence of hemosiderin in the hepatic cells. When advancing, a mass formation of hemosiderin is markedly noticeable around the lobule.

Hemochromatosis is quite often accompanied by hepatocellular carcinoma, which occurs three times more frequently in hemochromatosis than in liver cirrhosis. The clinical symptoms of hemochromatosis are skin pigmentation, diabetes mellitus, and liver cirrhosis. Pigmentation of the exposed skin is severe, and hard and enlarged swelling of the liver is observed in 90% of the cases; diabetes mellitus is recognized in 80%.

Although there is no defined treatment for hemochromatosis, repeating phlebotomy may allow the patients' survival time to be prolonged. The main fatal causes are hepatic coma, cardiac failure, and hepatic carcinoma.

2.8 Liver Abscess

Sequence of Diagnostic Imaging.

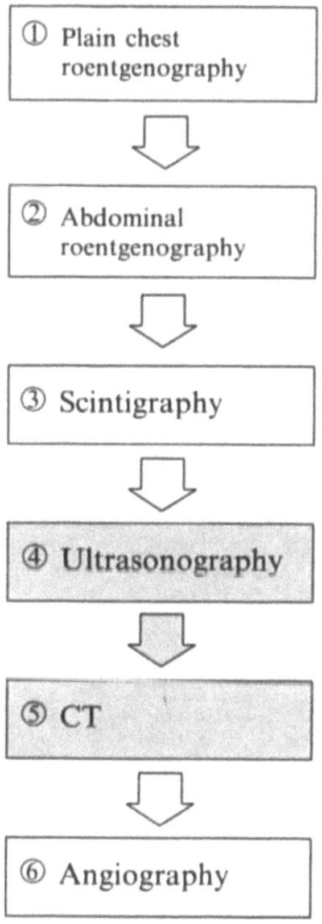

Patient. A 44-year-old woman.

Main Complaint. Fever, chill, general fatigue, and nausea.

History. Not specified.

Present Status. The patient has remittent fever and nausea associated with chill, pain in the right upper quadrant, and cough. A swollen liver is palpated 5 FB below the right costal margin. The patient has tenderness on pressure and percussion in the right upper quadrant with elevation of the upper limit of liver dullness.

Laboratory Data.

SGOT	142 mU/ml	↑
SGPT	206 mU/ml	↑
SGOT/SGPT	0.69	<1
ALP	363 mU/ml	↑
LDH	492 mU/ml	Normal
WBC	$19\,700/mm^3$	↑
Erythrocyte sedimentation	87 mm/h	↑
CRP	6+	↑

Purpose of Diagnostic Imaging. To detect the source of infection in the liver.

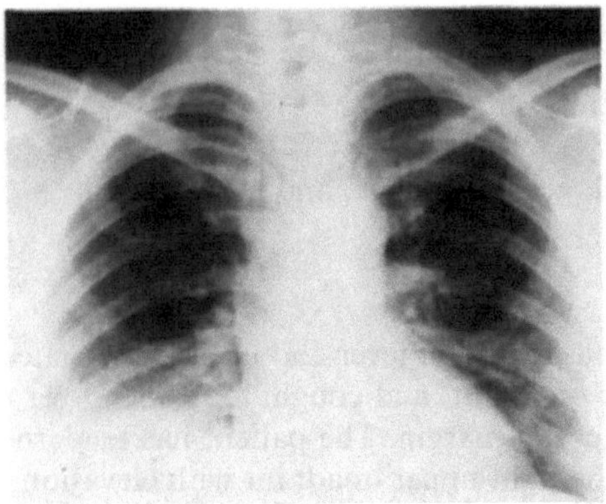

① Plain chest roentgenogram: A minor fissure is slightly thickened and separated, but normal in height. Elevation of the diaphragm, flattening of the costophrenic angle, and pooling of pleural effusion are observed.

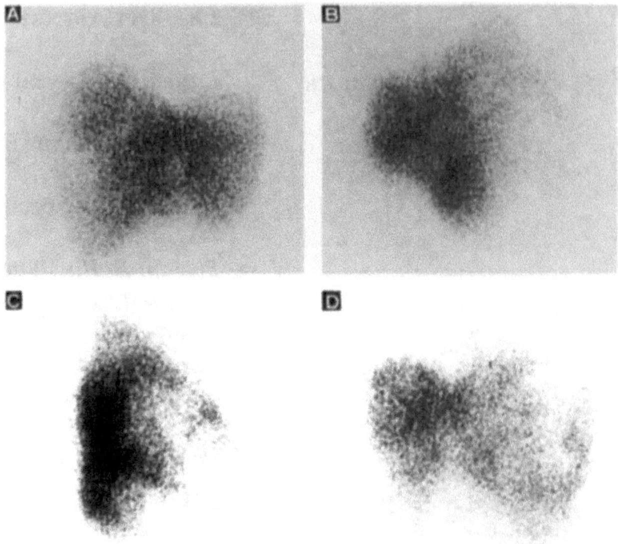

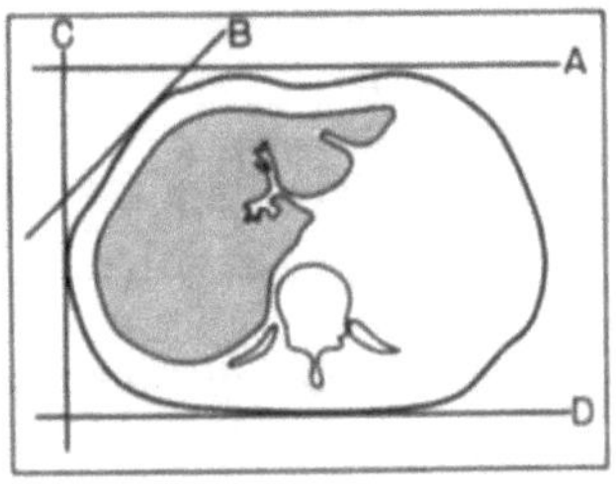

③ Scintigram
A Frontal view
B Right oblique view in 45°
C Right lateral view
D Posterior view
Liver scintigram (^{99m}Tc-phytate): Images of multiple defects in the lateral part of the right lobe are shown.

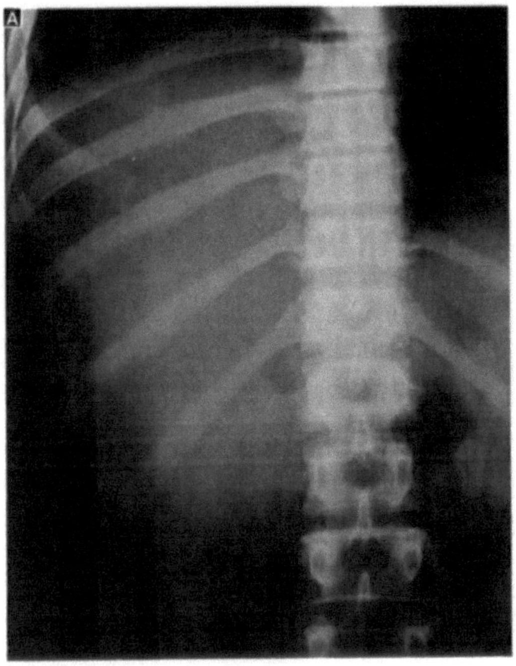

② Abdominal roentgenogram
A Plain abdominal roentgenogram: Swelling of the right lobe of the liver and pleural effusion are seen.

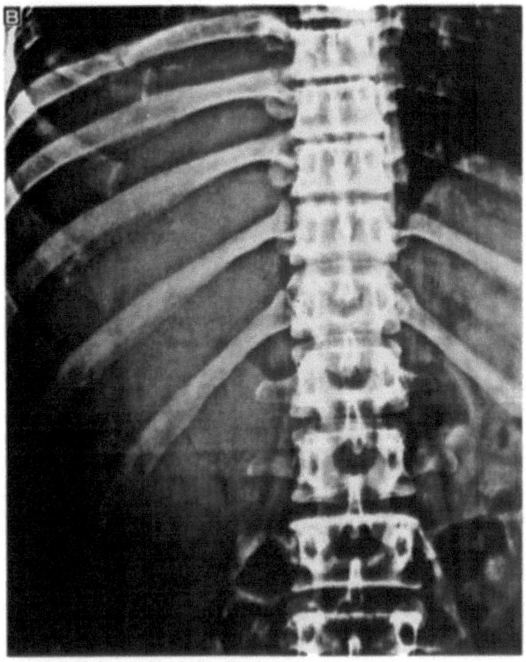

B Highly effective radiogram: A large translucency in the right lobe is visualized which cannot be observed on the plain roentgenogram.

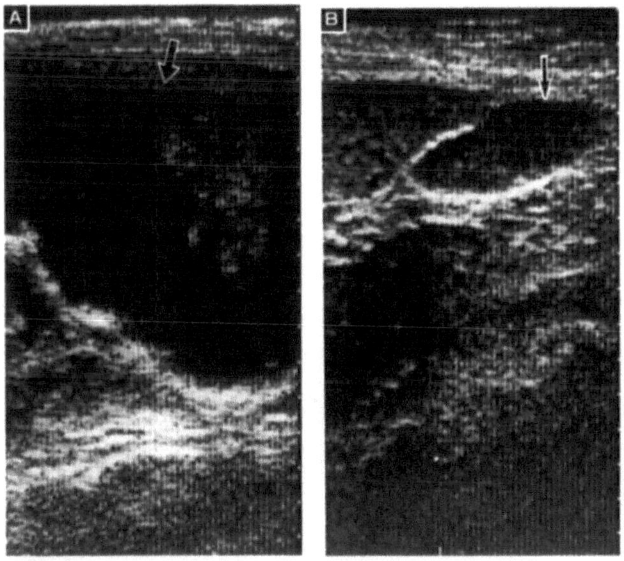

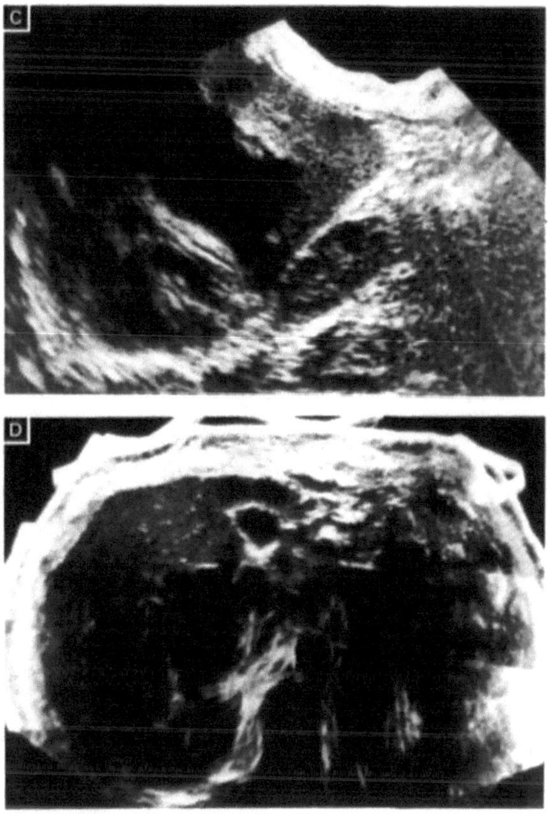

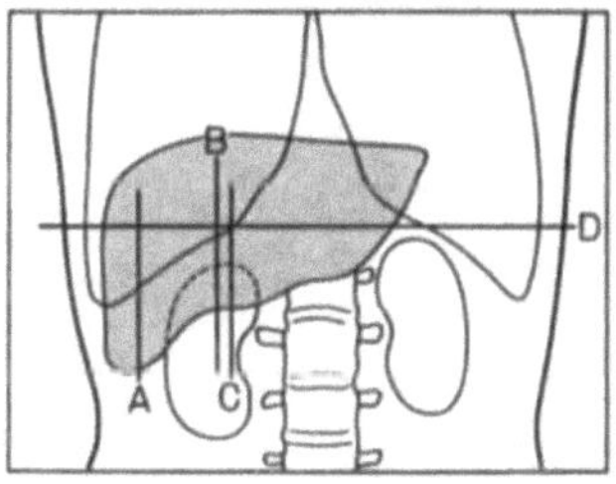

❹ Ultrasonogram
A, B Linear electronic scanning image: A large unechoic area with irregular contour is observed in the right lobe of the liver (→). No abnormality is seen in the gallbladder (→) and common bile duct.
C, D Contact compound scanning image: An unechoic region characterized by a multiple and multilocular image is observed with a clear septum.

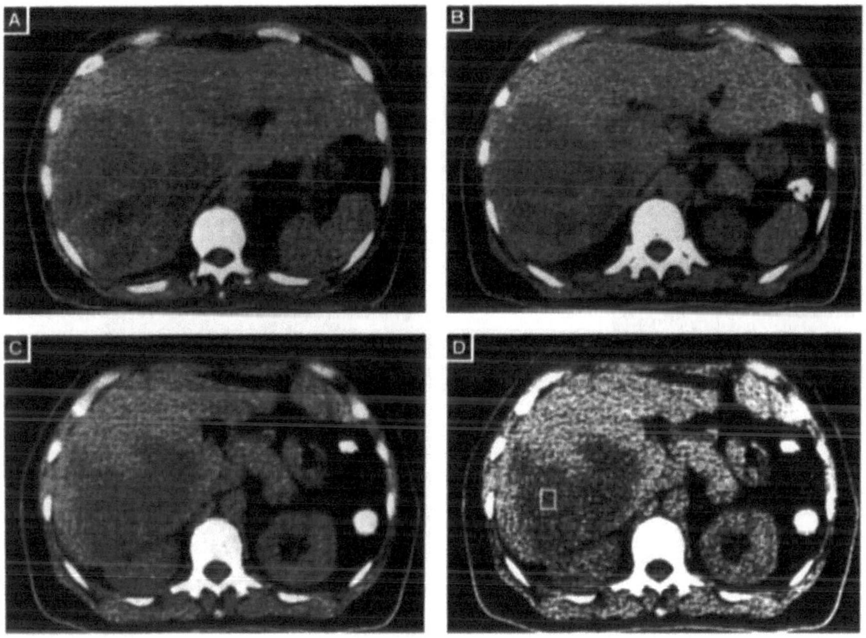

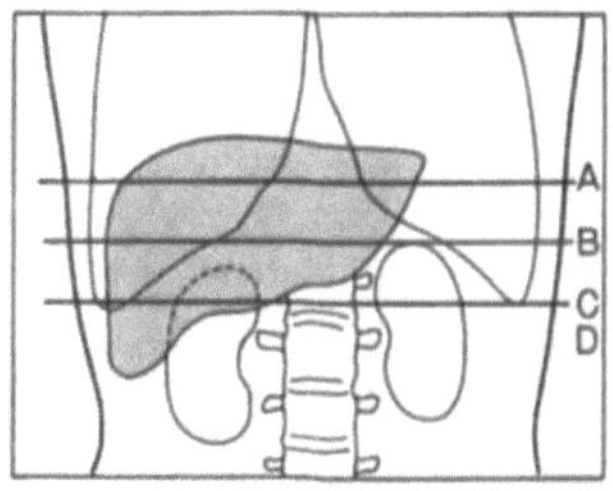

❺ CT image
A large low-attenuation area characterized by a multilocular image and a clear septum are observed. The CT number of the low-attenuation area is 14.1 HU and is higher than the water.

⑥ Angiography

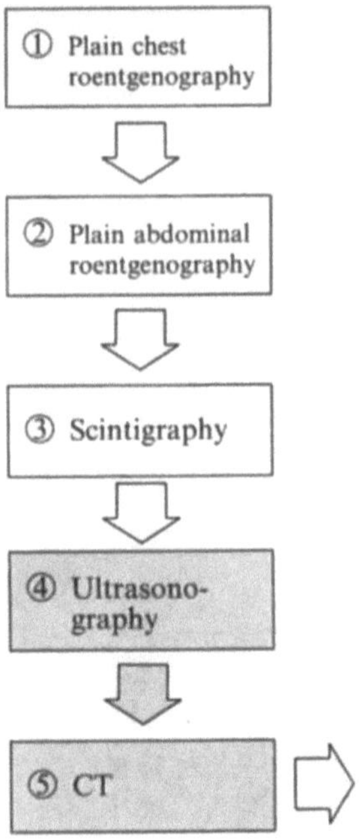

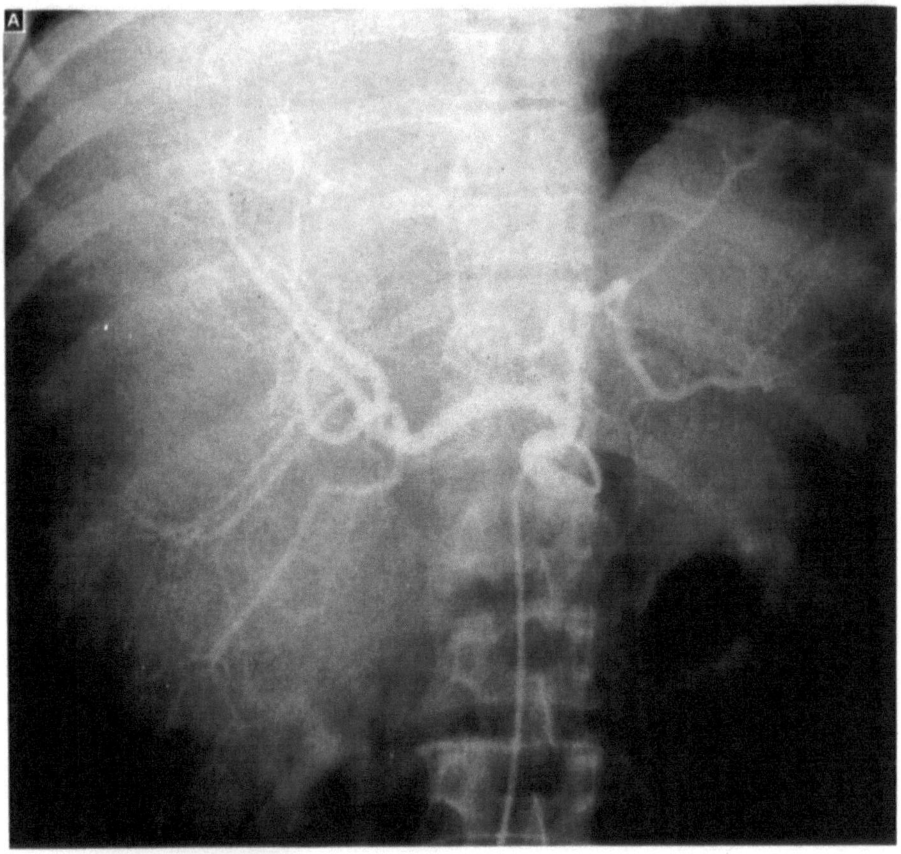

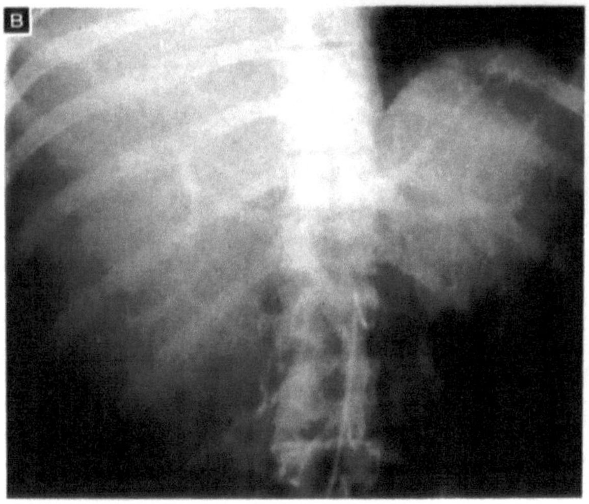

⑥ Angiogram
A, A′ Stereoscopic celiac arteriogram (arterial phase): Hypervascularity surrounding the avascular area is seen in the right lobe of the liver. Irregularity of the vasculature is not observed.
B Superior mesenteric arteriogram (venous phase): The portal vein runs around the avascular area. Interruption and occlusion of the portal vein are not observed.

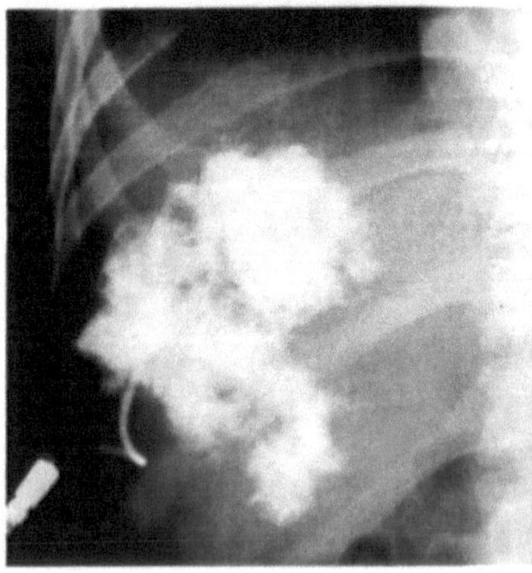

• Fistulography
Contrast medium is administered through the catheter after drainage. Abscesses comminicate with each other.

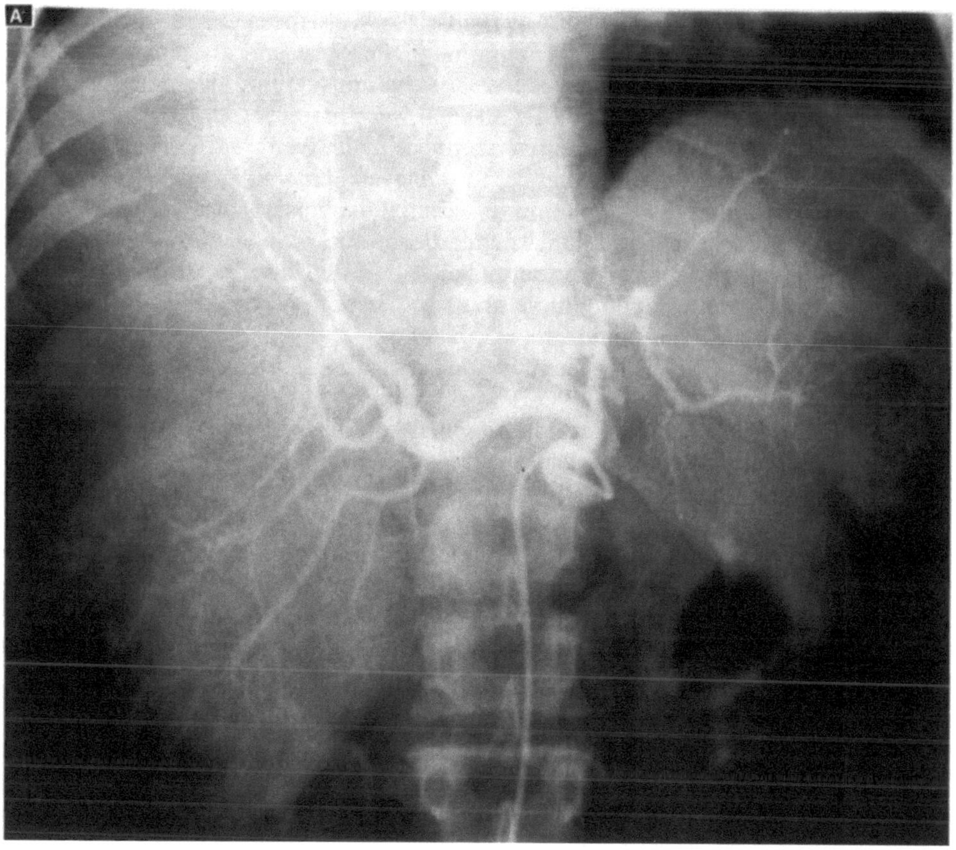

■ Treatment: Puncturing is performed under the guidance of ultrasound. Then a catheter is inserted to achieve drainage; 300 ml of drainage resulted in defervescence and the patient made good progress. Shown below are images after medical treatment.

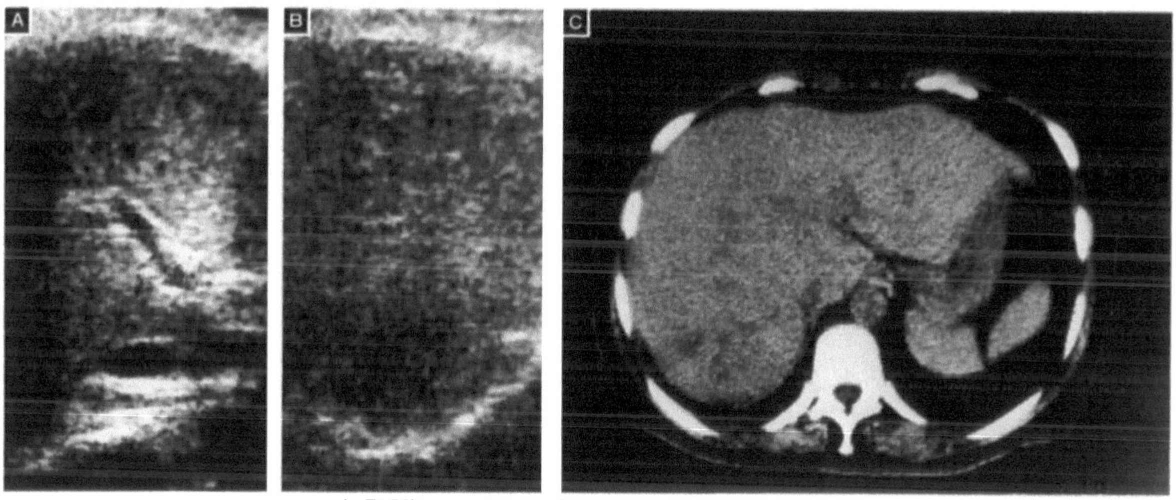

A, B Ultrasonogram: Linear electronic scanning image: 1 month after drainage, an abscess cannot be observed. **C** CT image: 2 months after drainage, only slightly low attenuation areas are observed.

Significance of Diagnostic Imaging. A liver abscess was suspected from the clinical symptoms and plain roentgenograms of the chest and abdomen. The liver scintigram also suggested a liver abscess, but definite diagnosis was impossible. Thus, ultrasonography and CT were required.

It is necessary to make a differential diagnosis from liver cyst, hydatid disease, and rarely hepatic carcinoma because they exhibit similar findings on ultrasonography and CT. A point for differential diagnosis is that a liver abscess shows a thickened wall and irregular contour, while a liver cyst exhibits a thin wall and regular contour. These findings, however, are not always clearly observable, and multiple small abscesses may sometimes be confused with parenchymal tumor.

Angiography is performed when a liver abscess is caused by malignant tumors or by unknown causes.

^{67}Ga-citrate is also useful for the diagnosis of massive liver lesion. However, differential diagnosis of liver abscess from malignant tumor is difficult because both cases show hot images.

General Matters Concerning Liver Abscess [26]. Liver abscesses are classified into pyogenic and amebic types, and in terms of formation can be divided into multiple and isolated types. Multiple pyogenic liver abscess is frequently caused by infection via the portal vein, hepatic artery, and bile duct.

Isolated pyogenic abscess is frequently chronically advanced with marked findings of a thickend wall of the abscess including granular formation. Infection routes are the portal vein, hepatic artery, neighboring organs, traumatic, and unknown routes. In two-thirds of pyogenic abscesses the pathogens are *Escherichia coli* and formerly *Staphylo-* and *Streptococcus aureus*. Recently, however, the use of antibiotics has changed the pattern of pathogens, causing an increase in anaerobic organisms and *Baccillus pyocyaneus*. In the case presented here, a gram-negative anaerobic organism was also detected.

Macroscopically, swelling of the liver is observed and sometimes misdiagnosed for multiple metastases to the liver accompanied by multiple abscesses. Hepatic cells occasionally necrotize into various sizes, and a large cavity with fusion of necrosis or honeycomb formation of a necrotic zone are seen.

For medical treatment, a large dose of an antibiotic agent is administered or a large abscess is drained. Conventionally, surgical drainage was performed, today percutaneous puncture drainage with ultrasound guidance to select the thick portion of the wall is also used.

Although the fatality rate is not high, dangerous conditions may develop depending on the kinds of pathogens and the time of definite diagnosis.

2.9 Hemangioma of the Liver

Sequence of Diagnostic Imaging.

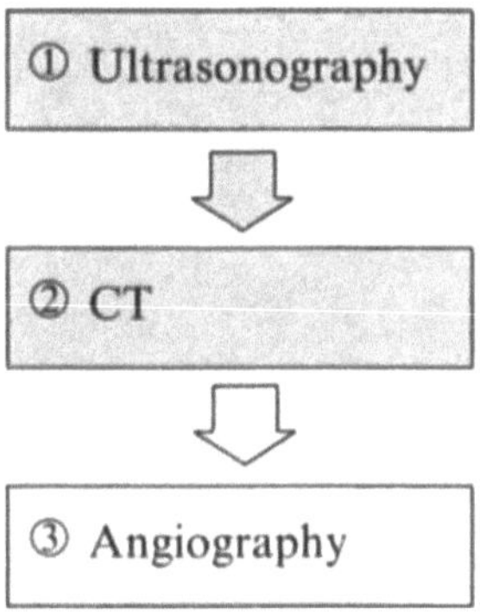

Patient. A 40-year-old man.

Main Complaint. Epigastralgia.

Present History. Epigastralgia occasionally for the past 3 years. He was hospitalized in the internal medicine department.

Present Status. The liver is not palpable. The patient experiences tenderness on pressure in the right hypochondrium.

Laboratory Data.

SGOT	29 mU/ml	Normal
SGPT	39 mU/ml	Normal
ALP	71 mU/ml	Normal
LDH	198 mU/ml	Normal
TTT	1 U	Normal
Total bilirubin	0.7 mg/dl	Normal
Direct bilirubin	0.1 mg/dl	Normal
AFP	3.5 mμg/ml	Normal

TTT, thymol turbidity test.

Purpose of Diagnostic Imaging. To examine the cause of epigastralgia.

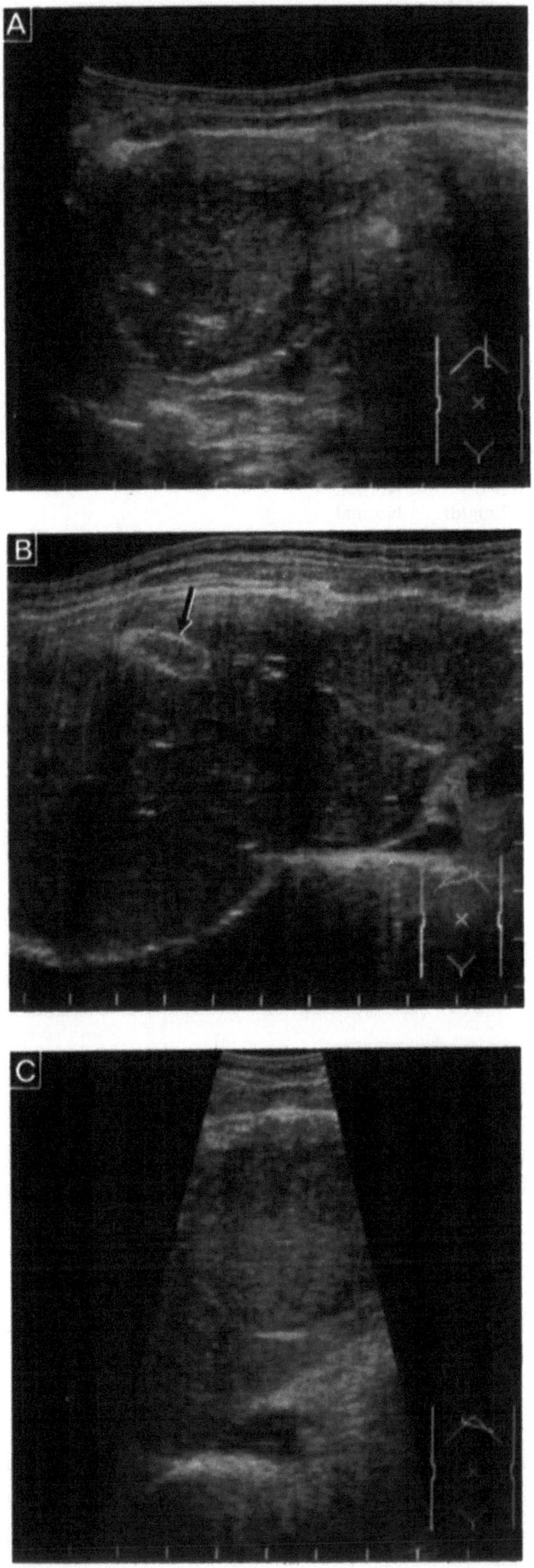

❶ Ultrasonogram
A, B Contact compound scanning (3.5 MHz)
C Sector electronic scanning (3.5 MHz)
Slight high echoic tumor 8 × 8 cm in size with lower echoic area within it is visualized in the lateral segment of the left lobe. It accompanies posterior echo enhancement. The gall-bladder is shrunken with a thickened wall (→).

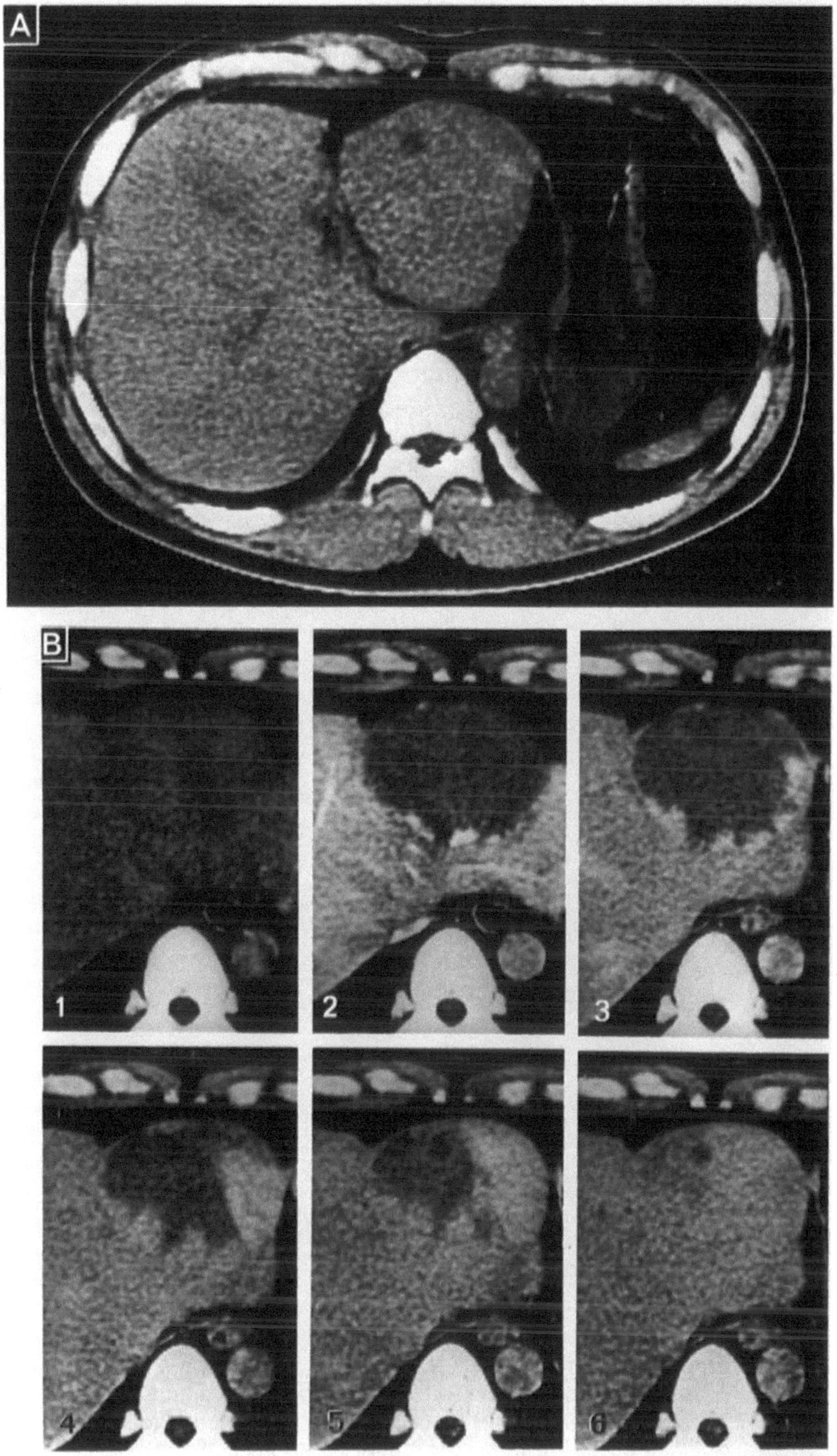

❷ CT image
A Precontrast scan
B Dynamic scan with bolus injection 1 Precontrast phase 2–6 Postcontrast phases 15 s (2), 70 s (3), 4 min (4), 10 min (5), and 20 min (6) after bolus injection
A tumor 8 × 8 cm in size with lower attenuation than the liver parenchyma is visualized in the lateral segment of the left lobe, and within it a much lower round attenuation area can be seen (**A**). On dynamic examination with a bolus injection of contrast media, the tumor gradually stains from the periphery to the center; 20 min after the injection (**B**), the tumor was almost completely stained except for the much lower attenuation area in the precontrast scan

③ Angiography

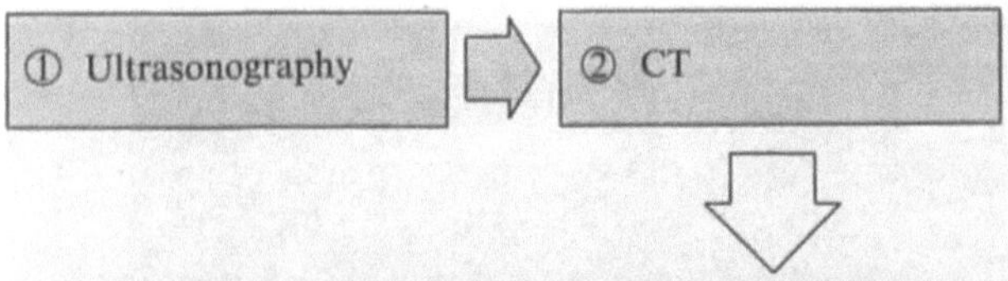

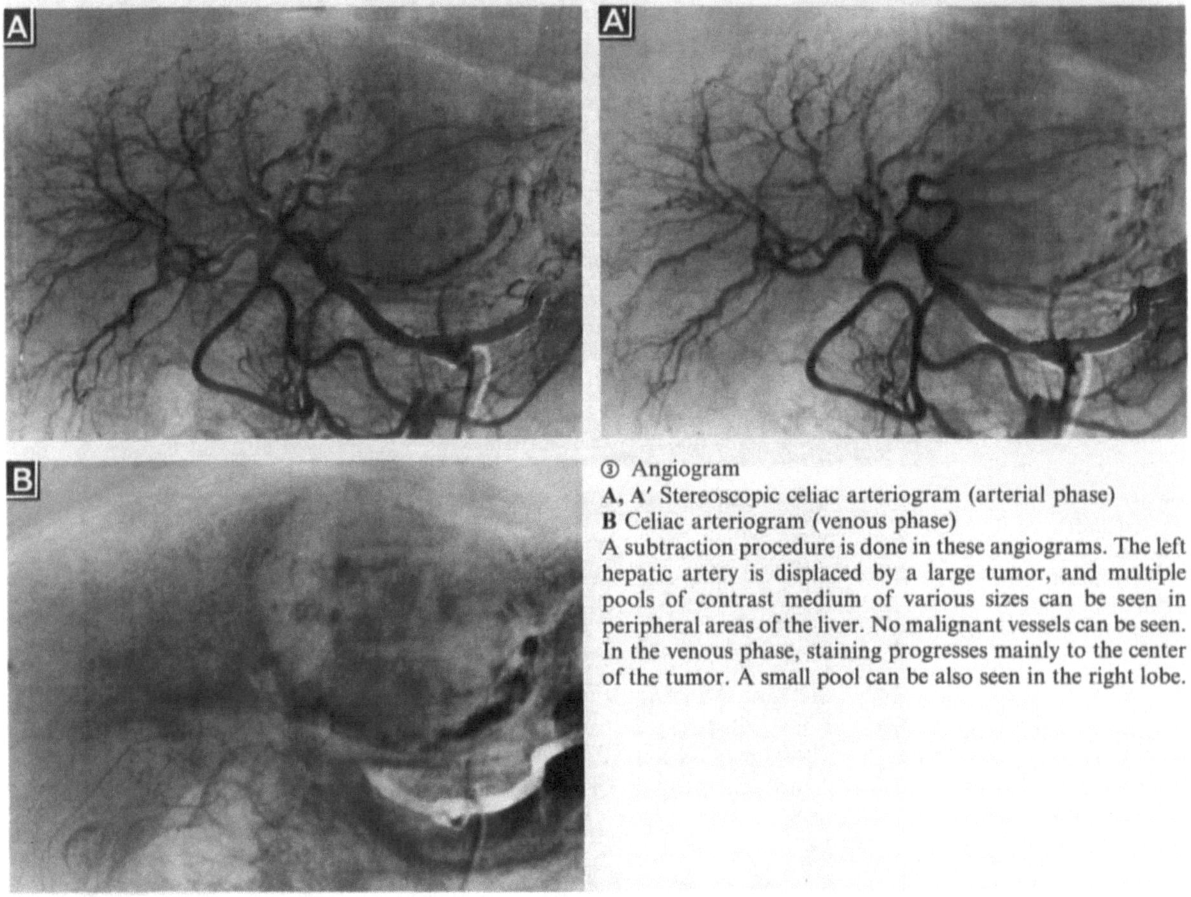

③ Angiogram
A, A′ Stereoscopic celiac arteriogram (arterial phase)
B Celiac arteriogram (venous phase)
A subtraction procedure is done in these angiograms. The left hepatic artery is displaced by a large tumor, and multiple pools of contrast medium of various sizes can be seen in peripheral areas of the liver. No malignant vessels can be seen. In the venous phase, staining progresses mainly to the center of the tumor. A small pool can be also seen in the right lobe.

Operative Findings. A left lateral lobectomy was performed with cholecystectomy. A cavernous hemangioma without malignancy was found. A small organized necrotic area was within the tumor. He has also cholecystitis with a gallstone.

Significance of Diagnostic Imaging. In this case, disorders of the biliary tract were suspected due to intermittent epigastralgia. Ultrasonography was performed first, and a tumor of the lateral lobe of the liver was detected unexpectedly.

CT with progressive scanning after bolus injection of contrast medium is very useful for the diagnosis of hemangioma. A characteristic finding of hemangioma is gradual staining from the periphery to the center.

Some authors maintain that the central area frequently remains unstained, but so far as our experience is concerned, a tumor is completely stained when it is small in size. Angiography may be necessary when the tumor is not completely stained in the delayed contrast CT scan.

General Matters Concerning Hepatic Hemangioma [22]. Hepatic hemangioma is the most frequent among benign tumors of the liver, representing 0.7%–9% of autopsies, performed following death from a liver tumor. Among all hemangioma cases, 19% occur in the liver. The sex distribution ratio between males and females is 1:1.3–6, and hemangioma occurs more frequently in people above 40 years than under 40 years of age.

Hepatic hemangioma is classified into capillary and cavernous. Cavernous hemangioma is more common. In most cases, hepatic hemangioma is single. Multiple hemangioma occurs in 10% of all cases. Generally, it is under 5 cm in diameter and rarely exceeds 30 cm. The tumors have clear boundaries, but capsules are not observable.

When a hemangioma becomes large thrombus develops inside it and then cicatrization and fibrosis occur. Fibrosis originates in the center of the tumor, occasionally causing entire hardening or calcification. Generally, cavernous formation is observed in the blood-filled sinuses, which are histologically surrounded with septum consisting of connective tissue.

Correlation between hemangioma and female hormones is suspected, because of its frequent occurrence in pregnancy.

Usually no symptoms appear, but in some cases marked enlargement of the tumor or involvement of other organs may occur. Rarely, severe bleeding may also take place. Treatment is by surgical resection, but radiation therapy may be effective in large or multiple types.

2.10 Hepatoblastoma

Sequence of Diagnostic Imaging.

① IVP
⇩
② Scintigraphy
⇩
③ CT
⇩
④ Angiography

Second Examination

① Ultrasonogram
⇩
② CT
⇩
③ Angiography

Patient. A 7-month-old baby girl.

Main Complaint. Abdominal mass.

Present History. Seven months after birth, another clinic diagnosed the abdominal mass and the patient was hospitalized.

Present Status. A hard bosselated tumor with an irregular edge is palpated on the right upper abdomen.

Laboratory Data.

Blood		
SGOT	69 mU/ml	↑
SGPT	18 mU/ml	↓
LDH	849 mU/ml	↑
TC*	712 mg/dl	↑
TB	2.0 mg/dl	↑
AFP	over 10000 mμg/dl	↑
Hb	11.6 g/dl	normal
Platelet	44.2	↓
Urine		
VMA	(−)	

* Total cholesterol.

Purpose of Diagnostic Imaging. To identify the localization and differentiation of the abdominal mass.

First Diagnostic Imaging

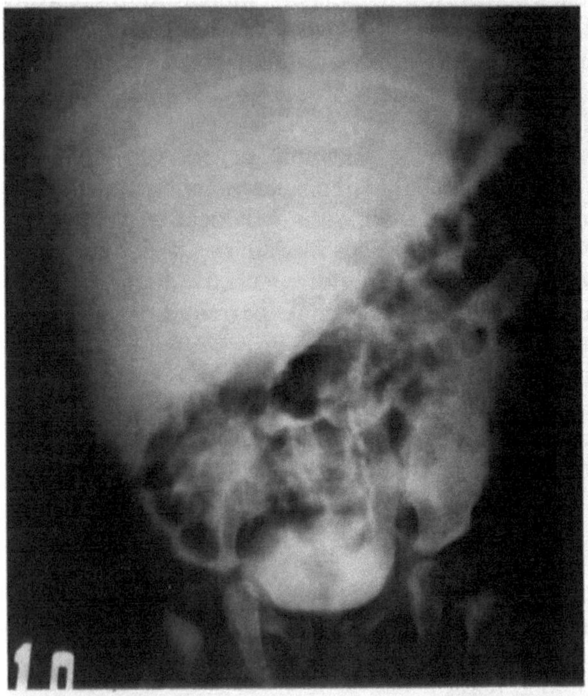

① IVP image
Localization and morphology of the kidney are normal but hepatomegaly is observed.

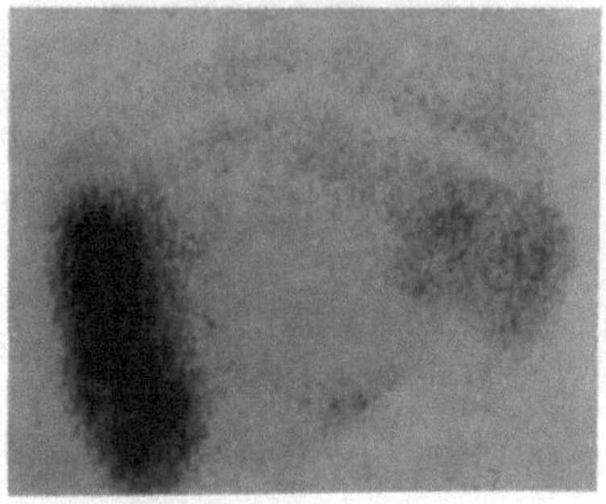

② Scintigram
Liver scintigram (^{99m}TC-phytate): A large defect area is seen in the central portion of the liver.

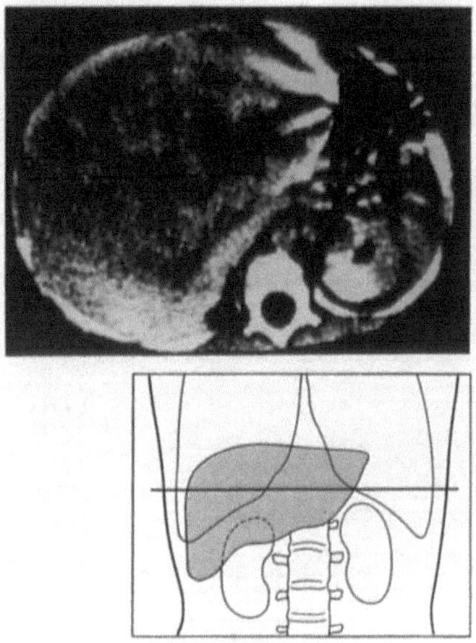

③ CT image
An irregular low-attenuation area expanding over both lobes of the liver is seen, but the CT number is 51 HU, suggesting a solid mass.

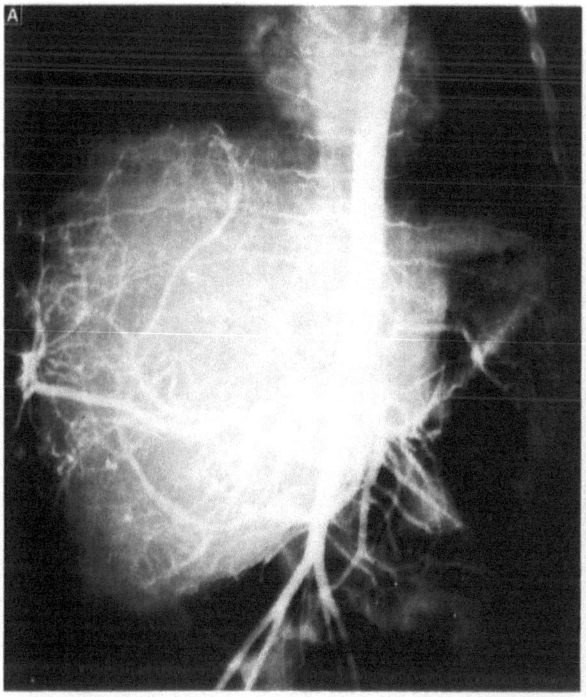

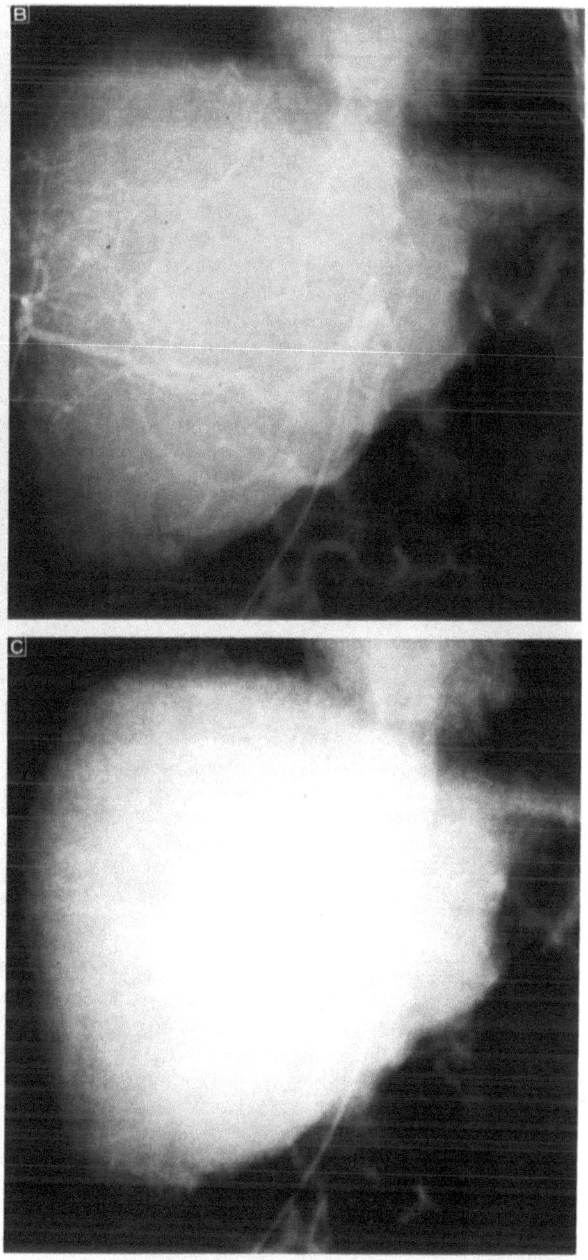

❹ Angiogram
A Abdominal aortogram (arterial phase): Hypervascular tomors in the liver are seen.
B Celiac arteriogram (arterial phase): Increased diameter of the right hepatic artery and its branches are angulate and tortuous in their course. In the capillary phase, the lateral inferior part of the right lobe remains normal while vivid tumor vessels, which run indirectly in a loop form, are seen in the right lobe. Additionally, vessels feeding the tumor branch off from the left hepatic artery, but this region is relatively hypovascular.
C Celiac arteriogram (venous phase): Clear pooling is not seen although mottled staining image is observed.

Progress. After inoperable hepatoblastoma was diagnosed vincristine and adriamycin were administered intravenously. Since the tumor was decreased in size, diagnostic imaging was performed again 3 months later, and a palliative operation was determined to be possible.

Second Diagnostic Imaging

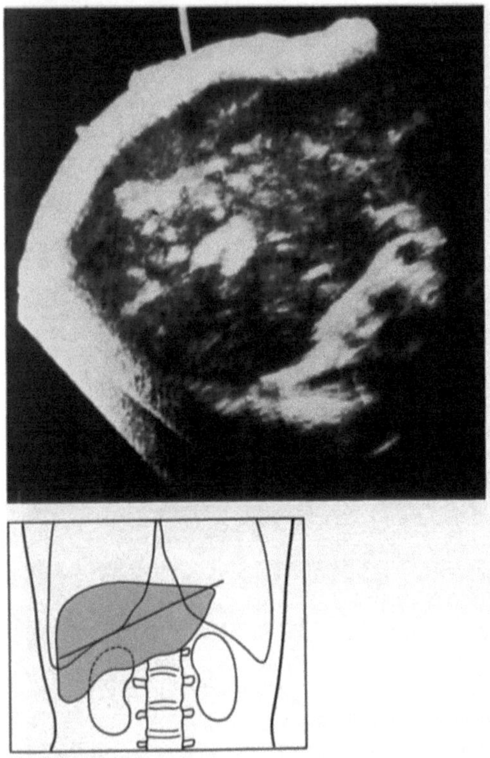

① Ultrasonogram
Contact compound scanning: Several inhomogeneous echogenic masses are observed in the liver.

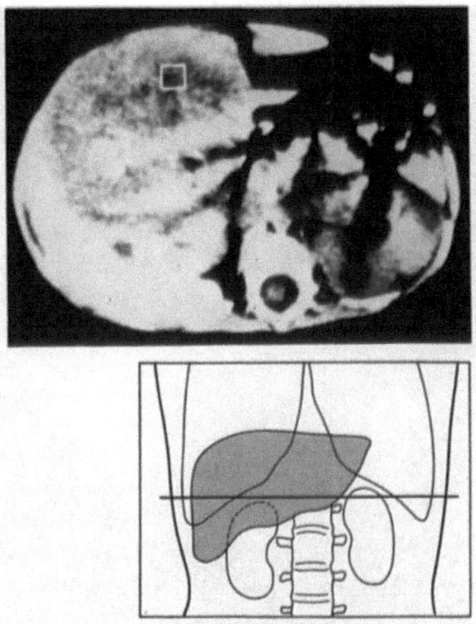

② CT
Although the tumor is decreased in size, an uneven low-attenuation area is seen in the central portion of the liver; the CT number is 29 HU in the lowest attenuation area.

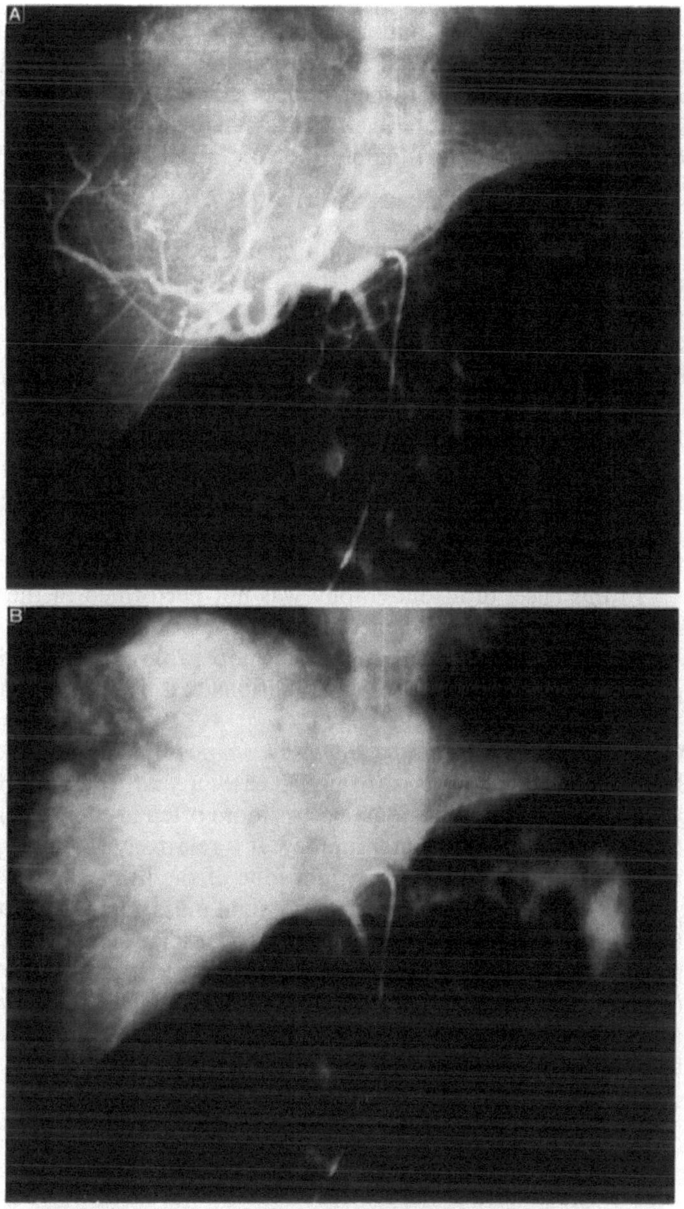

❸ Angiogram
A Celiac arteriogram (arterial phase): The right hepatic artery is reduced in diameter and the tumor is decreased in volume. The tumor is fed by the right and left hepatic arteries. The tumor is fist-sized and located in the central portion of the liver. In both lateral sides of the liver, normal tissue still remains. The tumor, consisting of multiple nodules, has abundant small vessels and occupies 80% of the volume of the liver.
B Celiac arteriogram (venous phase): Several vivid nodular staining images are seen.

Operative Findings. A tumor, located in the central portion of the liver, mainly occupies the medial segment of the left lobe. Normal tissue is seen in the lateral side of both hepatic lobes. Although trisegmentectomy was performed and the entire liver was resected except for the lateral segment of the left lobe, unfortunately the day after the operation, the patient suddenly died.

Histological Findings. A well-differentiated hepatoblastoma was determined and classified as stage III (T_3, C_1, V_0, N_0, M_0).

Significance of Diagnostic Imaging. With liver scintigraphy and CT, the existence of a tumor in the liver was clearly indicated. Hepatoblastoma was strongly suspected since the case was an infantile malignant tumor in the liver. The tumor was identified from angiography.

Although a diagnosis of infantile hepatoblastoma could be suspected from an increasing level of AFP and total cholesterol and a palpable mass, angiography contributed greatly toward definite diagnosis and indication for operation.

In this case, ultrasonography was not performed in the first series of imaging examinations. Generally, however, ultrasonography and CT are beneficial for tracing the progress of inoperable cases. In this respect, CT performed in the first set of examinations can be regarded as valuable.

General Matters Concerning Hepatoblastoma [4]. In Japan, the frequency of hepatoblastoma is approximately 30 cases a year, often in infants under 2 years of age. Hepatoblastoma occurs more often in early infancy and hepatocellular carcinoma in later infancy. It is relatively more frequent in males and notably originates in the right lobe of the liver.

The main symptoms are an abdominal mass and gastrointestinal symptoms such as abdominal pain with fever. Jaundice often appears in the latest stage. The clinical findings are an increase in the levels of AFP, LDH (especially L_4 and L_5), total cholesterol, and SGOT, very occacionally accompanied by liver dysfunction. Urine cystathionine is positive and sometimes platelets may increase.

2.11 Hepatocellular Carcinoma

Sequence of Diagnostic Imaging.

① Scintigraphy

⇩

② CT

⇩

③ Angiography

Patient. A 52-year-old woman.

Main Complaint. Not specified.

Present Status. There is hepatomegaly, and the patient is under medical treatment for liver cirrhosis and diabetes mellitus.

Laboratory Data.

SGOT	73 mU/ml	↑
SGPT	45 mU/ml	↑
ALP	30 mU/ml	Normal
LDH	219 mU/ml	Normal
γ-GTP	208 mU/ml	↑
ZTT	13.6 U	↑
TTT	11.0 U	↑
HBs Ag	(−)	
HBs Ab	(+)	
AFP	2007.4 mμg/dl	↑

Purpose of Diagnostic Imaging. For the prior 2 years, the patient has been medically treated for liver cirrhosis. Recently, the level of AFP increased, and hepatic carcinoma was suspected.

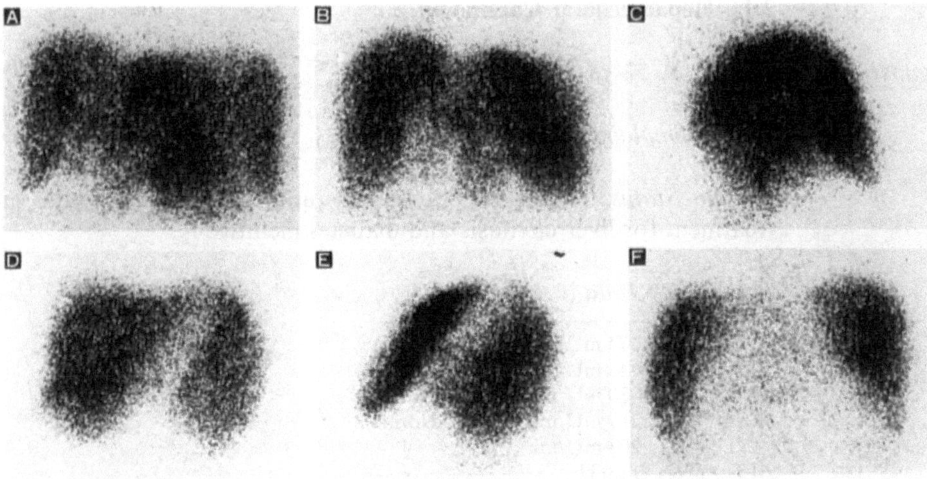

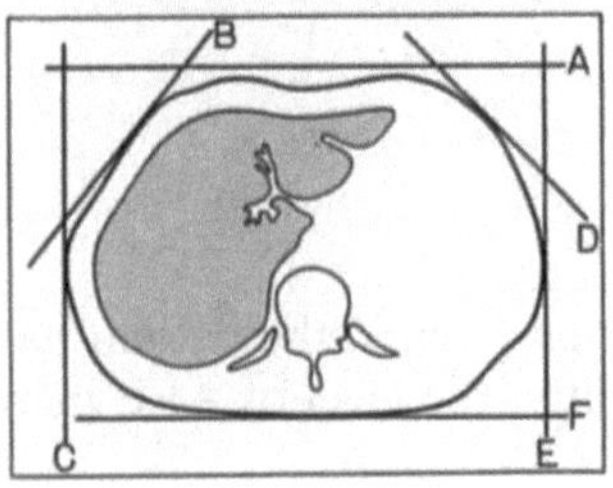

① Scintigram
A Frontal view
B Right anterior oblique view
C Right lateral view
D Left anterior oblique view
E Left lateral view
F Posterior view

Swelling of the left hepatic lobe, increasing uptake of RI into the spleen and particularly by the bone marrow, splenomegaly, and inhomogeneous image of the liver are characteristic findings of liver cirrhosis. However, a space-occupying lesion cannot be clearly seen.

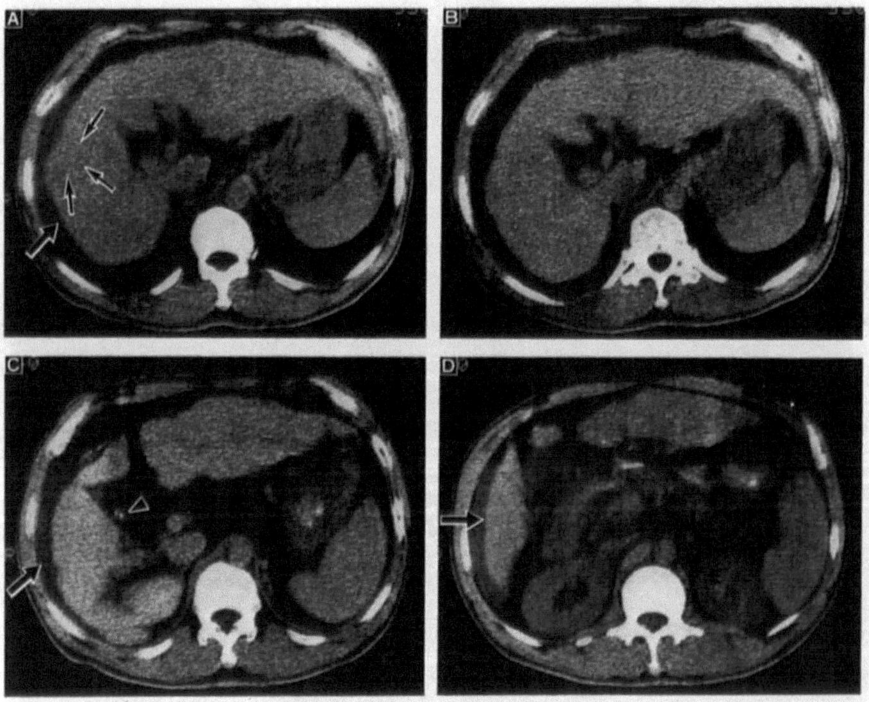

② CT image
A, D Before contrast enhancement
B, C After contrast enhancement

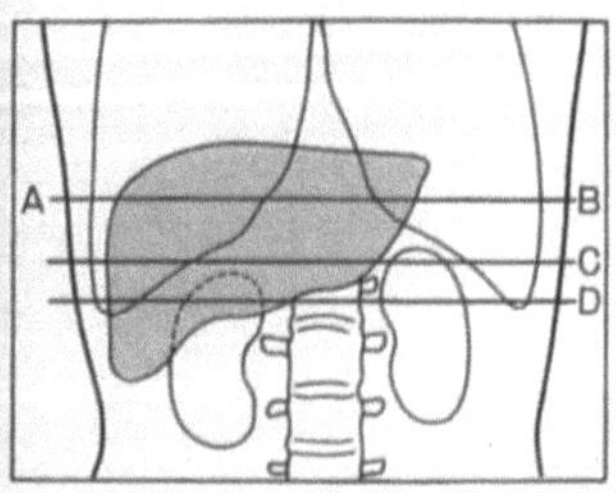

Atrophy of the right lobe, swelling of the lateral segment of the left lobe, uneven surface of the liver, splenomegaly, and ascites (→) are seen. In the superior lateral region of the right lobe, a lower attenuation area than surrounding the liver (→) is observed corresponding to the prominent portion. This region, however, is not clearly seen after contrast enhancement by the drip infusion method. No findings suggesting space-occupying lesions are observed in any other areas. A stone image (▶) is seen in the gallbladder. After contrast enhancement, varices are visualized posterior to the stomach.

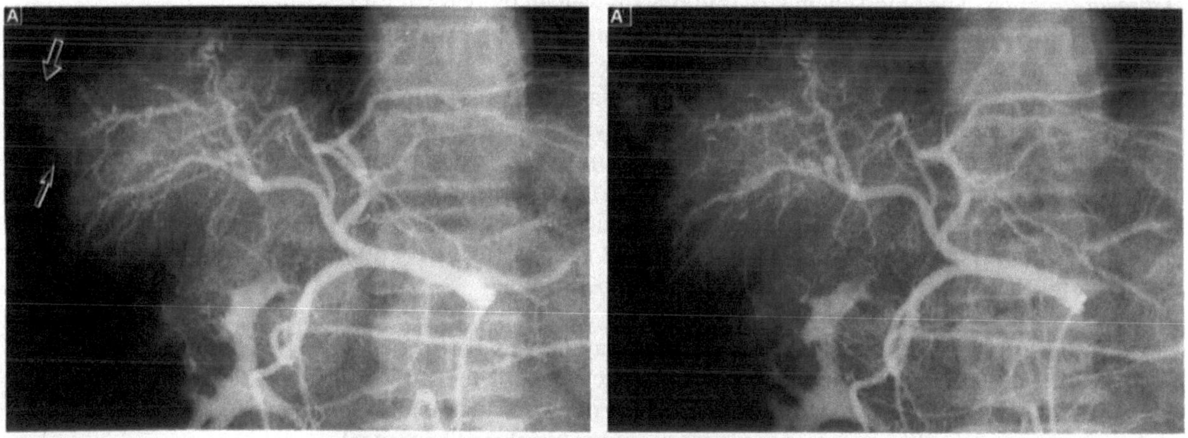

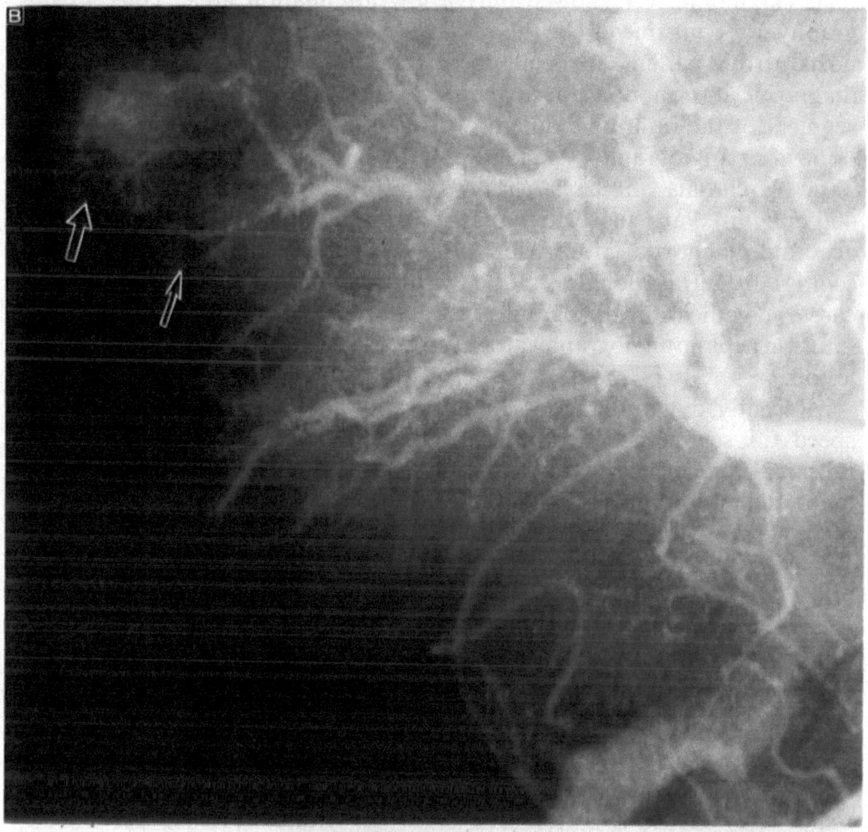

❶ Angiogram
A, A′ Stereoscopic common hepatic arteriogram (arterial phase)
B Magnification common hepatic arteriogram (arterial phase)
C Superior mesenteric arteriogram (venous phase)

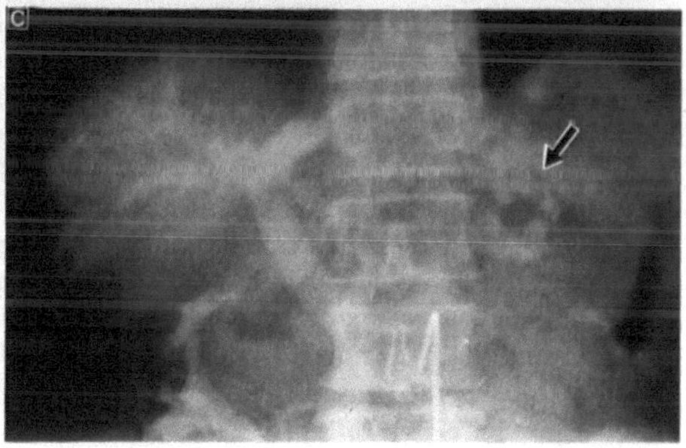

The right hepatic artery is angulated and tortuous, showing characteristic images of liver cirrhosis. In the left lobe, vessel stretching due to compensatory swelling is demonstrated. A vessel fedding the tumor 1.8 × 2.5 cm in size is demonstrated in the lateral side of the posterior segmental branch of the right hepatic artery. Irregular tumor vessels and staining image are observed (→). A smaller tumor (→) is observed just inferior to the above-mentioned tumor. The coronary vein and clear varices in the cardiac portion of the stomach are seen (→) in the venous phase. However, disorders of the intrahepatic portal venous tract cannot be observed on this angiogram.

Clinical Progress. The blood chemistry findings showed an increase of GOT up to 139 mU/ml, GPT to 92 mU/ml, and AFP to 3500 mμg/ml 1 month after the examination just before the operation.

From laparotomy, nodules about 5 mm in diameter caused by liver cirrhosis were detected on the surface of the liver with a finding of ascites. Lobectomy was impossible due to the advancement of the liver cirrhosis; only a probe biopsy was performed. Histopathologically, the case was a well-differentiated hepatocellular carcinoma. For medical treatment, radiation therapy was performed with 3000 rad of cobalt gamma rays, with poor results, and the patient died 4 months after the operation.

Significance of Diagnostic Imaging. Diagnostic imaging was performed to identify the existence of hepatic carcinoma suspected from the rapid increase in the level of AFP while following up the progress of liver cirrhosis. A liver scintigram could not detect the location of the suspected hepatocellular carcinoma. CT showed only a low attenuation area. Thus, angiography was confirmed to be the valuable diagnostic technique for the diagnosis of this patient. Also, ultrasonography could not provide accurate diagnostic information due to poor visualization of the superior lateral segment of the right lobe due to obstruction by the lung although it was done after angiography. Angiography is essential for the diagnosis of hepatic carcinoma in cases with a notably high level of AFP (over 400 mμg/ml). Particularly in the case of a tumor under 1–2 cm in diameter, accurate diagnostic information cannot be obtained from either a liver scintigram, ultrasonogram, or CT with conventional techniques. In such cases, magnification angiography, ultraselective hepatic arteriography, and infusion hepatic angiography are necessary to demonstrate the pathological lesion.

Recently, dynamic CT or CT angiography which is performed with high speed CT scanning under intravenous bolus injection or under arterial injection is regarded to enable detection of small hepatic carcinoma as a high-attenuation image. Thus, these are valuable techniques in cases with high levels of AFP.

General Matters Concerning Hepatocellular Carcinoma [2, 3, 8, 9, 14, 16, 20, 22, 29]. Primary hepatic carcinoma is classified into hepatocellular carcinoma originating from the liver cells, cholangioma from the bile duct cells, and their mixed type, in addition to infantile hepatoblastoma. In Japan, the frequency of hepatocellular carcinoma is high, accounting for 70%–80% of all primary hepatic carcinoma. The statistics for 1975 report 2824 cases of hepatocellular carcinoma in Japan. The sex distribution ratio between males and females is 3–4:1. The occurrence ratio is 15–25 per 100000 persons and rapidly increases after 45 years of age. Hepatocellular carcinoma ranks sixth highest among malignant neoplasms in autopsy cases.

The etiology of hepatocellular carcinoma is considered to be closely associated with hepatitis B virus because the hepatitis B antigen is positive in 40%–50% of patients. It is regarded that in many cases hepatocellular carcinoma occurs after advancement of liver cirrhosis. Around 80% of the cases are associated with liver cirrhosis, while 30%–40% of liver cirrhosis are accompanied by hepatocellular carcinoma. Hepatocellular carcinoma associated with liver cirrhosis is frequently the B and B′ type of Miyake's classification.

Conventionally, the macroscopic classification of hepatic carcinoma by Eggel (1901) has been used: (a) massive, (b) nodular, and (c) diffuse. The nodular type, which includes various sized tumors, is most frequent and represents 50%–60% of all cases. The massive type in which a large tumor occupies the hepatic lobe accounts for 30%–40%, and the diffuse type in which small nodules exist diffusely is the least frequent, representing slightly over 10% based on autopsy results. However, according to clinical data, massive tumor is the most frequent, the nodular type is the second, and the diffuse type is the least frequent. This difference is regarded as being caused by intrahepatic metastasis of the massive tumor as tumor growth propresses, making it difficult to differentiate between the nodular type and the massive type. At any rate, resectability is high at 30%–40% in the massive type, and around 5% in nodular type, while the diffuse type is almost impossible to resect. In hepatocellular carcinoma, the tumor often generates into the right lobe of the liver.

Histologically, Edmondson's calssification is commonly used with I–IV types related to cell differentiation.

Grade I is probably best reserved for those areas in grade II carcinomas where the difference between the tumor cells and hyperplastic liver cells is so minor that the diagnosis of carcinoma rests upon the demonstation of more aggressive growths in other parts of the neoplasm. This condition resembles benign adenoma. In grade II carcinoma, a well-differentiated type, the cells show a marked resemblance to normal hepatic cells. The nuclei are larger and more hyperchromatic than normal but the cytoplasm is abundant and acidophilic. The lumina of acini are often filled with bile. In grade III carcinoma, the nuclei are larger and more hyperchromatic than those of grade II. These nuclei occupy a relatively greater proportion of the cell. Bile and acinar formation are noted less frequently. In grade IV carcinoma, a poorly differentiated type, the nuclei are intensely hyperchromatic and occupy the greater part of the cell. The cytoplasm is often scanty and contains fewer granules. The trabeculae are difficult to find. Actually, these types coexist in many cases.

In *The General Rules for the Clinical and Pathological Study of Primary Liver Cancer* by the Liver Cancer Study Group of Japan [5], small liver cancer is defined as under 2 cm in maximum diameter on liver scintigraphy. Even small liver cancer does not always have a good prognosis due to associated cirrhosis.

At present, metastasis of primary hepatic carcinoma is frequent because it is not detected in an early stage. Based on autopsy findings, the rate of metastases is about 66% in hepatocellular carcinoma and 86% in cholangioma. In both cases, the rate of metastases to the lung is 40%–50%, to the lymph nodes 35%–52%, and 17%–33% of cases are a direct extension to the peritoneum, which is more frequently metastasis from cholangioma. Hepatocellular carcinoma tends to infiltrate into portal or hepatic veins, i.e., tumor thrombus, and occurs in about 10% of all cases. Intrahepatic metastasis of hepatocellular carcinoma is also frequent. However, carcinoma may originate multicentrically in the liver. Thus, multiple tumor in the liver is difficult to be differentiated from intrahepatic metastasis or multicentrically originating cancer.

Initial symptoms of primary hepatic carcinoma are discomfort, pain, and fullness of the abdomen, anorexia, and general fatigue. When diagnosed, many cases are in an advanced stage, and the liver swelling is detected in 90% of cases. Feverescence may also be observed during the clinical course.

Primary hepatic carcinoma is complicated by bleeding from esophageal varices in about 20% of cases and gastric ulcer in 10%. Also, tumor rupture into the abdominal cavity is found in 3%–6% and bloody ascites in 12%–13%. Liver abscess is a complication in about 10% of cholangioma and in about 1% of hepatocellular carcinoma.

A laboratory finding of hepatocellular carcinoma is positive serum AFP. In AFP measurement, radioimmunoassay (RIA) is the most sensitive enabling the measurement of AFP to within 2 mμg/ml. With RIA, 90% of the cases of hepatocellular carcinoma show high values of AFP, and 80% of the cases exceed 1000 mμg/ml. The level of AFP may also be high in cases of diffuse hepatocellular diseases, occasionally exceeding 1000 mμg/ml. However, with progressive measurement, a high level of AFP is obtained continuously in hepatocellular carcinoma, while it is measured transitionally in diffuse hepatocellular diseases becauses the abnormal increase of AFP is caused by regeneration of liver cells. In diffuse hepatocellular diseases, a high level of AFP hardly continues over 3–6 months. However, in cases of AFP levels over 400 mμg/ml, examination is necessary to identify the existence of hepatocellular carcinoma.

In cases of chronic hepatitis or liver cirrhosis, a sudden increase in the level of AFP during continuous observation of slightly abnormal AFP of 100–200 mμg/dl may suggest the existence of liver carcinoma. Thus, it is necessary to precisely examine for the presence of hepatocellular carcinoma. In such cases, however, frequently the cancer has already advanced. In cholangioma, the level of AFP is below 100 mμg/dl or negative in most cases. In metastatic liver carcinoma, AFP turns to positive in 30%–40% of cases, but rarely exceeds 400 mμg/dl. As for the relationship between hepatitis B antigen (HBs Ag) and AFP, a positive ratio of AFP in hepatocellular carcinoma with positive HBs Ag is higher compared to that with negative HBs Ag, suggesting that patients with positive HBs Ag are to be regarded as a high risk group who tend to hepatocellular carcinoma.

Primary hepatic carcinoma is clinically misdiagnosed as extrahepatic bile duct carcinoma in about one-third of cases and may also be misdiagnosed as metastatic carcinoma of the stomach, pancreas colon, and lung. Forty percent of primary carcinoma cases are overlooked due to liver cirrhosis accompanying hepatic carcinoma. Another 40% was misdiagnosed as another cancer with metastasis to the liver.

Surgical resection is the only radical treatment, but in cases of adults in Japan, many are accompanied by liver cirrhosis making resection impossible. Additionally, the cancer itself has already advanced in many cases; thus, the resectability of hepatocellular carcinoma is a little over 20%. Resectability of cholangioma is about 21% and that of hepatoblastoma is comparatively high at about 50% because it is not accompanied by liver cirrhosis and the massive type is common. In many cases of hepatic carcinoma, the patient dies 5 months after the appearance of symptoms. In resected cases, two-thirds of the patients die within 1 year. The most fatal cause is recurrence of the cancer. The 5-year survival rate is 5%–20% in cases of successful operations. In hepatoblastoma, the 5-year survival rate is high, exceeding 60%.

Chemotherapy plans with anticancerous agents are by intravenous injection and by continuous intra-arterial infusion. In addition, one injection using the technique of angiography is also employed. At any rate, these techniques only increase the survival rate a littles.

Transcatheter embolization therapy using angiography has also been carried out recently. This procedure proved to be effective in reducing the tumor volume. The cumulative survival rate of patients with unresectable hepatocellular carcinoma was 44%–52.6% at 1 year, 20.3%–29% at 2 years, and 15% at 3 years.

2.12 Hepatocellular Carcinoma

Sequence of Diagnostic Imaging.

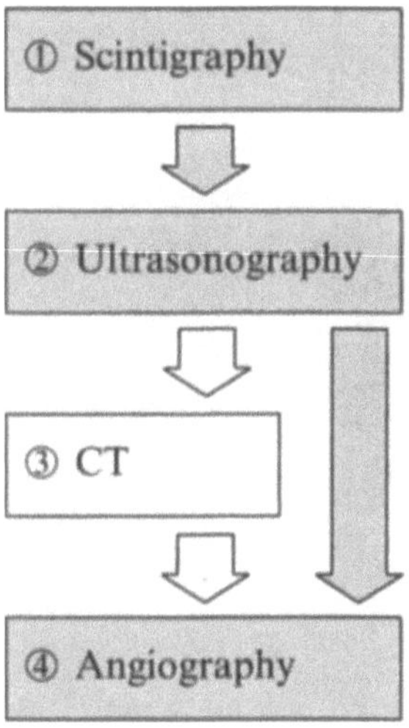

Patient. A 77-year-old woman.

Main Complaint. Abdominal mass.

History. Pulmonary tuberculosis at 60 years of age. Ingestion of alcohol is about 300 ml of beer a day.

Present History. Ten years prior, a mass the size of a ping-pong ball on the right side superior to the navel was noticed but neglected. For the past 3 years, the mass has gradually grown with dull pain appearing during fatigue or deep respiration. The patient had acute pain a week prior and was admitted to another clinic and then referred to our hospital.

Present Status. The liver is palpated 4 FB below the right costal margin. A hard guitar-shaped mass is palpable at the epigastrium, which moves on respiratory and is easily mobile. Jaundice, ascites, palmar erythema, and vascular spider are not observed.

Laboratory Data.

SGOT	57 mU/ml	↑
SGPT	22 mU/ml	Normal
ALP	186 mU/ml	↑
LDH	268 mU/ml	↑
γ-GTP	95 mU/ml	↑
Cho E	380 U/dl	Normal
Total bilirubin	6.8 mg/dl	Normal
Direct bilirubin	0.5 mg/dl	Normal
ZTT	5.1 U	Normal
AFP	78.5 mμg/dl	↑
HBs Ag	(−)	
CEA*	(−)	

* Carcinoembryonic antigen.

Purpose of Diagnostic Imaging. To identify the origin of the abdominal mass.

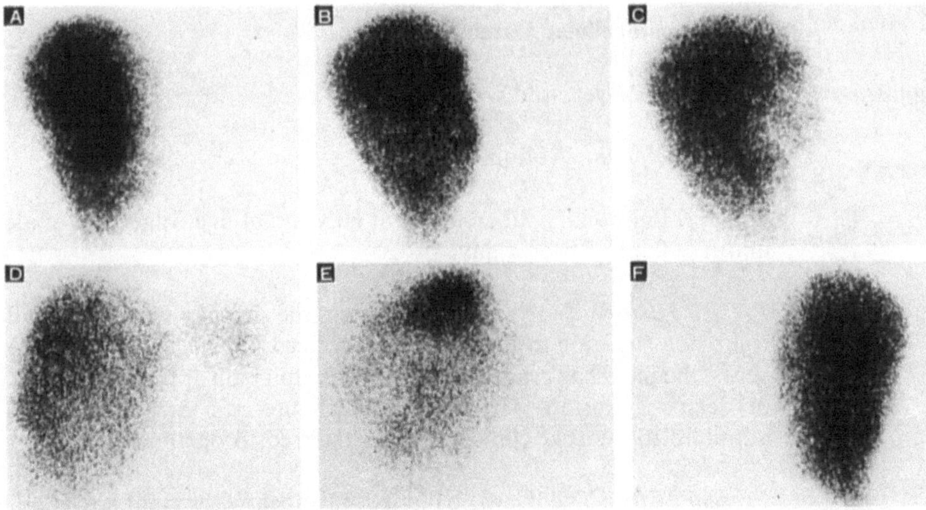

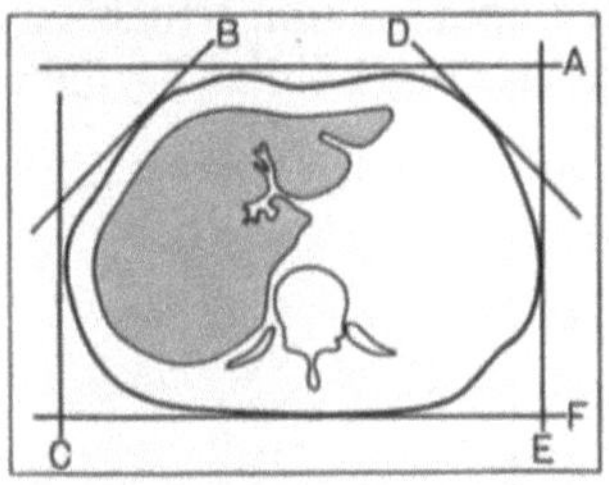

❶ Liver scintigram
Images of a defect is observed almost entirely in the left lobe of the liver.

A Frontal view
B Right anterior oblique view
C Right lateral view
D Left anterior oblique view
E Left lateral view
F Posterior view

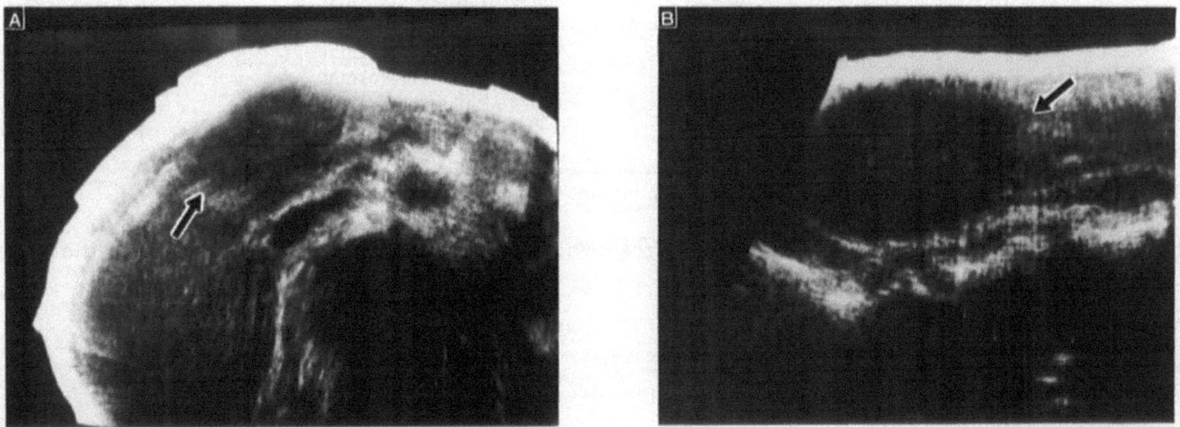

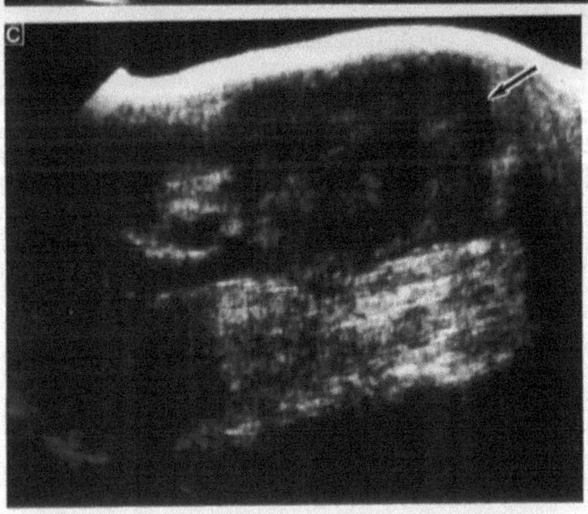

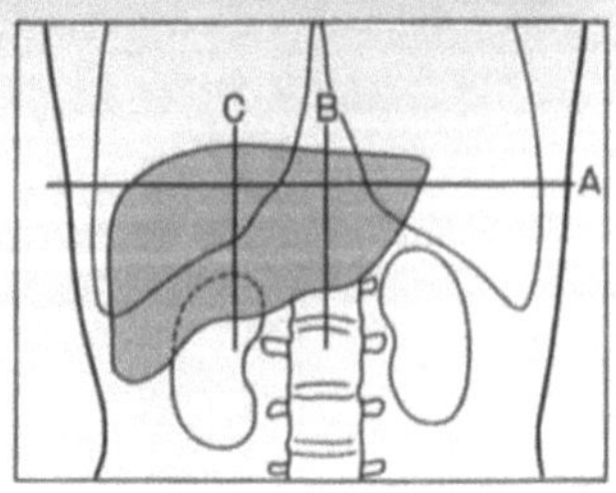

❷ Ultrasonogram
A–D Contact compound scanning: Two masses are visualized on the ultrasonograms. One occupies the left hepatic lobe (→) and the other is prominent out of the liver (→). Both masses show low internal echo images including lower echoic areas suggesting necrosis. The prominent mass moves inferior to the liver and becomes separated from the liver in the sitting position.

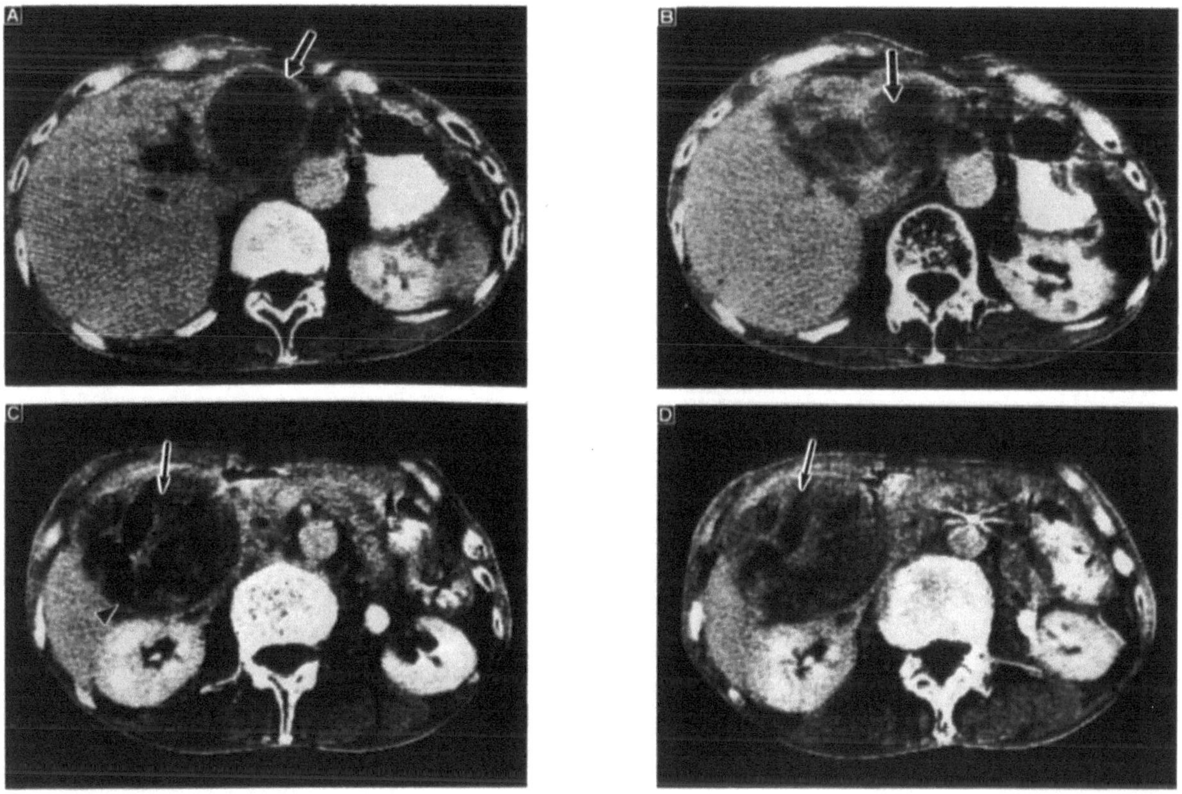

③ CT images
A–D After contrast enhancement
The CT image shows a round low-attenuation area with clear contour (→) in the left lobe and another larger round low-attenuation area (→) at the lower portion of the mass. A capsule of the mass (▶) separates the right hepatic lobe and the right kidney. Necrosis is more severe in the lower one. Multiple cysts are visualized in the right kidney.

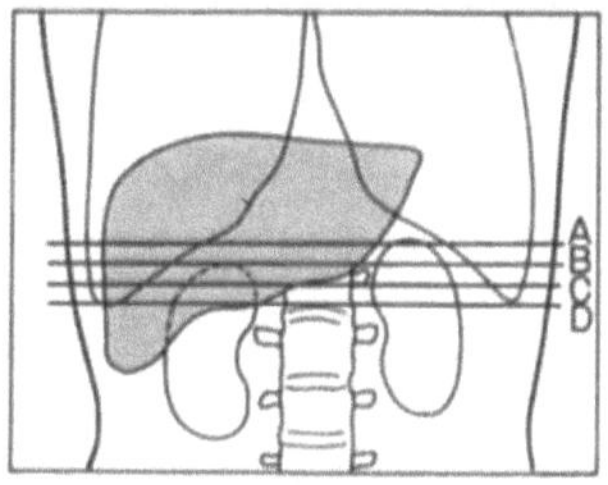

④ Angiography

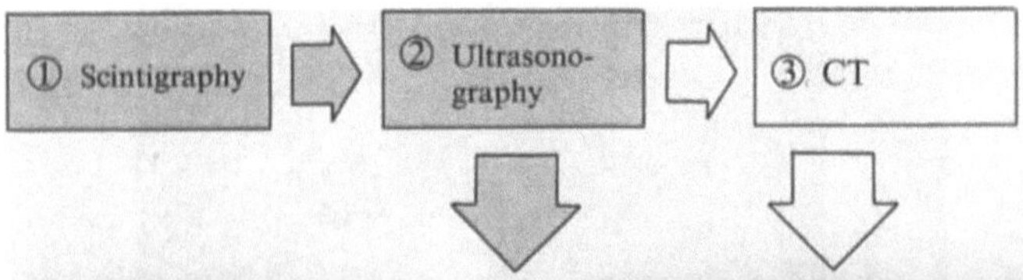

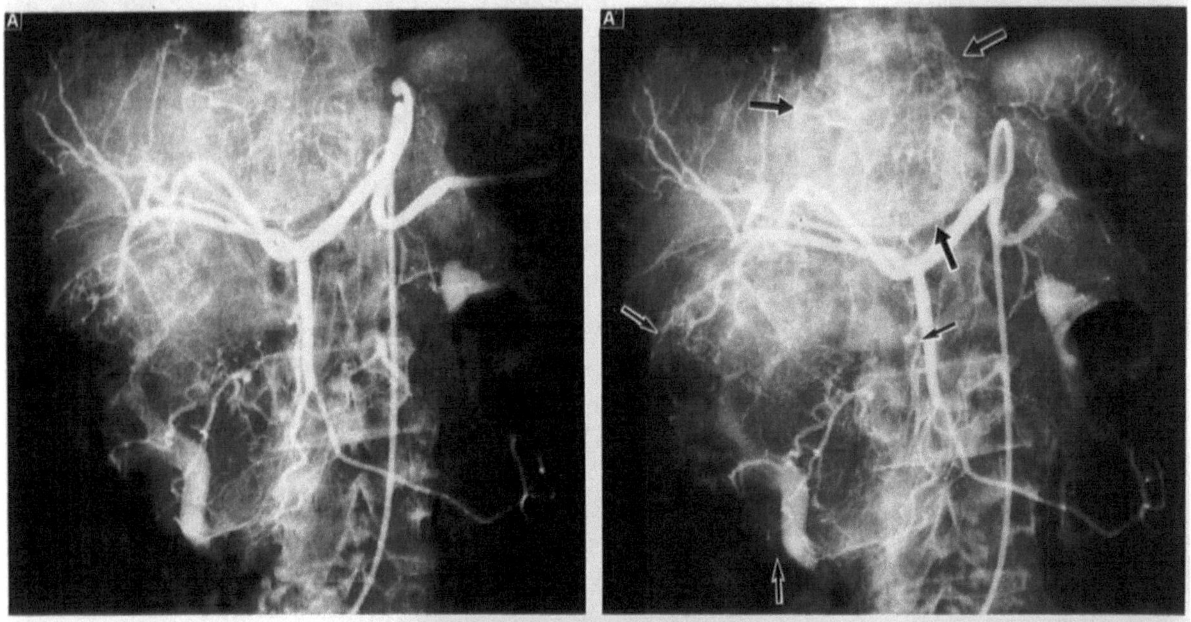

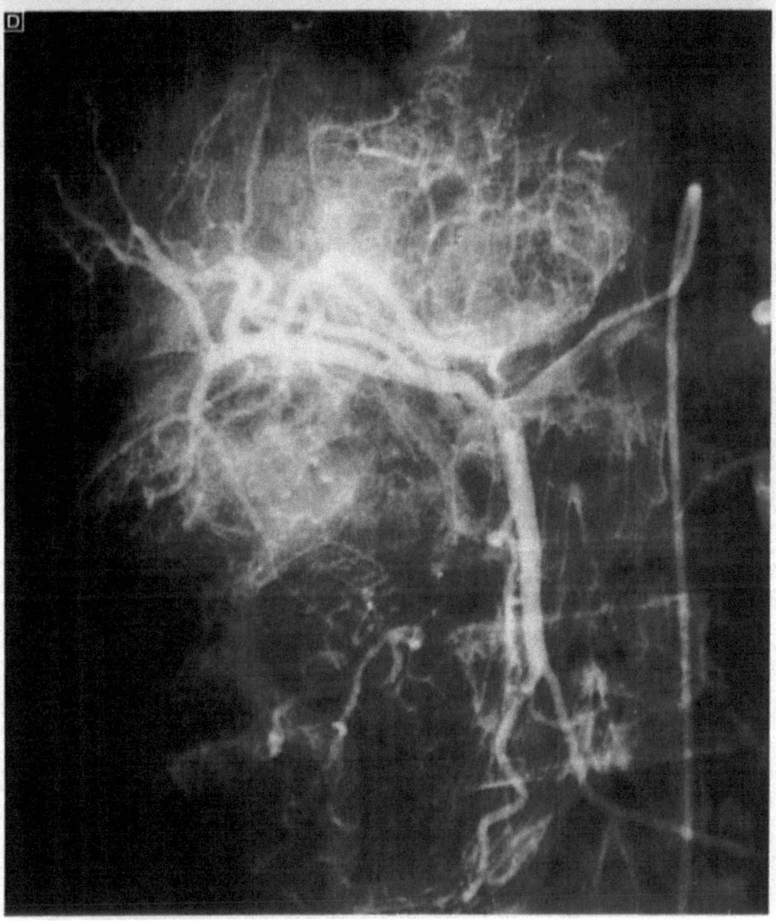

❹ Angiogram
A, A′ Stereoscopic common hepatic arteriogram (arterial phase)
B Common hepatic arteriogram (capillary phase)
C Superior mesenteric arteriogram (portal phase)
D, D′ Stereoscopic magnification common hepatic arteriogram (arterial phase)
The two masses (➞, →) are fed by the left hepatic artery. Tumor-feeding arteries branch from the thick capsule-feeding artery and show encasement. The tumors are gradually stained from the capillary to the venous phase, although they are not clearly seen. A hypovascular area suggests necrosis, and no arterioportal shunt is observed. The left portal branch is not opacified.

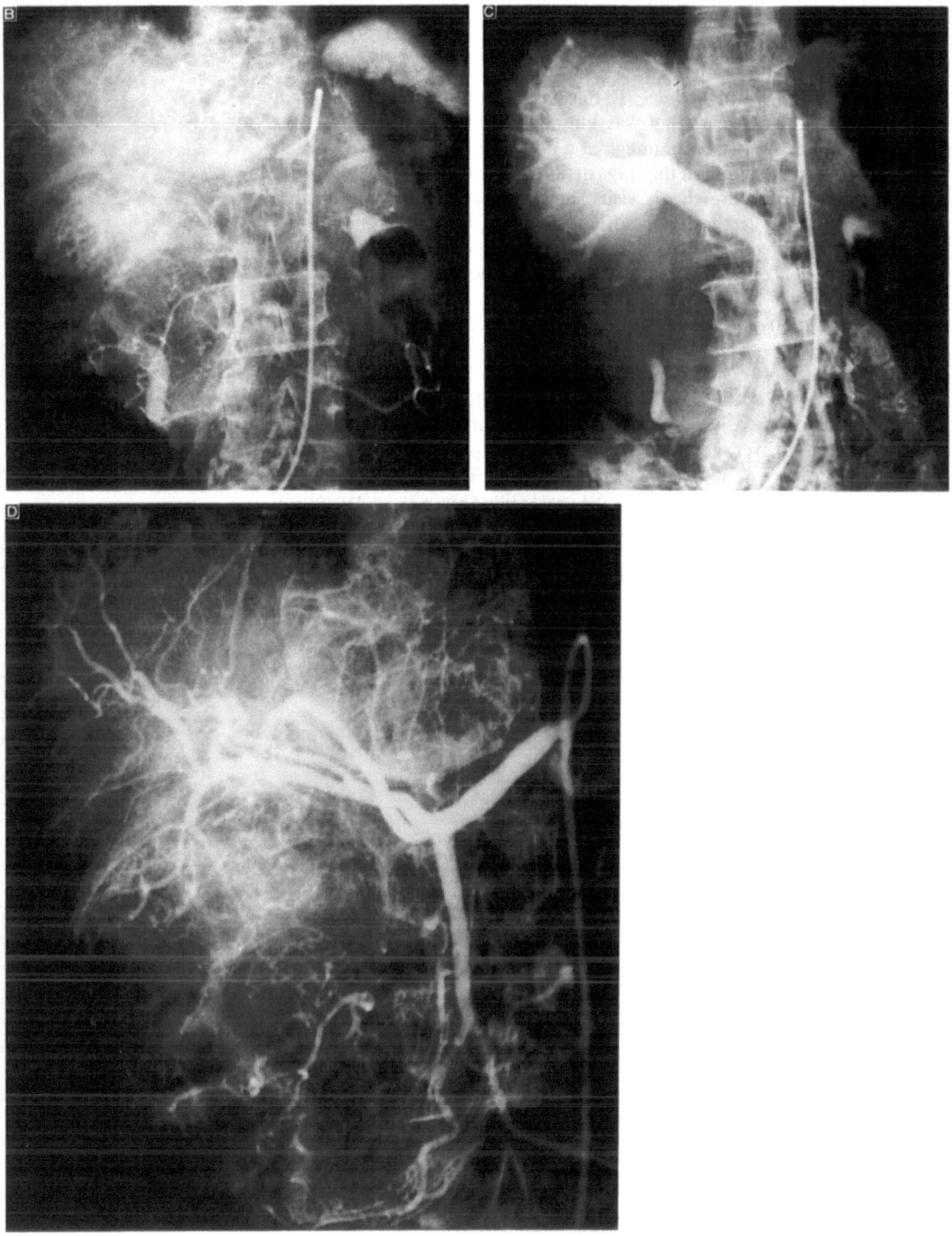
B
C
D

Operative Findings. Two guitar-shaped tumors with irregular surfaces, each 8 × 8 cm and 8 × 11 cm in size, are observed in the left side of the falciform ligament without communicating with each other. Both tumors are encapsulated. No liver cirrhosis can be observed. There is no metastasis to the surrounding lymph nodes. Histologically, both tumors are hepatocellular carcinoma and type I–II in Edmondson's classification. The lower larger tumor is regarded as a pedunculated tumor and diagnosed as primary carcinoma of the slow growing type.

Significance of Diagnostic Imaging. In this case, identification of the origin of the tumor at the epigastrium was initially required. Although a liver scintigram can demonstrate an image of a defect in the left lobe, the relationship between the tumor at the epigastrium and that in the left lobe is not ascertainable. CT can also clearly visualize the tumor, but the relationship of the lower tumor with the liver is difficult to determine. Ultrasonography, where scanning direction is freely selectable, is superior to CT and liver scintigraphy when observing the relationship of the tumor at the epigastrium with the liver and examining the solidity of the tumor in the left lobe. Needless to say, angiography is ultimately required.

General Matters Concerning Pedunculated Hepatic Carcinoma [6, 17, 18, 23, 31].There have been only ten cases of pedunculated hepatic carcinoma reported in Japan where it is decribed as originating in the accessory hepatic lobe or the ectopic liver tissue. Eggel's macroscopic classification (massive, nodular, diffuse) is not applicable to pedunculated hepatic carcinoma. Although liver cirrhosis accompanies most cases, this case was an exception. A slow-growing hepatoma has a capsule formation and belongs to type I–II of Edmondson's classification. Although identification in clinics is impossible, this case is suspected to have had a long history with the tumor growing during the previous 10 year or the massive accessory hepatic lobe having cancerated in 3 years.

2.13 Cholangiocarcinoma

Sequence of Diagnostic Imaging.

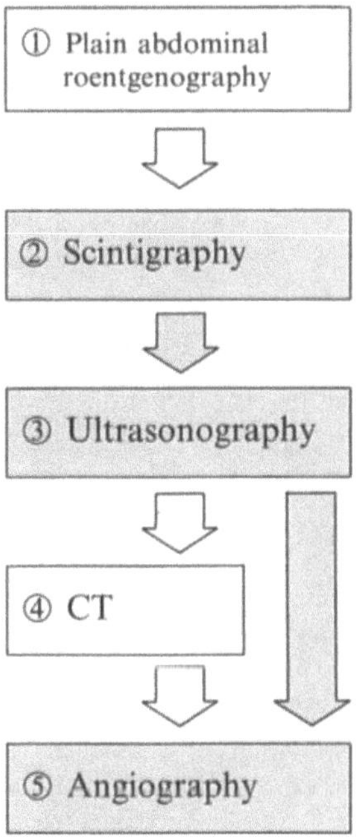

Patient. An 83-year-old man.

Main Complaint. Anorexia and left hypochondralgia.

Present Status. The liver is palpated 5 FB from the epigastrium with tenderness on pressure.

Laboratory Data.

SGOT	26 mU/ml	Normal
SGPT	17 mU/ml	Normal
ALP	118 mU/ml	↑
LDH	225 mU/ml	Normal
γ-GTP	35 mU/ml	Normal
Cho E	277 U/dl	Normal
ZTT	3.3 U	Normal
Total bilirubin	0.6 mg/dl	Normal
AFP	33.2 mμg/dl	↑

Purpose of Diagnostic Imaging. Precise examination of the swollen liver.

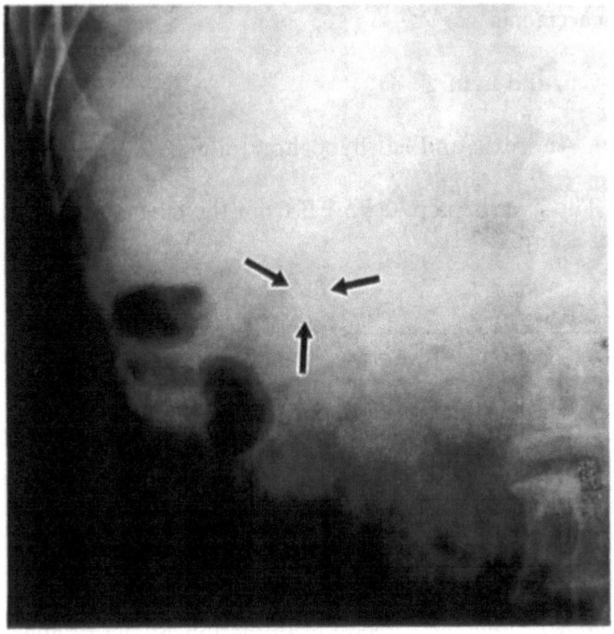

① Plain abdominal roentgenogram
Calcification is seen at the right costal margin (→) suggesting a gallstone.

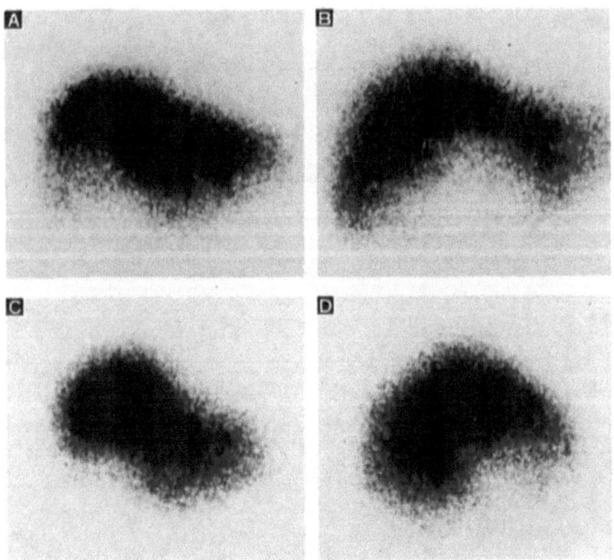

❷ Scintigram
A Frontal view
B Right anterior oblique view at 45° angle
C Right anterior oblique view at 30° angle
D Right lateral view
Liver scintigram: Swelling of the left hepatic lobe and an image of a defect inferior to the right lobe are seen.

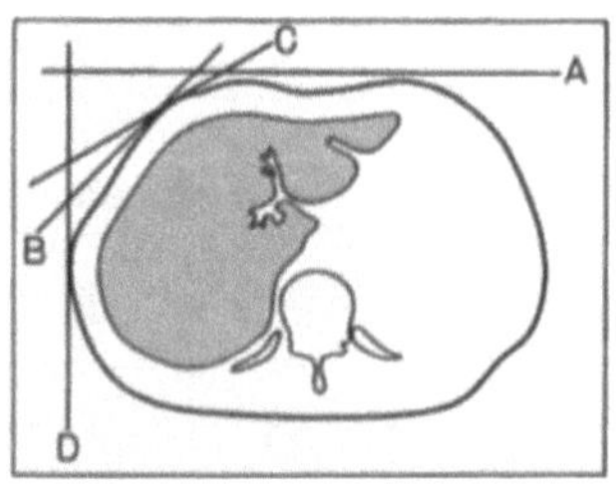

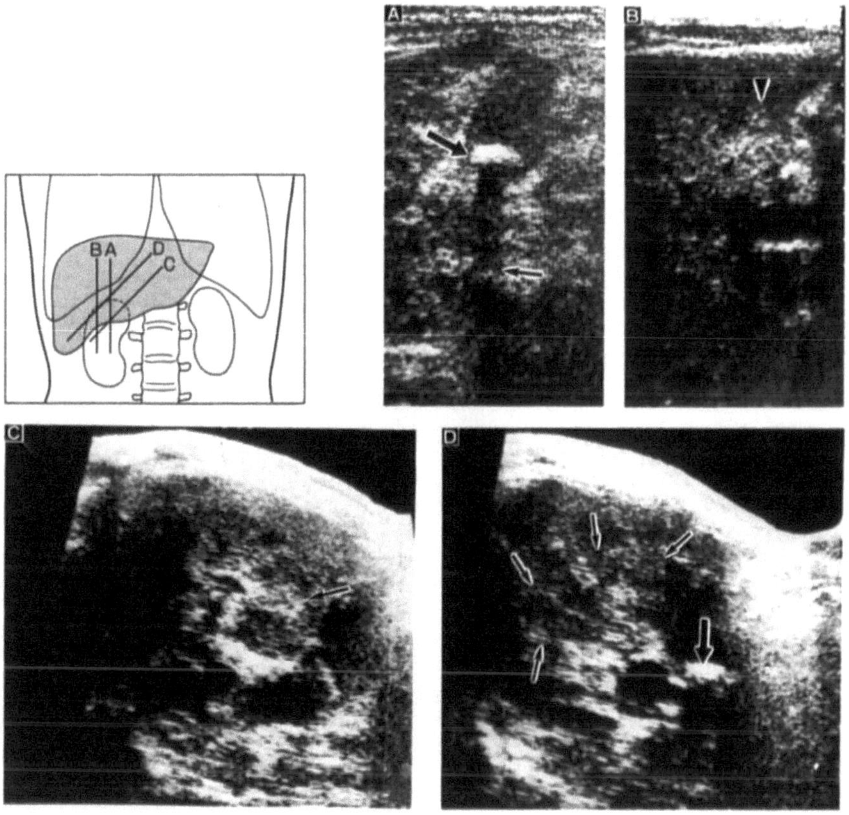

❸ Ultrasonogram
A, B Linear electronic scanning
A stone (→) in the gallbladder accompanied by acoustic shadow (→) and a slightly high echogenic tumor (▶) in the anterior part of the lower segment of the right lobe are visualized.
C, D Contact compound scanning
A stone in the gallbladder (→) and a tumor with inhomogeneous echo level (→) anterosuperior to the stone are seen.

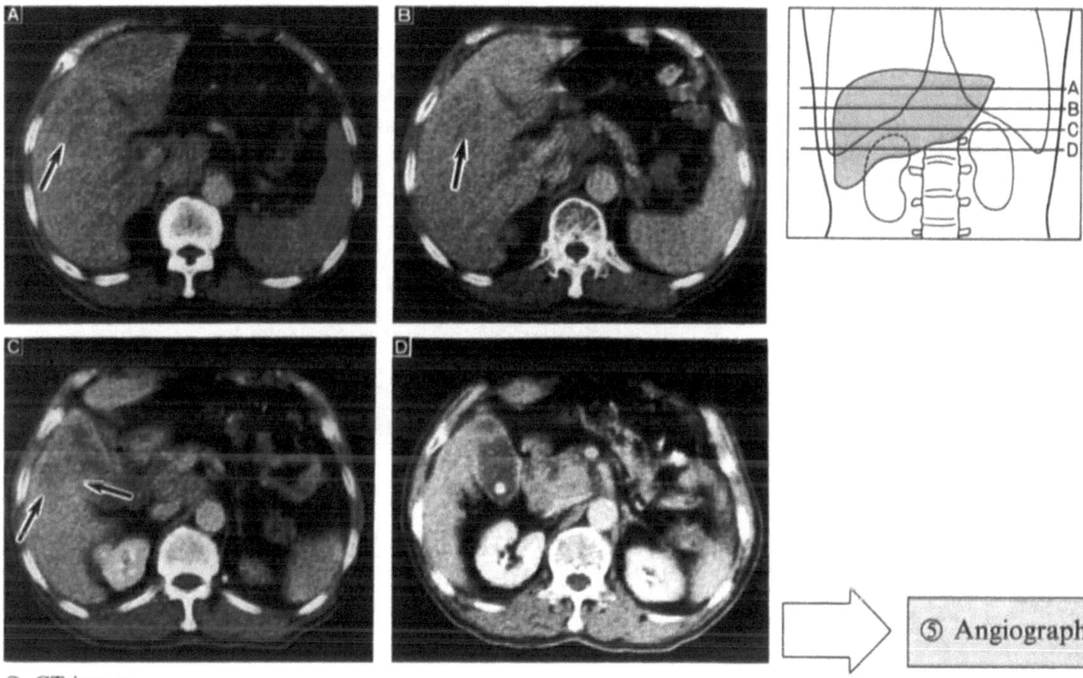

⑤ Angiography

④ CT image
A–D After contrast enhancement
A Low-attenuation area (→), anteroinferior part in the right hepatic lobe, is adjacent to the gallbladder at the lower portion. The smooth wall of the gallbladder including a gallstone is observed. Metastasis to the lymph node is also visualized anterior to the inferior vena cava.

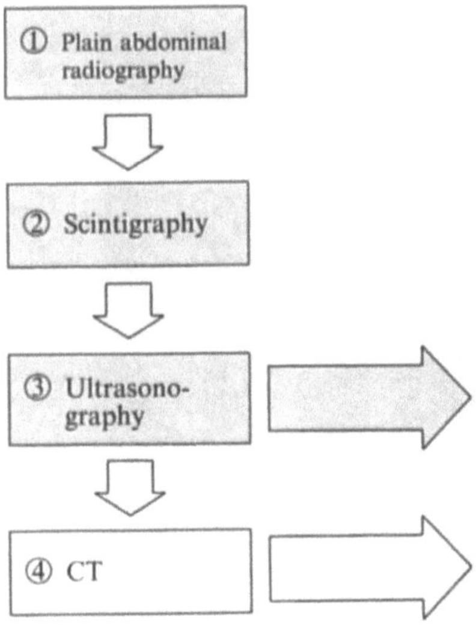

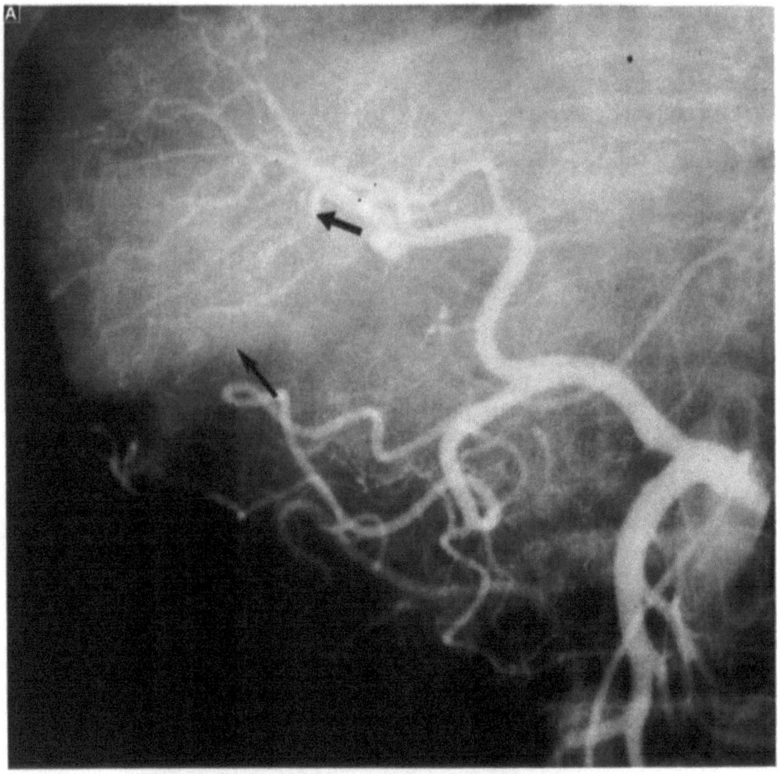

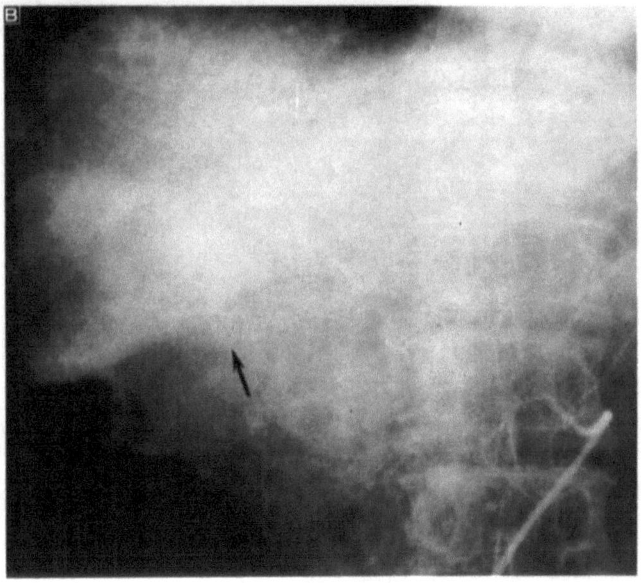

❺ Angiogram
A, A′ Stereoscopic right hepatic arteriogram (arterial phase)
B Right hepatic arteriogram (venous phase)
C Superior mesenteric arteriogram (venous phase)
The right hepatic artery branches from the superior mesenteric artery, and its branches show encasement (→), hypervascularity (→), and irregularity at the more distal side (**A, A′**). This portion is gradually stained during the venous phase (**B**, →), and obstruction is seen in the right inferior branch (→) of the intrahepatic portal vein (**C**). Arterioportal shunt is not observed.

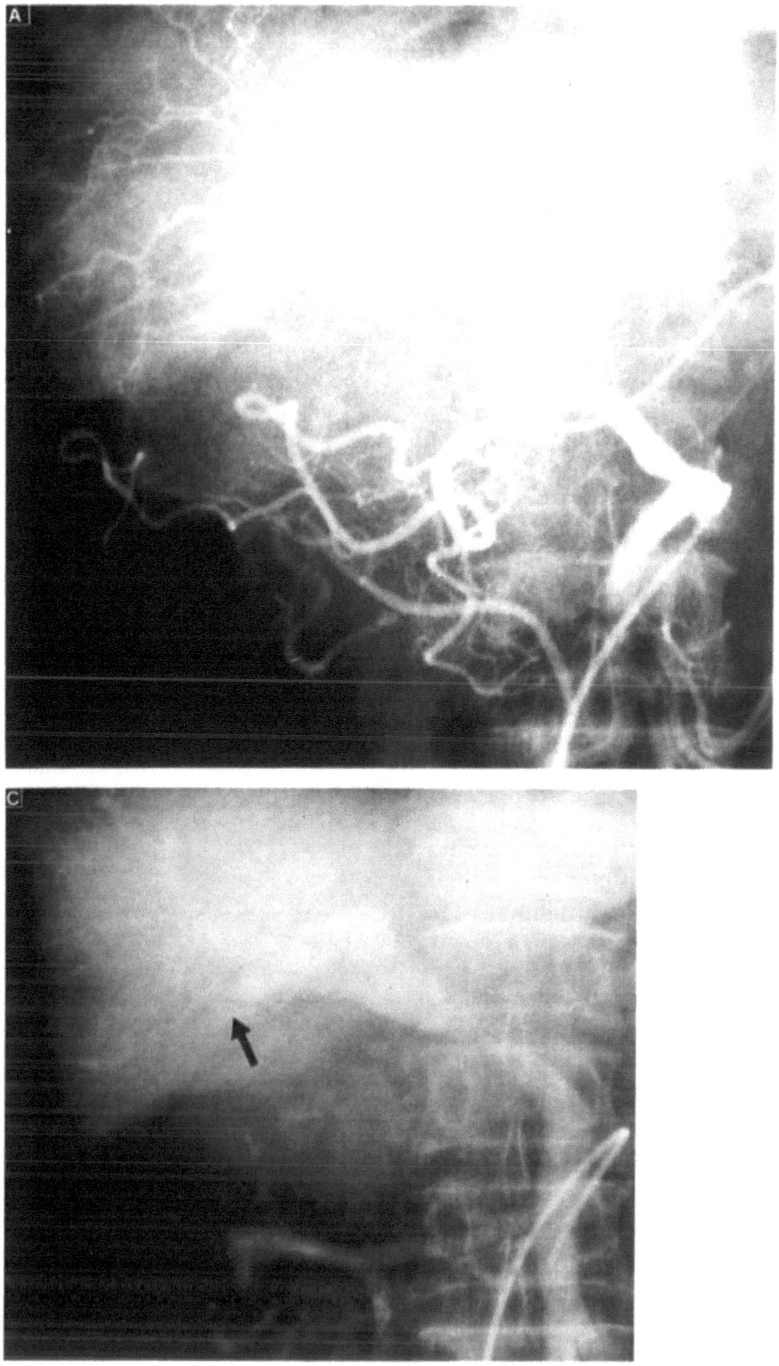
A
C

Final Diagnosis. Cholangiocarcinoma was determined by autopsy.

Significance of Diagnostic Imaging. Ultrasonography can provide sufficient information to confirm the existence of the defective portion detected from the liver scintigram and examine the solidity of the mass. Especially at the lower portion of the right hepatic lobe, the mass can be visualized in almost all cases. Qualitative diagnosis is carried out with angiography, but sometimes distinguishing from undifferentiated hepatocellular carcinoma characterized by hypovascularity or metastatic liver tumor may be difficult. A correct diagnosis of primary hepatic carcinoma during the initial examination is low at 33.3% in cases of intrahepatic cholangioma [12]. Qualitative diagnosis with ultrasonography or CT is difficult. With magnification angiography, irregularity of the periportal artery and neovascularity are visualized permitting easy diagnosis. Thus, magnification angiography is regarded as a valuable technique.

General Matters Concerning Cholangiocarcinoma [22]. Cancer of the biliary tract originates from the intra- or extrahepatic bile duct, without any histological difference between them. Generally, carcinoma that originates from the intrahepatic bile duct containing the porta hepatis is called cholangioma and included in primary hepatic carcinoma. Cholangioma arising from small radicles of the intrahepatic bile ducts is named the peripheral type, and that generating from the major intrahepatic bile ducts near the porta hepatis is called the hilar type. The latter is more common. Clinically, jaundice appears earlier in the hilar type than in the peripheral type; thus, the hilar type can be discovered earlier.

The frequency of the cholangioma is one-sixth to one-seventh that of hepatocellular carcinoma. There is no sexual difference. Cholangioma is more frequent in older people than hepatocellular carcinoma. The rate of accompanying liver cirrhosis is 10%–20%, and there is no association with liver cirrhosis except in biliary cirrhosis. Also, a relationship with HBs Ag has not been observed. Even if the level of AFP is elevated, it is under 100 mμg/ml and almost always negative.

Histologically, cholangioma is similar to adenocarcinoma of the extrahepatic bile ducts, but sometimes it cannot be differentiated from metastasis to the liver originating from the extrahepatic bile duct or pancreas. Also, in cases of extension to the gallbladder fossa, differentiation from primary gallbladder carcinoma may be difficult.

The success rate of medical treatment and the prognosis are poor. Resectability is poor at 10%–20%. In inoperable cases, administration of anticancerous agents results in a mean survival period of about 3 months.

2.14 Liver Metastasis (Cacinoma of the Rectum)

Sequence of Diagnostic Imaging.

① Scintigraphy
⇩
② Ultrasonography
⇩
③ CT
⇩
④ Angiography

Patient. A 47-year-old woman.

Main Complaint. Notspecified.

Present History. Two months prior, the patient was operated on for rectal carcinoma.

Present Status. The liver is hard and palpable 3 FB from the epigastrium, with tenderness on pressure.

Laboratory Data.

SGOT	79 mU/ml	↑
SGPT	51 mU/ml	↑
ALP	213 mU/ml	↑
LDH	255 mU/ml	↑
γ-GTP	52 mU/ml	↑
Cho E	460 U/dl	Normal

Purpose of Diagnostic Imaging. To detect liver metastasis.

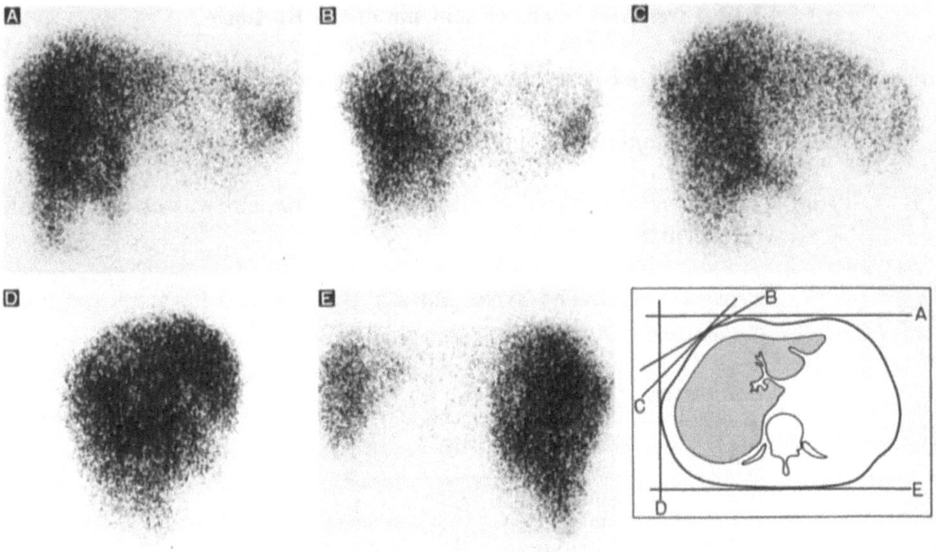

❶ Scintigram
A Frontal view
B Right anterior oblique view at 30° angle
C Right anterior oblique view at 45° angle
D Right lateral view
E Posterior view
Multiple defects are seen in both the right and left lobes of the liver.

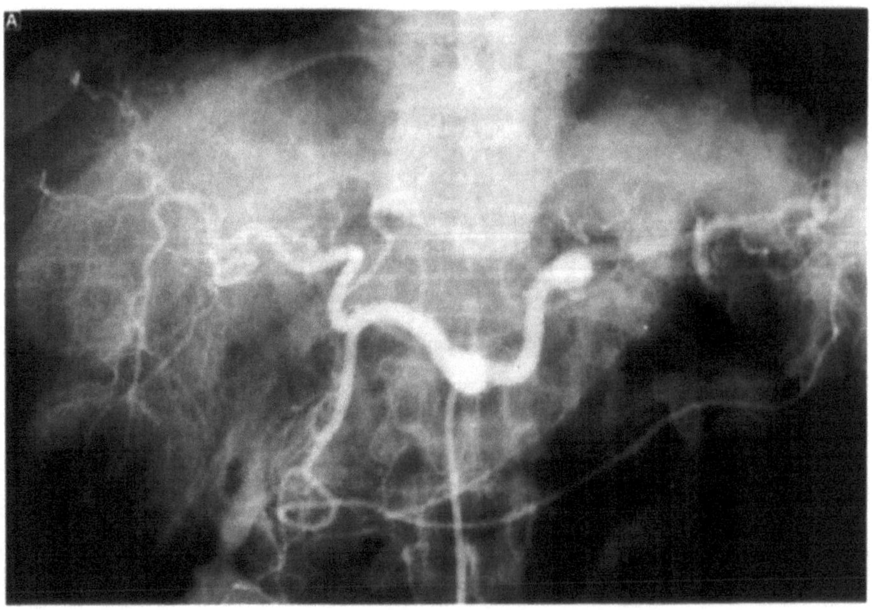

④ Angiogram (A)
A, A′ Stereoscopic celiac arteriogram (arterial phase)

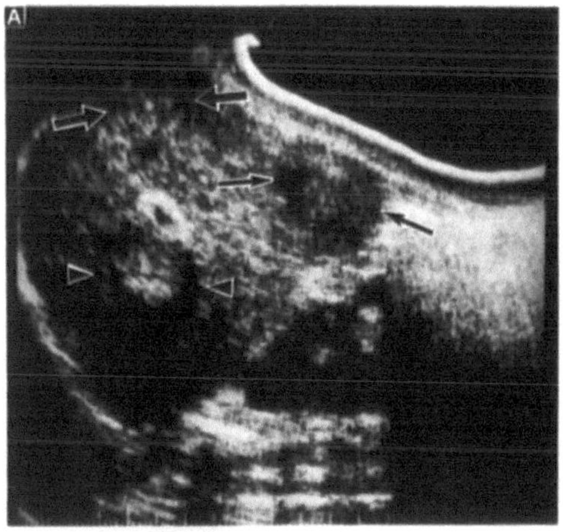

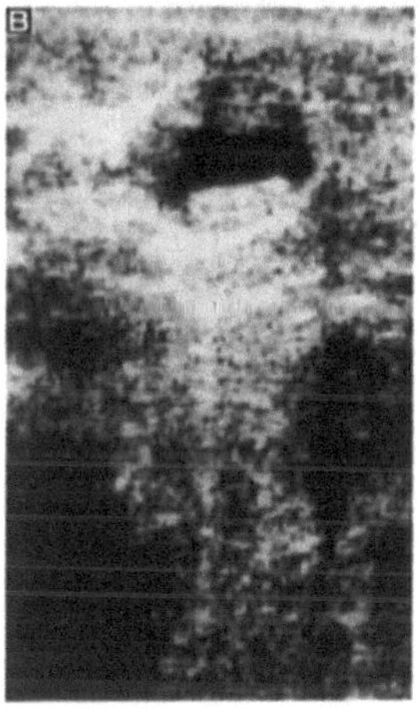

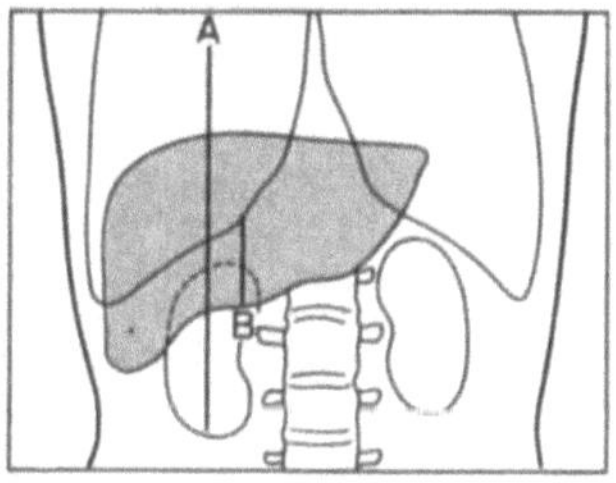

❷ Ultrasonogram
A Contact compound scanning
B Linear electronic scanning

Multiple space-occupying lesions are observed in both the right and left lobes. Particularly in the lateral part of the right lobe, a high echoic image (→) in the upper anterior portion, a low echoic image (→) in the lower anterior portion, and a tumor of the bull's-eye type (▶) in the posterior portion are observed. A stone is seen in the gallbladder.

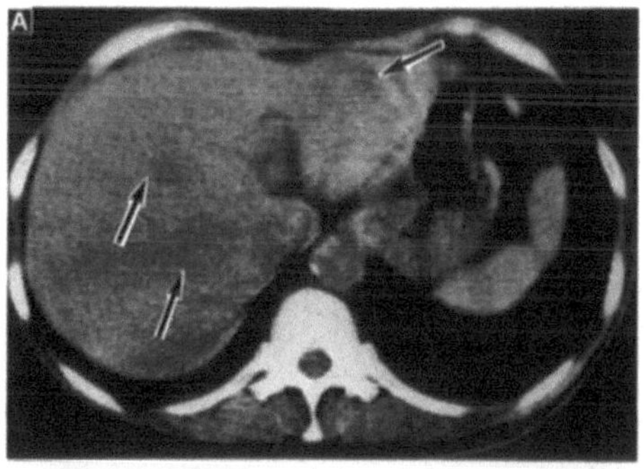

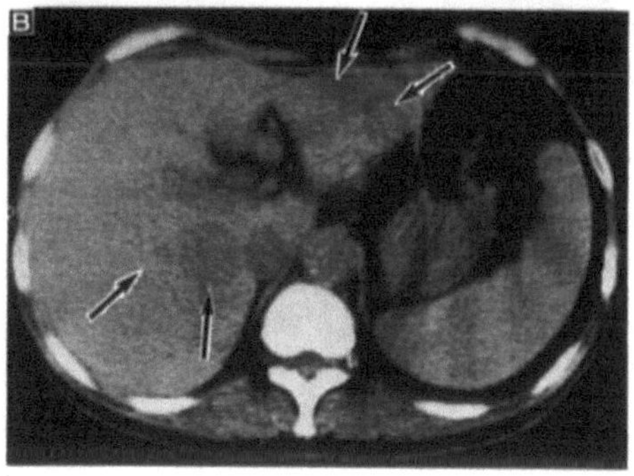

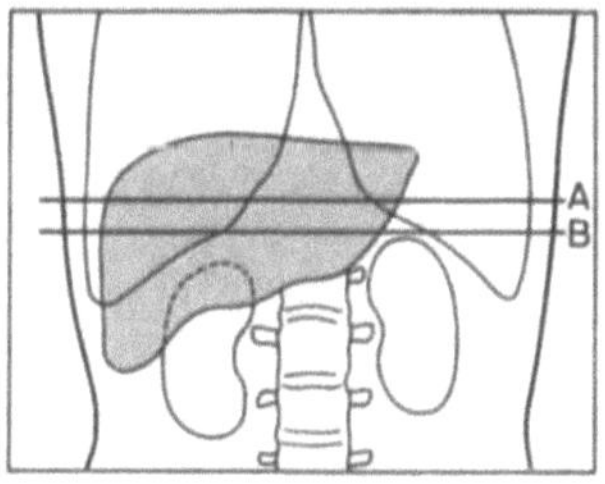

❸ CT image
Low-attenuation areas (→) of various sizes are seen in both the right and left lobes of the liver.

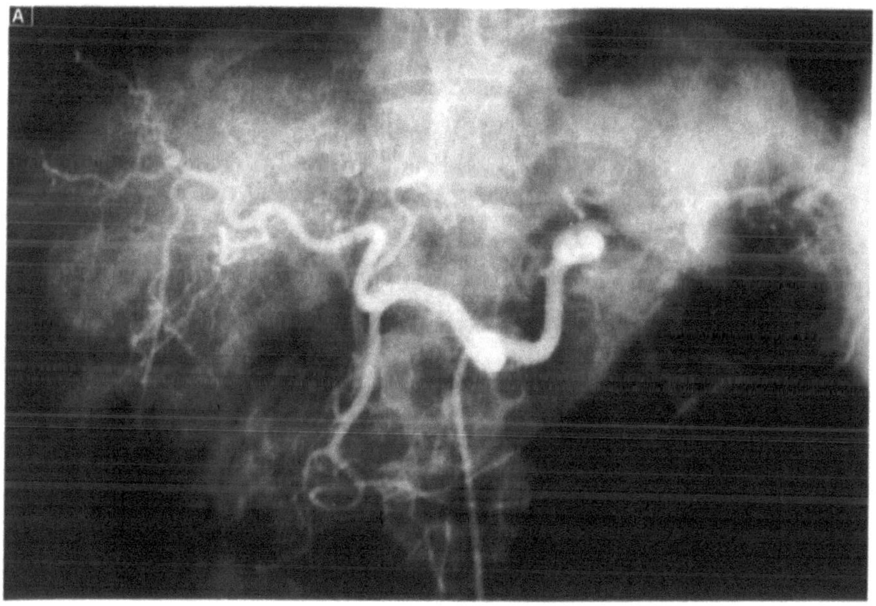

④ Angiography (BB′, CC′)

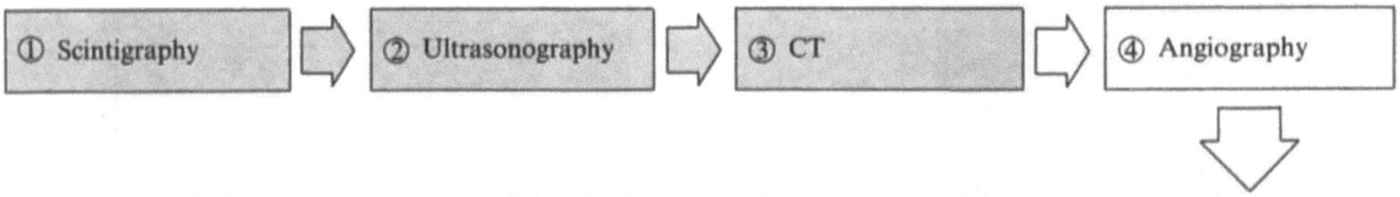

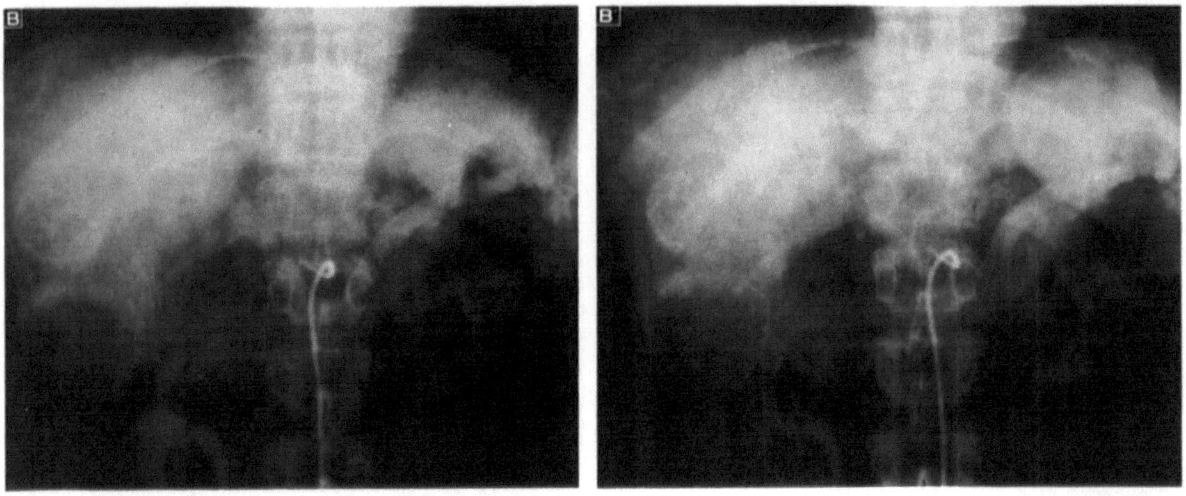

④ Angiogram (B, C)
B, B′ Stereoscopic celiac arteriogram (venous phase)
C, C′ Stereoscopic superior mesenteric arteriogram (venous phase, after prostaglandin administration)

Medical Treatment. Arterial infusion of mitomycin C 20 mg through a catheter was performed during angiography. The results were poor. Therefore, 3 months later, mitomycin 20 mg was injected intra-arterially and the angiogram was photographed.

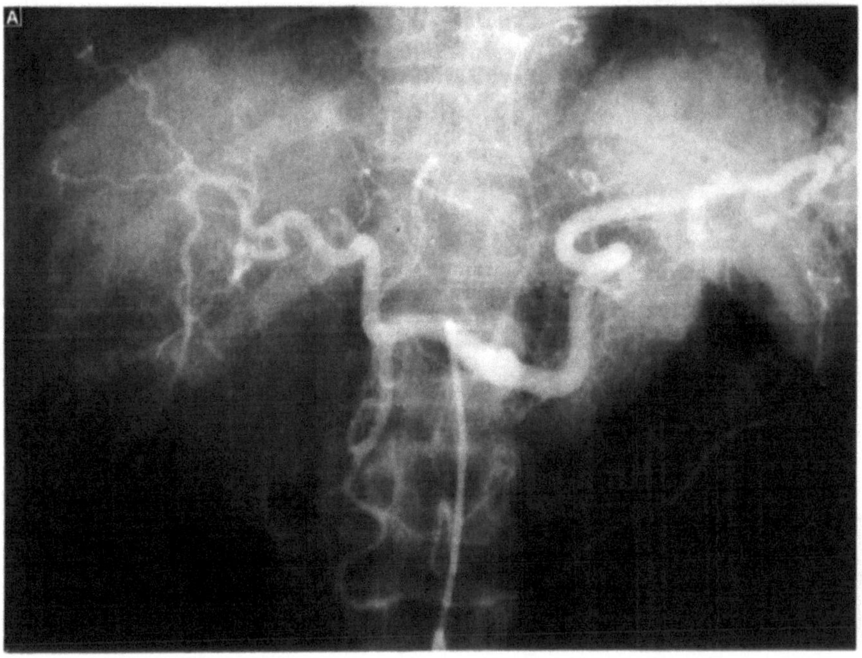

Angiogram (after 3 months)
A, A′ Stereoscopic celiac arteriogram (arterial phase)
The arteriogram obtained after 3 months shows the tumor increased in size.

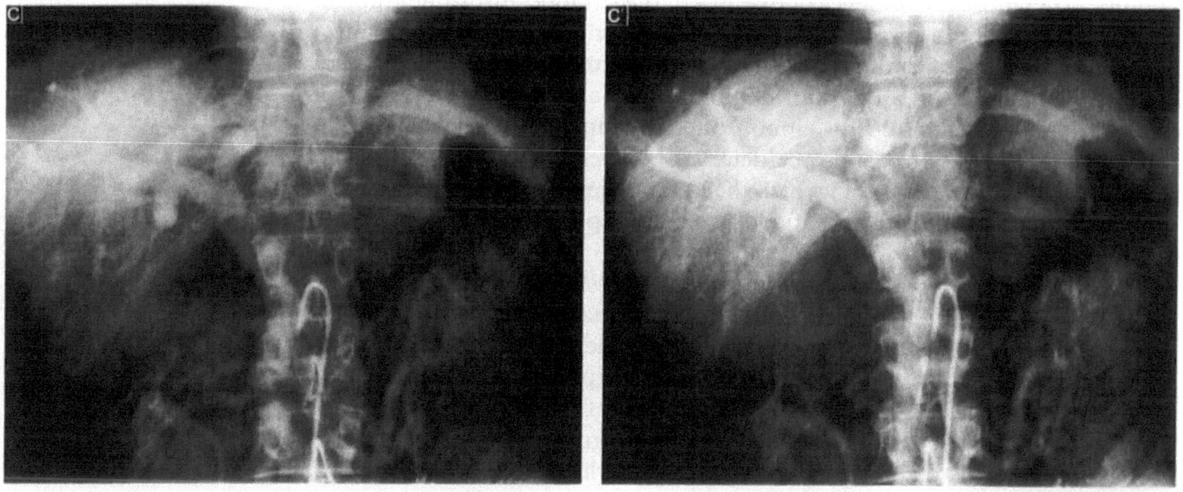

From the celiac arteriogram, in the early arterial phase, the vessels present in the capsule and tumors of various sizes are visualized in the liver, and they are gradually stained from the capillary to the venous phase. A large tumor in the left lobe is not clearly seen. In the portal phase, the right portal branch is compressed by the tumor without occlusion.

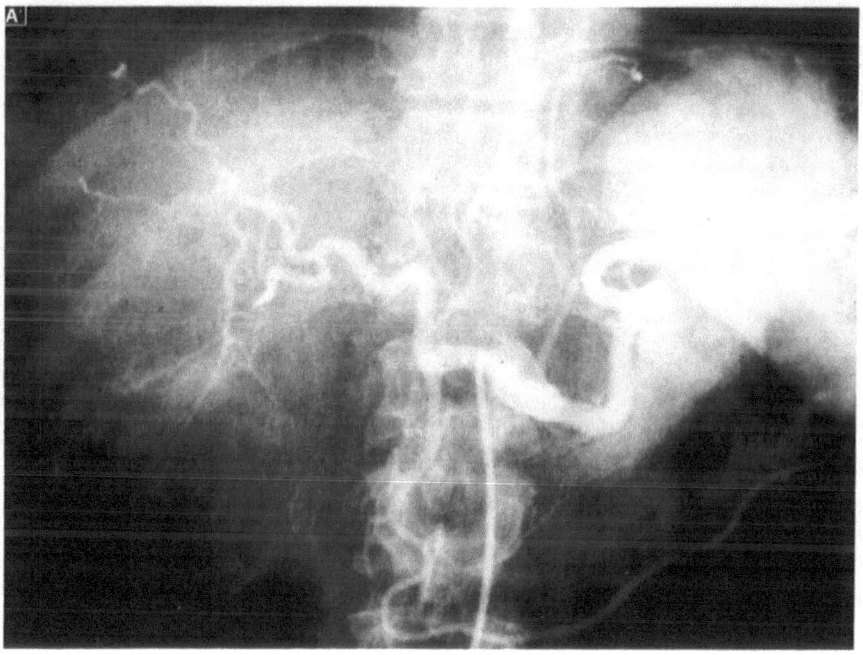

Significance of Diagnostic Imaging. Quantitative identification can be done from any examination, but in this case, metastasis in the left lobe was not clearly determined by angiography. This is not only because of a lack of technical skill in angiography but also because visualization of space-occupying lesions in the left lobe is sometimes difficult. In terms of the ability to diagnose the presence of diseases in the left lobe, ultrasonography and CT may be more appropriate. Angiography is not regarded as valuable except in cases in which other possibilities besides metastasis are suspected or with the purpose of a one-shot treatment with anticancerous agents by intra-arterial infusion and for embolization treatment. In cases in which space-occupying lesions cannot be detected by liver scintigraphy, ultrasonography, or CT, i.e., cases in which the lesion is small in size or located in the upper part of the right hepatic lobe, angiography is required.

General Matters Concerning Metastatic Liver Carcinoma. Metastasis to the liver is diagnosed in one-half to one-third of cancer patients, frequently from cancer of the digestive organs, the lungs, or the breast. In other words, hematogenous metastasis via the portal vein or hepatic artery is common, and lymphatogenious metastasis from carcinoma of the stomach, pancreas, and cervix uteri is not frequent. Direct extension from surrounding organs sometimes may also take place. The nature of cirrhotic liver means that it is rarely accompanied by metastasis.

2.15 Hepatic Injury

Sequence of Diagnostic Imaging.

① Scintigraphy

⇩

② Angiography

Second Diagnostic Imaging (4 months later)

① Scintigraphy

⇩

② Angiography

Patient. A 6-year-old boy.

Main Complaint. Abdominal pain.

Present History. The patient was hit by a circular saw and hospitalized the next day complaining of abdominal pain and nausea.

Present Status. The abdomen is slightly swollen with abrasion in the abdominal wall.

Laboratory Data.

WBC	$17700/mm^3$	Slightly ↑
RBC	$345 \times 10^4/mm^3$	↓
Hb	9.7 g/dl	↓
Platelet	$28.3 \times 10^4/mm^3$	Normal
SGOT	over 1500 mU/ml	↑
SGPT	1500 mU/ml	↑
LDH	1000 mU/ml	↑
Total protein	6.0 g/dl	Normal
Na	125 mμg/l	↓
K	4.7 mμg/l	Normal
Cl	86 mμg/l	↓
CRP	(3+)	↑

Purpose of Diagnostic Imaging. To identify the presence of hepatic injury.

First Stage of Diagnosis

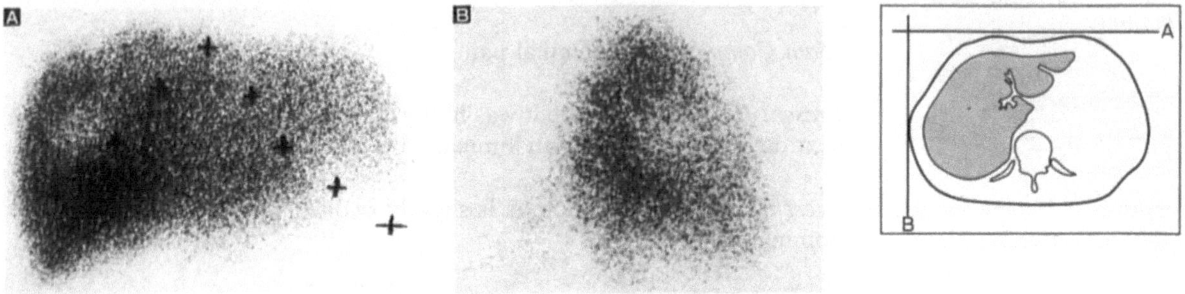

① Liver scintigram with ^{99m}Tc-phytate: A cold area in the right hepatic lobe is observed.
A Frontal view
B Right lateral view

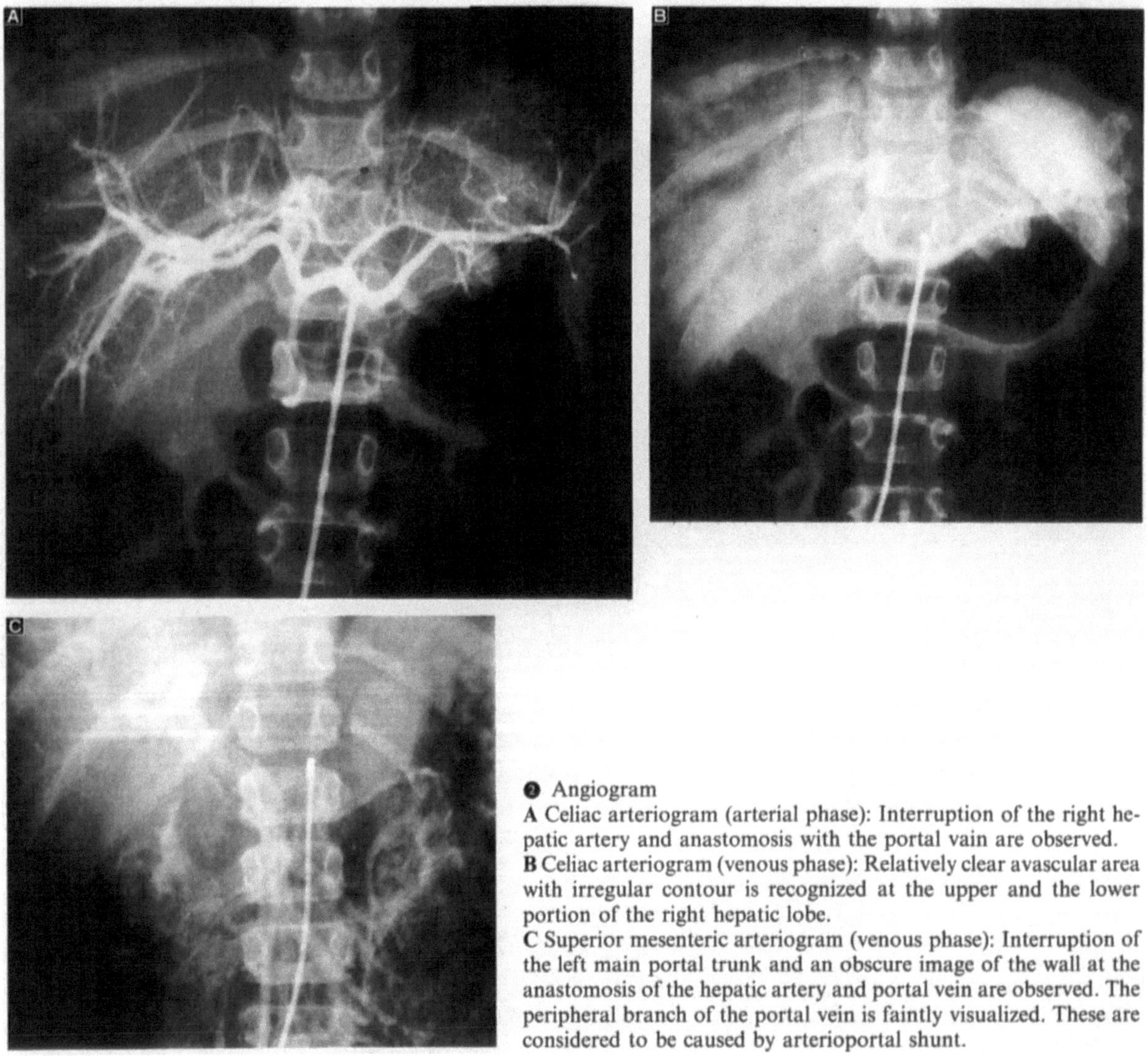

❷ Angiogram
A Celiac arteriogram (arterial phase): Interruption of the right hepatic artery and anastomosis with the portal vain are observed.
B Celiac arteriogram (venous phase): Relatively clear avascular area with irregular contour is recognized at the upper and the lower portion of the right hepatic lobe.
C Superior mesenteric arteriogram (venous phase): Interruption of the left main portal trunk and an obscure image of the wall at the anastomosis of the hepatic artery and portal vein are observed. The peripheral branch of the portal vein is faintly visualized. These are considered to be caused by arterioportal shunt.

Second Stage 4 Months Later

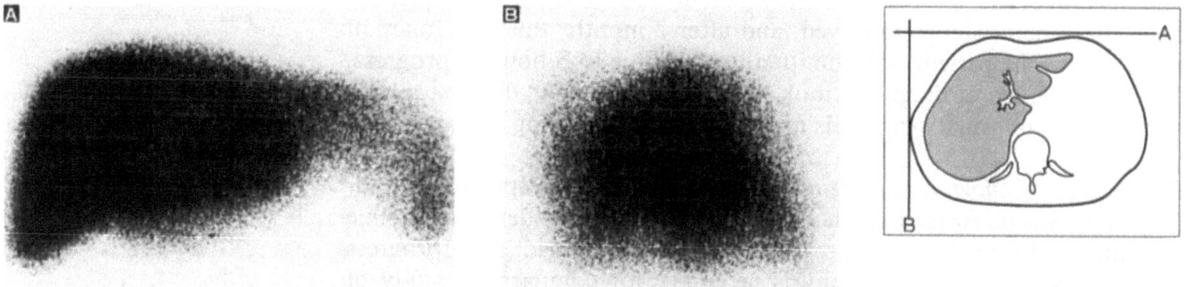

① Liver scintigram with ^{99m}Tc-phytate: Slightly obscure, decreased lesions are visualized on both images.
A Frontal view
B Right lateral view

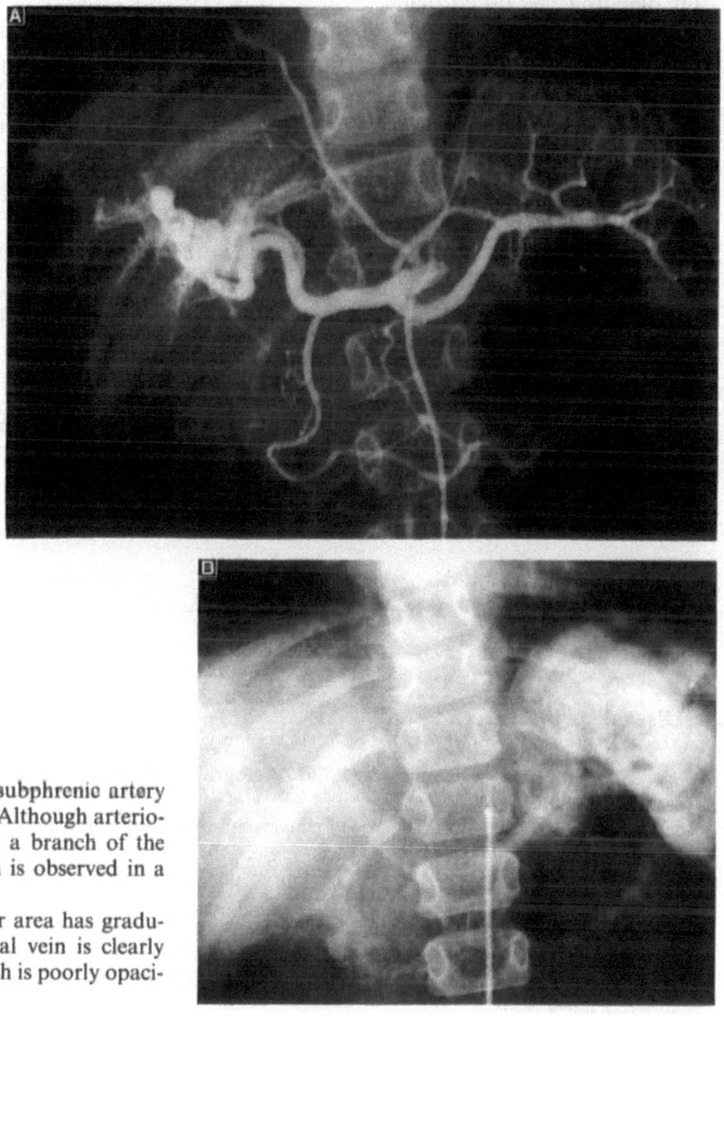

② Angiogram
A Celiac arteriogram (arterial phase): Dilated subphrenic artery with a part running into the liver is observable. Although arterio-portal shunt has decreased, the liver is fed by a branch of the portal vein with anastomosis. Pseudoaneurysm is observed in a portion.
B Celiac arteriogram (venous phase): Avascular area has gradually decreased. The major branch of the portal vein is clearly visualized, and the intrahepatic peripheral branch is poorly opacified due to arterioportal blood shunting.

Clinical Procedure. After hepatic injury was diagnosed, blood transfusion and infusion solution were given to observe progress. Bloody effusion in the right pleural cavity was observed transitionally and gradually disappeared. Then the general status improved, and after 2 months the liver function normalized. The patient was admitted to the clinic to follow up progress. The second stage of diagnosis took place 4 months after the first angiography. No abnormal symptoms appeared in the following 3 years.

Significance of Diagnostic Imaging. Hepatic injury was suspected and angiography was performed the day after hospitalization to detect a possible bleeding condition. No findings of bleeding were obtained; thus, progress was observed. Liver scintigraphy is necessary for comparative study of progress.

In cases of hepatic injury, a plain abdominal roentgenogram visualizes elevation of the right diaphragm, increasing distance between the right abdominal wall and intestine, disappearance of psoas shadow and liver contour shadow, and dilated intestine caused by intra-abdominal bleeding. On a liver scintigram, the pathological lesion is demonstrated as an image of low uptake or of a defect. With ultrasonography, the bleeding area is shown as a cystic unechoic area, but is sometimes accompanied by internal echoes or movable echoes in the direction of gravity due to debris. CT demonstrates the bleeding area as a low-attenuation portion except soon after bleeding has taken place.

Angiography is essential to study the location and extent of the injury [1, 30]. Extension, stenosis, interruption of the intrahepatic major arterial branches, leakage of the contrast medium, and arteriovenous shunting are observable in the arterial phase, and the venous phase visualizes an avascular area and after a while an aneurysm.

General Matters Concerning Hepatic Injury [19]. Symptoms of hepatic injury are abdominal pain, pallor, tenderness on pressure, lack or decrease of abdominal sound, hypotension, and tachycardia. Laboratory findings are leukocytosis, anemia, elevation of SGOT, SGPT, and alkaline phosphatase, which are transitional and proportional to severeness. Especially the elevation of SGPT and ALP suggest intrahepatic injury.

Complications are caused by injury of other organs or the hepatic injury itself, which causes infection (abscess, sepsis), cholangitis, gastrointestinal hemorrhage, ileus, hemobilia, etc.

References

A: Disease of the Liver

1. Boijsen E, Judkins, MP, Simay A (1966) Angiographic diagnosis of hepatic rupture. Radiology 86:66–72
2. Edmondson HA, Steiner PE (1954) Primary carcinoma of the liver. A study of 100 cases among 48900 necropsies. Cancer 7:462–503
3. Eggle H (1901) Über das primäre Carcinom der Leber. Beitr Z Pathol Anat Allg Pathol 30:506–604
4. Exelby PR, Filler RM, Grosfeld JL (1975) Liver tumours in children in the particular reference of hepatoblastoma and hepatocellular carcinoma: American academy of pediatric surgical section survey, 1974. J Pediat. Surg 10:329–337

5. Liver Cancer Study Group of Japan (1983) The general rules for the clinical and pathological study of primary liver cancer. Kanehara Shuppan, Tokyo
6. Gyotoku Y, Sugihara H, Amagasaki T, Mori I, Kinoshita I (1980) An autopsy case of pedunculated liver cell carcinoma and its review (in Japanese). Jpn J Cancer Clin 26:92–96
7. Ichida F (1974) Clinical statistics of liver cirrhosis in Japan (in Japanese). Jpn J Clin Med 32 [Suppl]: 376–383
8. Imaeda T, Senda K, Kato T, Asada S, Suzuki M, Ishigaki T, Yamawaki Y, Doi H (1978) Analysis of 30 hepatocellular carcinoma cases detected during the observation period for chronic hepatitis or liver cirrhosis (in Japanese). Nippon Acta Radiol 38:1073–1094
9. Ishikawa K (1976) Follow-up survey of primary hepatic cancer in Japan (in Japanese). Acta Hepatologica Japonica 17:460–465
10. Ito H, Toda T, Kishikawa T, Yamaguchi S, Kani A, Funabiki T, Aoki H, Arai M, Shamoto M, Takeuchi J, Yokoi K, Miyata T, Matsuyama K (1979) A case of mesenchymal hamartoma of the liver with a review of the reported cases in Japan (in Japanese). J Jpn Soc Pediat Surg 15:997–1003
11. Ito S, (1977) Fatty liver (in Japanese). In: Yoshitoshi Y, Nakao K, Yamaga S, et al (eds) Handbook of internal medicine vol 23. Nakayama Shoten, Tokyo, pp 7–44
12. Kido C, Mori R (1976) Angiography of primary liver cancer (in Japanese). Stomach Intestine 11:1591–1603
13. Kamegaya K (1978) Liver cirrhosis (in Japanese). In: Yoshitoshi, Y, Nakao K, Yamaga S, et al (eds) Handbook of internal medicine, vol 22B. Nakayama Shoten, Tokyo, pp 3–110
14. Kobayashi K, Kumagai M, Kameda S, Sugimoto T, Suzuki K, Nishimura K, Kato Y, Sugioka G, Hatoori N, Takeuchi J (1980) Hepatoma development during long term frollow-up period of liver cirrhosis (in Japanese). Acta Hepatol Japonica 21:1581–1586
15. Kuroishi T, Tominaga S, Hirose K (1981) Cancer mortality in Japan (in Japanese). Jpn J Cancer Clin 27:421–515
16. Nakamura H, Oi H, Tanaka T, Hori S, Tokunaga K, Yoshioka H, Kuroda C, Okamura J, Sakurai M, Taguchi T (1984) Treatment of hepatic tumours by transcatheter chemo-embolization with gelatin sponge (in Japanese). Jpn J Cancer Chemother 11:789–797
17. Ninomiya F, Kawahara T, Yamaguchi G, Maruyama N, Motoori H, Nagata E, Tanikawa K, Arakawa M (1980) A case of pedunculated hepatoma (in Japanese). Acta Hepatol Japonica 21:1581–1586
18. Nishioka M, Nishimura H, Hayakawa M, Takenami T, Oka T, Akagawa E, Nawata J, Noda K, Fukumoto Y, Kan T, Fujii R, Mizuta M, Takemoto T (1977) Clinical course on patients with primary hepatocellular carcinoma surviving longer one year (in Japanese). Acta Hepatol Japonica 18:548–553
19. Maemura K, Sugimoto H, Yoshida T, Sugimoto T (1979) Central hematoma of the liver (in Japanese). Surg Therapy 41:536–541
20. Obata H, Tamiya, M, Hayashi N, Hisamitsu T, Motoike Y, Nara S, Takemoto T, Takasaki K, Muto H, Amo T, Suzuki S, Kobayashi S (1976) Development of hepatocellular carcinoma on the ground of chronic liver diseases. Prospective study in 59 cases of liver cirrhosis (in Japanese). Acta Hepatol Japonica 17:335–347
21. Oda T, Suzuki H, Oka H (1980) Liver disease (in Japanese). Chugai Igaku, Tokyo
22. Okuda K, Peters RL, (1976) Hepatocellular carcinoma. Wiley New York
23. Omanik, S, Jablonsky I (1972) Pedunculated accessory hepatic lobe. Arch Surg 105:792–794
24. Ota K, Endo H (1977) Liver cirrhosis (in Japanese). In: Yamagata S, Kosaka K, Masuda M, Ishii K (eds) Handbook of clinical gastroenterology, vol 3. Kanehara Shuppan, Tokyo, pp 205–231
25. Shiraishi T (1977) Hemochromatosis (in Japanese). In: Yoshitoshi Y, Nakao K, Yamagato S, et al (eds) Handbook of internal medicine, vol 23. Nakayama Shoten, Tokyo, pp 66–78
26. Takino T (1977) Liver abscess (in Japanese). In: Yoshitoshi Y, Nakao K, Yamagata S, et al (eds) Handbook of internal medicine, vol 23. Nakayama Shoten, Tokyo, pp 189–222
27. Tohyama J, Ishigaki T, Ishikawa T, Niwa K, Banno T, Mizutani M, Makino N, Mizutani H, Kamata N, Imagunbai N, Sakuma S (1982) Comparative study of scintigraphy, ultrasonography and computed tomography in the evaluation of liver tumours (in Japanese): J Med Imagings 2:882–889

28. Wittenberg, J, Fineberg HV, Black EB, Kirkpatrick RG, Shaffer DL, Ikeda MK, Ferruci JR Jr (1978) Clinical efficacy of computed body tomography. Am J Roentgenol 131:5–14
29. Yamada, R, Sato M, Kawabata M, Nakatsuka, H, Nakamura K, Takashima T (1983) Hepatic artery embolization in 120 patients with unresectable hepatoma. Radiology 148:397–401
30. Yamamoto S, Shigeki S, Aikawa N, Sudo M, Hiramatsu K, Ido K (1976) Abdominal angiography of the abdominal injuries (in Japanese). J Clin Surg 34:637–649
31. Zeniya M, Aizawa Y, Akiba M, Sato N, Asukata I, Saegusa M, Kameda H, Sugawara K (1978) A case of hepatocellular carcinoma followed up for more than 2 years 6 months (in Japanese). Acta Hepatol Japonica 19:393–398

B: Diagnostic Imaging of Diseases of the Biliary Tract

1 Procedure

There are various means of diagnostic imaging of the biliary tract, such as plain abdominal roentgenography, excretory cholecystocholangiography, percutaneous transhepatic cholangiography (PTC), endoscopic retrograde cholangiopancreatography (ERCP), angiography, ultrasonography, and CT. Recently, noninvasive and easy to operate ultrasonography has been used initially, especially applied as a screening examination, instead of oral cholecystography for the diagnosis of gallbladder stones. Also, in the differentiation of jaundice between obstructive or nonobstructive, ultrasonography is performed first instead of PTC. PTC can be done with safety and accuracy under the guidance of ultrasound.

Figures 1 and 2 show examination procedures for cases in which disease of the gallbladder and obstructive jaundice are suspected. The significance of angiography in malignant neoplasm of the biliary tract is not high compared to that of the liver or pancreas since angiography can only provide definite findings in advanced cases and no clear findings can be obtained in the early stages of cancer. As shown in Fig. 5.24 in Chap. 5, an early stage of cancer may be demonstrated with magnification angiography. Such cases, however, are rarely diagnosed and the effectiveness of magnification angiography has not yet been proved.

In malignant neoplasm of the biliary tract, early detection is difficult and radical medical treatment is impossible in many cases if examination is after the appearance of jaundice. Takemoto and Fuji [17] reported 85 cases of early stages of gallbladder cancer in Japan, and Tsunoda et al. [20] reported 37 cases of cancer of the biliary tract at an early stage. Nevertheless, cases diagnosed before operation were 10 gallbladder cancer and 25 cancer of the biliary tract. Diagnostic means in these cases were mostly a combination of ERCP with PTC and ultrasonography. Even without jaundice, if disease of the biliary tract is suspected from clinical or laboratory findings, an examination should be performed to obtain pisitive identification. Independent of the presence of jaundice, a lack of dilatation of the bile duct on the ultrasonogram doses not always mean there is no obstruction, and early cancer is one condition in which, this appearance is found; selection of examination procedures is therefore difficult.

Diagnostic imaging must be performed sufficiently utilizing statistical data concerning the disease, such as symptoms, frequency in age groups, morbidity, and annual transition of the disease in addition to considering efficacy of each examination and discomfort to patients.

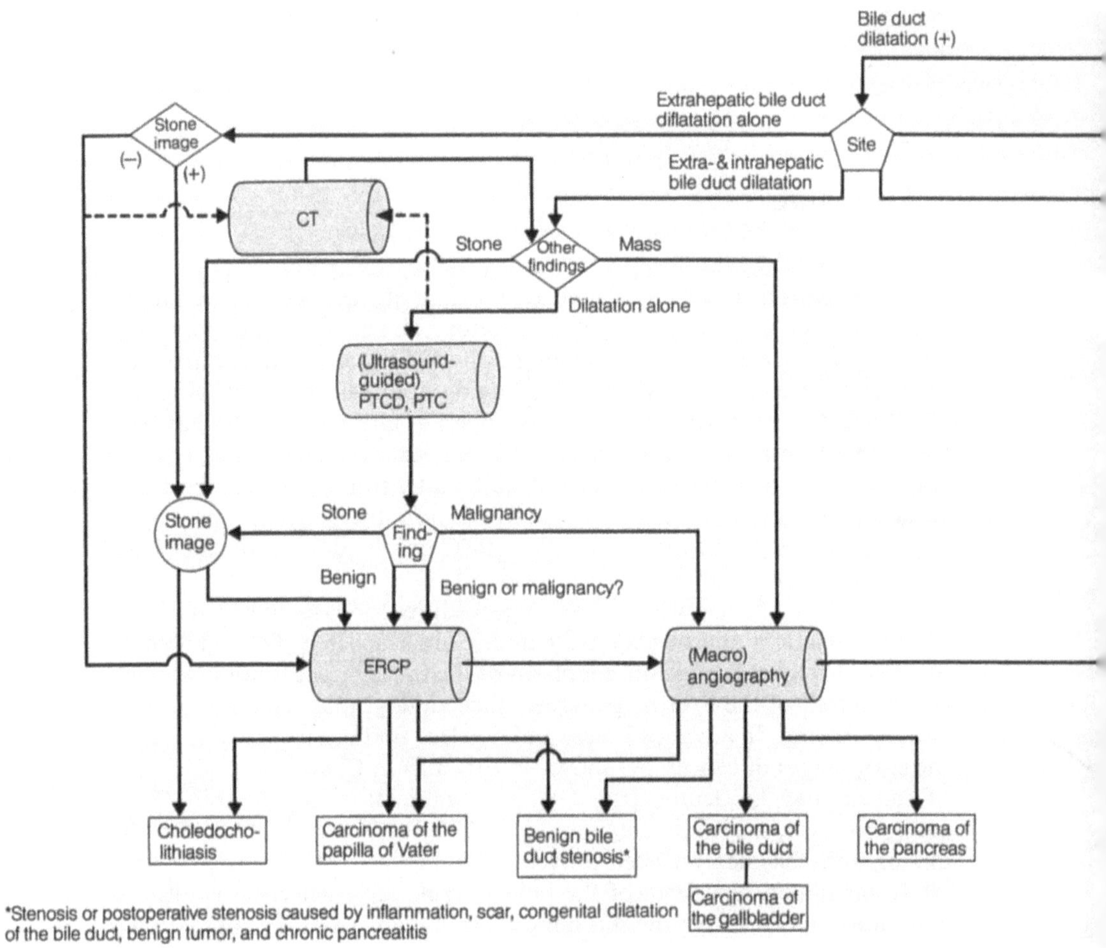

Fig. 1. Procedure of diagnostic imaging in jaundice

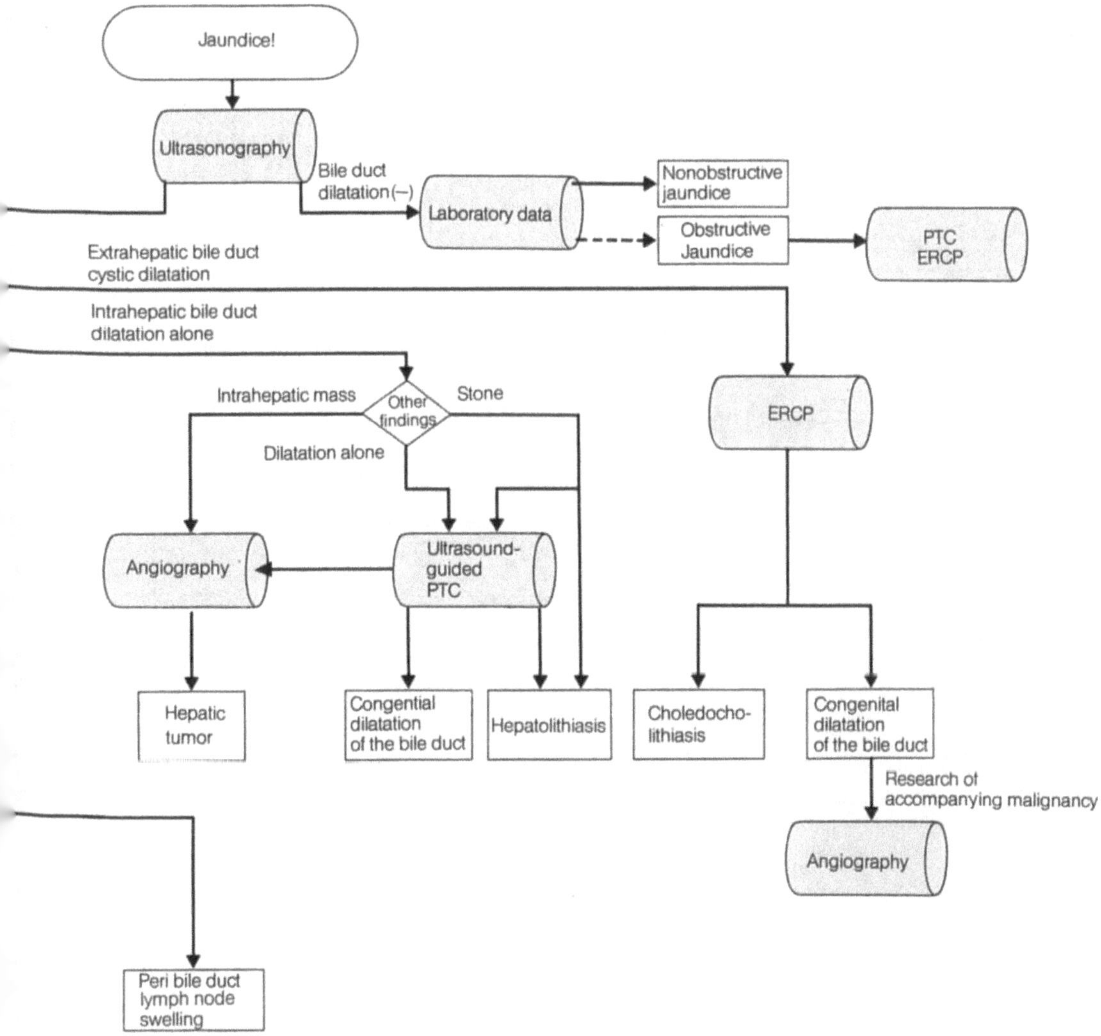
Jaundice!
Ultrasonography
Bile duct dilatation (–)
Laboratory data
Nonobstructive jaundice
Obstructive Jaundice
PTC ERCP
Extrahepatic bile duct cystic dilatation
Intrahepatic bile duct dilatation alone
Intrahepatic mass
Other findings
Stone
Dilatation alone
ERCP
Angiography
Ultrasound-guided PTC
Hepatic tumor
Congential dilatation of the bile duct
Hepatolithiasis
Choledocho-lithiasis
Congenital dilatation of the bile duct
Research of accompanying malignancy
Angiography
Peri bile duct lymph node swelling

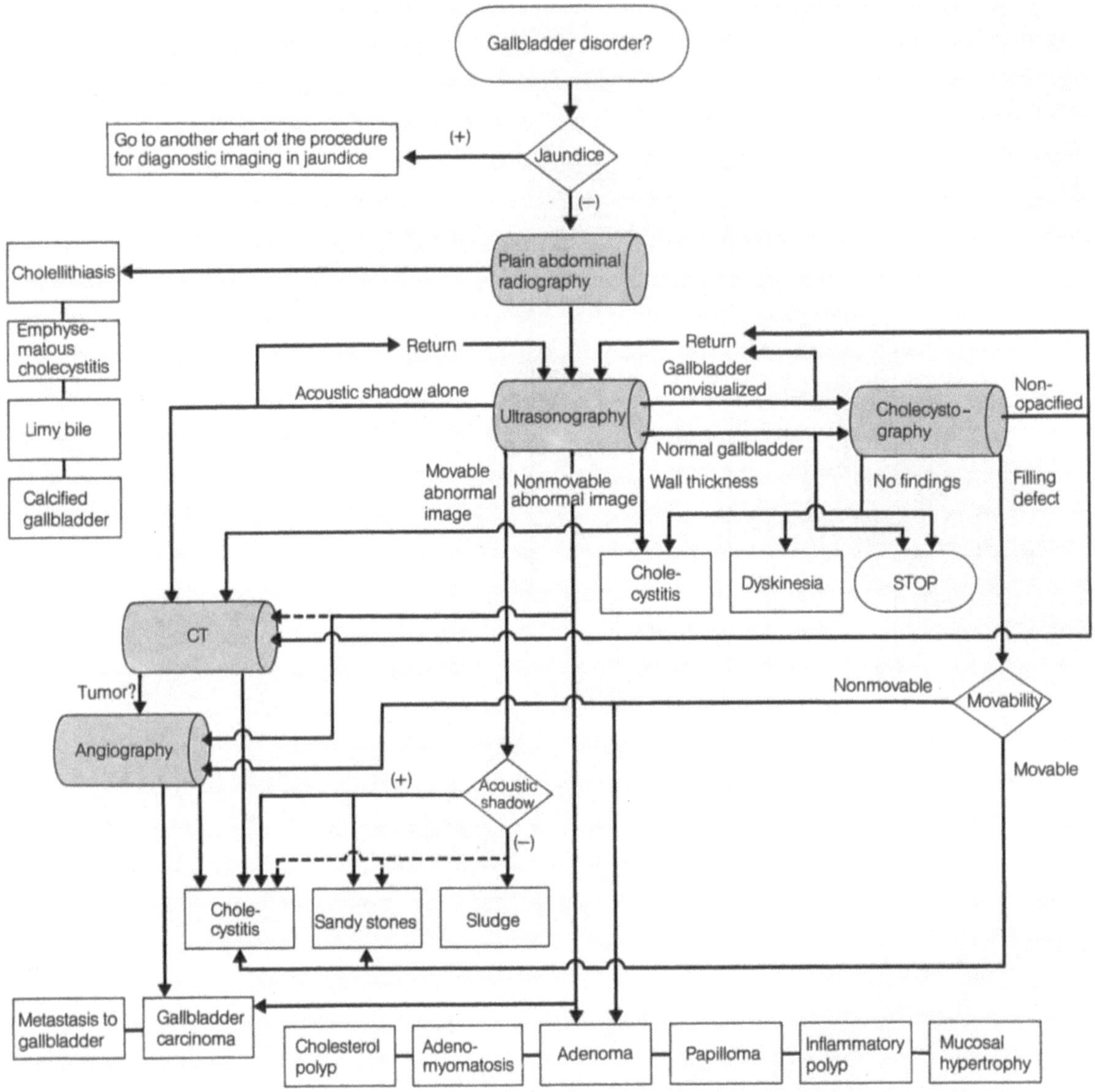

Fig. 2.. Procedure of diagnostic imaging in suspected gallbladder diseases

Recently, the appearance of gallstones in adults has been increasing annually. Carcinoma of the biliary tract increases in higher age groups. Diseases of the biliary tract are more frequent among females. The occurrence ratio of females/males was 0.76 in 1970 compared to 0.94 in 1965, and therefore frequency in females is increasing (Fig. 3) [3].

In females, mortality from diseases of the biliary tract is increasing in cancer of the biliary tract and decreasing in inflammatory diseases, such as choledocholithiasis, cholecystitis, and cholangitis (Fig. 4), with an increase in the occurrence of cancer of the biliary tract.

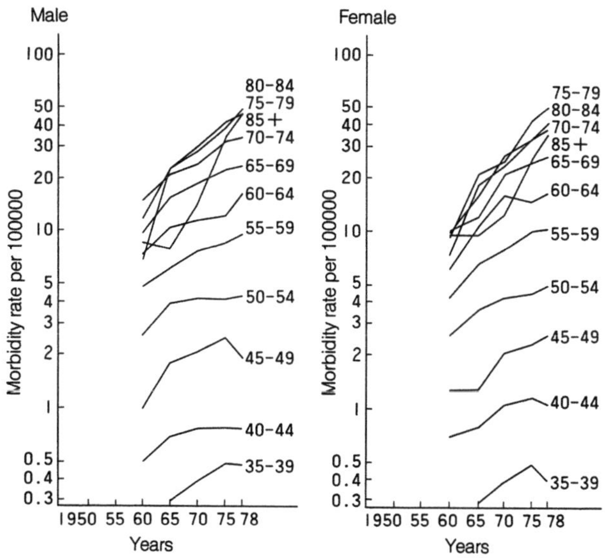

Fig. 3. Morbidity rate of biliary tract carcinoma by ages [26]

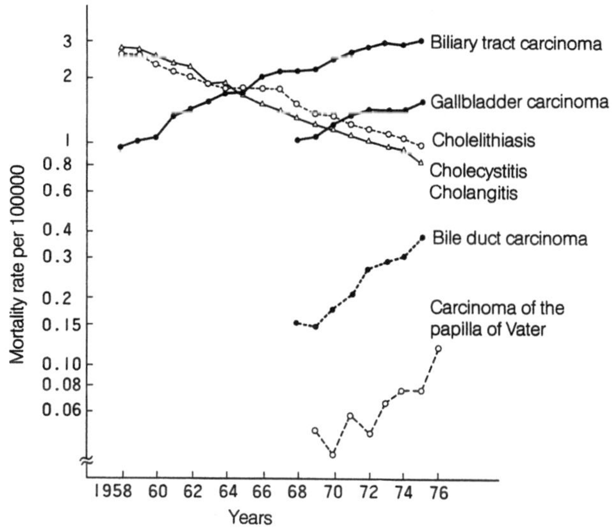

Fig. 4. Mortality rate of biliary tract diseases in females [26]

Over 4% of adults suffer from cholelithiasis. According to Kameda's statistical projection method [6], of 70000000 people over the age of 20 in Japan, 4% or 2800000 people will develop gallstones, and of these people 16%, or 470000, will undergo cholecystectomy and 2330000 will not. Among 2330000, about 70%, or 1630000, will spend their lives with a silent stone, 18%, or 420000, will have cancer of the biliary tract, and 12%, or 280000, will die due to gallstone or cholangitis. The relationship between cancer of the biliary tract and gallstones or cholangitis is well-known. Early diagnosis of cancer of the biliary tract necessitates positive detection of patients with a gallbladder stone. In order to achieve that, mass examinations with ultrasonography are recommended for women over 40 years of age, who are the high-risk group for cholelithiasis and gallbladder cancer.

2. Cases

2.1 Hepatolithiasis and Choledocholithiasis

Sequence of Diagnostic Imaging.

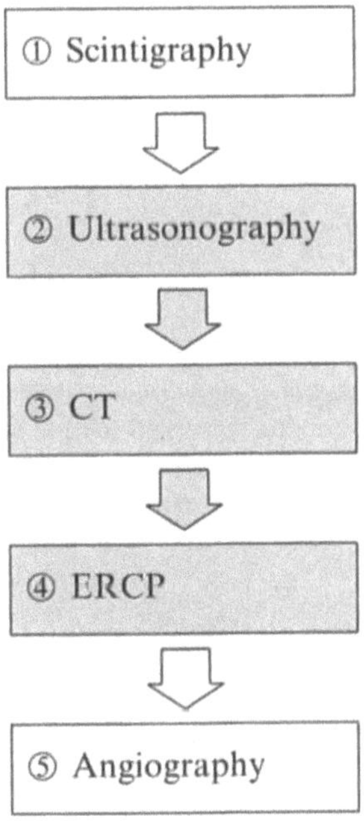

Patient. A 55-year-old woman.

Main Complaint. Fever, jaundice, and right hypochondralgia.

Present History. Jaundice was noticed 1 month prior. After 20 days, the patient had fever (40.7° C) and pain in the right costal portion; the fever lasted for 3 days. The patient was admitted to another clinic and medically treated. Fever and jaundice disappeared, but the patient was admitted to our clinic for further examination.

Laboratory Data.

SGOT	54 mU/ml	↑
SGPT	106 mU/ml	↑
ALP	193 mU/ml	↑
LDH	189 mU/ml	Normal
γ-GTP	134 mU/ml	↑
Cho E	558 U/dl	Normal
ZTT	6.9 U	Normal
Total bilirubin	1.0 mg/dl	Normal
Serum amylase	113 IU/l	Normal
Urine amylase	380 IU/l	Normal

Purpose of Diagnostic Imaging. To analyze the cause of jaundice.

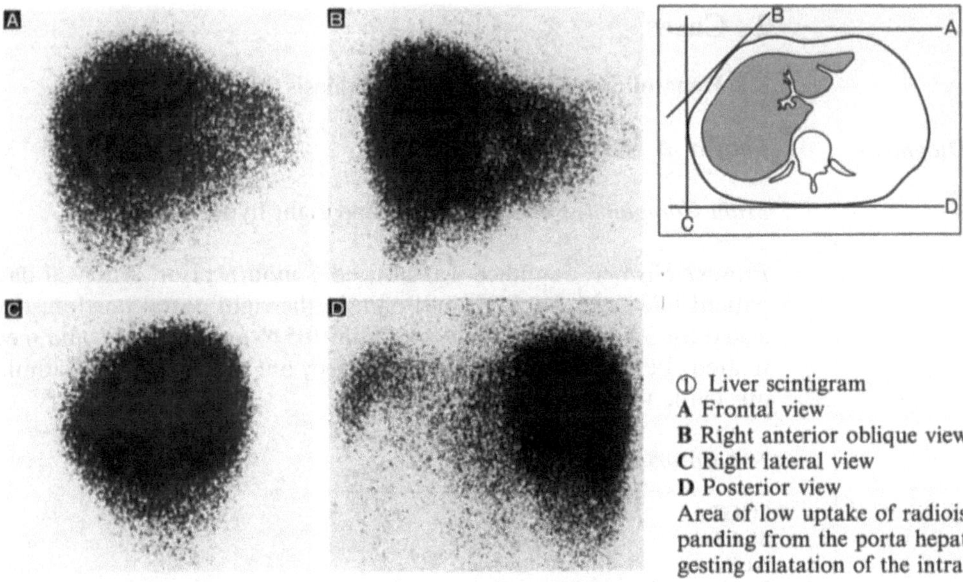

① Liver scintigram
A Frontal view
B Right anterior oblique view
C Right lateral view
D Posterior view
Area of low uptake of radioisotope is visualized expanding from the porta hepatis to the left lobe suggesting dilatation of the intrahepatic bile duct.

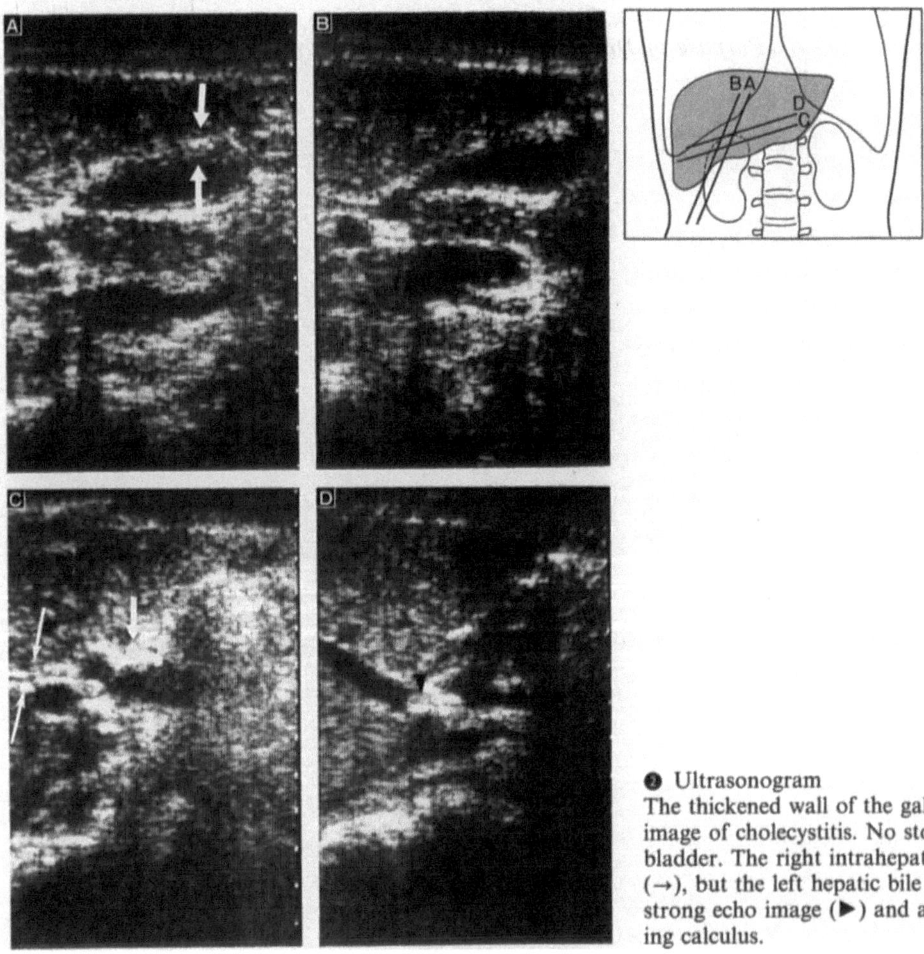

❷ Ultrasonogram
The thickened wall of the gallbladder (→) shows an image of cholecystitis. No stone is observed in the gallbladder. The right intrahepatic bile duct is not dilated (→), but the left hepatic bile duct is visualized with a strong echo image (▶) and acoustic shadow, indicating calculus.

❸ CT images
A, C, E Before contrast enhancement
B, D, F After contrast enhancement
Multiple high-attenuation shadows exist in the left hepatic lobe, suggesting stones (→). Gas images are seen in the bile duct (→), which become clearer after contrast enhancement.

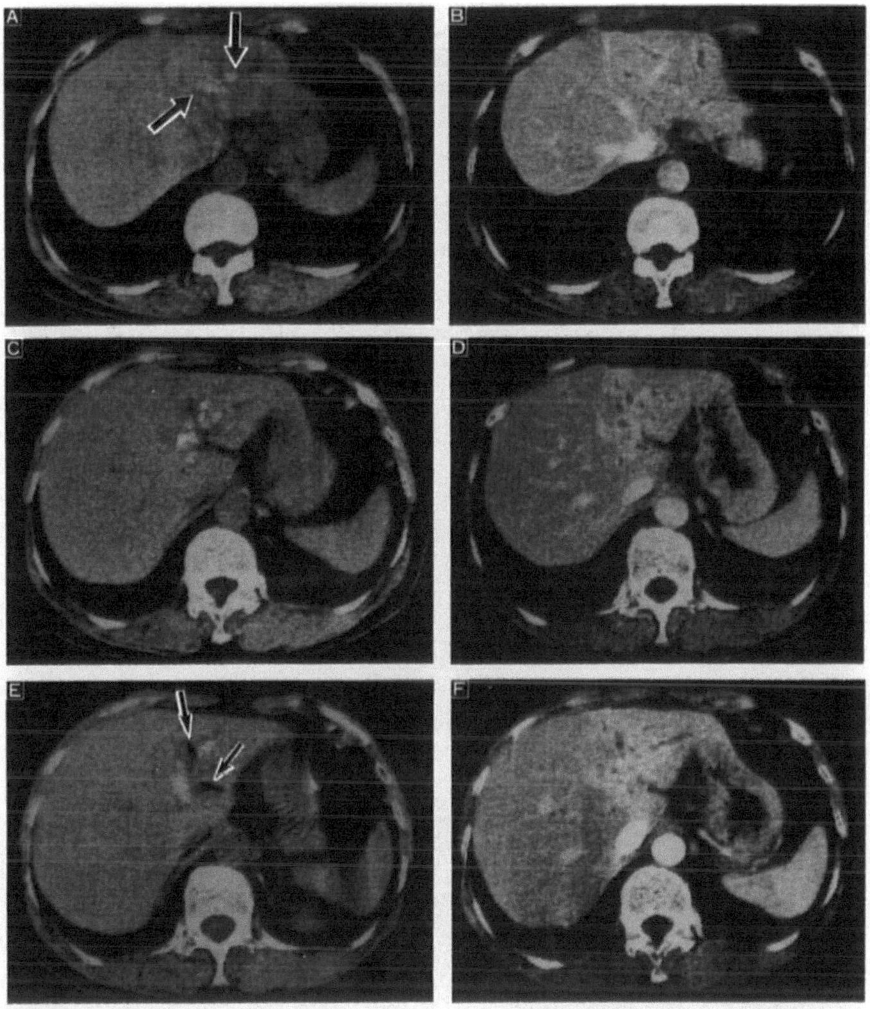

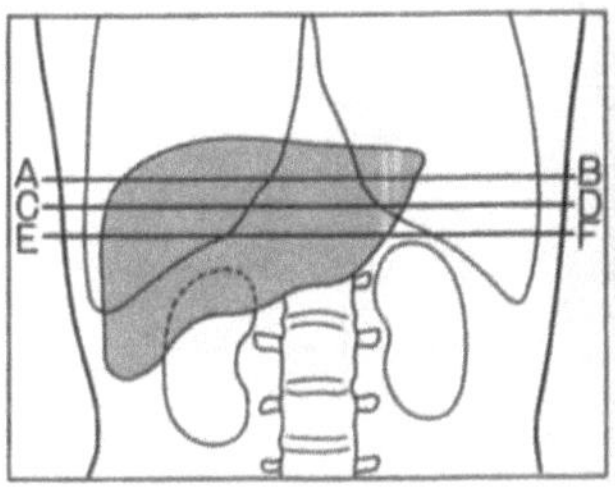

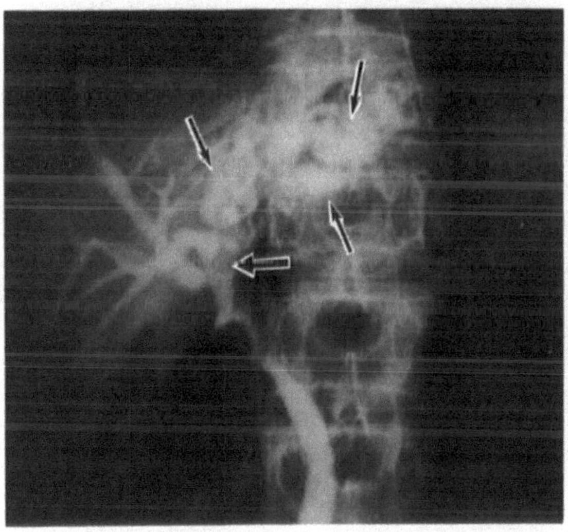

❹ ERCP
The left hepatic bile duct is stenosed in its origin and poorly opacified. At the distal portion, multiple stones are observed (→). A stones image is also seen in the common bile duct (→).

⑤ Angiography

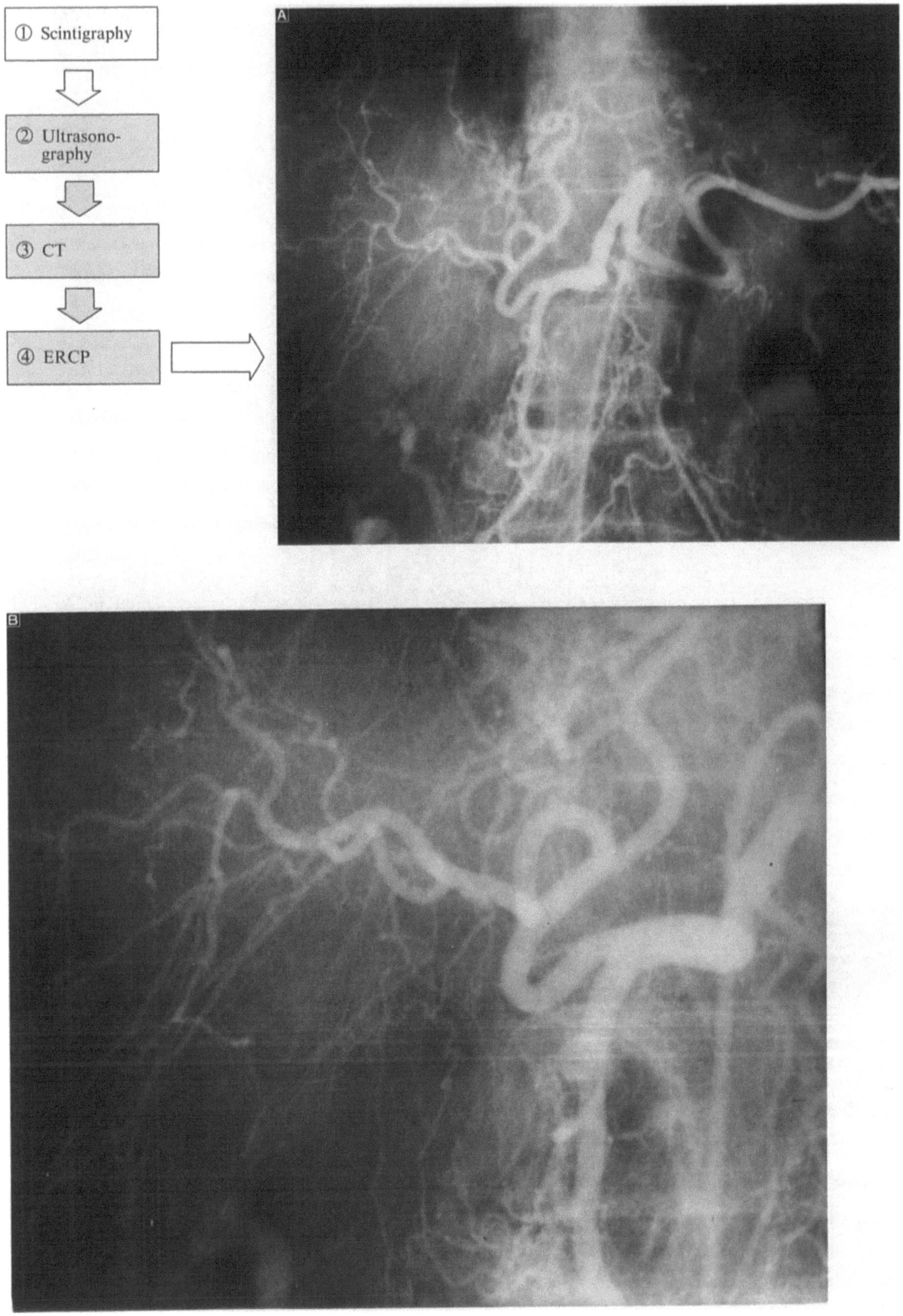
① Scintigraphy
② Ultrasono-graphy
③ CT
④ ERCP
A
B

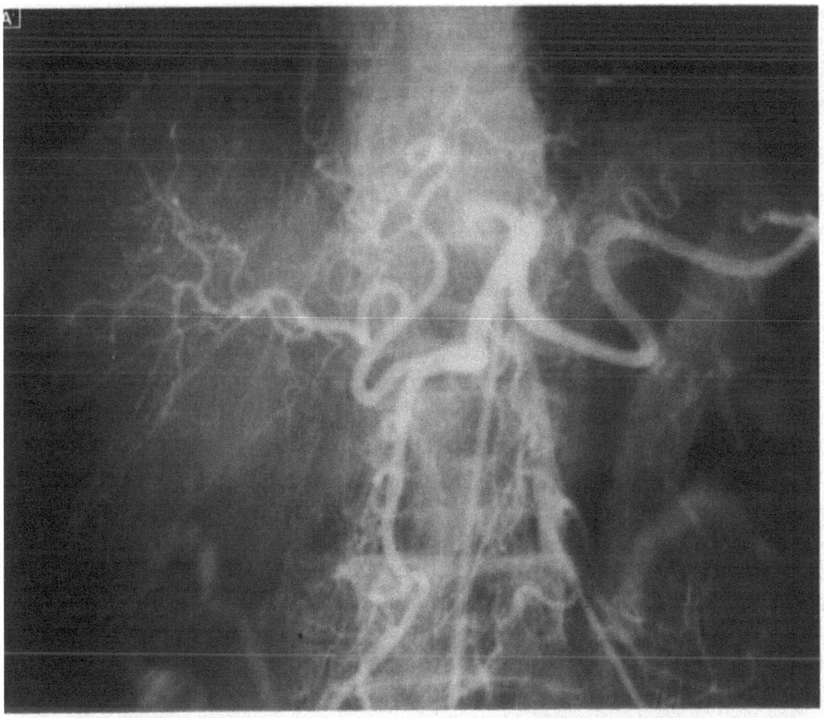

⑤ Angiogram
A, A′ Stereoscopic celiac arteriogram (arterial phase)
B Magnification celiac arteriogram (arterial phase)
C, C′ Stereoscopic superior mesenteric arteriogram (venous phase)
Branches to the medial segment of the left lobe show hypervascularity without malignant findings, suggesting an inflammatory disease. The portal vein shows no abdnormality.

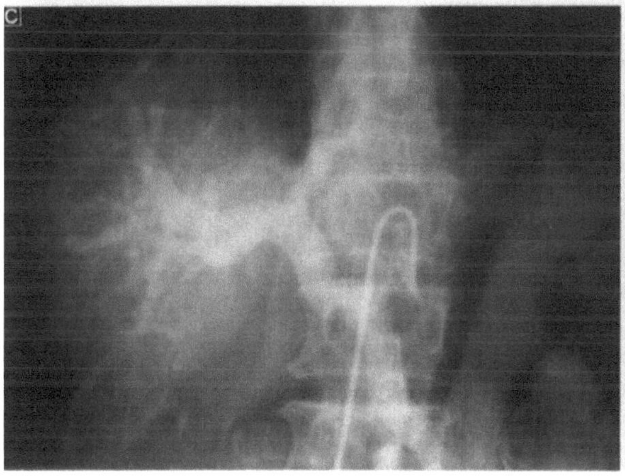

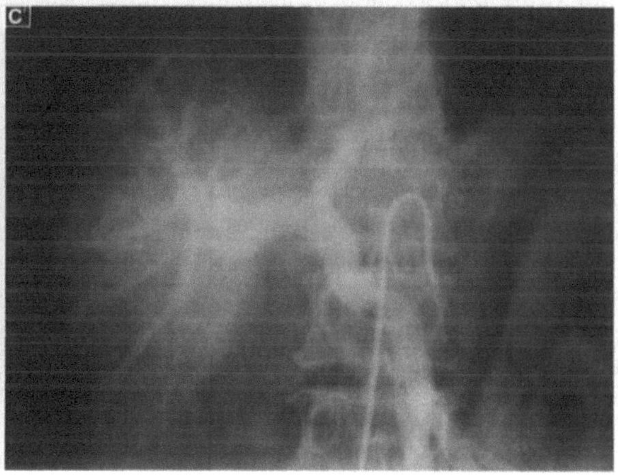

Operative Findings. Left hepatic lobectomy and cholecystectomy were performed. The left hepatic duct shows stenosis near its bifurcation, and the more distal branch is cystic and dilated with multiple stones inside. A stone the size of the tip of the little finger is observed in the common bile duct.

Significance of Diagnostic Imaging. Ultrasonography is useful in diagnosing intrahepatic stones. Particularly stones in the dilated intrahepatic bile duct are easily diagnosed. CT can also demonstrate a calcified stone as a high-attenuation area. However, to determine the operability and method of operation, examination of the intrahepatic bile duct with PTC and ERCP is required. Angiography may be performed to identify the existence of malignancy. In this case, ultrasonography or CT and ERCP are regarded as important examinations.

General Matters Concerning Hepatolithiasis [7, 12, 13]. The frequency of hepatolithiasis in Japan is regarded as high compared with Western society. Recently, it is said to be decreasing compared to before the world war II, and the frequency of hepatolithiasis is now 4–8% that of cholelithiasis in Japan. However, cholelithiasis is generally increasing, thus the absolute number is not decreasing. It is more frequent at 30–50 years of age there is no sex-related difference in incidence.

There are various reports about the classification of hepatolithiasis. Distinguishing is done by reference to localization of the stone or existence of stenosis and dilatation of the bile duct. Hepatolithiasis may also be divided into primary, which is caused by congenital factors of an intrahepatic stone, and secondary due to an extrahepatic bile duct stone. Hepatolithiasis is defined as a stone at the peripheral intrahepatic bile duct proximal to the right or left hepatic duct and consists mostly of calcium bilirubinate stone.

Hepatolithiasis is caused by stasis of bile juice and infection of the bile duct, and growth of the bile duct stone is accelerated by an anomalous connection and morphological abnormality of intrahepatic bile duct. Major clinical symptoms are abdominal pain, jaundice, and fever.

Accurate diagnosis of hepatolithiasis has been made possible by the use of PTC, ERC, ultrasonography, and CT. Generally, medical treatment consists of surgical operations, such as lithotomy and hepatectomy, and adjunctive operations, such as T-tube choledochal drainage, sphincteroplasty, and choledochoenterostomy.

2.2 Congenital Dilatation of the Bile Duct

Sequence of Diagnostic Imaging.

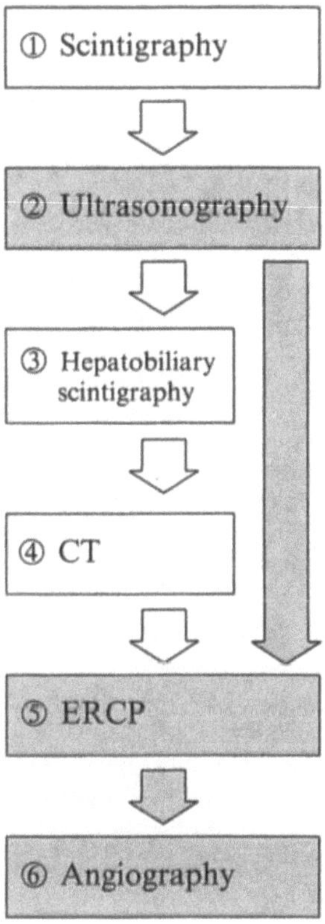

Patient. A 36-year-old man.

Main Complaint. Epigastralgia, nausea, and jaundice.

Past History. Cholecystitis at 10 and hepatitis at 22 years of age.

Present History. Sudden epigastralgia, nausea, and vomiting 1 year prior. Afterward similar symptoms appeared occasionally. Jaundice was detected in this examination.

Present Status. Not specified.

Laboratory Data.

SGOT	34 mU/ml	Normal
SGPT	29 mU/ml	Normal
ALP	72 mU/ml	Normal
LDH	136 mU/ml	Normal
γ-GTP	43 mU/ml	↑
Cho E	374 U/dl	Normal
Total protein	6.9 g/dl	Normal
ZTT	3.6 U	↓
Total bilirubin	1.1 mg/dl	Normal
Serum amylase	255 IU/l	Normal
Urine amylase	325 IU/l	Normal

Purpose of Diagnostic Imaging. Precise examination of the jaundice.

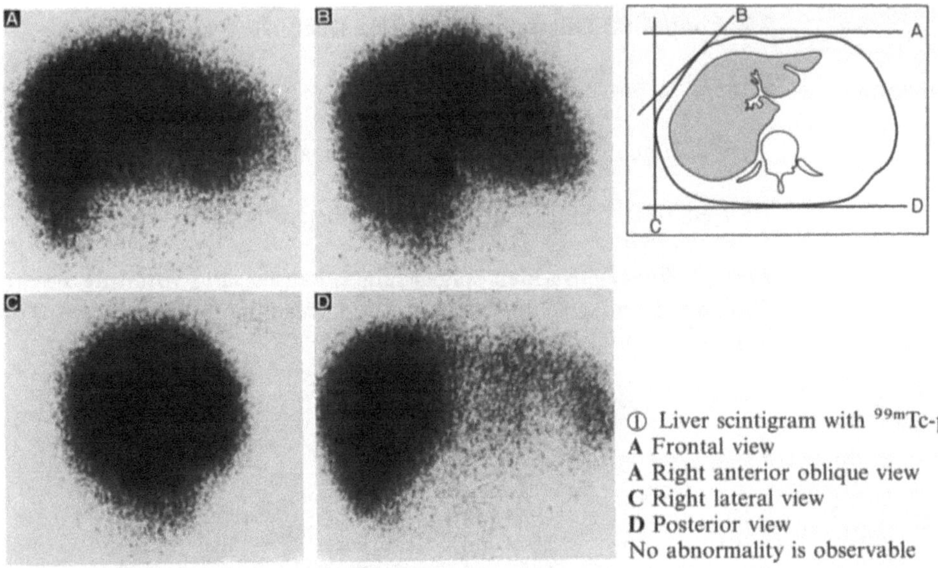

① Liver scintigram with ^{99m}Tc-phytate
A Frontal view
A Right anterior oblique view
C Right lateral view
D Posterior view
No abnormality is observable

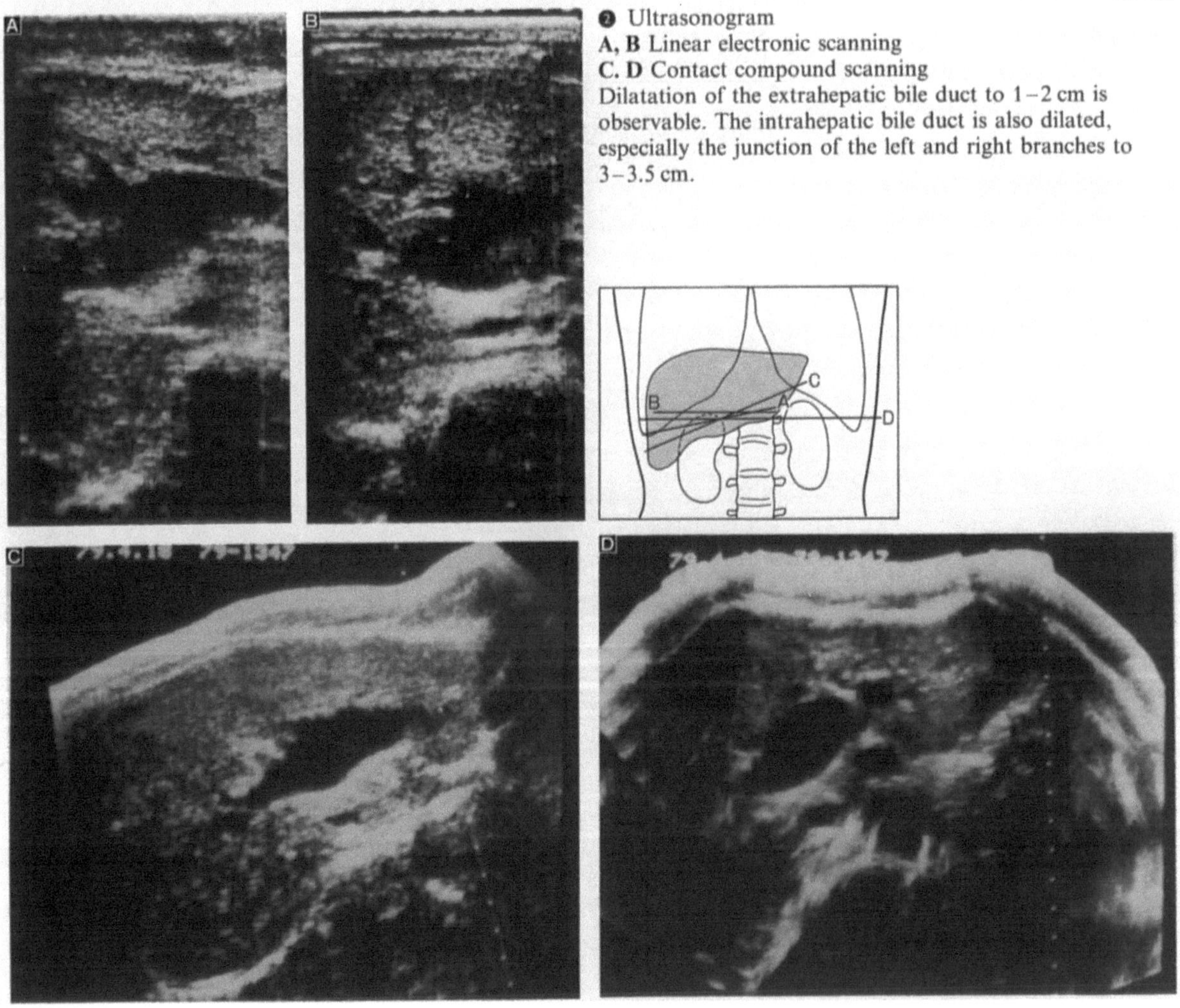

❷ Ultrasonogram
A, B Linear electronic scanning
C. D Contact compound scanning
Dilatation of the extrahepatic bile duct to 1–2 cm is observable. The intrahepatic bile duct is also dilated, especially the junction of the left and right branches to 3–3.5 cm.

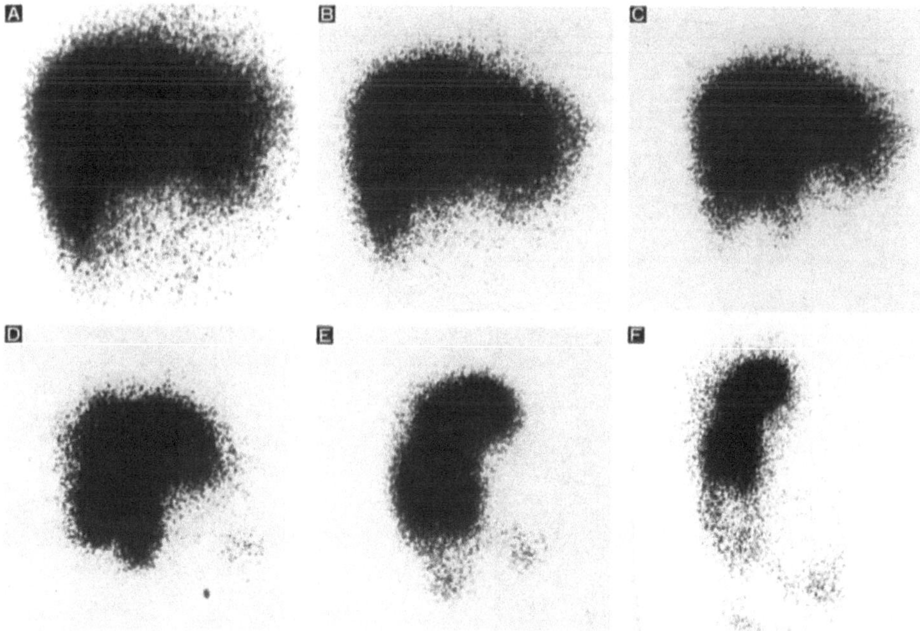

③ Hepatobiliary scintigram with ^{99m}Tc-HIDA
A After 10 min
B After 20 min
C After 40 min
D After 80 min
E After 150 min
F After 4 h
Twenty minutes after injection, only the liver is visualized, and the gallbladder and biliary tract are not visualized. After 30–40 min, massive uptake of radioisotope in the porta hepatis and dilated common bile duct are demonstrated. After 80 min, although uptake of radioisotope in the liver still remains, dilatation of the intra- and extrahepatic bile ducts and excretion of radioisotope to the intestine are clearly observable. After 4 h, uptake of radioisotope in the liver disappears, but that in the intrahepatic bile duct, hepatic duct, and extrahepatic bile duct still remain, indicating severe dilatation. Radioisotope was completely excreted into the intestine 6 h after the injection.

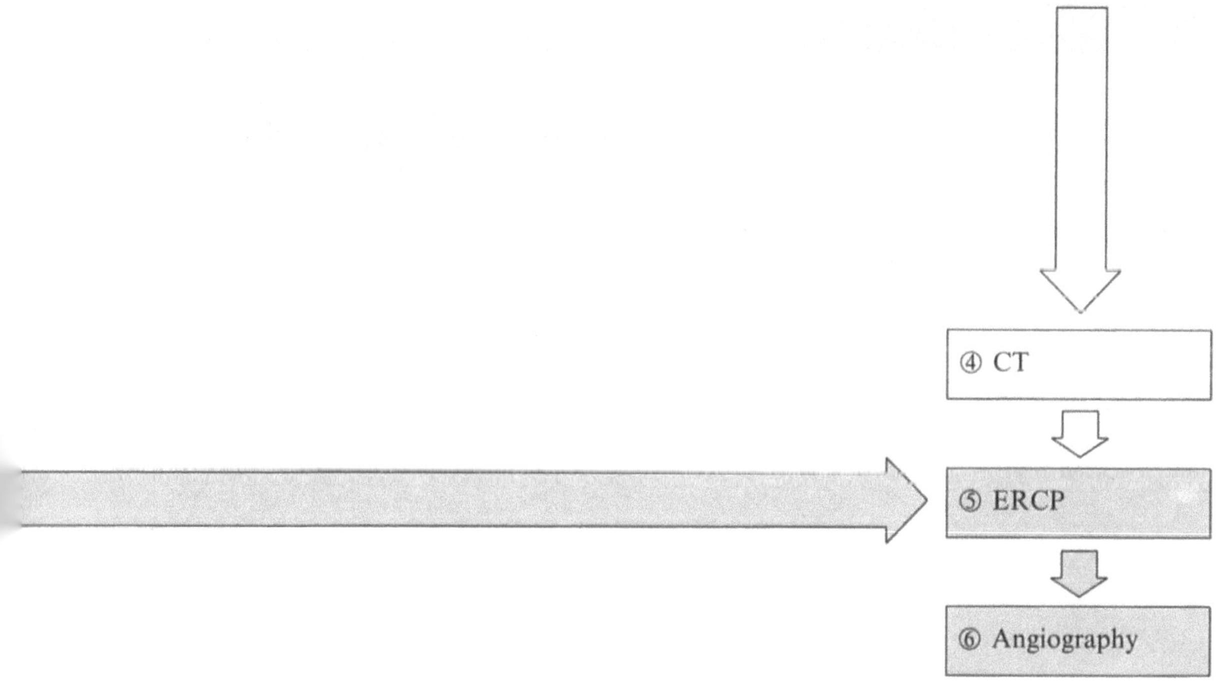

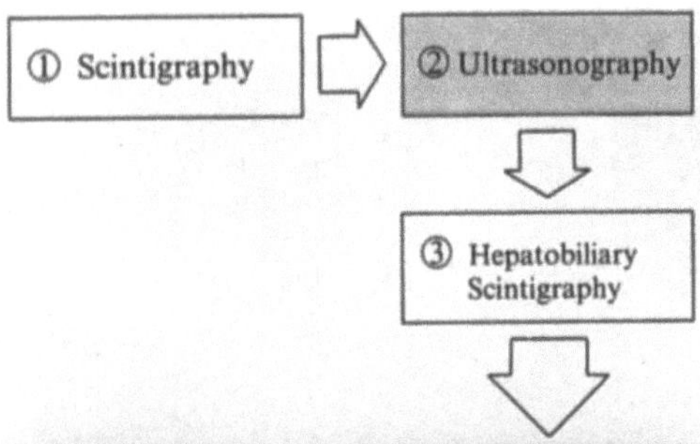
① Scintigraphy
② Ultrasonography
③ Hepatobiliary Scintigraphy

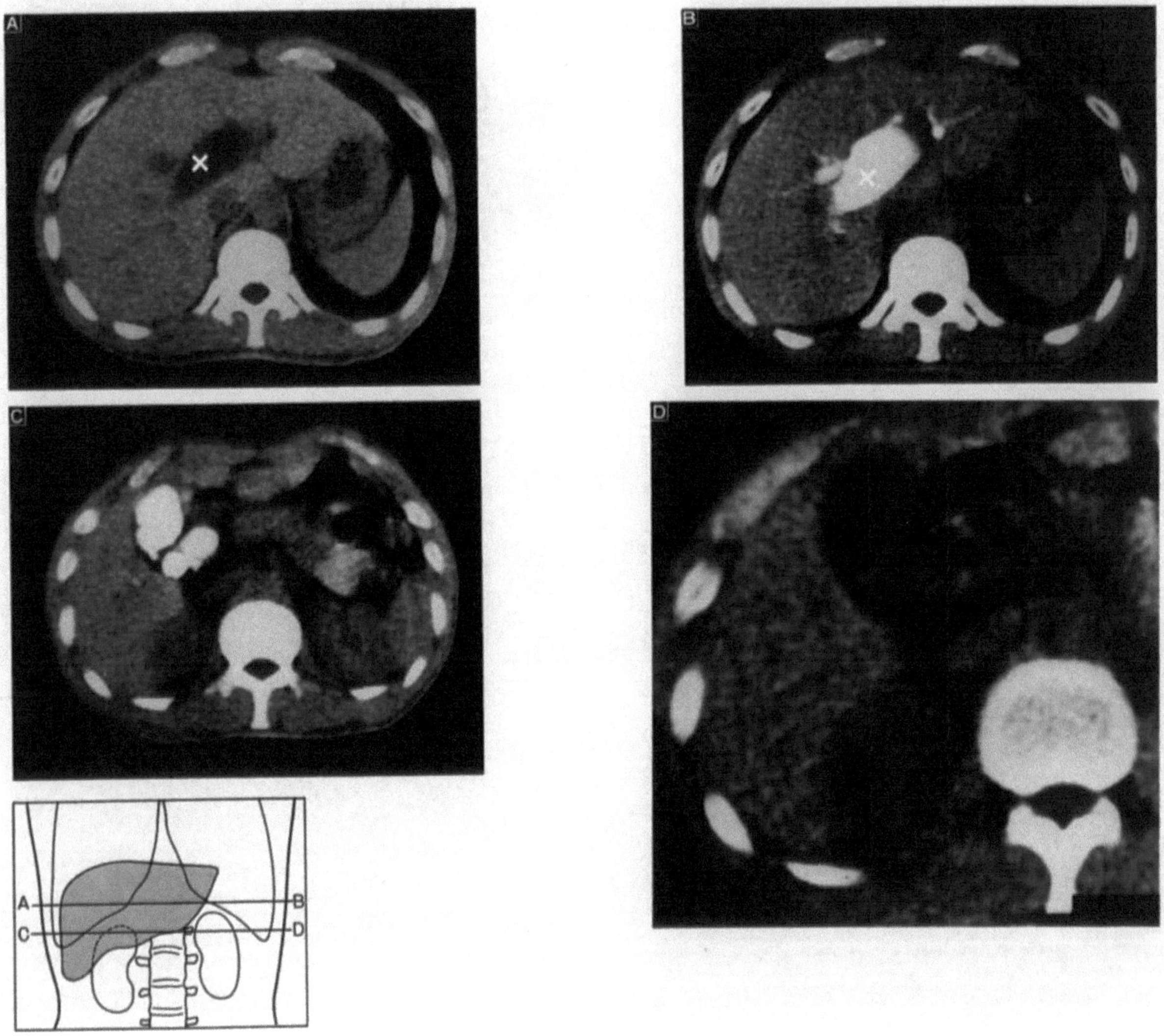
A
B
C
D

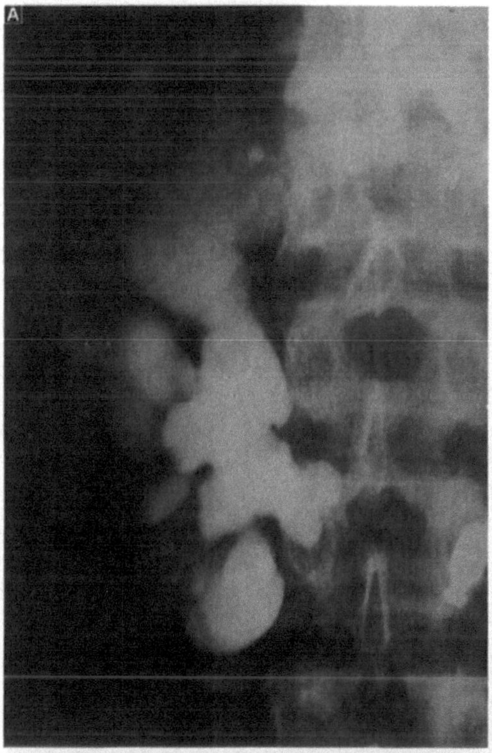

❺ ERCP combined with hypotonic duodenography
A Frontal view
B Right anterior oblique view
C Left anterior oblique view
D Frontal view

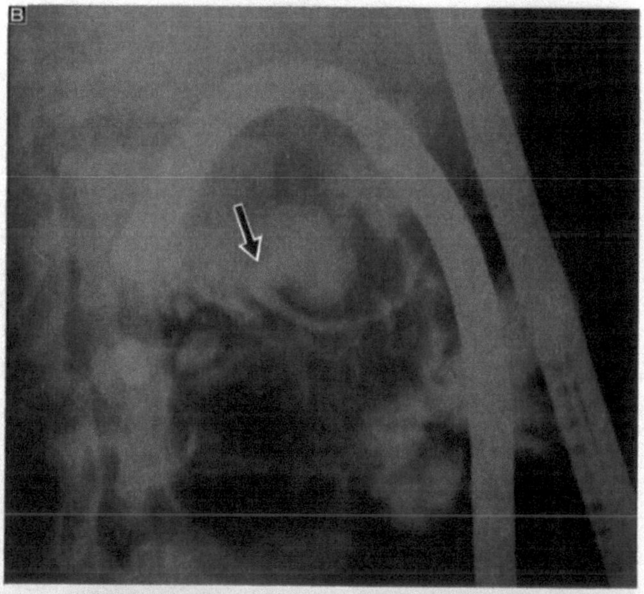

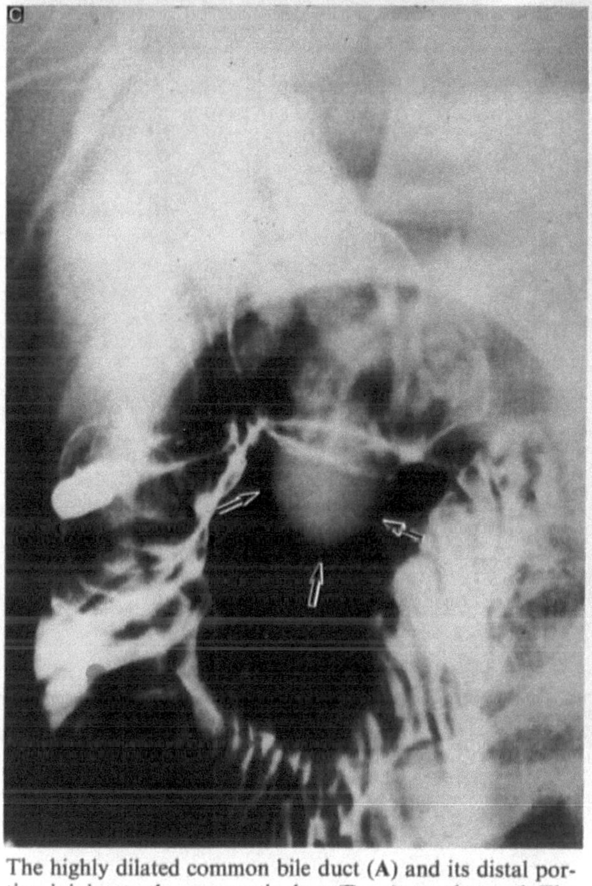

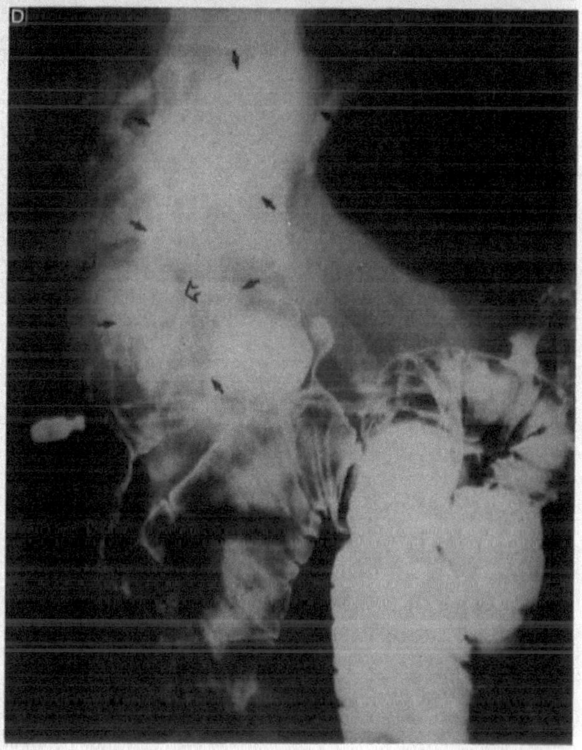

The highly dilated common bile duct (**A**) and its distal portion joining to the pancreatic duct (**B**, →) are observed. The gallbladder is normal in morphology (**C**, →), and cystic dilatation of the left hepatic duct is marked (**D**, →).

⑥ Angiography

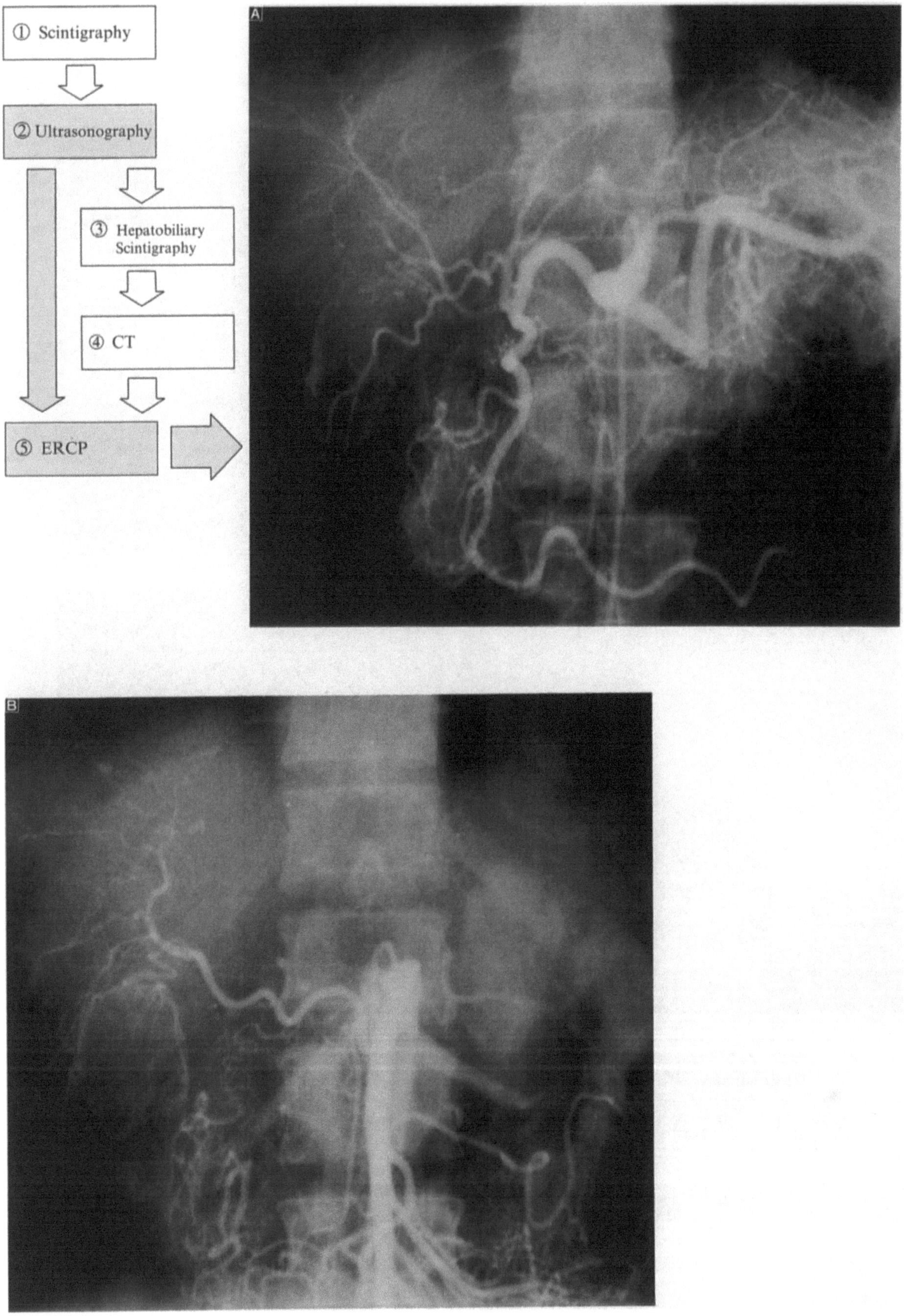
① Scintigraphy
② Ultrasonography
③ Hepatobiliary Scintigraphy
④ CT
⑤ ERCP
A
B

❻ Angiogram
A Celiac arteriogram (arterial phase)
B Superior mesenteric arteriogram (arterial phase)
C Magnification (× 3) celiac arteriogram (arterial phase)
D Superior mesenteric arteriogram (venous phase)
The cystic artery branches from the right hepatic artery, which itself branches from the superior mesenteric artery. Hypervascularity of the extrahepatic bile duct suggests dilatation of the bile duct without any malignant findings. The middle and left hepatic arteries are displaced from the porta hepatis to the left lobe where hypervasculatity of fine vessels is markedly seen, indicating dilatation of the intrahepatic bile duct. The portal vein is well visualized, but the left branch is displaced posteriorly at the bifurcation. No malignant findings are observed in the liver.

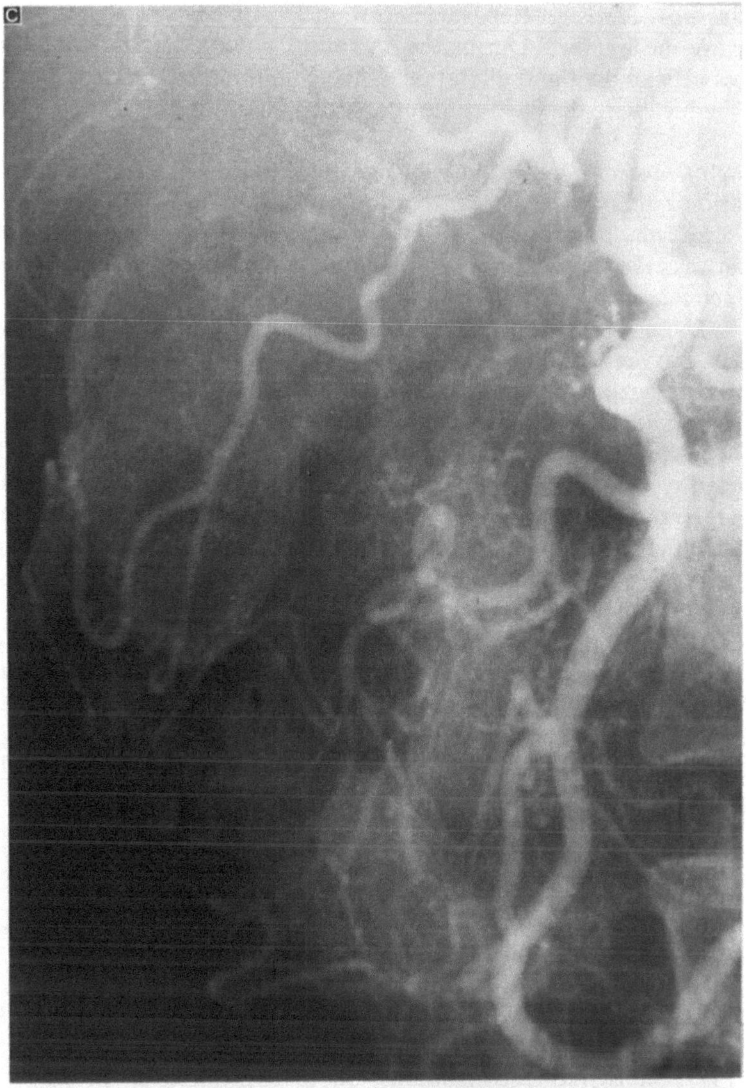

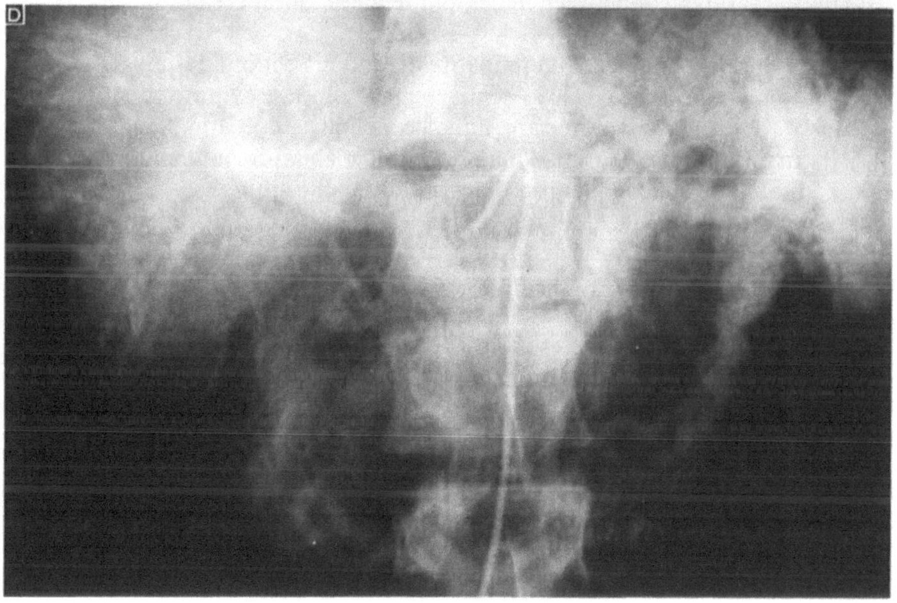

Operative Findings. Hepatojejunostomy (Roux-en-Y) was performed to improve the jaundice. During the operation, however, cystic dilatation of the left hepatic duct and dilatation of the common hepatic duct and common bile duct were detected without any malignant findings.

Significance of Diagnostic Imaging. Definitive diagnosis of congenital dilatation of the bile duct can be done with ERCP or PTC, which directly opacify the biliary tract. ERCP is required for studying the relationship between the pancreatic duct or for differentiation from dilatation of the bile duct caused by a stone.

The presence of disease can often be studied with CT or ultrasonography, but hepatobiliary scintigraphy is also useful. To identify the existence of a malignant tumor, which frequently accompanies congenital dilatation of the bile duct, angiography is desirable prior to the operation.

In case 2, cystic dilatation of the bile duct can be detected by ultrasonography, CT, and hepatobiliary scintigraphy; thus the presence of disease can be diagnosed with any of these techniques. ERCP is indispensable to study the condition of the entire biliary tract and to decide on the operation method. Angiography is also necessary for detection of accompanying malignant tumors.

General Matters Concerning Congenital Dilatation of the Bile Duct [1, 8, 9, 14]. Congenital dilatation of the bile duct is a localized cystic dilatation of the biliary tract including that conventionally called the congenital choledochal cyst. It is classified into three types by Alonso-Lej et al. [1]:

I = congenital cystic dilatation of the common bile duct
II = congenital diverticulum of the common bile duct
III = congenital choledochocele

Later, various classifications were made including multiple biliary cysts and intrahepatic cystic bile duct.

Congenital dilatation of the bile duct is regarded as rare in Western society, but relatively frequent in Japan. One-third of Alonso-Lej's reports are cases which occurred in Japan. Komi et al. [9] totaled 560 cases in Japan (1977). It is frequent in infants, about two-thirds of all cases. The sex distribution ratio is 1:4 between males and females, but it is said that there is less sex difference in infants.

Symptoms are jaundice, abdominal pain, and an abdominal mass as a triad, but only a little above 20% of cases show all these symptoms simultaneously. The main symptoms are jaundice, acholic stool, and swelling of the liver in infants, an abdominal mass in younger children, and abdominal pain and jaundice are frequent in older children and adults.

It is regarded as congenital, but cases with fusiform dilatation may also be acquired. Additionally, an anomalous connection between the distal end of the common bile duct and the pancreatic duct occurs with high frequency.

Internal treatment may result in the patient's death due to accompanying biliary cirrhosis or other complications (liver abscess and sepsis). Therefore, surgery is the treatment of first choice. Cancer of the bile duct may be present, necessitating a radical operation including cystectomy.

2.3 Primary Sclerosing Cholangitis

Sequence of Diagnostic Imaging.
Before the operation

① Ultrasonography
⇩
② PTC
⇩
③ Angiography

After the operation

① Scintigraphy
⇩
② CT
⇩
③ Angiography

Patient. A 70-year-old man.

Main Complaint. Jaundice and itching over the whole body.

Present History. Jaundice was diagnosed by another clinic 3 months prior, and had improved well with internal treatment. Jaundice appeared again 1 month prior and PTC was performed. He was admitted to this clinic with suspected carcinoma of the common hepatic duct.

Laboratory Data.

SGOT	49 mU/ml	↑
SGPT	42 mU/ml	↑
ALP	233 mU/ml	↑
LDH	137 mU/ml	Normal
Cho E	277 U/dl	Normal
γ-GTP	52 mU/ml	↑
Total bilirubin	12.9 mg/dl	Normal
Direct bilirubin	10.1 mg/dl	↑

Purpose of Diagnostic Imaging. Further examination of the jaundice.

Diagnostic Imaging Before the Operation

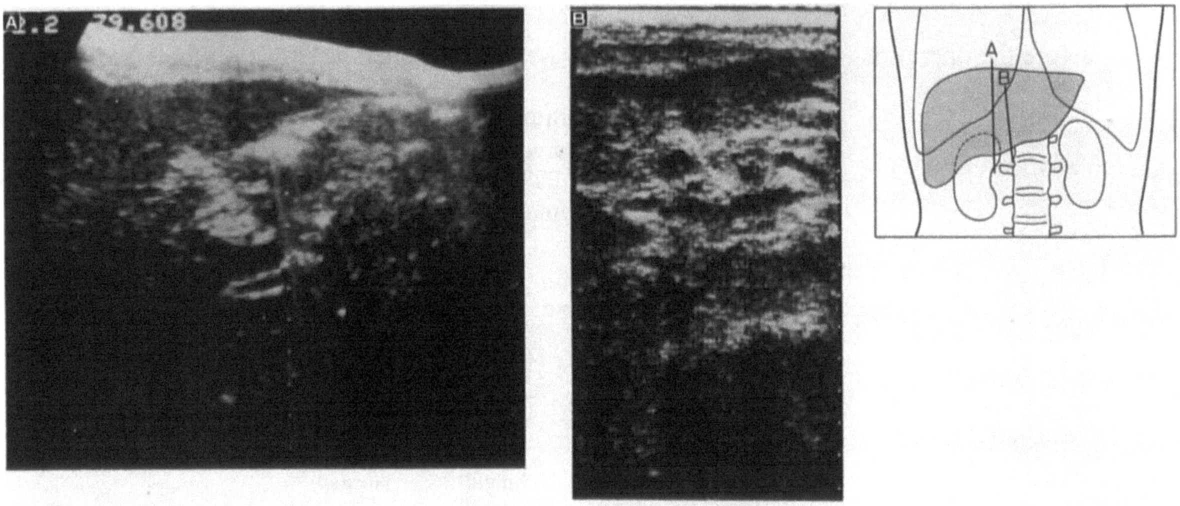

① Ultrasonogram
A Contact compound scanning
B Linear electronic scanning
An entirely inhomogeneous echogenicity is observable including partial spotty strong echoes. Dilatation of the intrahepatic bile duct or findings of tumor are nonexistent.

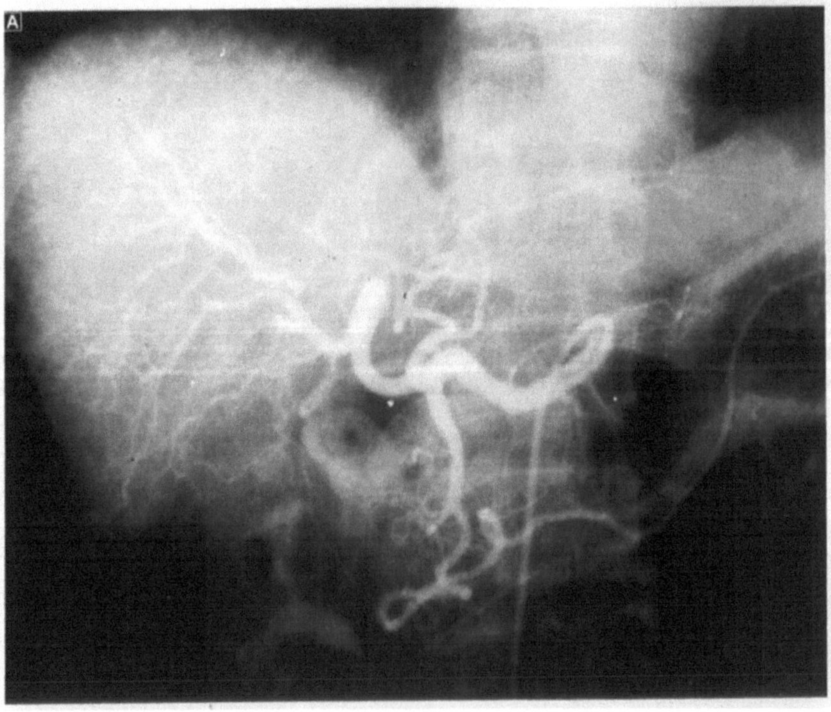

❷ Angiogram
A, A′ Stereoscopic celiac arteriogram (arterial phase)
Opacification was achieved by inserting a catheter into the common hepatic artery. Encasement of the right hepatic artery at the bifurcation and an entirely swollen liver are observed.

❷ PTC
Stenosis of the right hepatic duct (→) and lower common bile duct (→) are observed.

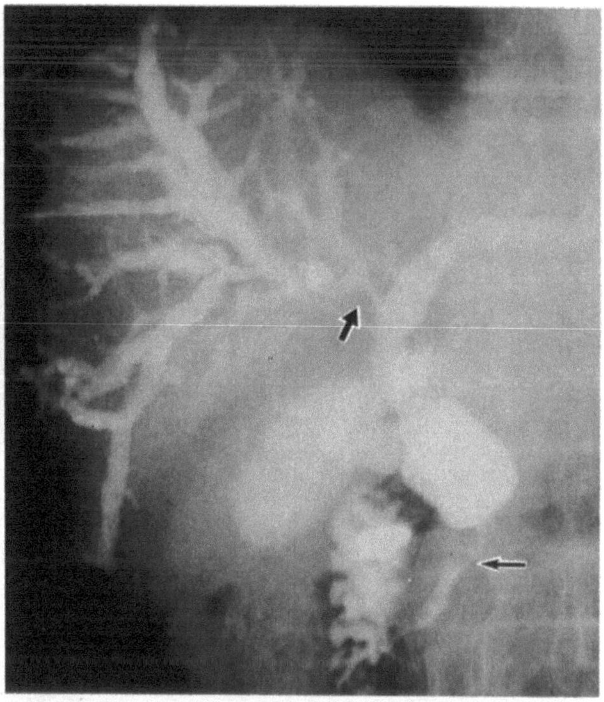

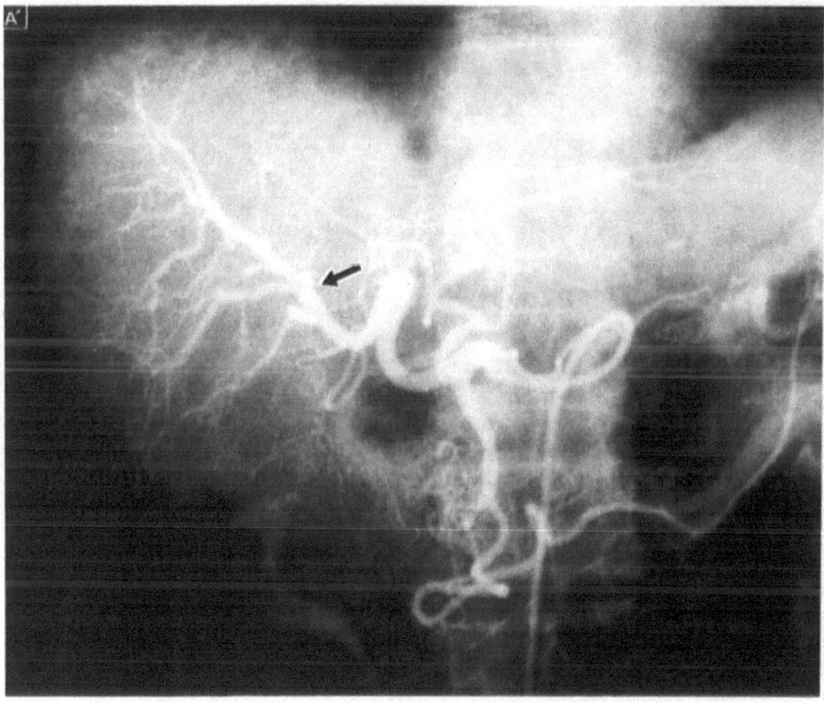

③ Angiography (B, C)

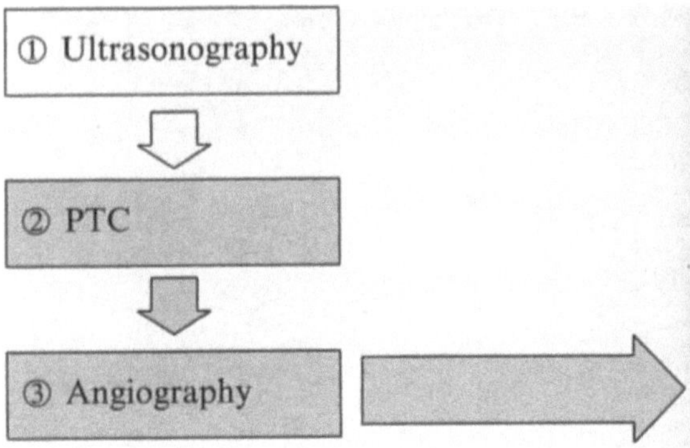

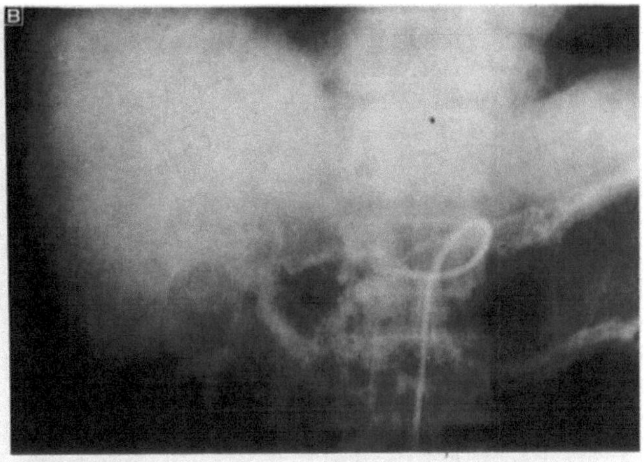

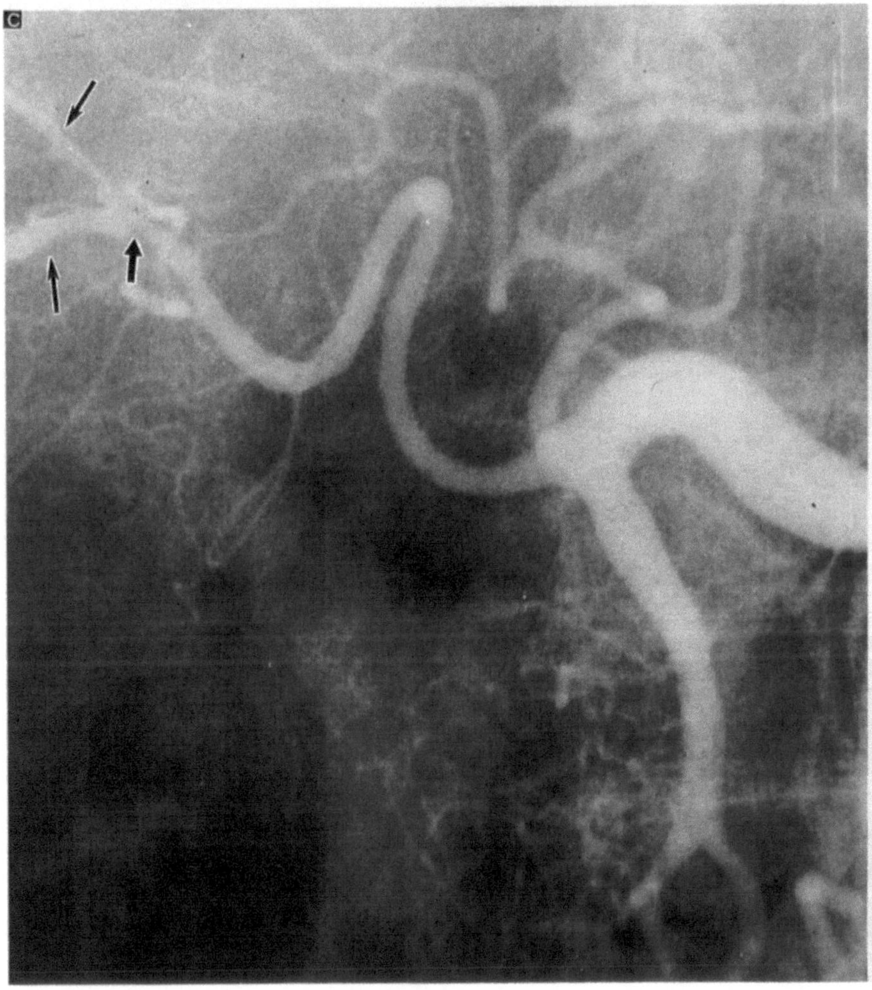

B Celiac arteriogram (venous phase)
C Magnification celiac arteriogram
The hepatogram phase (**B**) is homogeneously opacified throughout. The magnification celiac arteriogram (**C**) apparently shows stenosis (→) and poststenotic dilatation (→) of the right hepatic artery. No abnormality is observed in the periportal artery. Malignancy cannot be ruled out on these angiograms.

① Hepatobiliary scintigram with ^{99m}Tc-HIDA
A After 30 min
B After 45 min
C, D After 60 min
There are no abnormalities except slightly delayed excretion of contrast medium in the bile duct.

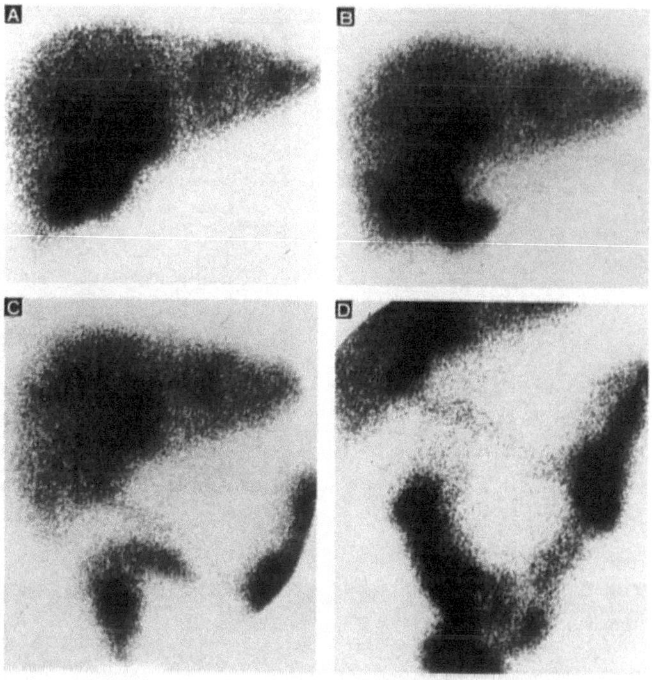

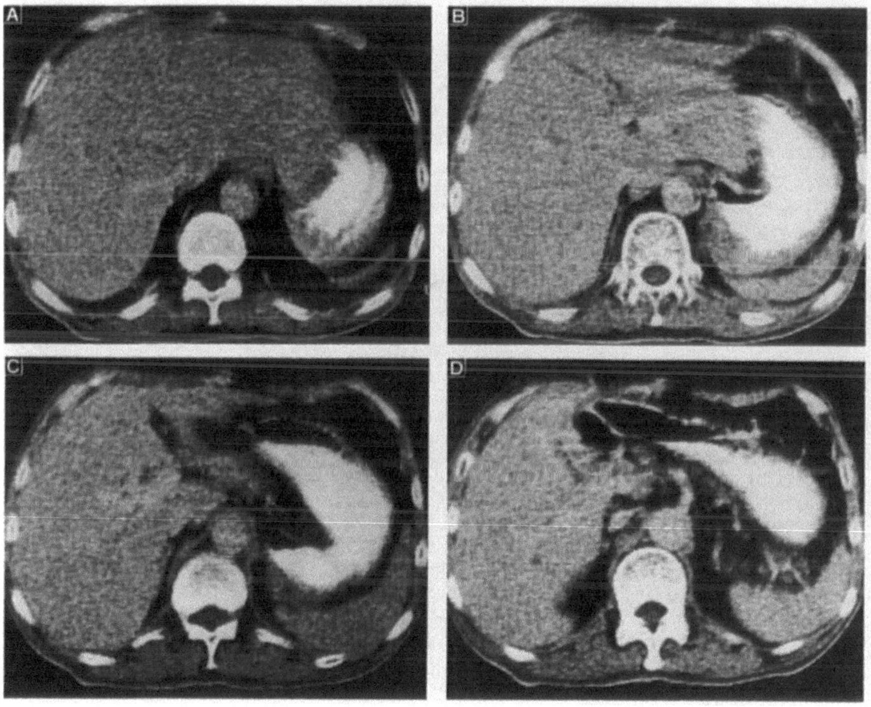

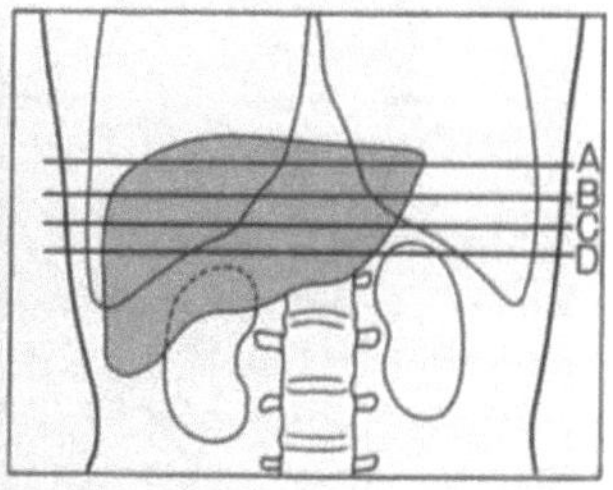

② CT image
After contrast enhancement, dilatation of the intrahepatic bile duct and a finding of tumor in the porta hepatis are not observed. Varices exist in the stomach.

③ Angiography

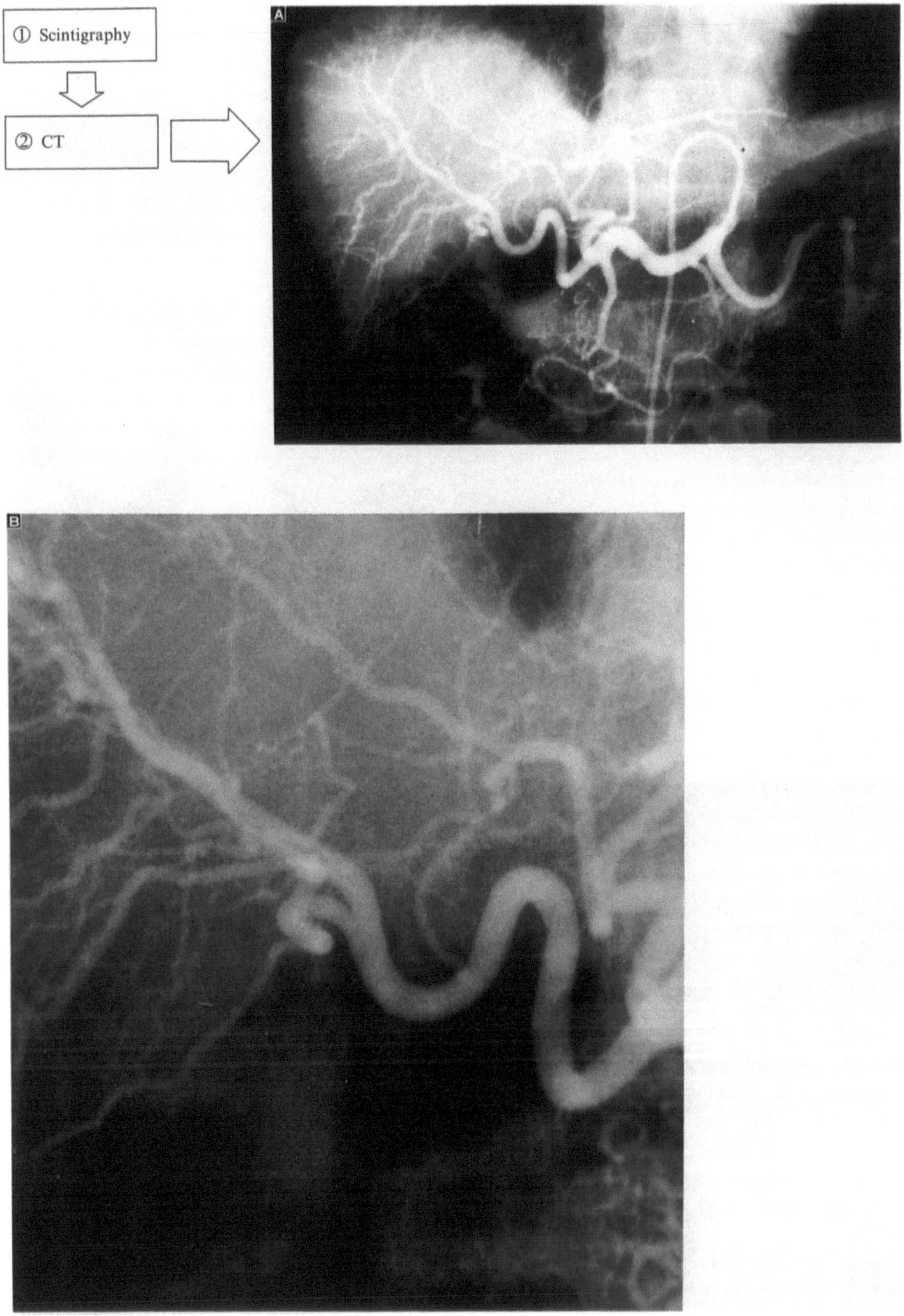
① Scintigraphy
② CT
A
B

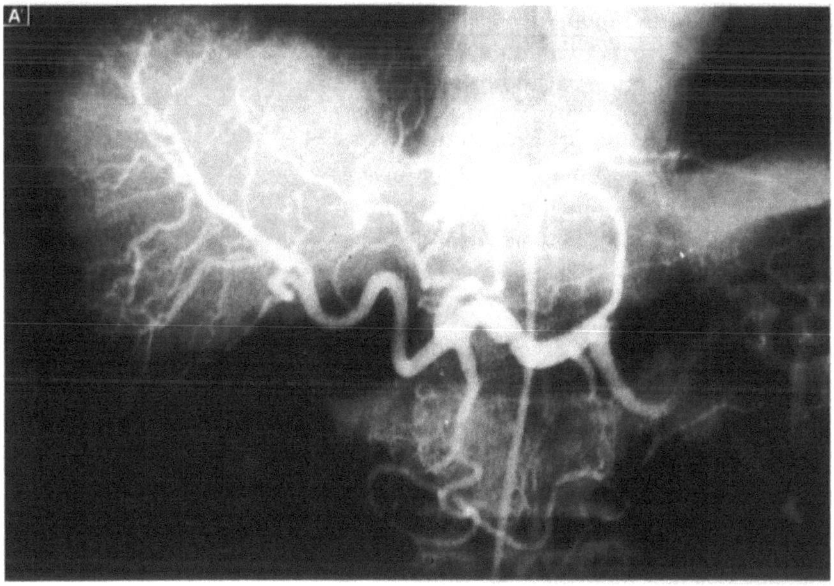

❸ Angiogram
A, A' Stereoscopic celiac arteriogram
B Magnification celiac arteriogram
The stenosis observed at the bifurcation of the right hepatic artery before the operation is not seen, and the swelling of the liver has almost disappeared. Spasms due to the inserted catheter are observed in the common hepatic artery (**A, A'**). Stenosis is also not seen on the magnification angiogram (**B**), and the periportal artery runs and branches normally.

Operative Findings. Adhesion of the gallbladder, bile duct, and intrahepatic bile duct and severely hardened right and left main hepatic ducts suggested carcinoma. Thus, cholecystectomy, resection of the hepatic duct at the porta hepatis, and choledochojejunostomy were performed. The wall had thickened from the left and right main hepatic ducts to the common bile duct, and inflammatory proliferation mainly consisting of fibrosis and plasmacytes was marked without any malignant findings.

Treatment. The therapy consisted of a corticosteroid injection into the bile duct.

Significance of Diagnostic Imaging. Precise examination of jaundice should be started with ultrasonography. In this case, however, PTC had already been performed in another clinic; thus, ultrasonography was actually undertaken after PTC. During ultrasonography, the dilatation of the intrahepatic bile duct cannot be seen because of PTC drainage, and no tumor image is observable in the porta hepatis. Angiography visualized abnormality of vessels at the porta hepatis, and in preoperative diagnosis opinion varied on its cause between inflammation and cancer. Angiographic findings are insufficient to diagnose cancer compared to marked findings on PTC. Krieger et al. [10] reported cholangiogram findings as follows:

> Stricture is the characteristic radiographic feature and involves the extrahepatic bile ducts and intrahepatic biliary radicles with variable length of the stricture, ranging from uniform involvement of the extrahepatic bile ducts to short focal strictures of the hepatic ducts with sparing of the common bile duct. Involvement of the intrahepatic ducts is characterized by obliteration of the smaller biliary radicles, giving a "pruned tree" appearance with luminal irregularities and beading of the bile ducts. Another important finding is the absence of marked dilatation of the intrahepatic ducts proximal to a stricture of the extrahepatic bile ducts due to the inflammatory fibrosis of the walls of the intrahepatic ducts.

However, differentiation with only PTC is not always easy, and definite diagnosis may be possible from a magnification angiogram without abnormality in addition to the PTC.

General Matters Concerning Primary Sclerosing Cholangitis [2, 11,16]. The primary sclerosing cholangitis which causes obstructive jaundice is a rare disease among benign biliary strictures. The stricture is caused by thickening of the bile duct wall, and diffuse inflammatory sclerosis of the bile duct wall is observed over a broad region. Thus, a hard and stringy bile duct is palpated. It is frequent in those over 40 years of age and a sex difference is nonexistent. There are many different theories about its causes, such as bacterial, viral, autoimmunity, or bile juice infection, but so far none have been confirmed. Many cases are accompanied by ulcerative colitis. The diagnostic criteria as stated by Schwartz are as follows:

1. Diffuse thickening of the extrahepatic bile duct
2. No surgical history of the bile duct
3. No bile duct stone or tumor

However, Longmire [11] queries the accuracy of these criteria.

Preoperative diagnosis may occasionally be possible from PTC and ERCP findings, but frequently differentiation from bile duct carcinoma is difficult. Furthemore, even histologically, differentiation from the well-differentiated sclerosing carcinoma of the bile duct may be difficult [2].

Internal steroid administration is regarded as effective for medical treatment, but actually in many cases, after determining bile duct carcinoma in preoperative examinations, surgery is frequently performed.

2.4 Carcinoma of the Gallbladder

Sequence of Diagnostic Imaging.

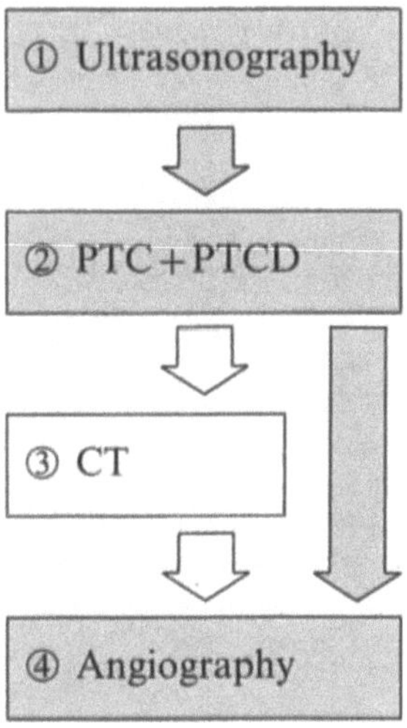

Patient. A 78-year-old woman.

Main Complaint. General fatigue and jaundice.

Present History. Above-mentioned symptoms of the past 2 weeks. The patient was hospitalized in the internal medicine department.

Present Status. Severe jaundice and tenderness on pressure at the epigastrium without palpability of the mass.

Laboratory Data.

SGOT	219 mU/ml	↑
SGPT	125 mU/ml	↑
ALP	1280 mU/ml	↑
LDH	306 mU/ml	↑
γ-GTP	213 mU/ml	↑
Cho E	244 U/dl	Normal
ZTT	4.6 U	Normal
Total bilirubin	26.8 mg/dl	↑
Direct bilirubin	21.3 mg/dl	↑
Serum amylase	69 IU/l	↓

Purpose of Diagnostic Imaging. To differentiate the jaundice and detect its causes.

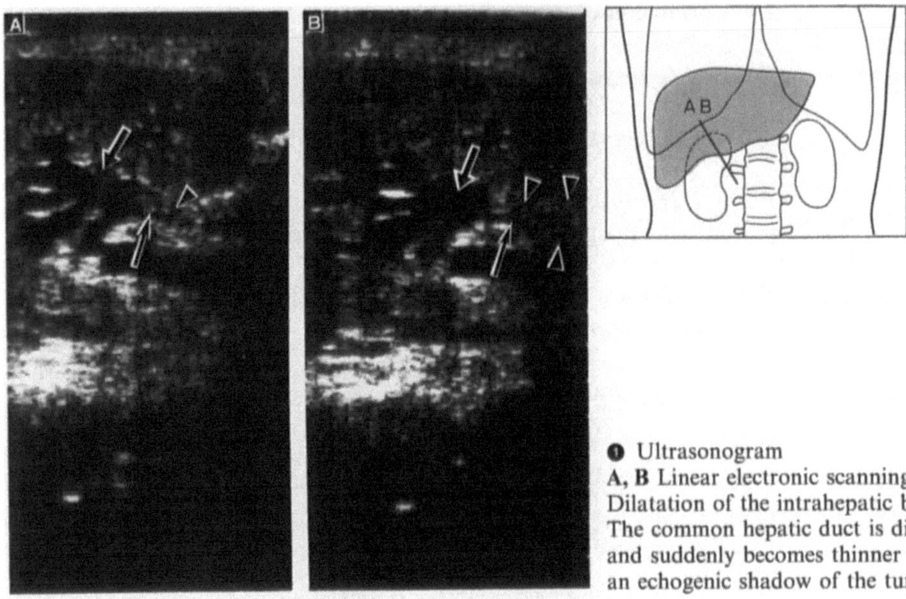

❶ Ultrasonogram
A, B Linear electronic scanning
Dilatation of the intrahepatic bile duct is marked (→). The common hepatic duct is dilated at the proximal side and suddenly becomes thinner and irregular (→) where an echogenic shadow of the tumor is seen (▶).

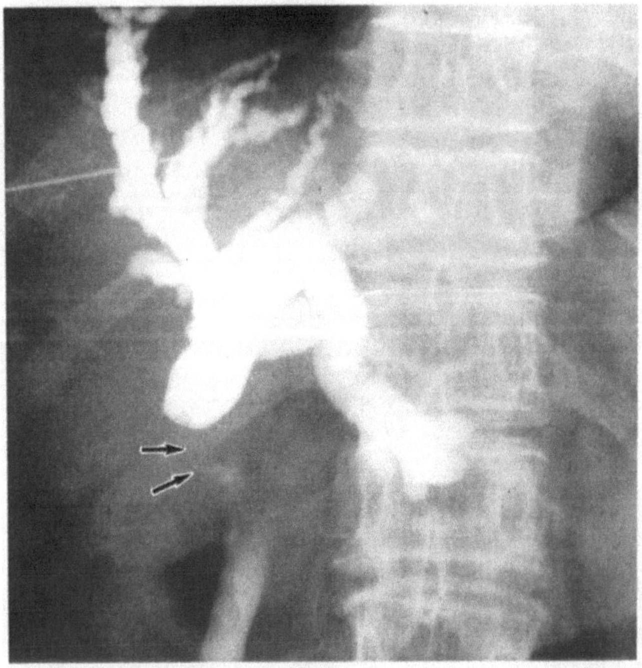

❷ PTC + PTCD
Dilatation of the intrahepatic bile duct and common hepatic duct and stenosis (→) at the joining point of the common hepatic duct, common bile duct, and cystic duct are visualized. The gallbladder and cystic duct are nonopacified.

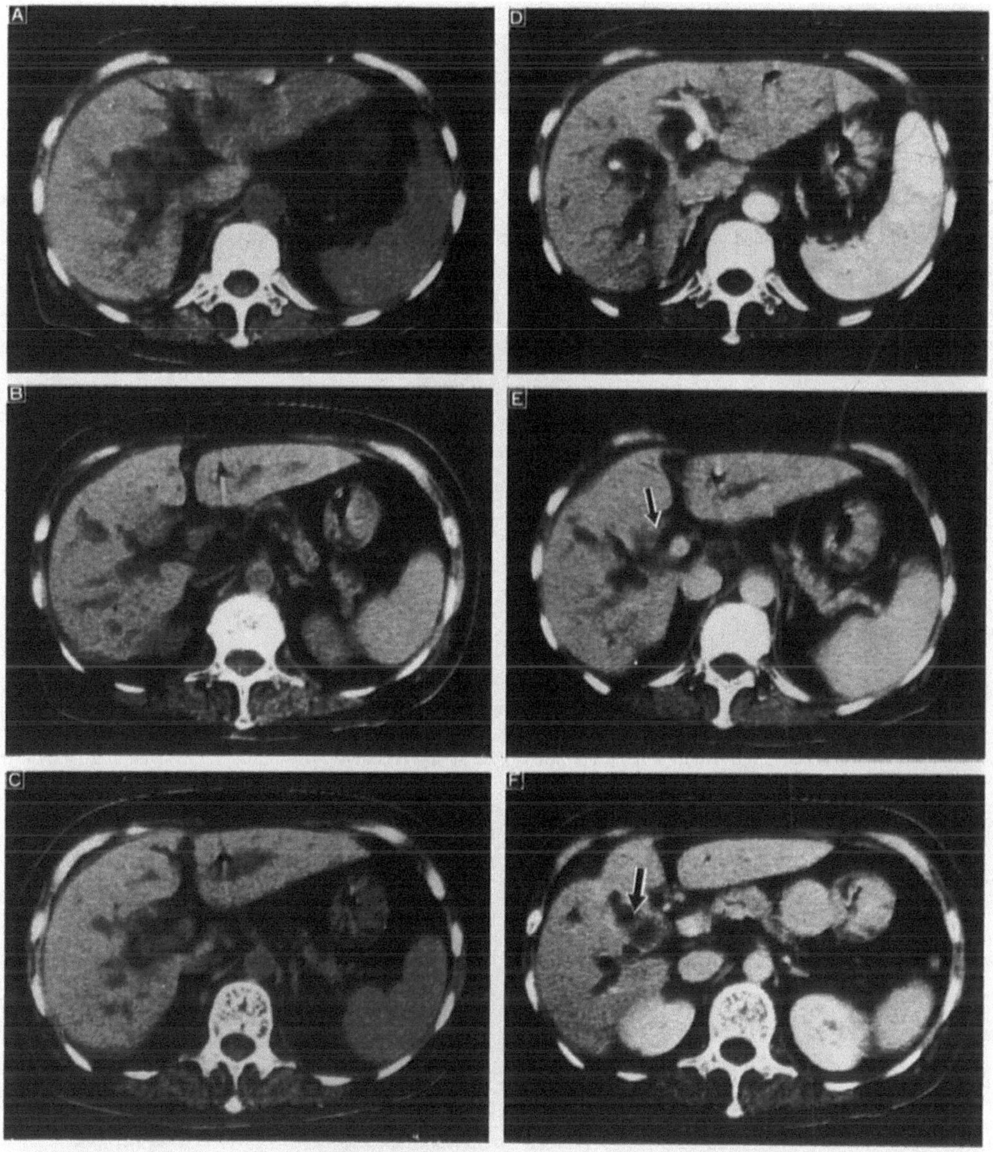

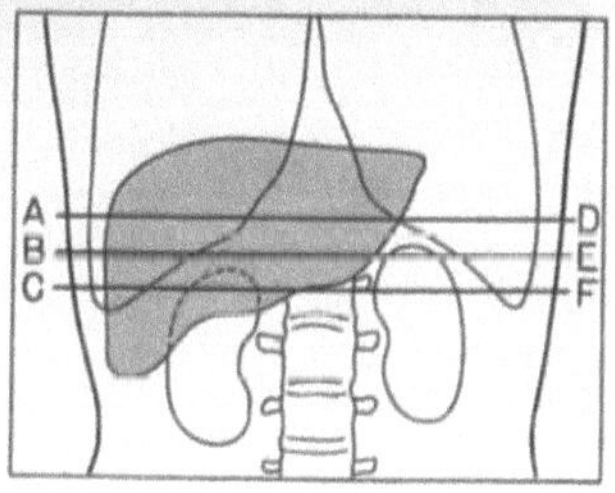

③ CT image
A, B, C Before contrast enhancement
D, E, F After contrast enhancement
The intrahepatic bile duct is markedly dilated. A low-attenuation area which is different from dilatation of the bile duct is recognized by contrast enhancement (→).

④ Angiography

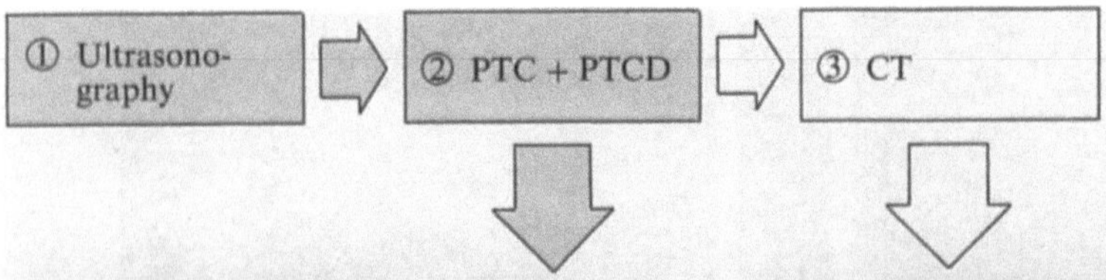

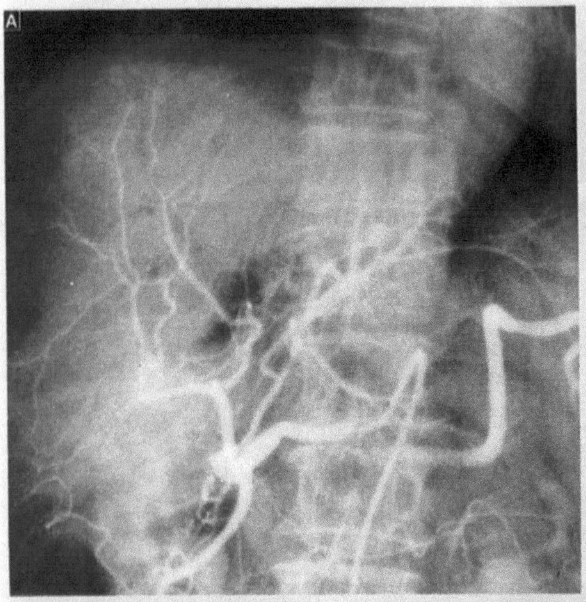

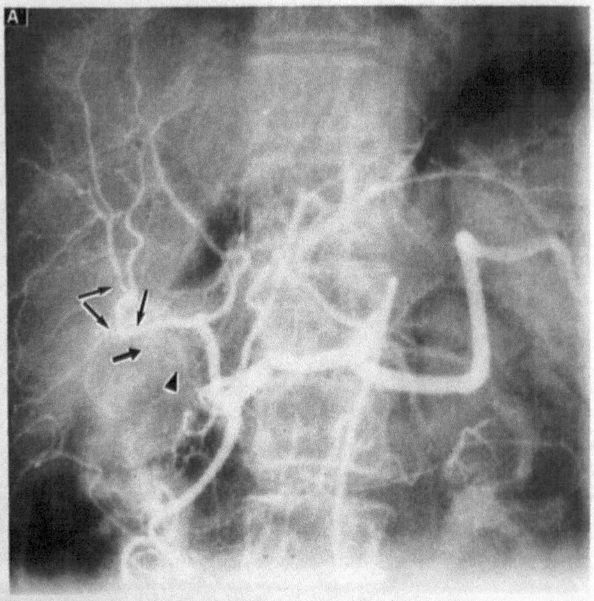

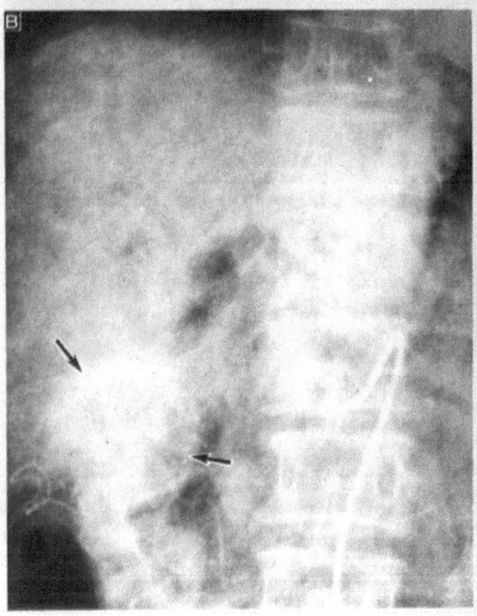

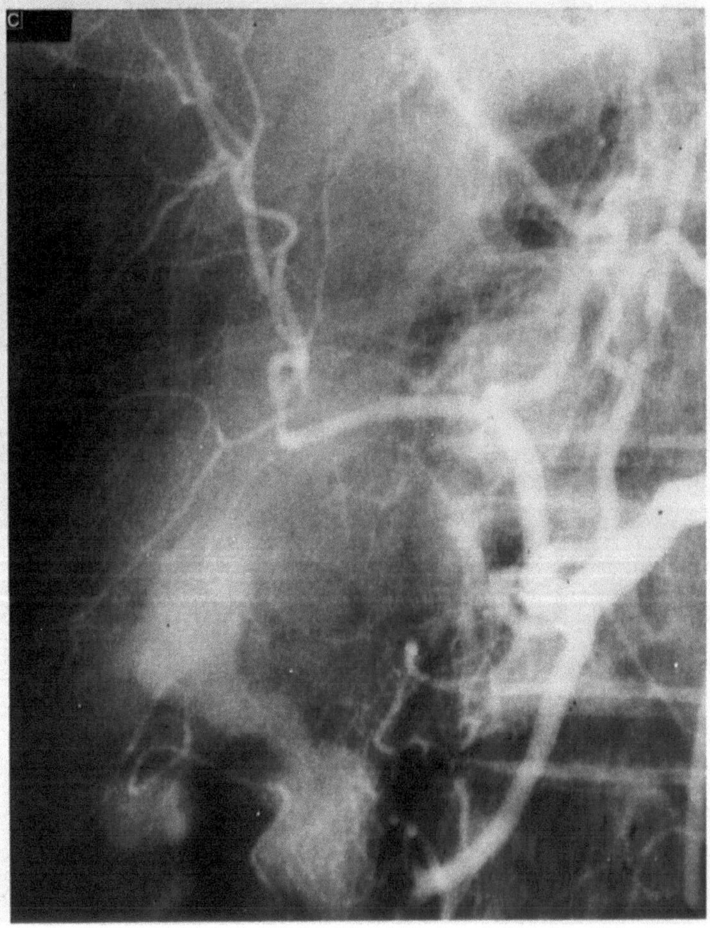

❹ Angiogram
A, A′ Stereoscopic common hepatic arteriogram (arterial phase)
B Common hepatic arteriogram (capillary phase)
C Magnification (×3) common hepatic arteriogram (arterial phase)
D Superior mesenteric arteriogram (venous phase)
E Celiac arteriogram (arterial phase)
F Celiac arteriogram (venous phase)

Encasement of the right hepatic artery, particularly severe at the bifurcation to the anterior and posterior segments is seen (**A**) (→). The cystic artery is irregular and obstructed just after its origin (→). Air in the extrahepatic bile duct allows its feeding artery to be well identified with neovascularity and irregularity (▶). In the capillary phase (**B**), a highly stained image is seen at the periphery of the common bile duct, which is opacified by air (→). It can be observed precisely with threefold magnification arteriography (**C**). No infiltration is shown in the portal venous system (**D**). A hypervascular mass (→) can be visualized in the lesser curvature of the body of the stomach by celiac arteriography (**E, F**).

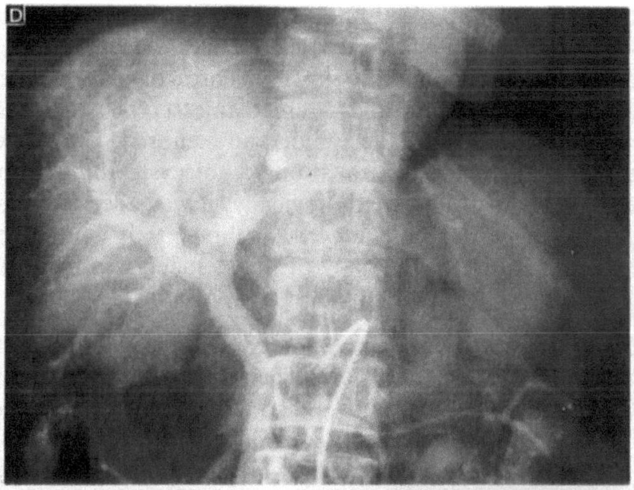

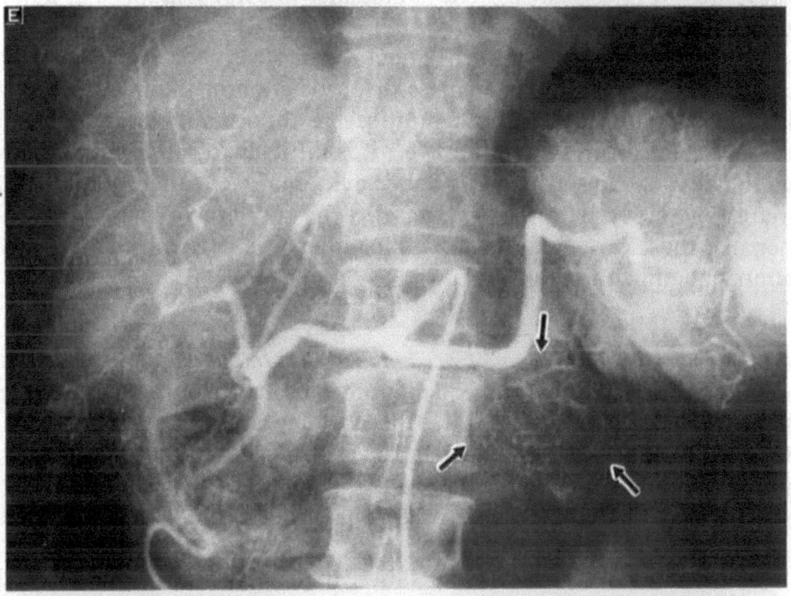

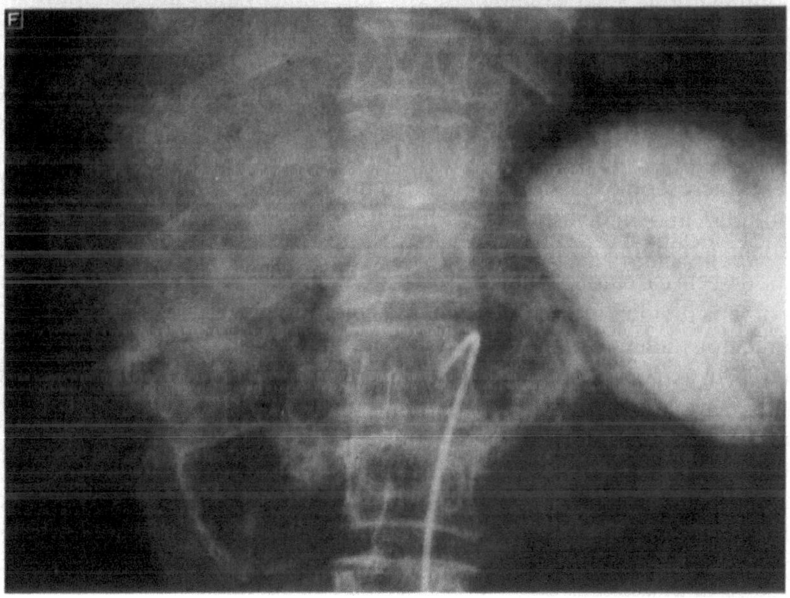

Operative Findings. A tumor at the porta hepatis infiltrating into the descending portion of the duodenum was detected. The gallbladder is attached to the tumor, resulting in its entire displacement by caner including two stones of 8 mm and 5 mm diameter. The extrahepatic bile duct is partially invaded by the tumor and stenosed. Complete resection of the tumor was impossible; thus, only cholecystectomy with T-tube drainage was performed. Histopathologically, it was adenocarcinoma and primary carcinoma of the gallbladder. A submucosal tumor of walnut size in the lesser curvature of the body of the stomach was identified as leiomyoma.

Significance of Diagnostic Imaging. Ultrasonography was performed just before PTC and PTCD for suspected obstructive jaundice based on data from clinical examinations. Obstructive jaundice was easily detected from ultrasonograms, and stenosis of the common bile duct with an echogenic mass was also recognized. However, examination of the distal area was prevented by intestinal gas. The gallbladder was not visualized as a normal nonechoic image.

With PTC, stenosis of the bile duct is demonstrated, indicating a malignant tumor. Generally, in stenosis or obstruction of the bile duct by gallbladder carcinoma, PTC shows more severe abnormality in the right side of the bile duct. In this case, however, it is difficult to differentiate between gallbladder carcinoma and bile duct carcinoma. With angiography, abnormality of the cystic artery was marked in addition to that of the porta hepatis, thus, carcinoma of the gallbladder was determined. CT did not contribute much for this diagnosis.

General Matters Concerning Carcinoma of the Gallbladder [4, 15, 19]. Carcinoma of the gallbladder is frequent in the 60s age group and more often in females (male:female = 1:2–3). Tominaga reported that the mortality rate from gallbladder carcinoma in Japan is at a peak in the 75–84 year age bracket and that the male:female ratio is 0.46. It has also been reported that the frequency of carcinoma of the gallbladder is 0.6%–0.7% of a total number of autopsies.

Carcinoma of the gallbladder shows almost no clinical symptoms; thus, complications such as cholelithiasis and cholecystitis are generally attendant. There are many reports concerning the relationship with cholelithiasis, which state that carcinoma of the gallbladder is accompanied by cholelithiasis in 50%–60% of cases and that this rate is less frequent than in Western society. Furthermore, gallbladder stones are associated with carcinoma of the gallbladder in 2%–7% of all cases.

Macroscopic classification of carcinoma of the gallbladder is papillary, nodular, and an invasive type, which is most common. Histopathologically, adenocarcinoma is most frequent and occasionally adenoachantoma, squamous cell carcinoma and anaplastic carcinoma also occur. Adenocarcinoma is divided into papillary adenocarcinoma, scirrhous carcinoma, and mucinous adenocarcinoma in terms of growing pattern and histopathology. An extension pattern of the tumor is metastasis to neighboring organs such as the liver, omentum, diaphragm, and colon in addition to lymph node metastasis. The route of metastasis is direct invasion; lymphatic metastasis, dissemination, and perineural and intraductal extension are also common. Among these, metastasis to the liver, especially to the gallbladder fossa, is frequent. Metastasis to the common bile duct may take place often via intraductal invasion of primary carcinoma of the neck of the gallbladder or cystic duct; rarely, metastasis to the bile duct by lymph node metastasis in the hepatoduodenal ligament may occur.

Radical resectability is only 20%–30% and prognosis is poor; almost all patients die within 2 years. The 5-year survival rate is 6.4% of resected cases. Recently, however, trials to improve radical resection have been carried out including performance of extended right lobectomy and pancreato-duodenectomy.

2.5 Carcinoma of the Common Bile Duct

Sequence of Diagnostic Imaging.

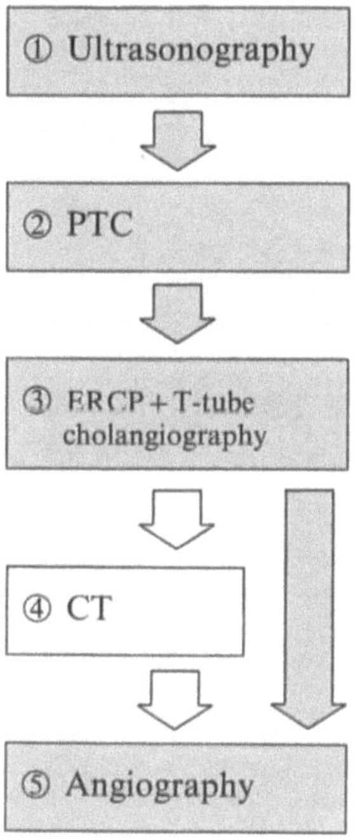

Patient. A 74-year-old man.

Main Complaint. General fatigue, abdominal discomfort, and jaundice.

Present History. The above-mentioned symptoms appeared 2 months prior. The patient was admitted to the department of radiology for precise examination.

Present Status. No symptoms other than jaundice.

Laboratory Data.

SGOT	80 mU/ml	↑
SGPT	105 mU/ml	↑
ALP	45.8 U	↑
LDH	320 mU/ml	↑
ZTT	4.0 U	Normal
Total bilirubin	14.0 mg/dl	↑
Direct bilirubin	7.5 mg7dl	↑
HBs Ag	(–)	

Purpose of Diagnostic Imaging. Differentiation of jaundice.

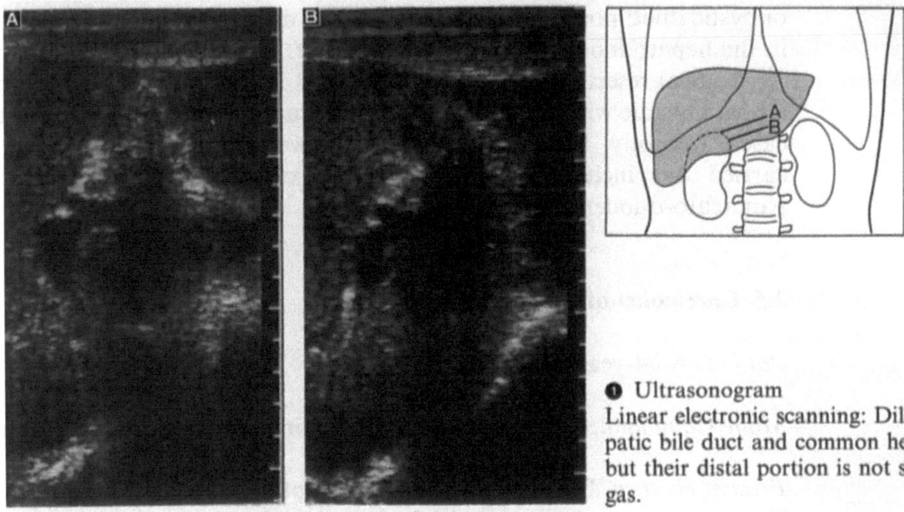

❶ Ultrasonogram
Linear electronic scanning: Dilatation of the intrahepatic bile duct and common hepatic duct is observable, but their distal portion is not seen due to intestinal gas.

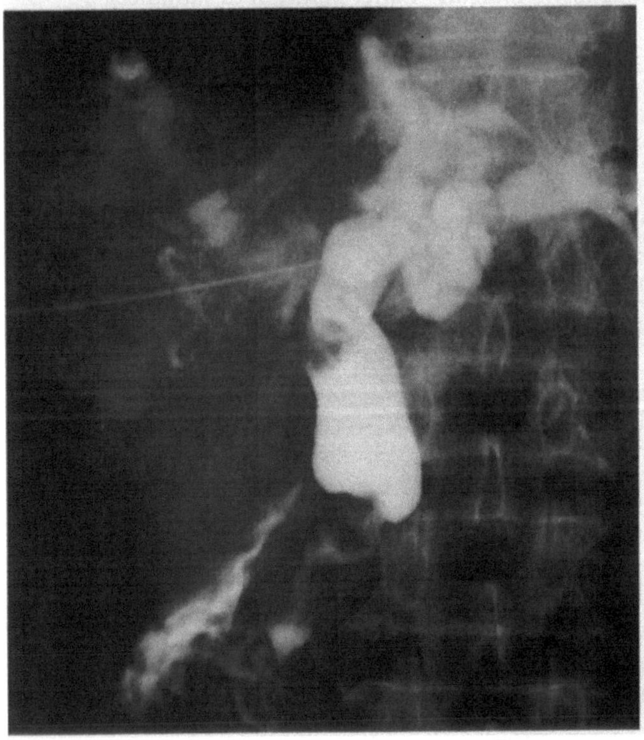

❷ PTC
Partial stenosis of the lower common bile duct is visualized. The gallbladder is nonopacified

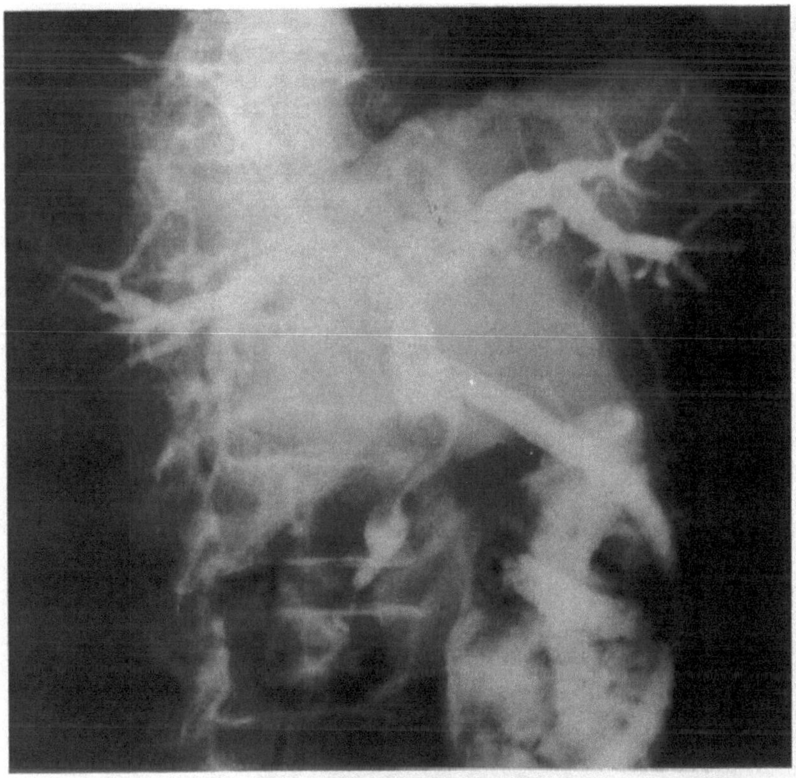

❸ ERCP + T-tube colangiography: Stenosis of the lower common bile duct suggests a tumor of the prominent type. No abnormal finding of the pancreatic duct is seen.

⑤ Angiography

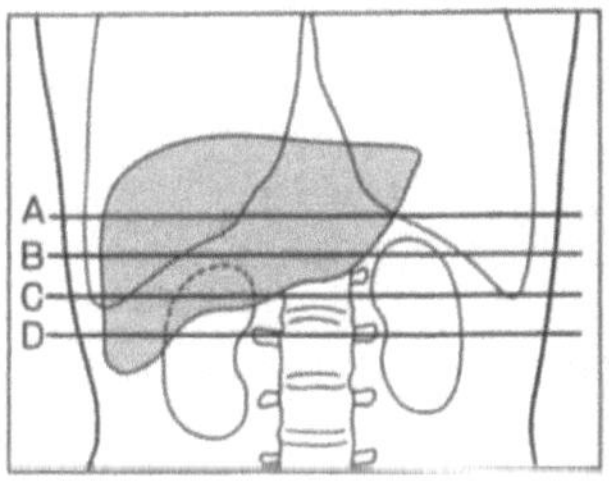

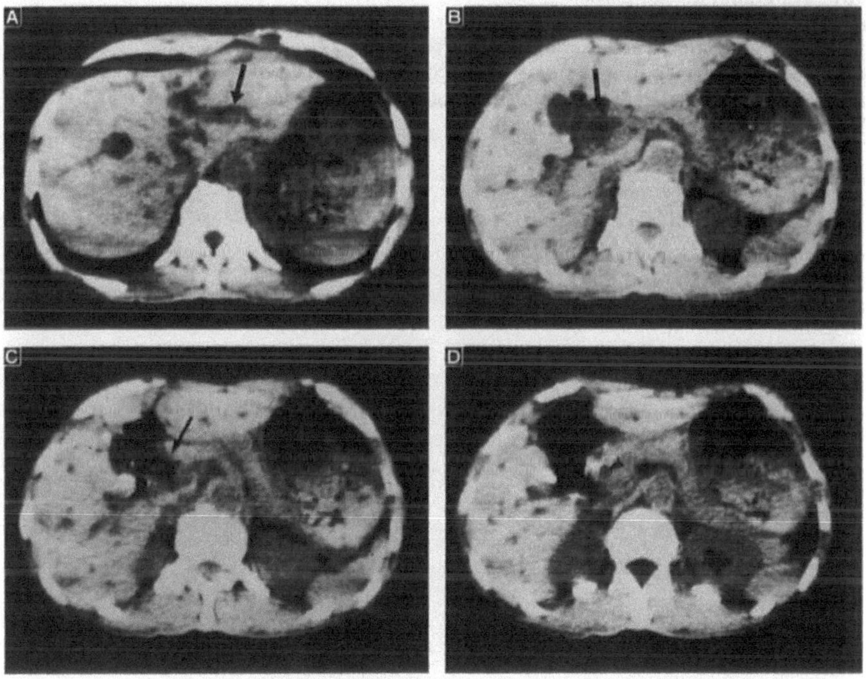

④ CT image
Dilated intra- and extrahepatic bile ducts (→) show irregular dilatation at a part of the head of the pancreas (→), but at more distal portion no dilatation is observed (▶). In the head of the pancreas, no tumor image is seen and a stone exists in the gallbladder.

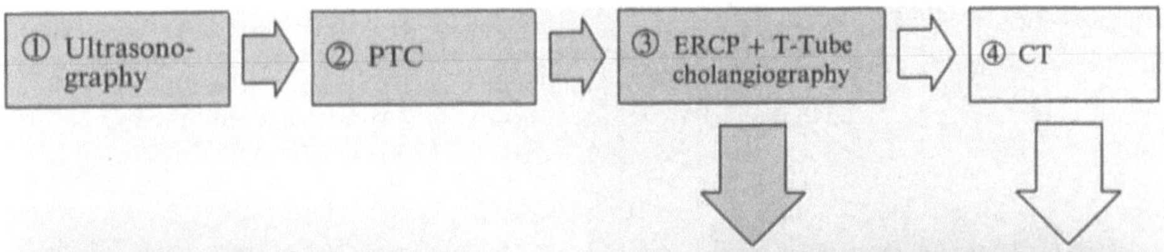

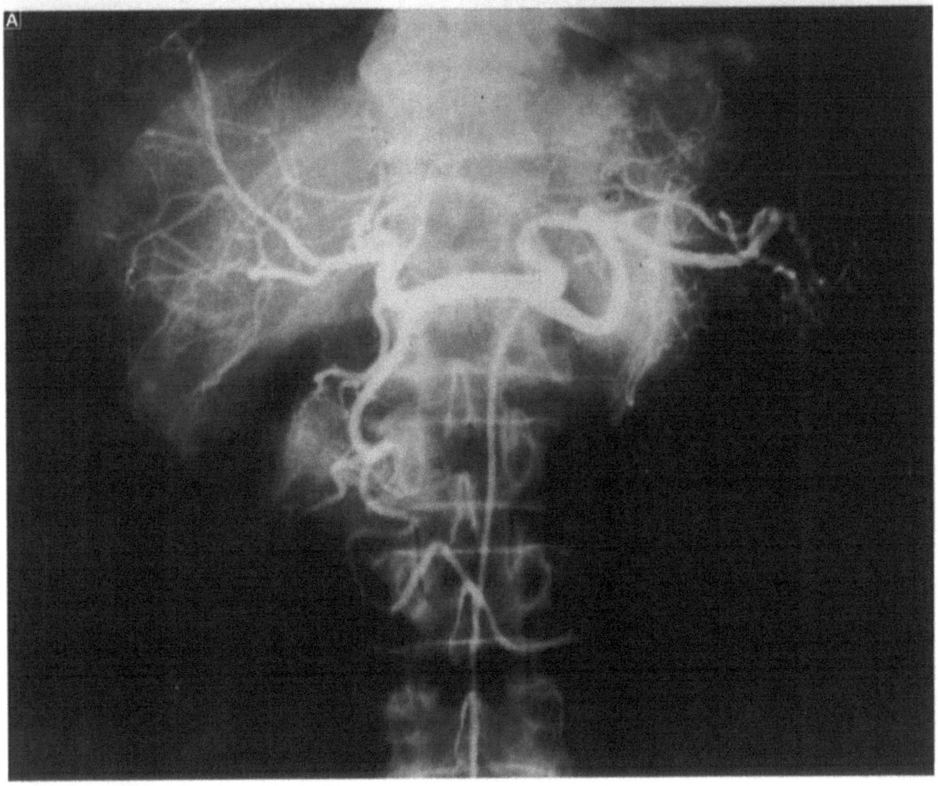

❺ Angiogram
A Celiac arteriogram (arterial phase)
B Magnification gastroduodenal arteriogram (arterial phase 1)
C Magnification gastroduodenal arteriogram (arterial phase 2)
Fine neovascularity showing irregularity is observed from the lower portion of the common bile duct to the porta hepatis, and a similar finding is seen in the intrahepatic branches at the porta hepatis, suggesting infiltration to the liver.

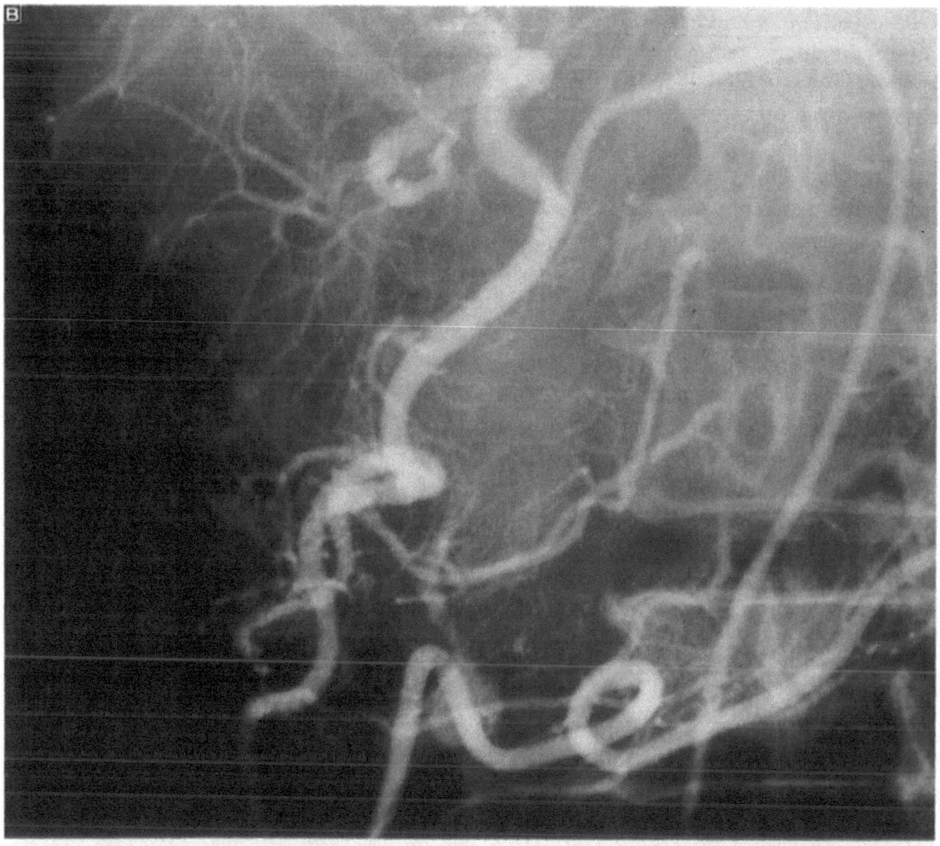
B

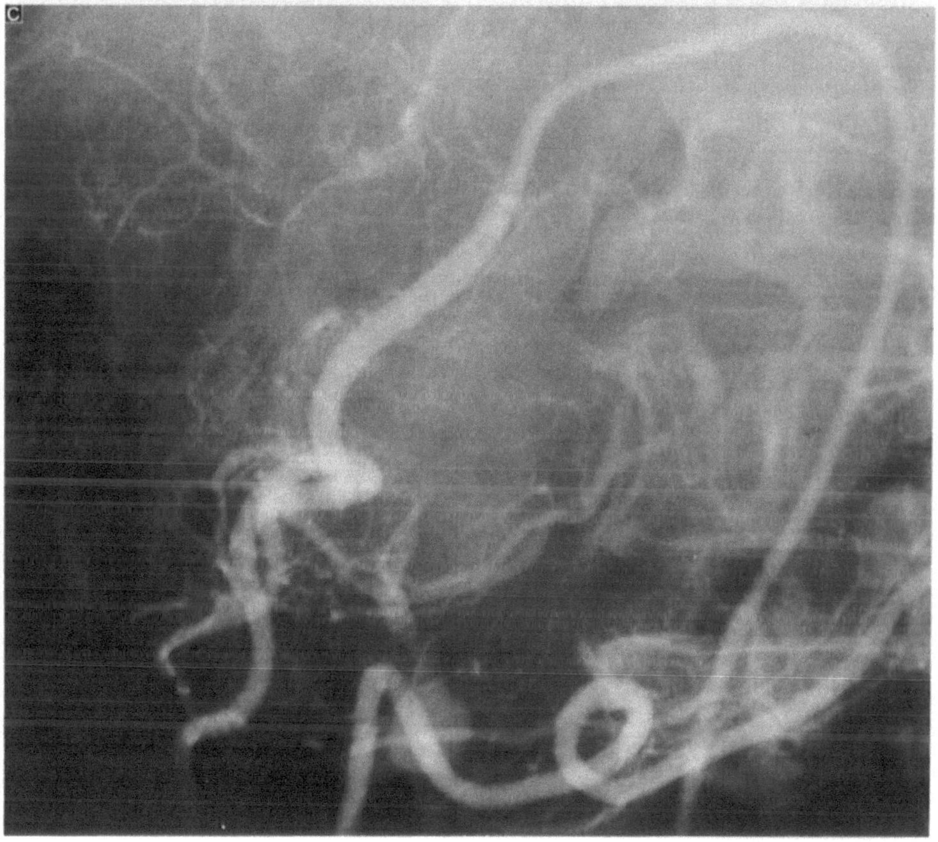
C

Operative Findings. Pancreatoduodenectomy and extended resection of the hilar bile duct detected a primary adenocarcinoma originating from the lower common bile duct, which is a nodular infiltrative type prominent toward the lumen and deeply infiltrating into the muscle layer. There was no invasion into the pancreatic parenchyma, but the tumor infiltrated upward into the bile duct lumen, then to the right hepatic duct. Cancer cells were detected at the resected edge. Therefore, radical resection of the tumor could not be achieved.

Significance of Diagnostic Imaging. Although obstructive jaundice was detected from an ultrasonogram, further diagnostic information could not be obtained because of insufficient ultrasonic examination. With PTC, irregular stenosis of the lower portion of the common bile duct suggested carcinoma. CT also demonstrated irregular dilatation of the lower portion of the common bile duct and no abnormality at the head of the pancreas; thus carcinoma of the bile duct was suspected.

With angiography, infiltration of the carcinoma extending to the porta hepatis was detected; thus, an extended resection was not possible. Identification of obstructive jaundice is easily done with ultrasonography, but demonstration of the lower portion of the common bile duct itself is difficult due to obstruction by intestinal gas and because the common bile duct is not parallel to the portal vein at this portion. In this respect, CT may sometimes be superior to ultrasonography. However, PTC and ERCP provide the most information in the lumen [18], and angiography is excellent in diagnosing infiltration to the wall and away from the lumen.

General Matters Concerning Carcinoma of the Bile Duct [5, 19, 21]. The extrahepatic bile duct extends from the right and left main hepatic ducts to the perforating portion of the wall of the duodenum. Carcinoma of the bile duct most frequent originates in the common bile duct, secondly in the portion between the right and left hepatic ducts and the common hepatic duct, then at the joining point of the common hepatic duct, common bile duct, and cystic duct. The rate of frequency is about one-fourth that of carcinoma of the gallbladder; it is more frequent in males. The male-to-female mortality ratio for carcinoma of the bile duct in Japan is 1.08. Patients are admitted to a hospital complaining of jaundice as a subjective symptom. The rate of accompanying stones is 20%–30% which is less frequent than in carcinoma of the gallbladder.

Histologically, 80%–90% of carcinoma of the bile duct is adenocarcinoma, and especially mucocellular adenocarcinoma; adenosquamous cell carcinoma, squamous cell carcinoma, and anaplastic carcinoma may occur. Macroscopically, it is classified in nodular, infiltrative, and papillary types. The former two types have rich interstitial fibrotic elements. The growth pattern is divided into the diffuse type which infiltrates along the wall and the nodular type. The rate of resectability is best, at 50%–70%, in carcinoma of the lower portion of the bile duct, next best, with 30%–50%, in carcinoma of the middle portion, and lowest (10%–20%) in carcinoma of the upper portion of the bile duct. In carcinoma of the lower portion of the bile duct, resection associated with the head of the pancreas is possible in cases with extraluminal infiltration. Even in cases with infiltration along the wall, resection can often be carried out. On the other hand, however, surgery is difficult in cases of carcinoma of the upper portion of the bile duct with infiltration to the liver parenchyma or the hepatic duct. The resectability of the nodular and papillary types of macroscopic classification is high, but that of the infiltrative type is low. The 5-year survival rate is relatively high at 40% – 50% in carcinoma of the lower portion of the bile duct and low in that of the middle and upper portions of the bile duct. Inoperable cases are treated by reducing jaundice, such as by PTC drainage and cholangiojejunostomy. Additionally, radiation therapy is carried out temporarily, and recently intraoperative radiotherapy and intracavitary irradiation of the bile duct are also performed.

2.6 Carcinoma of the Common Hepatic Duct

Sequence of Diagnostic Imaging.

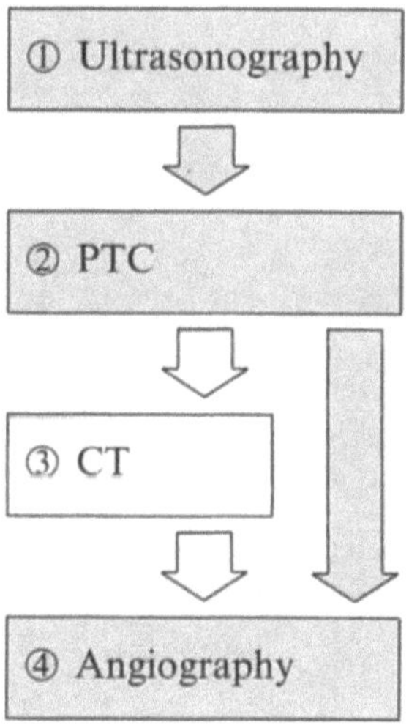

Patient. A 56-year-old man.

Main Complaint. Right hypochondralgia and jaundice.

Present History. The right hypochondralgia occurred 1 1/2 months prior, then jaundice appeared after 2 weeks. Obstructive jaundice was diagnosed by another hospital, and the patient was admitted to our hospital for further examination.

Present Status. No abnormalities except for jaundice.

Laboratory Data.

SGOT	57 mU/ml	↑
SGPT	48 mU/ml	↑
ALP	229 mU/ml	↑
LDH	264 mU/ml	↑
Total bilirubin	10.4 mg/dl	↑

Purpose of Diagnostic Imaging. Differentiation of jaundice and identification of the primary disease.

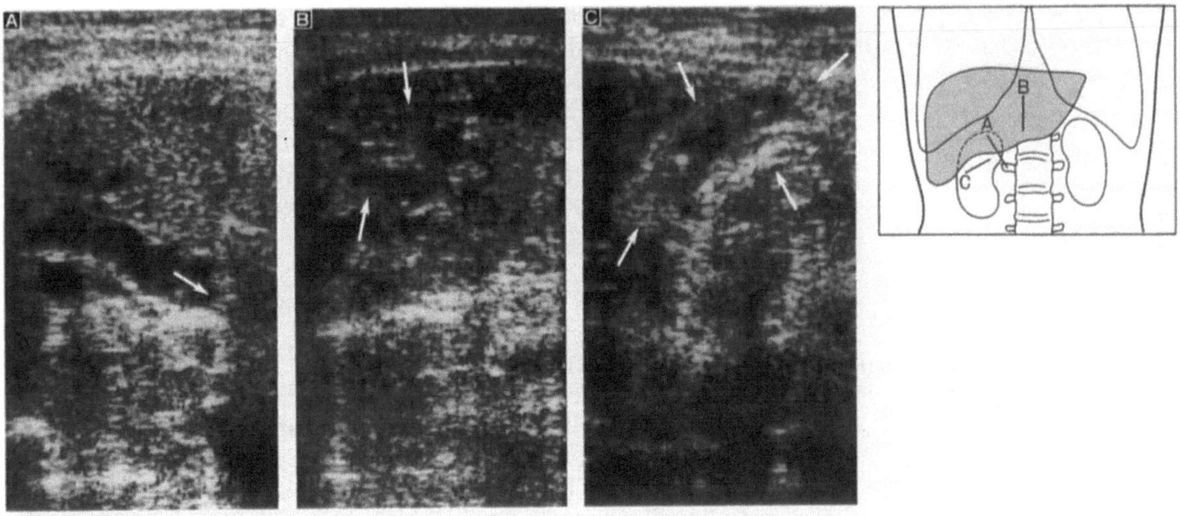

❶ Ultrasonogram
A–C Linear electronic scanning
The common hepatic duct is dilated and obstructed at the porta hepatis (**A**, →). The intrahepatic bile duct is markedly dilated (**B**, →). Entire atrophy of the gallbladder (**C**, →) and its wall thickened to 7–8 mm are observed.

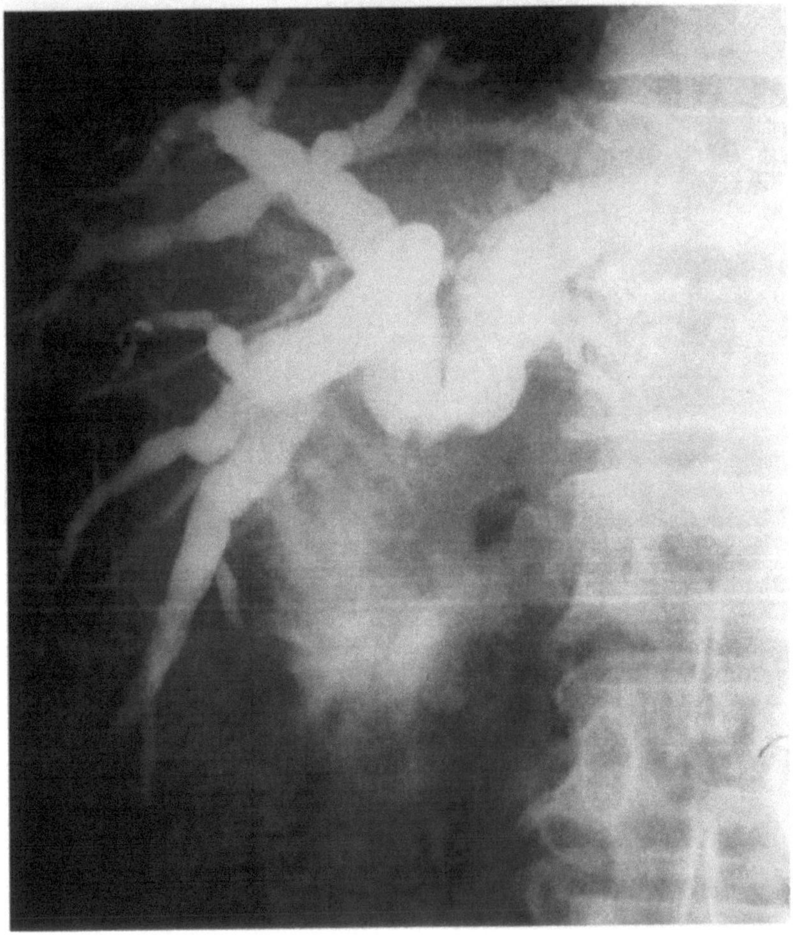

❷ PTC
Obstruction of the common hepatic duct at the porta hepatis is observed.

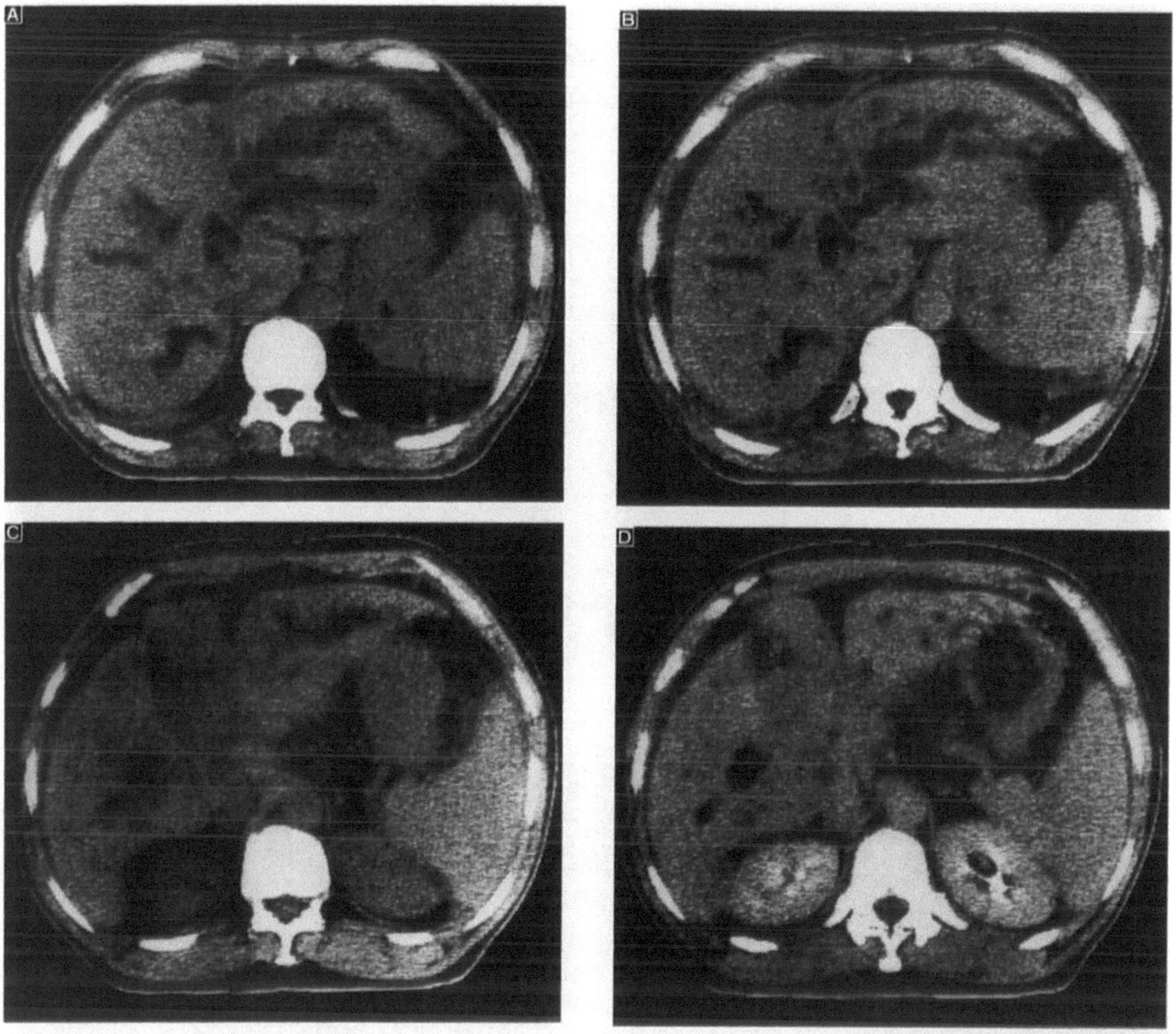

③ CT
A, C Before contrast enhancement
B, D After contrast enhancement
The intrahepatic bile duct is markedly dilated, but the dilated hepatic duct is not observed below the porta hepatis, suggesting a tumor. However, the extent of the tumor is not apparent. Atrophy of the gallbladder is observable.

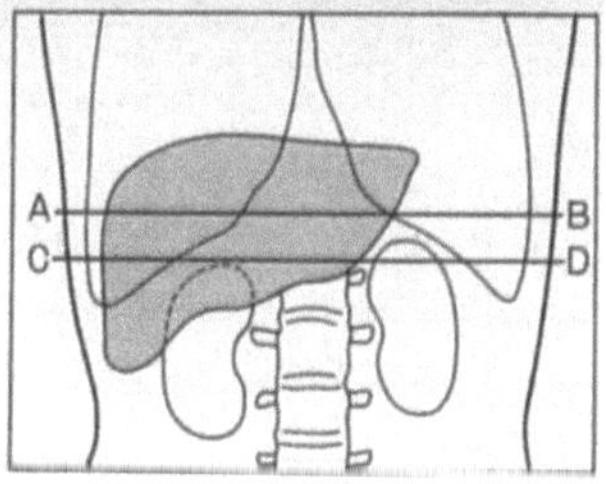

④ Angiography

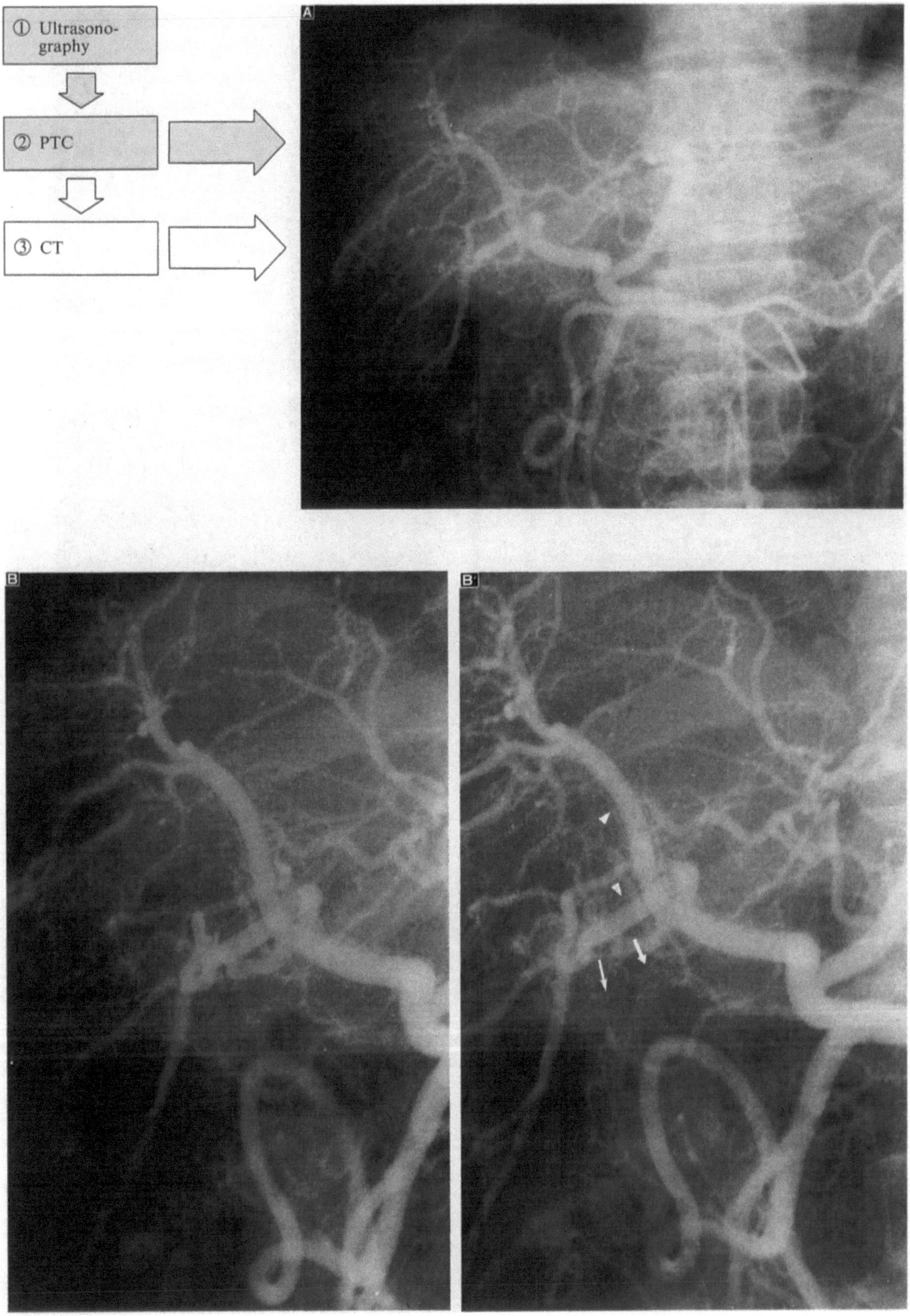
① Ultrasonography
② PTC
③ CT
A
B
B'

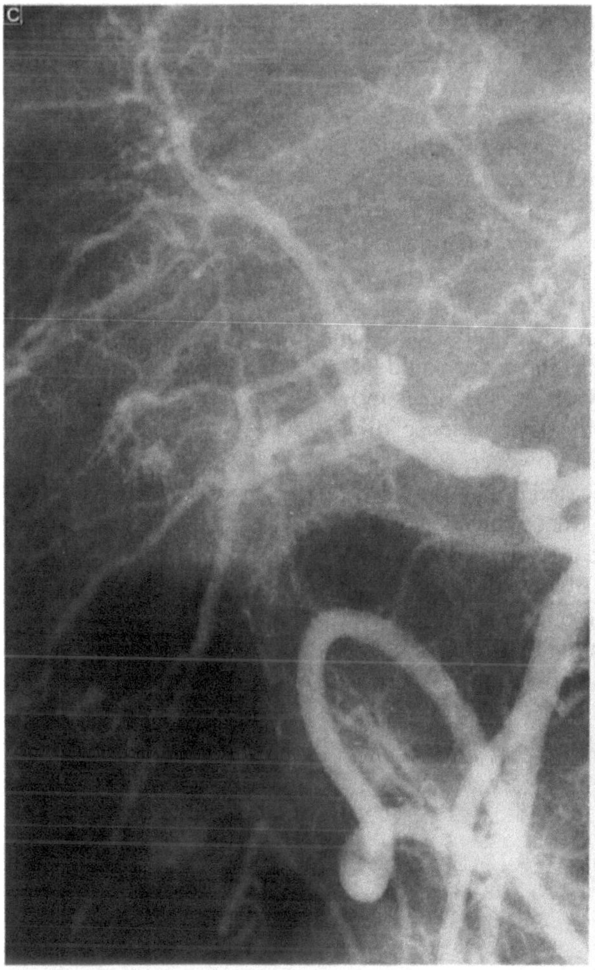

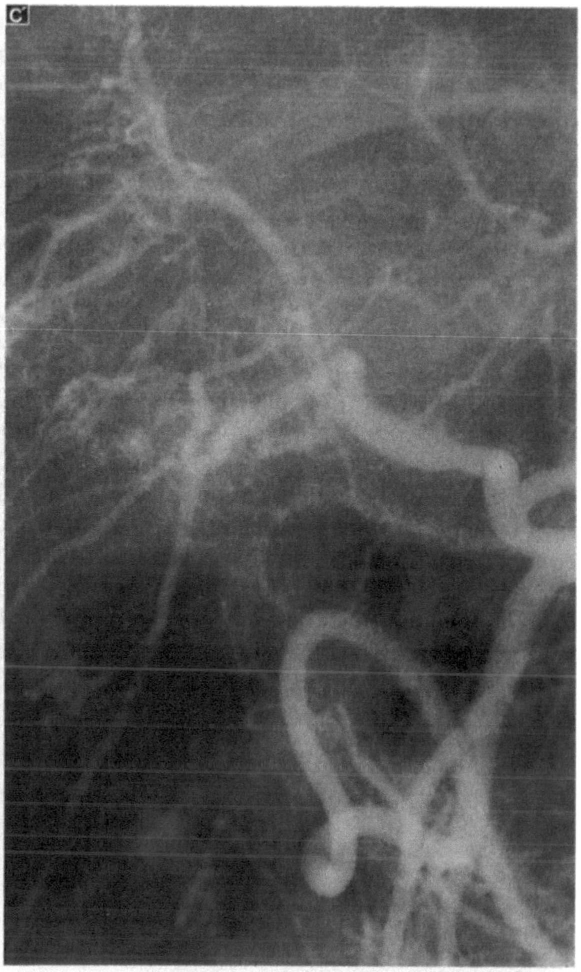

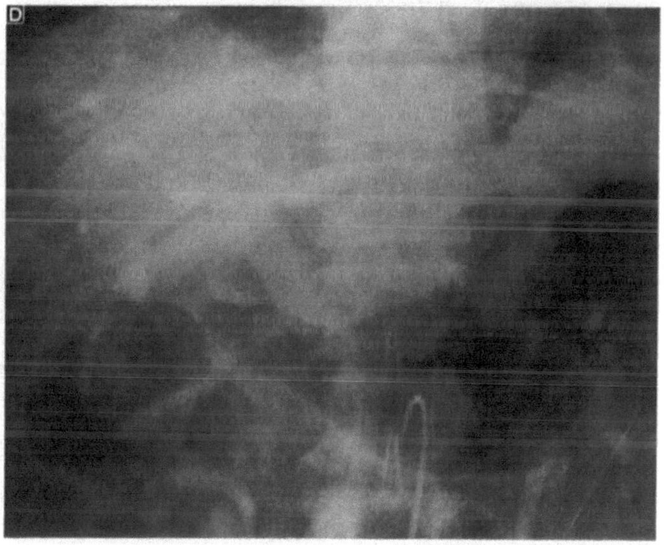

❻ Angiogram
A Common hepatic arteriogram (arterial phase)
B, B′ Stereoscopic magnification common hepatic arteriogram (arterial phase)
C, C′ Stereoscopic magnification common heptic arteriogram (arterial phase after arterial injection of noradrenalin)
D Superior mesenteric arteriogram (venous phase)
The pericholedochal arterial plexus is visualized clearly, and with magnification (**B**) it shows irregularity at the distal side of the porta hepatis (→). Atrophy of the gallbladder and an inflammatory change of the cystic artery (→) are observed. Noradrenalin administration (**C**) causes contraction of the intrahepatic and cystic arteries, but the irregularity observed in **B** is more clearly visualized. Also, the periportal arteries are clearly seen due to dilatation of the intrahepatic bile duct (**B**, →). No abnormality of the portal vein is observed (**D**).

Operative Findings. Hepatojejunostomy was performed. A nodular infiltrative type of carcinoma of the hepatic duct (adenocarcinoma) 2×0.8 cm in size and slightly infiltrating to the serosa was found. A metastasis to the supero-posterior pancreaticoduodenal lymph node was detected. The gallbladder exhibited chronic cholecystitis, and although no malignant findings were observed, infiltration of cancer cells was observed to a small extent in the cystic duct. Extension or metastasis to the liver and pancreas and infiltration into the hepatic artery or portal vein were not present.

Significance of Diagnostic Imaging. PTC identified the obstruction caused by a tumor at the porta hepatis suspected from an ultrasonogram. Although the presence of a tumor was suggested from CT, its extent could not be revealed by CT. If the bile duct can be sufficiently observed, ultrasonography is superior to conventional CT in diagnosing the presence of a tumor of the upper part of the bile duct. Dynamic CT, however, could give more information. Magnification angiography indicated malignant findings in a part of the peripheral artery of the bile duct which feeds the common hepatic duct, allowing carcinoma of the bile duct to be diagnosed. However, a chronic inflammatory change was also observed in the cystic artery, making differentiation from carcinoma of the bile duct difficult. In this case, diagnosis with angiography was made possible by the presence of infiltration of cancer to the serosa.

General Matters Concerning Carcinoma of the Bile Duct. See Sect. B. 2.5.

References

B. Disease of the Biliary Tract

1. Alonso-Lej F, Rever WB Jr, Pessagno DJ (1959) Cangenital choledochal cyst, with a report of 2, and on analysis of 94 cases. Int Abst Surg 108:1–30
2. Altmeier WA, Gall EA, Culberston WR, Inge WW (1966) Sclerosing carcinoma of the intrahepatic (hilar) bile ducts. Surgery 60:191–200
3. Aoki K, Sasaki R (1982) The epidemiology of cancer of liver, biliary tract and pancreas in Japan (in Japanese). Jpn J Clin Med 40:8–14
4. Beltz WR, Condon RE (1974) Primary carcinoma of the gallbladder. Ann Surg 180:180–184
5. Evander A, Predlund P, Hoevels J, Ihse I, Bengmark S (1980) Evaluation of aggressive surgery for carcinoma of the extrahepatic bile duct. Ann Surg 191:23–29
6. Kameda, H (1974) Clinical statics of cholelithiasis and cholecystitis in Japan (in Japanaese). Jpn J Clin Med 32 [Supp]: 402–414
7. Kameda H (1980) Recent trend of intrahepatic gall stones (in Japanese). Biliary Tract Pancreas 1:1425–1428
8. Komi N (1975) Anomalous arrangement of the pancreaticobiliary duct in the congenital dilatation of the biliary duct (in Japanese). Operation 29:73–83
9. Komi N, Kashiwagi Y, Ikeda N (1977) The etiology of congenital dilatation of the bile duct (in Japanese). Jpn J Pediatr Surg 9:1101–1108
10. Krieger J, Seaman WB, Porter MR (1970) The roentgenologic appearance of sclerosing cholangitis. Radiology 95:369–375
11. Longmire WP Jr, (1978) When is cholangitis sclerosing? Am J Surg 135:312–320
12. Maki T, Sato T, Matsushiro T (1972) A reappraisal of surgical treatment for intrahepatic gallstones. Ann Surg 175:155–165
13. Nakayama F, Furusawa T, Nakama T (1980) Hepatolithiasis in Japan: Present status. Am J Surg 139:216–220

14. Oi I, Hara T (1977) Abnormal connection between the choledocus and the pancreatic duct in case of congenital choledochal cyst examined by endoscopic pancreatocholangiography (in Japanese). Jpn J Pediatr Surg 9:1121–1129
15. Piehler JM, Crichlow RW (1978) Primary carcinoma of the gallbladder. Surg Gynecol Obstet 147:929–942
16. Schwartz SI, Dale WA (1958) Primary sclerosing cholangitis, review and report of six cases. Arch Surg 77:439–451
17. Takemoto T, Fuji T (1982) Definition and diagnosis of early cancer of the biliary tract – From the clinical viewpoint – (in Japanese). Stomach Intestine 17:613–618
18. Takeuchi T, Miyaji M, Ito K, Katagiri K, Ito M, Kozuka M, Goto K (1977) Diagnosis of biliary tract neoplasms (in Japanese). Stomach Intestine 12:717–732
19. Tominaga S (1980) An epidemiological study on cancer of the biliary passage in Japan (in Japanese). Biliary Tract Pancreas 1:1611–1622
20. Tsunoda T, Otsu T, Shinozaki T, Misael O J et al. (1981) A study of two patients with early bile duct carcinoma (in Japanese). Biliary Tract Pancreas 2:747–751
21. Tsuchiya R, Tsunoda T, Harada N, Nishimura R, Ito T (1977) Surgical treatment for carcinoma of the extrahepatic bile duct (in Japanese). Stomach Intestine 12:733–743

C: Diagnostic Imaging of Diseases of the Pancreas

1 Procedure

During diagnosis of diseases of the pancreas, ultrasonography and CT both contribute a great deal to the exact demonstration of the morphology of the pancreas. In acute pancreatitis, CT can provide information on the extent of swelling of the pancreas, the presence of hemorrhage or necrosis, the formation of an abscess or pseudocyst, extrapancreatic extension of inflammation, and furthermore, progressive observation is also possible. Although ultrasonography can also demonstrate the degree of swelling of the pancreas and the presence of an abscess or pseudocyst, visualization of the pancreas itself is frequently difficult due to intestinal gas produced during an acute attack; thus, in this respect CT is superior to ultrasonography. Figure 1 shows the sequence of examination in cases with suspected diseases of the pancreas excluding acute pancreatitis. Despite the fact that ultrasonography and CT are important as screening examinations, ERCP in chronic pancreatitis and ERCP and angiography in carcinoma of the pancreas are highly significant in terms of localization of diseases and qualitative diagnosis [10].

In carcinoma of the pancreas, similar to malignant tumor of the biliary tract, many cases are advanced at the time of diagnostic imaging and therefore often cannot save the lives of patients. In this respect, the value of diagnostic imaging is not high, and the value of CT and ultrasonography is dependent upon how they can be used in screening examinations.

The annual mortality rate (per 100 000 people) of pancreatic disordes in Japan has increased to 0.06 (65 people) in 1974 from 0.02–0.03 (23 people) in 1960. That of acute pancreatitis is almost the same, 0.5–0.6 (516 people) in 1960 and 0.5–0.7 (652 people) in 1974. That of carcinoma of the pancreas has increased two to three times, from 1.7–2.5 (1975 people) in 1960 to 4.1–5.8 (5402 people) in 1974 [11].

Etiological factors of acute pancreatitis are alcohol abuse in 46.5% (male 60.6%, female 4.6%), cholelithiasis in 13% (male 6.7%, female 31.5%) and an episode of acute pancreatitis in 6.3% (male 6.7%, female 5.1%) [20].

The risk factors for the occurrence of pancreatic carcinoma are smoking and fatty diets [5]. Although the relationship between pancreatolithiasis and carcinoma of the pancreas can be considered, chronic pancreatitis and carcinoma of the pancreas are not regarded as having much relationship. Detection of a group at high risk for carcinoma of the pancreas is regarded as quite difficult.

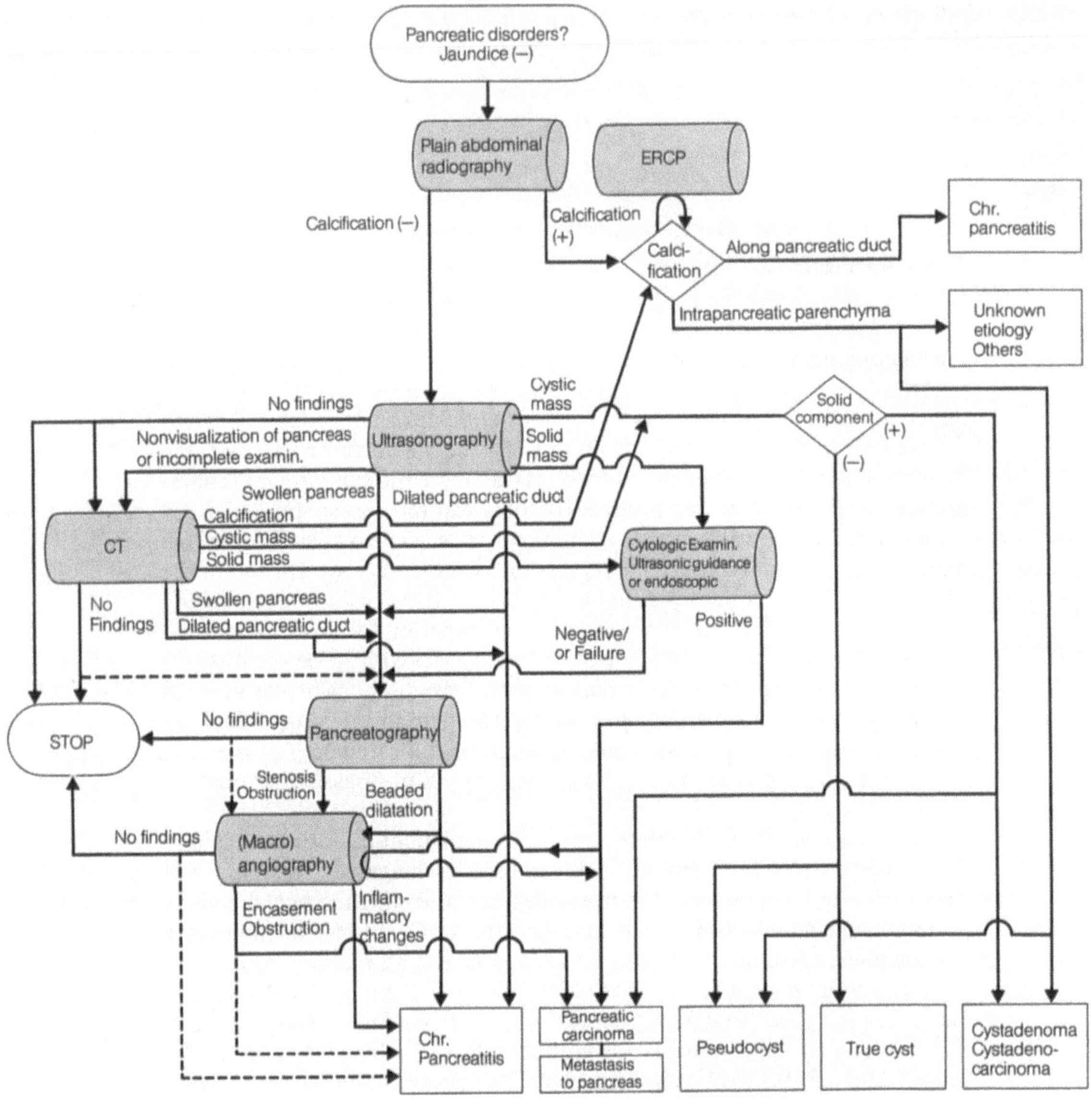

Fig. 1. Procedure of diagnostic imaging in suspected pancreatic disorders except for acute pancreatitis

2 Cases

2.1 Acute Pancreatitis

Sequence of Diagnostic Imaging.

① CT

Patient. A 59-year-old man.

Main Complaint. Epigastralgia and vomiting.

Present History. Epigastralgia suddenly appeared in the morning and got worse with vomiting 11 days prior to the first CT examination. It was not improved by pentazocine and an anticholinergic agent so that the patient was admitted to the department of surgery.

Present Status. Muscular rigidity and resistance at the epigastrium. Blumberg's sign is negative.

Laboratory Data.

	1st day	2nd day	6th day	11th day	20th day
SGPT (mU/ml)	33 (Normal)	–	32 (Normal)	13 (Normal)	20 (Normal)
Serum amylase (IU/l)	2030 (↑)	256 (Normal)	90 (Normal)	130 (Normal)	126 (Normal)
Serum glucose (mg/dl)	–	159 (↑)	99 (Normal)	97 (Normal)	–
White cell count (/mm^3)	18100 (↑)	23100 (↑)	15600 (↑)	10700 (↑)	7800 (Normal)

Purpose of Diagnostic Imaging. To study the morphology of the pancreas.

11 days after attack

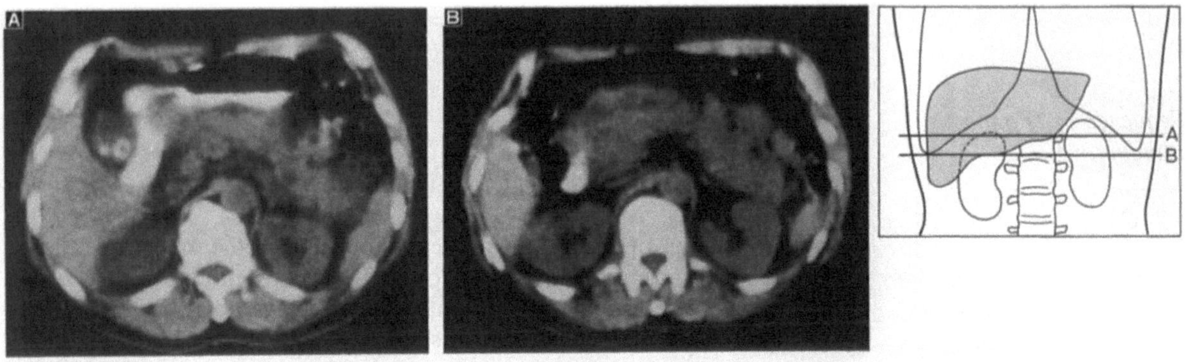

❶ CT image
An entirely swollen pancreas with an obscure contour is observed including partial low-attenuation areas. The mass shadow, compressing the duodenum, is visualized protruding from the head of the pancreas. The gallbladder is highly attenuated and a stone can be seen.

21 and 25 days after attack

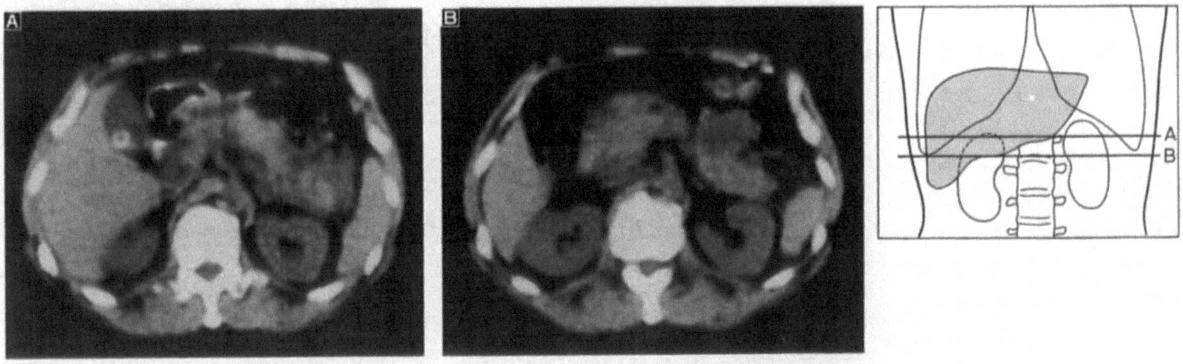

❷ CT image 21 days after attack

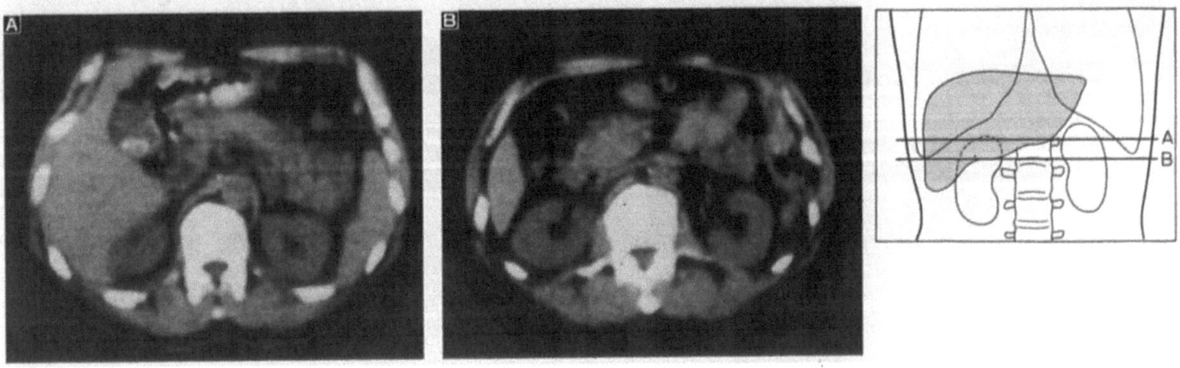

❸ CT image 25 days after attack
The pancreas is reduced in size and the attenuation value is normalized. The inflammatory mass in the head of the pancreas still exists but is reduced. A cystic change can be seen in the tail of the pancreas.

48 days after attack and
22 days after operation

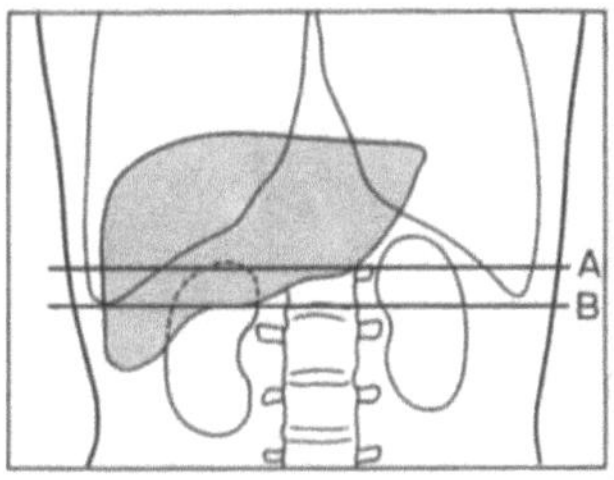

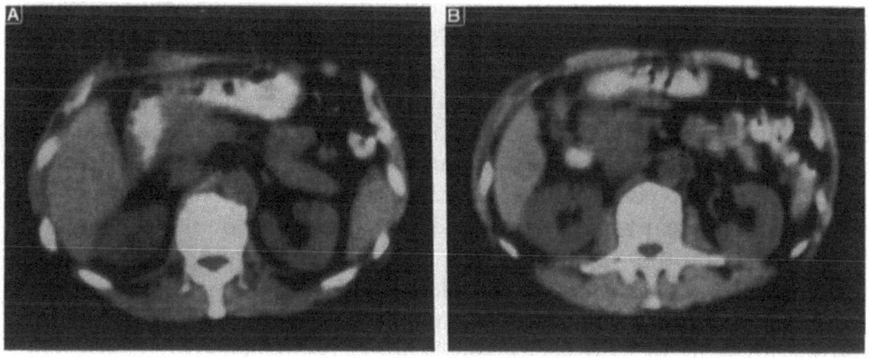

❹ CT image 48 days after attack and 22 days after operation
Although the pancreas is normal in size and attenuation value, an inflammatory mass in the head and tail of the pancreas is observed.

Clinical Progress. After acute pancreatitis was diagnosed from clinical examination data, rest and fasting were ordered and then administration of Gabexate mesilate and transfusion were performed. Cholelithiasis was detected from CT taken 11 days after the attack. Confirming that pancreatitis was caused by cholelithiasis, and surgery was carried out.

Operative Findings (Cholecystectomy). In the head of the pancreas, severe inflammatory changes, marked swelling, and tight adhesion with the gastric antrum were detected. An abscess 4 cm in diameter existed anterior to the hepatoduodenal ligament forming a fistula with the head of the pancreas. Also, in the body and tail of the pancreas, severe inflammatory changes, marked swelling, hardening, and adhesion with neighboring organs were recognized. The gallbladder was swollen with tension including dense bile juice and 80 stones (3 stones 1 cm in diameter, 4 stones 5 mm and, 73 stones 1–2 mm).

Significance of Diagnostic Imaging. In cases of acute pancreatitis, ultrasonography and CT are only useful for studying the morphological state of the pancreas without the patients suffering. However, accumulation of intestinal gas in acute pancreatitis prevents visualization of the pancreas by ultrasonography so that often only CT is applicable for diagnostic imaging. CT demonstrated not only swelling of the pancreas but also hemorrhage, an inflammatory mass, and an abscess. Pseudocyst formation can be studied by observation of the progress. The CT number decreases in cases of severe edema.

General Matters Concerning Acute Pancreatitis [9, 22]. Pancreatitis is classified into (a) acute pancreatitis, (b) relapsing acute pancreatitis, (c) chronic relapsing pancreatitis, and (d) chronic pancreatitis, according to the pattern of its progress. Acute pancreatitis is defined as an acute attack without relapsing or sequelae and relapsing acute pancreatitis as an acute attack accompanied by recurrence which heals once its cause is removed. The rate of frequency in Japan is about 0.2% of all hospitalized patients, and it often appears in the age group of 30- to 50-year-olds.

Regarding its pathogenesis, acute pancreatitis is caused by autodigestion of the pancreas due to destruction of the protective mechanism by enzyme-activated causes, such as cholelithiasis, alcohol, abdominal trauma, operation of abdominal organs, diseases of the duodenum or papillary portion, and mumps.

Histopathologically, acute pancreatitis is divided into acute interstitial edematous pancreatitis, which is a mild type and represents the majority of cases of acute pancreatitis, and acute necrotizing hemorrhagic pancreatitis, which is a severe type and is often accompanied by shock. Acute interstitial edematous pancreatitis is characterized by marked interlobular edema and leukocytic infiltration and macroscopically by a pale and glass-colored, highly swollen pancreas due to the edema. The edema may remain in the pancreas, but with advancement it expands to neighboring organs or the retroperitoneum. In acute necrotizing hemorrhagic pancreatitis, characteristic findings are fat necrosis and hemorrhagic necrosis of the parenchyma. Fat necrosis not only expands over the surface of the pancreas but also to the mesenterium, intestine, and retroperitoneum. Necrosis of the parenchyma exists entirely or partially over the pancreas and occasionally extends to surrounding organs or the retroperitoneum. Generally, the necrotic region heals after cicatrization, but in cases of a large pathological lesion or long duration, necrotizing materials are not absorbed and an abscess or pseudocyst forms due to secondary infection.

Conservative treatment has been regarded to produce better results than radical treatment, but recently in cases where symptoms have not improved or there is accompanying cholelithiasis, abscess, or cyst formation, some physicians insist on performance of a positive surgical operation. The rate of progressing to chronic pancreatitis varies with reports (5%–57%).

2.2 Chronic Pancreatitis

Sequence of Diagnostic Imaging.

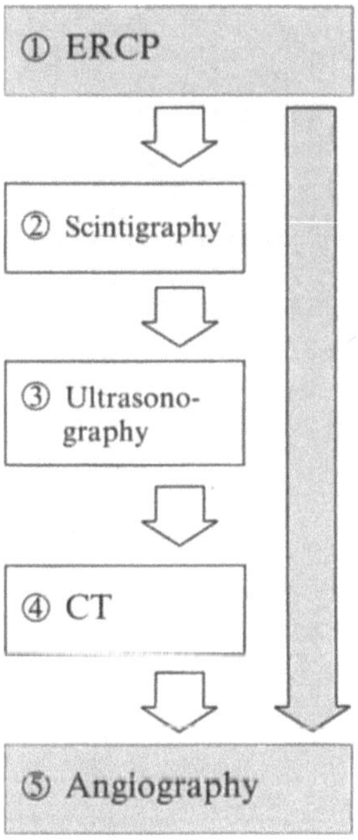

Patient. A 45-year-old man.

Main Complaint. Upper abdominal pain.

Present History: Occasional upper abdominal pain 2 weeks prior. The patient was admitted to another clinic, but the symptoms had not improved and the interval between pains had shortened and the duration of pain had gradually increased; thus, he was admitted to our hospital. Alcohol intake is about 650 ml of sake and three bottles of beer a day.

Laboratory Data.

SGOT	16 mU/ml	Normal	
SGPT	15 mU/ml	Normal	
ALP	76 mU/ml	Normal	
LDH	183 mU/ml	Normal	
γ-GTP	26 mU/ml	Normal	
Cho E	462 U/dl	Normal	
ZTT	4.7 U	Normal	
Total bilirubin	0.2 mg/dl	Normal	
Serum amylase	297 IU/l	Normal	
Urine amylase	511 IU/l	Normal	
AFP	20 under mμg/ml		Normal
HBS Ag	(−)		
Glucose tolerance test (venous blood)			
Fasting state	1 h	2 h	
93 mg/dl	170 mg/dl	143 mg/dl	diabetes mellitus type

Purpose of Diagnostic Imaging. To detect malignancy accompanied by chronic pancreatitis.

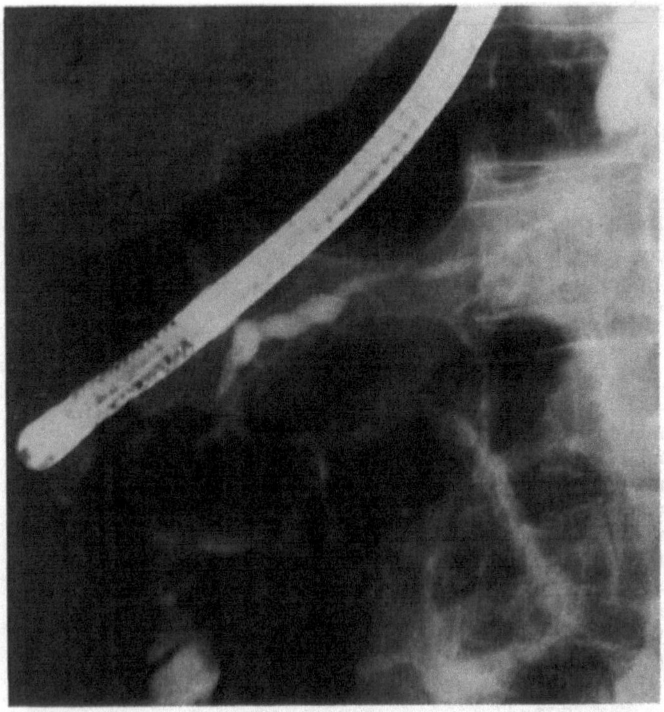

❶ ERCP
Dilatation and tortuosity of the main pancreatic duct suggesting chronic pancreatitis is observable.

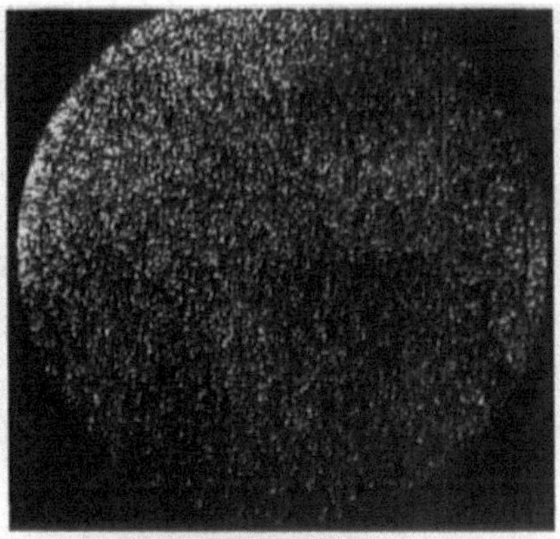

② Scintigram (^{75}Se-selenomethionine)
Inhomogeneous RI uptake indicative of chronic pancreatitis is seen.

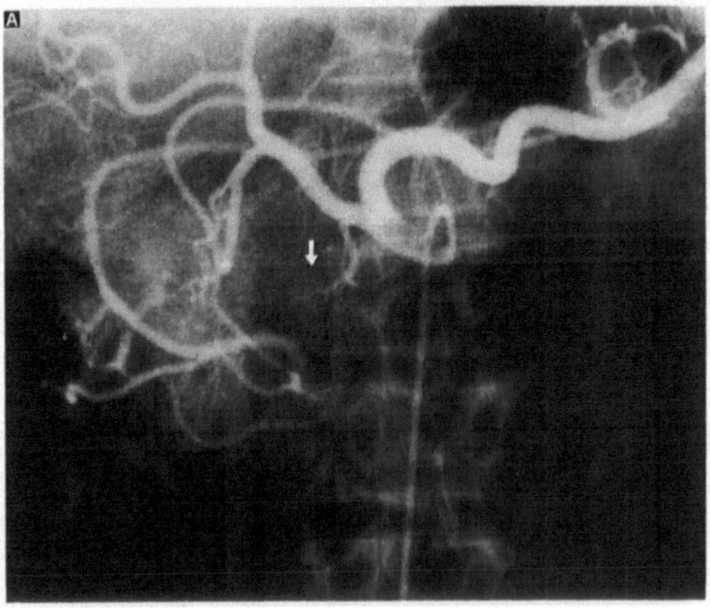

❺ Angiogram (I)
A, A′ Stereoscopic celiac arteriography (arterial phase)
A part of the vessels of the pancreatic arcades shows a beaded appearance. Irregularity and encasement of a portion of the branches from the dorsal pancreatic artery to the pancreatic arcades (→) are seen, but malignancy is not detected. The capillary phase visualizes a lightly stained pancreas. No abnormality is seen in the venous system.

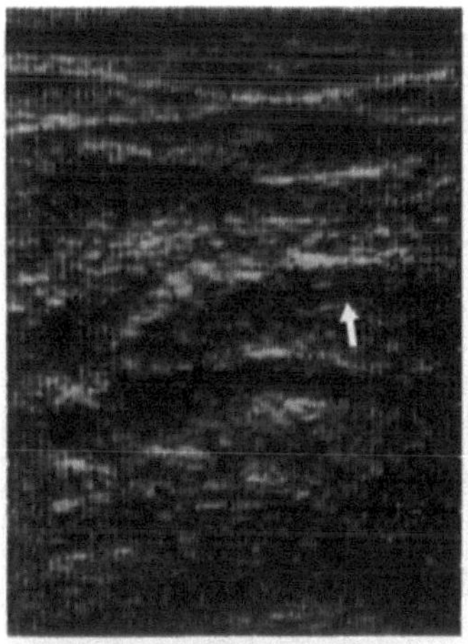

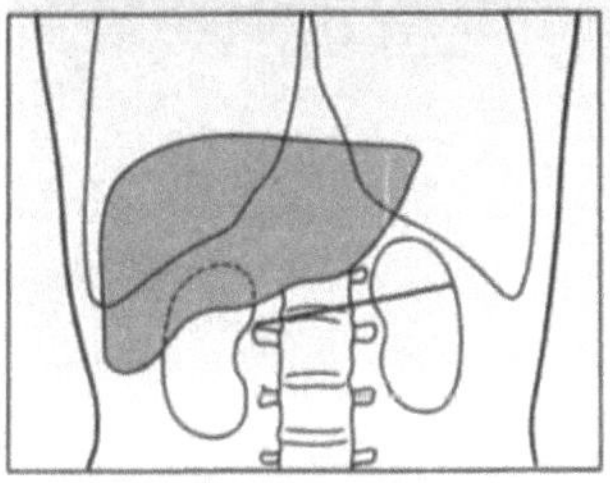

③ Ultrasonogram
Linear electronic scanning: Homogeneous echogenicity of the pancreatic parenchyma without swelling is observed, but dilatation of the main pancreatic duct (→) is visualized.

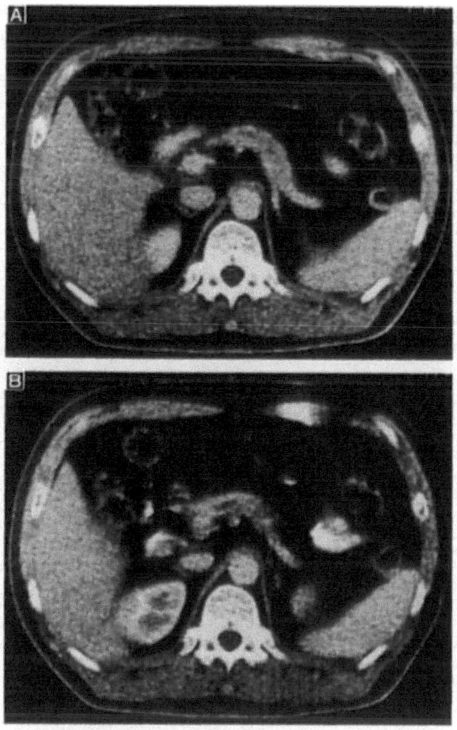

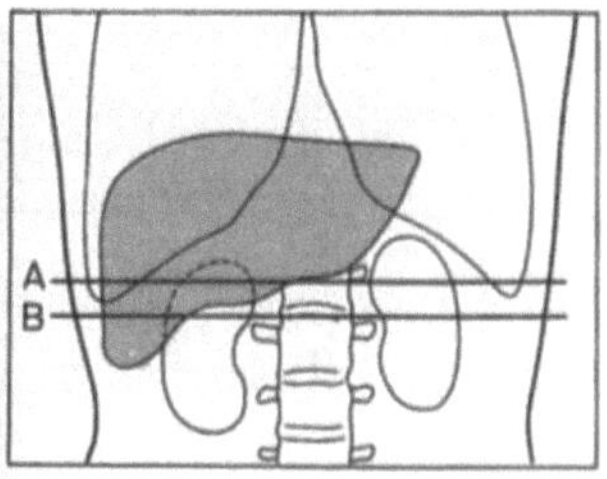

④ CT image
A smooth contour and no swelling of the pancreas including a low-attenuation zone indicative of dilated pancreatic duct are seen.

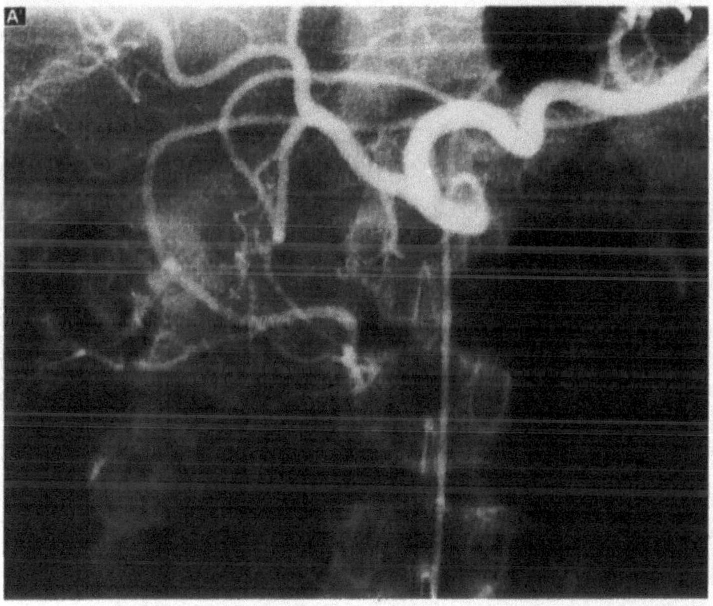

⑤ Angiography (II)

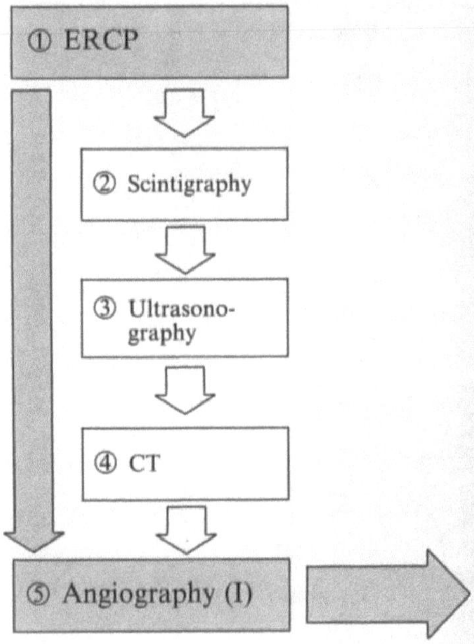

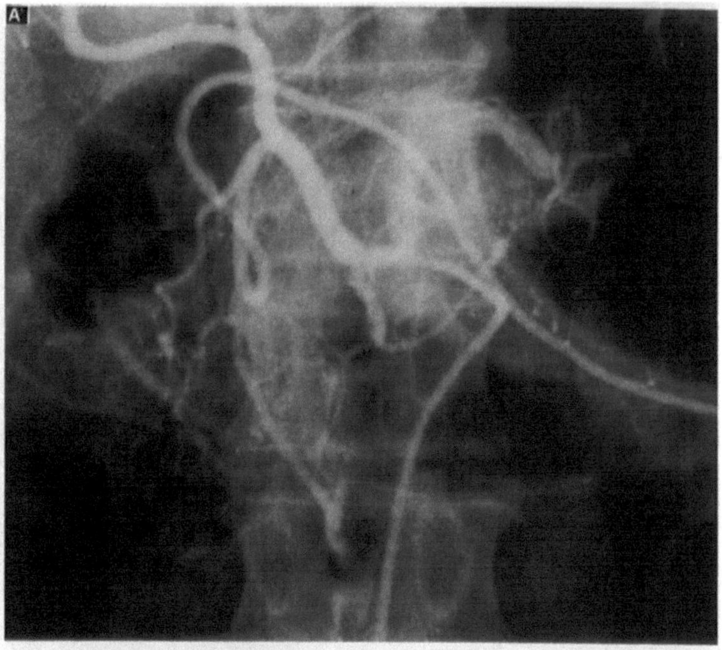

❺ Angiogram (II): 14 months after first angiogram
A, A′ Stereoscopic common hepatic arteriogram
B, B′ Stereoscopic magnification common hepatic arteriogram
Irregularity and encasement of the branches from the dorsal pancreatic artery to the pancreatic arcades as shown in the former angiogram are observable and also not regarded as malignant. A magnification angiogram allows clearer visualization of these findings.

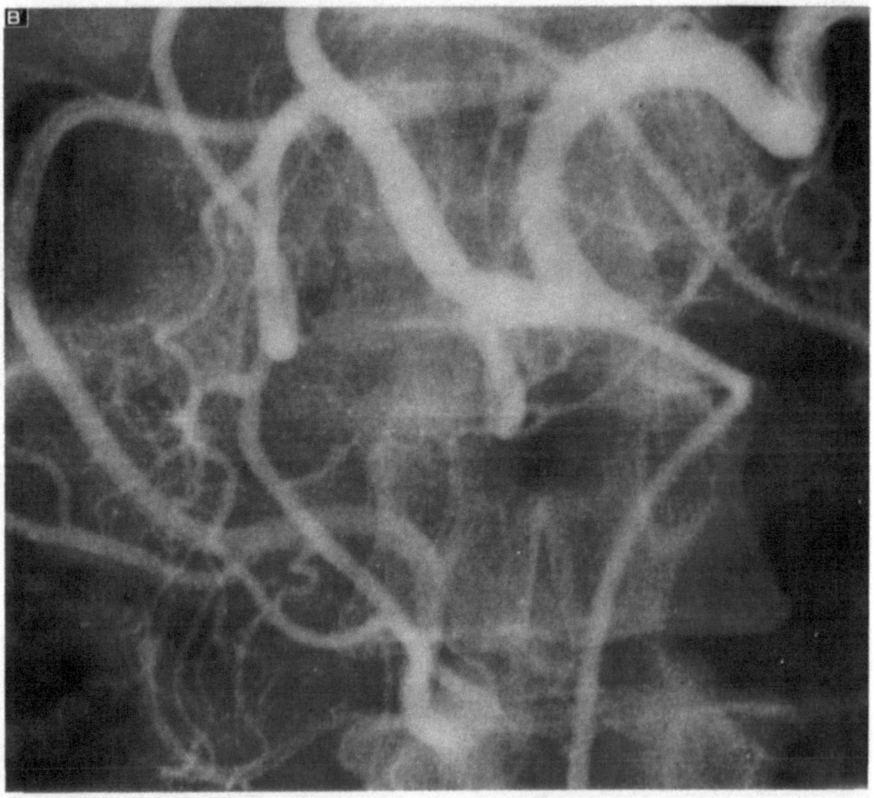

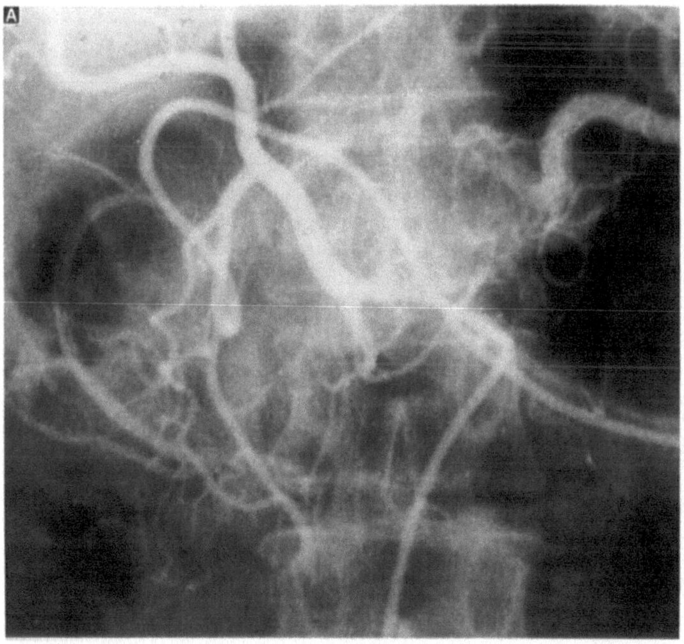
A

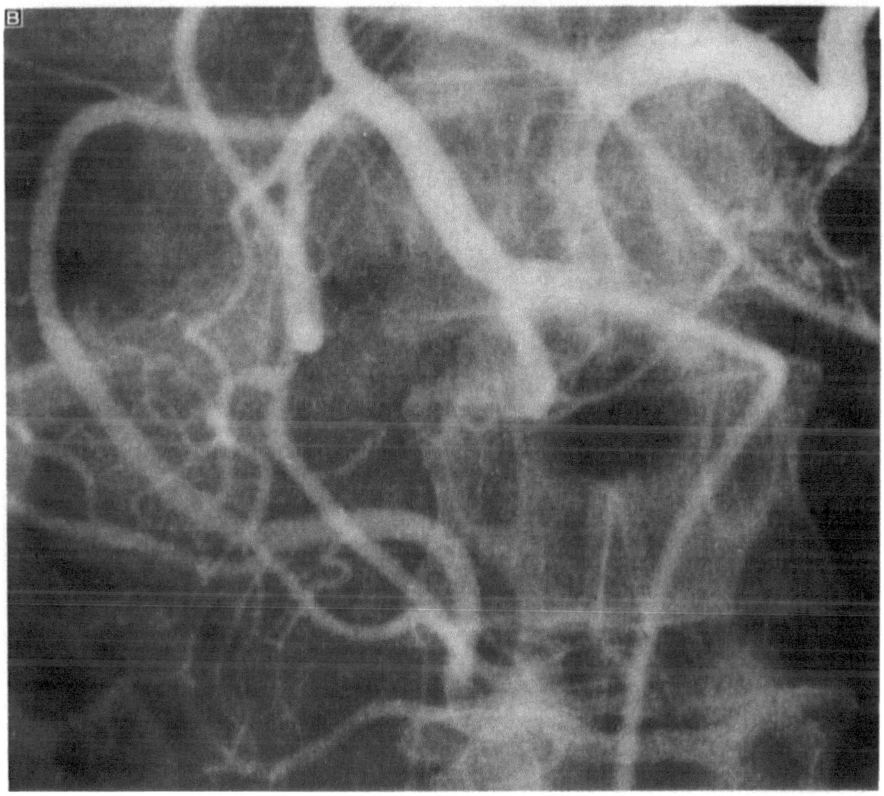
B

Clinical Progress. Carcinoma of the pancreas was ruled out, and cyst formation was not detected from examinations after hospitalization. Thus, the patient left the hospital 2 months after hospitalization and his progress was monitored. Epigastralgia disappeared by conservative treatment. However, 6 months after leaving the hospital, epigastralgia recurred and gradually became more severe and more frequent; thus, a year after leaving the hospital he was rehospitalized. ERCP, ultrasonography, and CT visualized dilatation of the pancreatic duct as before, and angiography showed no marked findings. The patient's progress was further monitored, and conservative treatment was undertaken.

Significance of Diagnostic Imaging. Differentiation between chronic pancreatitis and carcinoma of the pancreas is only achievable with angiography. In some cases, however, it may be difficult even with angiography. Small pathological lesions are diagnosed relying on slight changes of vessels; therefore, sufficient diagnostic imaging is indispensable. Additionally, the joint use of magnification angiography is desirable.

General Matters Concerning Chronic Pancreatitis [4, 19, 23]. Chronic pancreatitis is defined as localized or diffuse irregular fibrosis accompanied by characteristic findings, such as destruction or disappearance of pancreatic parenchymal cells, stenosis or dilatation of the pancreatic duct, or calculi formation in the pancreatic duct. An elemental histopathological finding is inflammatory cellular infiltration mainly composed of fibrosis and lymphocytosis. It is divided into intralobular and interlobular fibrosis in terms of the fibrotic portion, but the former is often accompanied by interlobular fibrosis. Furthermore, many abnormalities, such as various types of degeneration of exocrine glandular cells, metaplasia, regeneration, and hyperplasia of the epithelium of the pancreatic duct, narrowing or cystic dilatation of the pancreatic duct, pseudocyst formation, hyperplasia of fatty tissue, and atrophy, disappearance, and hyperplasia of the islets of Langerhans, are associated. Macroscopically, the early stage of chronic pancreatitis is basically characterized by slight fibrosis and lymphocyte infiltration; thus, despite swelling and hardness in consistency, the pancreas is not consistently hard. Solidity increases in proportion to the fibrous connective tissue. A disorder of the connective tissue between the lobule and interlobule results in an irregular surface and a more hardened pancreas. Further advancement of the disease gets rid of elasticity and causes a hard and contracted pancreas. Additionally, fibrotic thickening or adhesion of the capsule may occur.

The sex distribution ratio of chronic pancreatitis in Japan is 2–3:1 between males and females, and the frequency is 0.7%–2.1% of all hospitalized patients. The etiological factors of chronic pancreatitis based on a national investigation in Japan are alcohol in 46.5% (male 60.6%, female 4.6%) and cholelithiasis in 13% (male 6.7%, female 31.5%) of 1622 patients. Also, it is frequent in 30- to 40-year-olds.

Medical treatment in the early stage consists of internal treatment including pain countermeasures, diet therapy, and treatment of diabetes mellitus. Surgical treatment is employed in the following cases: (a) internal treatment of pain is inefficient, (b) calculus, pseudocyst, or abscess formation in the pancreas are complicated, (c) stenosis of the bile duct or diseases of the biliary tract are also present, and (d) carcinoma of the pancreas is suspected.

2.3 Chronic Pancreatitis (Pancreatolithiasis, Pseudocyst of the Pancreas)

Sequence of Diagnostic Imaging.

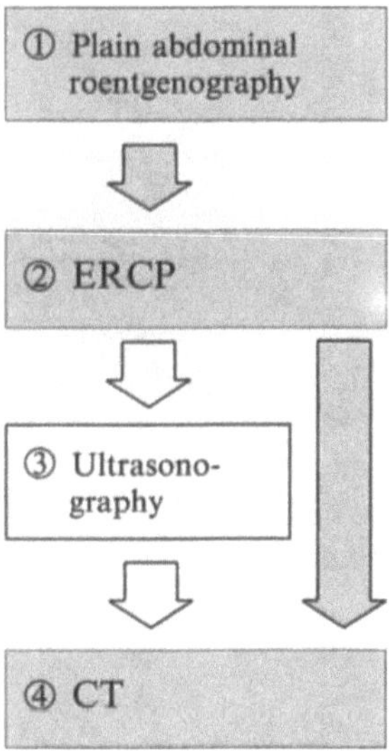

Patient. A 56-year-old woman.

Main Complaint. Left facial nerve palsy.

Present History. Left facial nerve palsy suddenly appeared 1 month prior and the patient was admitted to another hospital where diabetes mellitus was diagnosed; then further examination was performed in our hospital.

Past History. An episode of acute abdomen at 20 years of age. She has no history of trauma or alcohol abuse.

Present Status. No specific findings in the upper abdomen.

Laboratory Data.

SGOT	13 mU/ml	Normal
SGPT	5 mU/	Normal
LDH	225 mU/ml	Normal
ALP	8.2 mU/ml	↓
γ-GTP	3.9 mU/ml	Normal
Total bilirubin	0.4 mg/dl	Normal
Serum glucose	161.6 mg/dl	↑
Serum amylase	120 IU/l	Normal
PS test	3 factors decrease	

Purpose of Diagnostic Imaging. To precisely examine the pancreas and detect a malignant tumor.

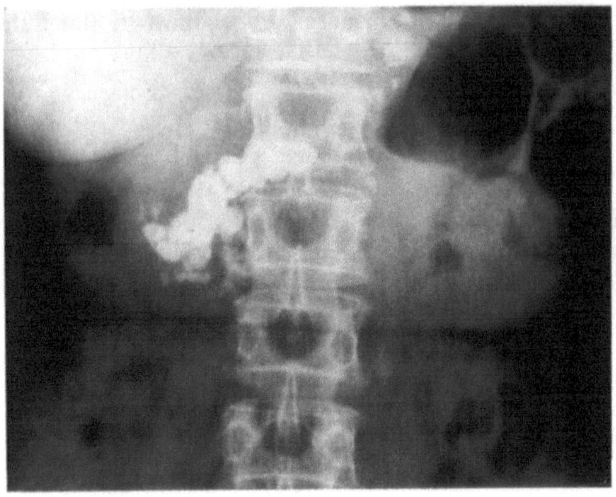

❶ Plain abdominal roentgenogram
Pancreatic calculi of various sizes are visualized from the head to the tail of the pancreas.

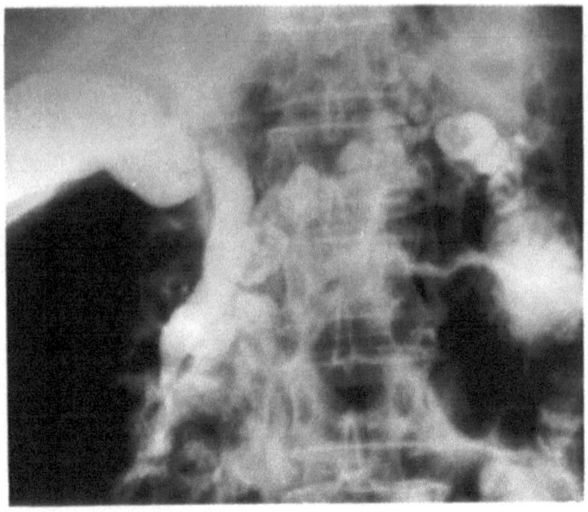

❷ ERCP
The pancreatic duct is poorly opacified.

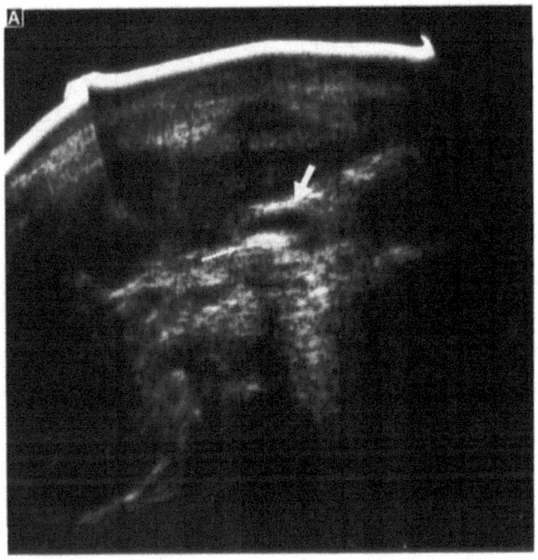

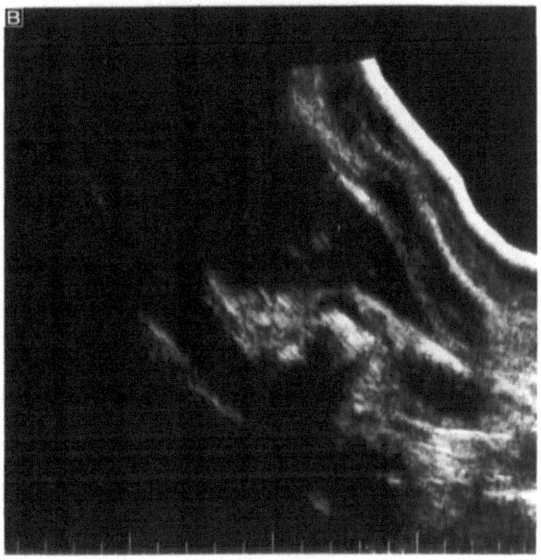

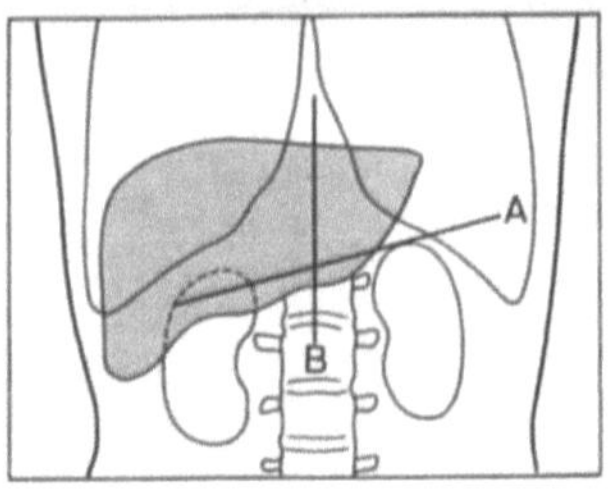

③ Ultrasonogram
A, B Contact compound scanning
The head and tail of the pancreas cannot be visualized due to intestinal gas. A cyst 2 × 1 cm in size (→) in the body of the pancreas and a strong echo of a stone behind it (→) accompanied by acoustic shadow are seen.

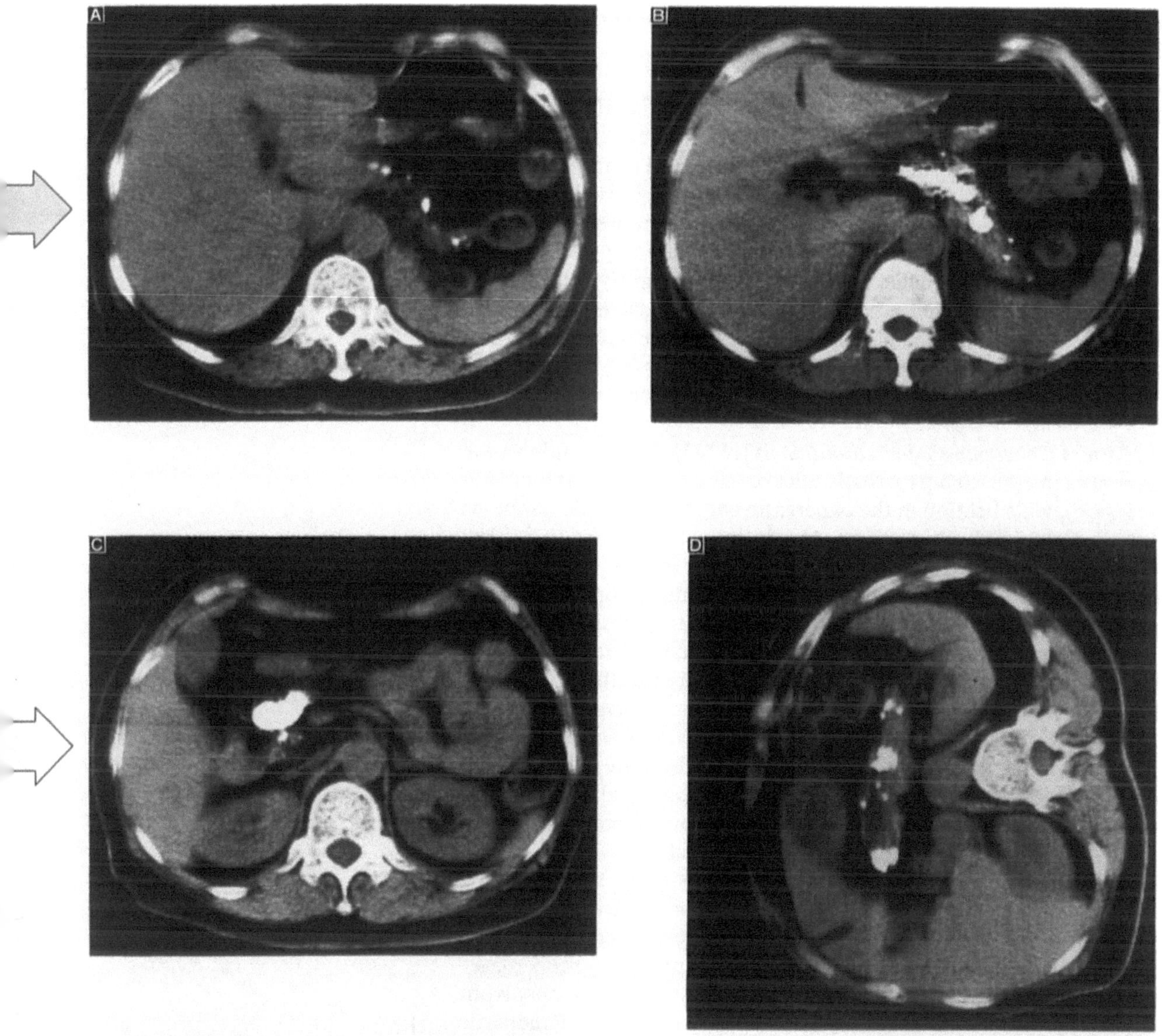

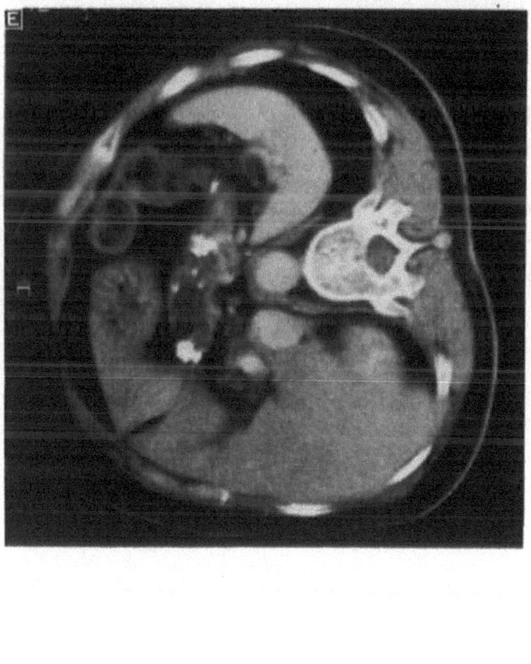

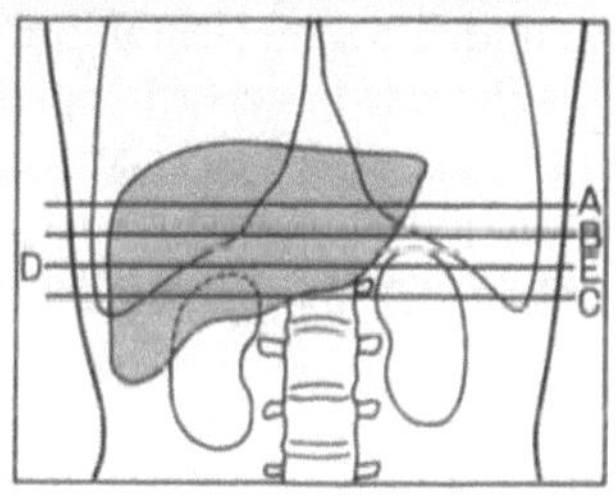

❹ CT image
A–D Plain CT
E After contrast enchancement
D, E Scanning in right lateral decubitus position
Stones are observed entirely from the tail to the head (**A–C**) of the pancreas. A pseudocyst 26 × 18 mm in size is seen in the head and other tiny scattered cysts exist with no contrast enhancement.

Clinical Progress. The patient has made fine progress and is now receiving outclinic treatment for diabetes mellitus.

Significance of Diagnostic Imaging. The presence of pancreatic calculi is easily detected with plain abdominal roentgenography, but ultrasonography and CT are both superior in studies of morphological changes, particulary where cysts exist in the pancreas. In cases with pancreatic calculi spread entirely over the pancreas, CT is preferred to ultrasonography because entire observation of the pancreas is sometimes prevented by the image of the pancreatic calculi and acoustic shadow in ultrasonography. Although in this case, ERCP did not offer satisfactory information, it is always performed regardless. If carcinoma is suspected from these examinations, angiography is required. In this case, however, angiography was not performed since no carcinoma of the pancreas was suspected.

General Matters Concerning Pancreatolithiasis [15, 23]. Calcification in the pancreas occurs in either the pancreatic duct or the pancreatic parenchyma (necrotic lesion). Calcification in the pancreatic parenchyma (false stone) is not frequent; thus, in chronic pancreatitis intraductal calcification (true stone) is carefully observed (pancreatolithiasis or chronic calcifying pancreatitis). The intraductal calcification distributes along the branches of the pancreatic duct. Diffuse distribution of the calcification entirely over the pancreas is observed in half the cases, and calcification localized in the head of the pancreas occurs in one-third of the cases. Pancreatolithiasis is classified into small, large, and mixed types in terms of stones demonstrated by plain abdominal roentgenography. The small type is closely associated with alcoholic pancreatitis, and large stones are detected in more than half the cases of nonalcoholic pancreatitis and are also frequent in idiopathic pancreatitis in females. Some stones not visible on a plain abdominal roentgenogram may be visualized as a filling defect by ERCP.

A pancreatic stone is made from calcium deposits on the laminated structure including collagen. This is gradually transformed from the mucoprotein plug (precursor of a stone) formed in the intercalated portion and small ducts in the lobules due to retention of the pancreatic juice.

This process takes place during migration of the mucoprotein plug from the small lateral side branches to the main pancreatic duct. Pancreatic stones are mainly comprised of calcium carbonate. They are more frequent in males, and the male:female ratio is 3.5:1, often in the 30 to 50-year age group. Of chronic pancreatitis patients, 40%–70% have pancreatic stones, and half the cases are heavy drinkers. Conversely, 90% of chronic alcoholic pancreatitis patients also have accompanying pancreatolithiasis. The frequency of pancreatolithiasis is high in local areas where protein ingestion is scarce.

In pancreatitis, the rate of accompanying diabetes mellitus is high at 70%–90%, and the prognosis is dependent upon the treatment of diabetes mellitus. Furthermore, pancreatitis is highly associated with carcinoma of the pancreas in 3%–25% of all cases.

2.4 Cyst of the Pancreas (Pseudocyst)

Sequence of Diagnostic Imaging.

① Plain abdominal roentgenography
⇩
② Ultrasonography
⇩
③ CT
⇩
④ ERCP
⇩
⑤ Angiography

Patient. A 62-year-old woman.

Main Complaint. Pain form the left side to the back.

Present History. Two years prior, the above symptom occurred two to three times a year, but since it disappeared within a day it was neglected. Recently, however, the symptom has appeared frequently and the patient was admitted to our hospital.

Present Status. Not a clear abdominal mass but some resistance was palpable in the left upper abdomen. Pleural bloody effusion was detected.

Past History. The patient has no history of alcohol abuse or trauma, but had an episode of pneumonia 30 years prior.

Laboratory Data.

SGOT	41 mU/ml	↑
SGPT	82 mU/ml	↑
ALP	42 mU/ml	Normal
LDH	231 mU/ml	↑
γ-GTP	11 mU/ml	Normal
Cho E	348 U/dl	Normal
Serum amylase	1030 IU/l	↑
Urine amylase	4446 IU/l	↑

Purpose of Diagnostic Imaging. A tumor of the pancreas was suspected from the clinical examination data, and an upper gastrointestinal tract examination at the time of hospitalization showed medial displacement of the great curvature of the stomach.

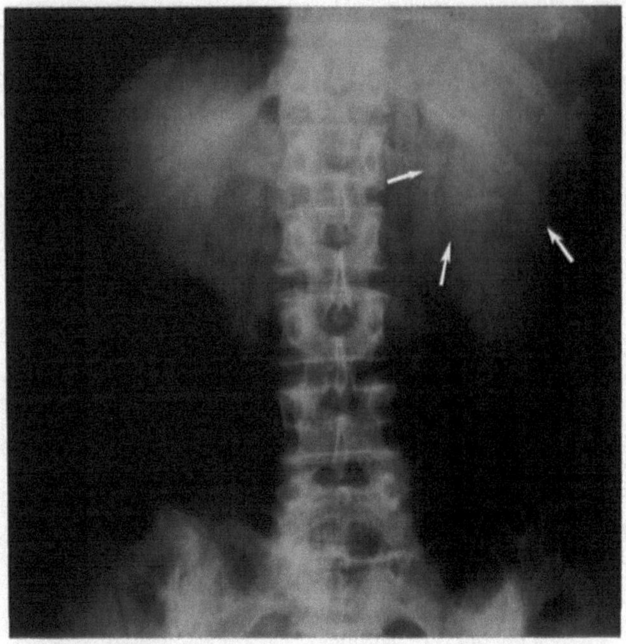

① Plain abdominal roentgenogram
A soft tissue density at the left upper abdomen is observable (→).

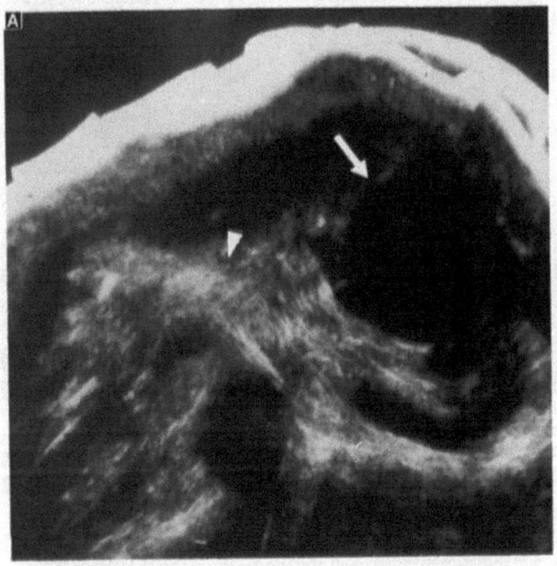

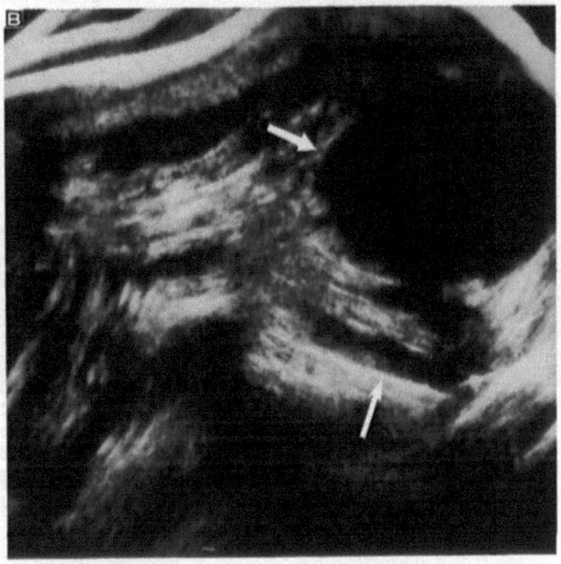

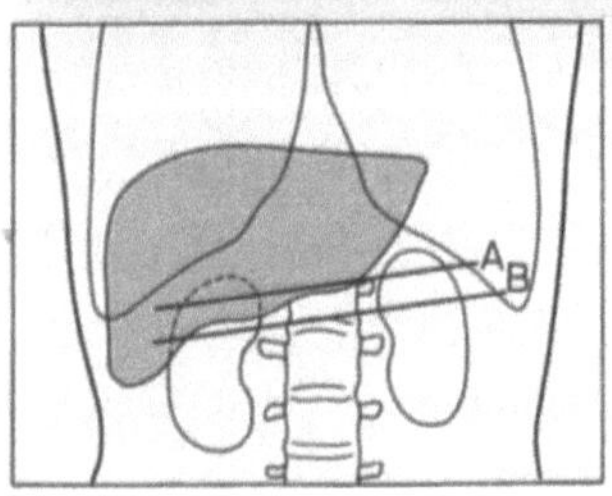

❷ Ultrasonogram
A, B Contact compound scanning
A cystic lesion with a relatively clear contour 8 × 8 cm in size is visualized in the tail of the pancreas (→). A solid mass is not observed. The left kidney (→) and the body of the pancreas (▶) are also seen.

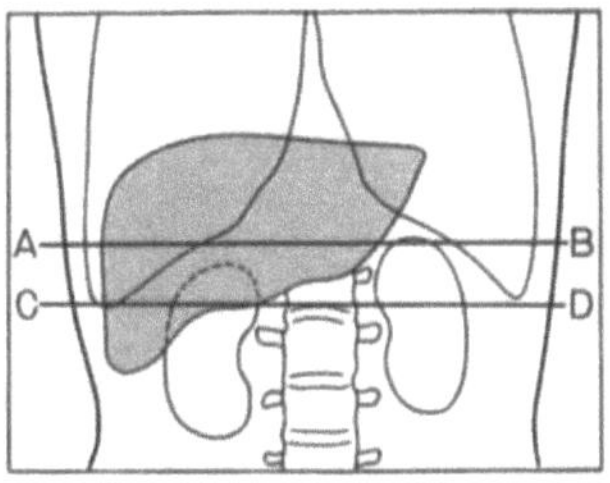

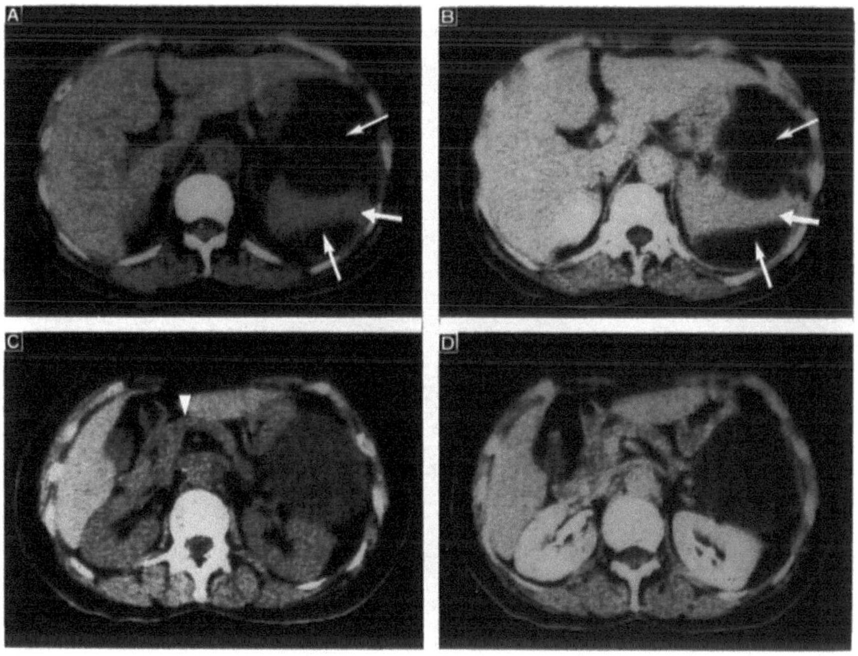

❸ CT image
A, C Before contrast enhancement
B, D After contrast enhancement
A and **B** show large and small cysts (→) with intervention of the spleen (→). The lower scanning slices (**C**, and **D**) clearly demonstrate the cysts originating from the tail of the pancreas (▶).

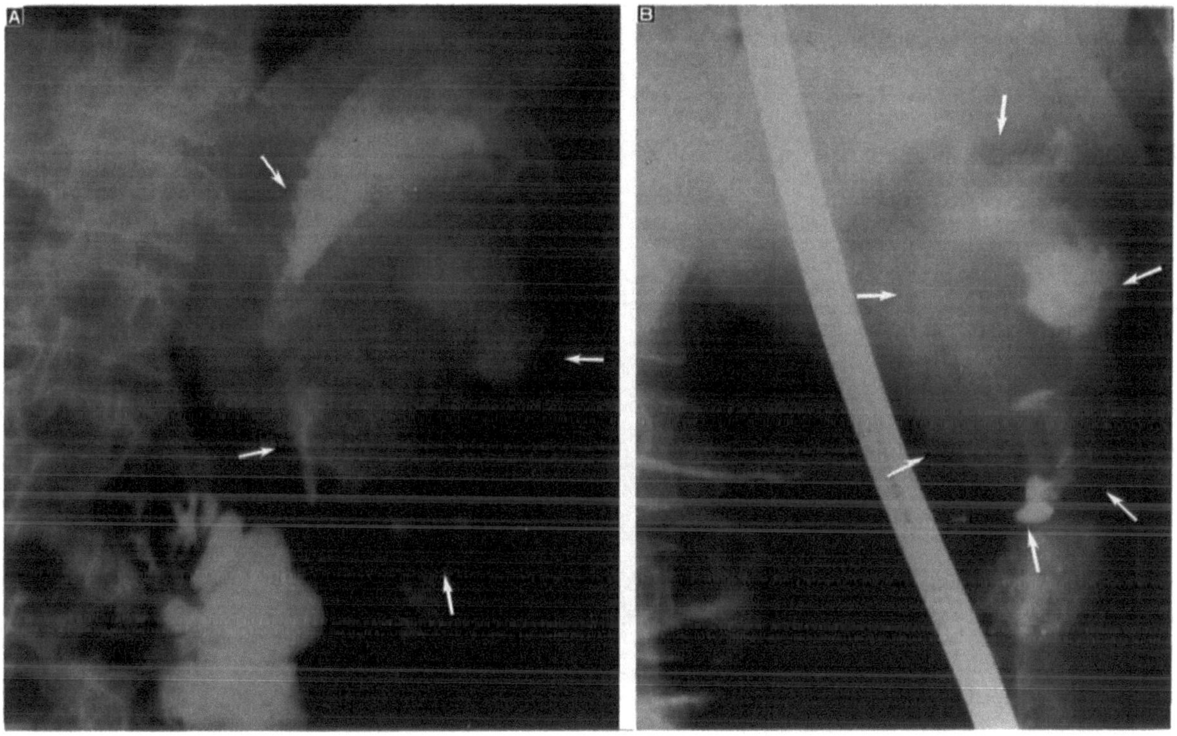

❹ ERCP
A Frontal view
B Right anterior oblique view
Pooling of contrast medium through the pancreatic duct into the cyst is visualized (→).

⑤ Angiography

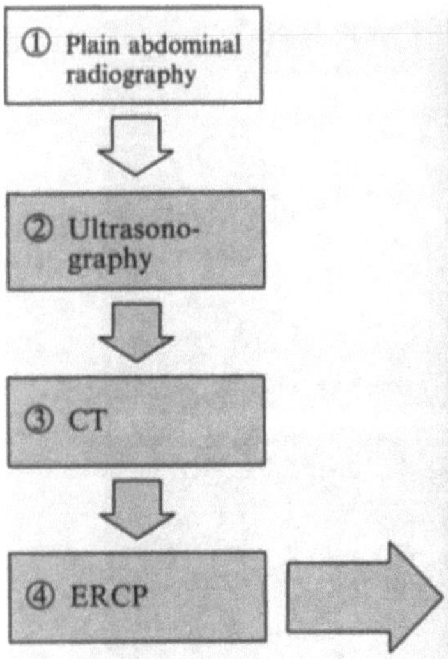
① Plain abdominal radiography
② Ultrasonography
③ CT
④ ERCP

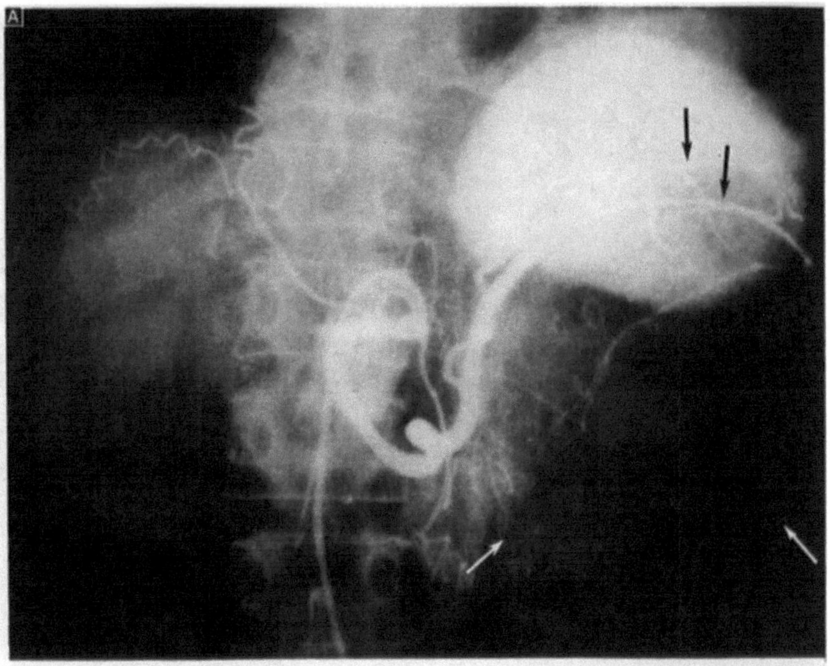
A

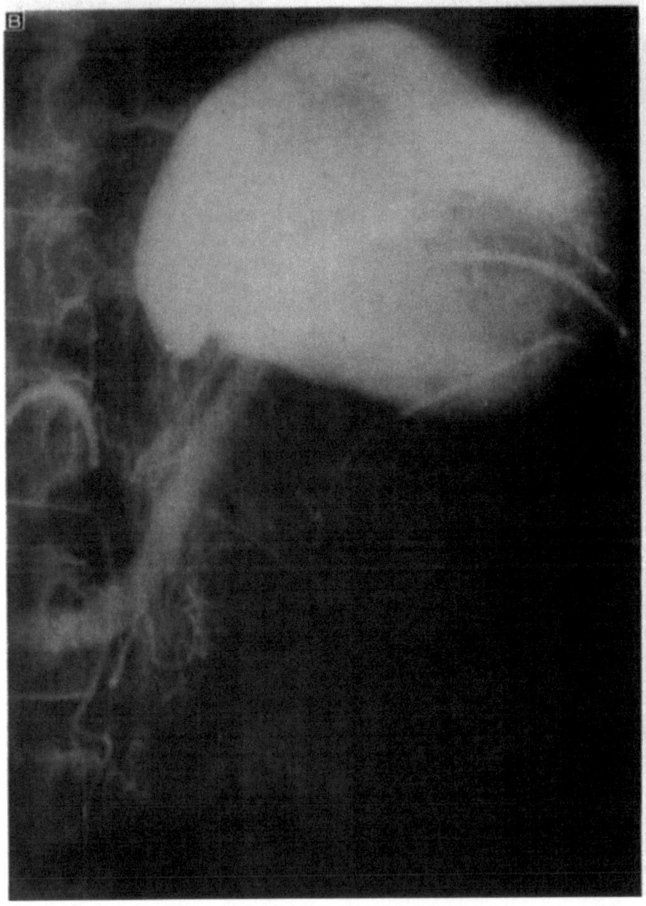
B

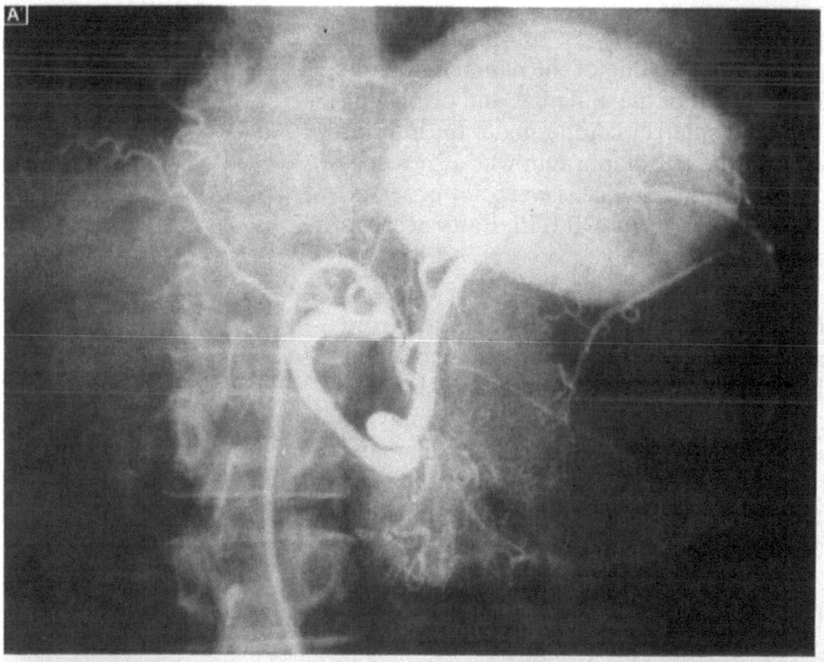

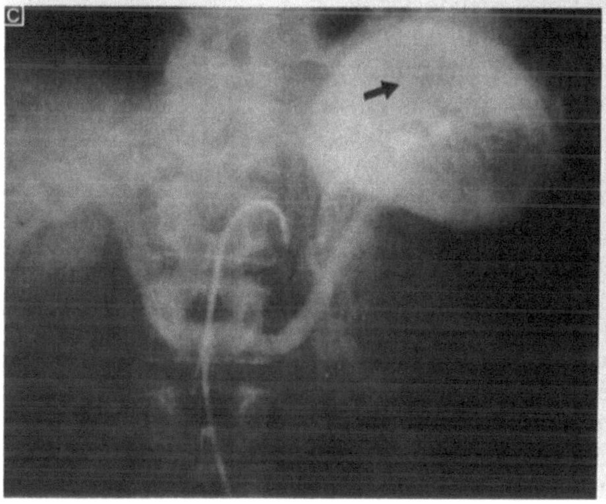

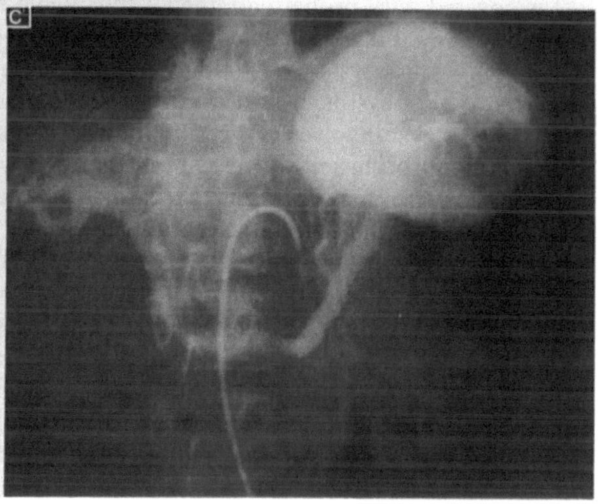

⑤ Angiogram
A, A′ Stereoscopic splenic arteriogram (arterial phase)
The splenic artery is displaced upward, and its peripheral branches and vessels in the tail of the pancreas increase and surround the tumor but do not extend inside the tumor (→).
B Magnification splenic arteriogram
Magnification allows the neovascularity of the fine vessels in the tail of the pancreas to be clearly visualized, but malignant findings or vessels extending into the tumor are not observed.
C, C′ Stereoscopic arteriogram (venous phase)
No abnormality of the splenic vein is observed. The contour of the cyst is lightly stained. A smaller defect in the splenogram superior to the large cyst suggests the existence of a small cyst in the spleen.

Operative Findings. A combined resection of the cysts, spleen, and tail of pancreas was performed. Slight edematous swelling of the pancreas including a fist-sized cyst originating from the tail of the pancreas and displacing the spleen upward was detected. Another small cyst adhering to the inferior surface of the left lobe of the liver and the left diaphragm was also recognized at the upper border of the spleen. Epithelial cells were not observed in the cyst. Amylase of the contents of the cyst is 98490 IU/l. Fatty necrosis in the pancreatic parenchyma was also detected.

Significance of Diagnostic Imaging. A cystic tumor is easily detected from ultrasonography and CT. In cases of huge cysts, identification of their origin may sometimes be difficult. In this respect, ultrasonography is superior to CT in terms of free selection of scanning direction. ERCP may be necessary to study the relationship between the cyst and the pancreatic duct. Determining whether the tumor includes only the cyst or both a cyst and solid component together may be possible with ultrasonography and CT, but if the result is uncertain, angiography is required.

General Matters Concerning Cyst of the Pancreas [2, 12, 13, 14]. Pancreatic cysts are divided into true cysts and pseudocysts. The inner wall of a true cyst is covered with proper endothelial cells while that of a pseudocyst is composed of granular tissue and fibrous connective tissue without endothelial cells. Pseudocysts are caused by trauma, inflammation, neoplasm, or parasites. A true cyst is classified into congenital and acquired types. An acquired true cyst involves cystic dilatation, called a "retention cyst," due to stenosis and occlusion of the pancreatic duct, which is also caused by inflammation, trauma, neoplasm, or parasites. Some scholars include the neoplastic cyst in the class of acquired true cysts.

Pseudocysts account for 60%–75% of all cases of pancreatic cysts, and many cases occur after inflammation or trauma. Destruction of pancreatic tissue by these inducers causes activation of trypsinogen and lipase resulting in necrosis and hemorrhage. The necrotic material accumulated in the omental bursa and retroperitoneal cavity are covered with fibrous tissue, and a cyst is produced. Pseudocysts are divided into intrapancreatic and extrapancreatic cysts. Extrapancreatic pseudocysts chiefly appear in the omental bursa or retoperitoneal cavity, but they may sometimes occur in the mediastinum, thoracic cavity, or neck. Though proximate to the spleen, it hardly ever ruptures into the spleen. Observation of the communication between a cyst and the pancreatic duct is dependent upon the case. A cyst is mainly unilocular, and sometimes has a septum. The wall is irregular in thickness and occasionally thickens to an extent of a few centimeters. The inner wall is uneven due to necrotic or granular tissues. It has bloody or serous contents, occasionally with floating or sedimentary necrotic tissue. The liquid substance is alkaline, frequently including a pancreatic enzyme, but activity is low and becomes lower with increasing lapse of time from development of the cyst.

The symptoms of a cyst in the pancreas depend on the causes. Abdominal pain and tenderness commonly appear in cases caused by pancreatitis. A tumor is palpable in 50%–90% of cases, but fluctuation is hardly ever recognized. Jaundice occurs in 10% of the cases.

A pseudocyst is spontaneously absorbed in cases in which absorption occurs before cystic wall formation or it forms an internal fistula by rupturing into the digestive tract. If not absorbed, the cyst grows until it affects the neighboring organs and produces symptoms; thus, surgical treatment is required. The fatality rate is high especially in cases with perforation into the abdominal cavity. Surgical treatment consists of a splenectomy, resection of the pancreas, or drainage, but pseudocysts often strongly adhere to neighboring organs, and therefore cystectomy is rarely possible.

2.5 Carcinoma of the Pancreas (Body and Tail)

Sequence of Diagnostic Imaging.

① CT

↓

② Ultrasonography

↓

③ ERCP

↓

④ Angiography

Patient. A 53-year-old female.

Main Complaint. Epigastralgia and back pain after meals.

Present History. Half a year prior, the patient was admitted to another hospital and carcinoma of the pancreas was suspected, but she refused surgery and it was neglected. Recently, the back pain became severe, and she was admitted to our hospital.

Present Status. Tenderness on pressure at the left upper abdomen without palpability of a mass. The liver is palpated 2 FB from the right hypochondrium.

Laboratory Data.

SGOT	24 mU/ml	Normal	
SGPT	23 mU/ml	Normal	
ALP	55 mU/ml	Normal	
LDH	141 mU/ml	Normal	
Cho E	355 U/dl	Normal	
γ-GTP	23 mU/ml	Normal	
Total protein	6.6 g/dl	Normal	
ZTT	6.4 U	Normal	
Total bilirubin	0.6 mg/dl	Normal	
AFP	1.0 mμg/ml	Normal	
HBs Ag	(−)		
Serum amylase	128 IU/l	Normal	
Urine amylase	216 IU/l	↓	
Glucose tolerance test (venous blood)			
Fasting state	1 h	2 h	
70 mg/dl	95 mg/dl	93 mg/dl	normal type

Purpose of Diagnostic Imaging. To obtain a definite diagnosis and assess the operability of carcinoma of the pancreas.

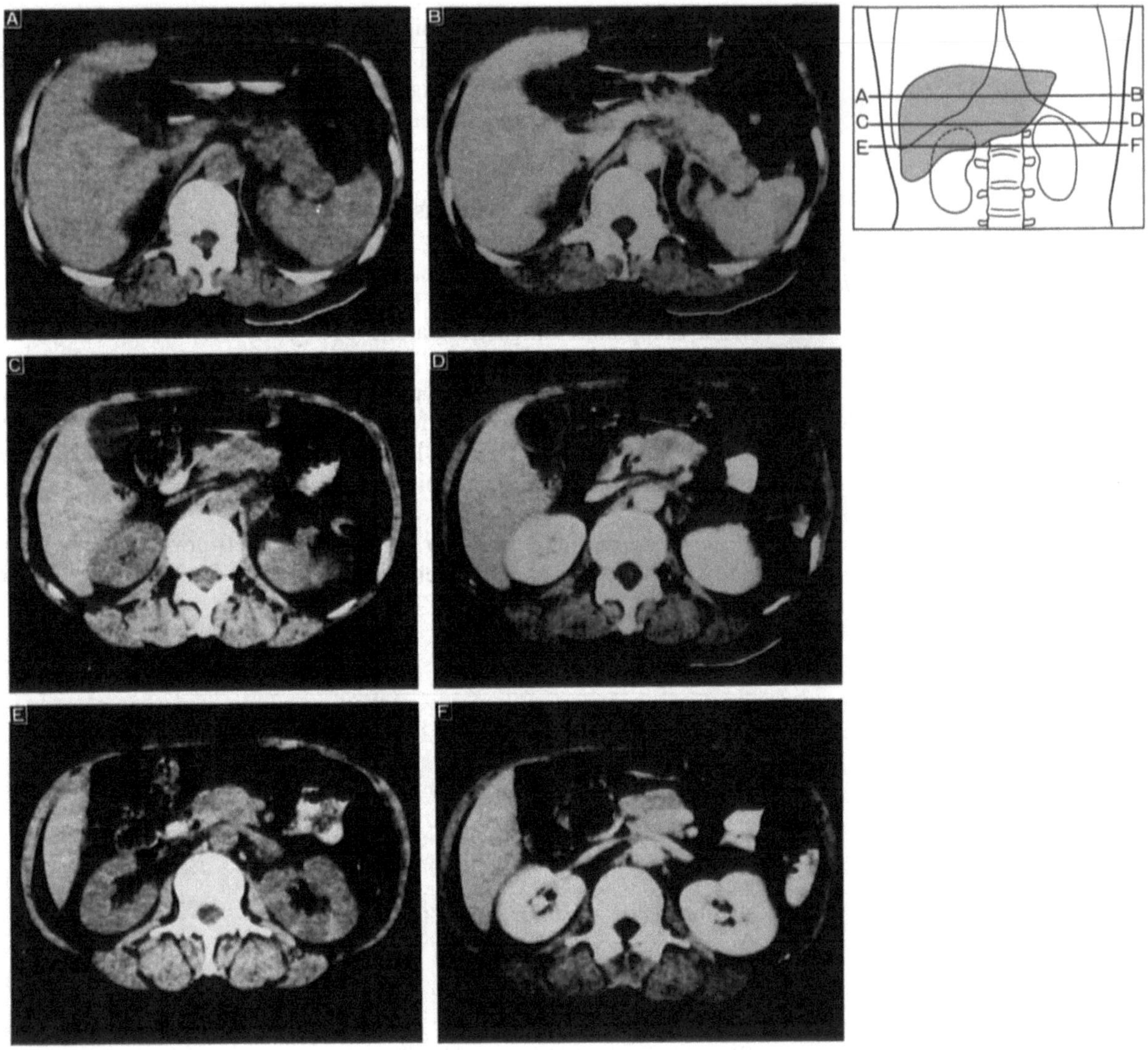

● CT image
A, C, E Before contrast enhancement
B, D, F After contrast enhancement
A tumor image with irregular contours is observable from the body to the tail of the pancreas. After contrast enhancement, the attenuation value of the pancreas increases, but that corresponding to the tumor does not rise. Marked posterior extension does not exist because a fat layer posterior to the pancreas is seen.

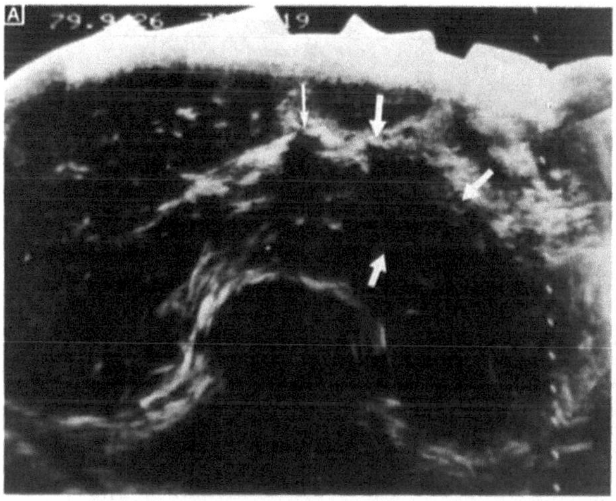

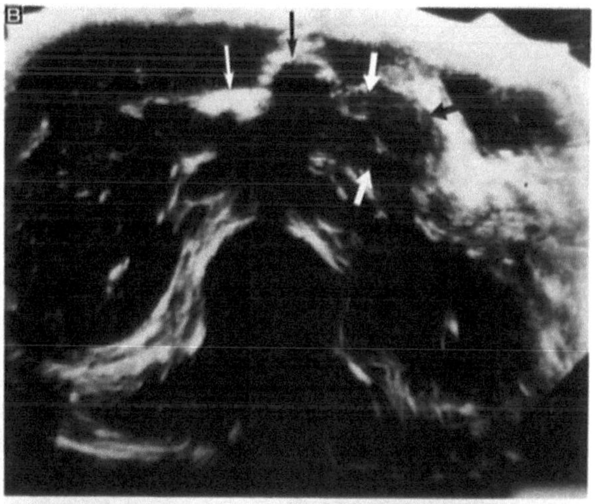

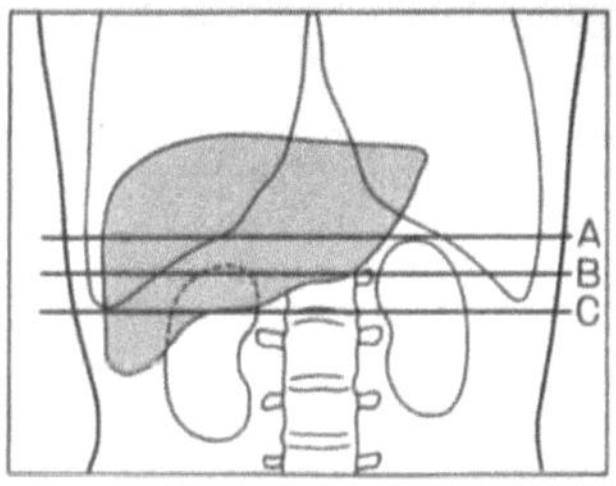

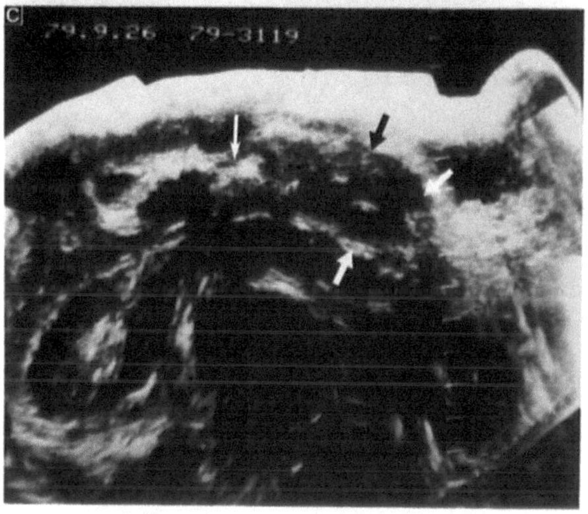

❷ Ultrasonogram
A–C Contact compound scanning
A tumor with inhomogeneous echogenicity is observed from the body to the tail of the pancreas (→). The body of the pancreas is poorly visualized due to intestinal gas (→). The head of the pancreas is normal.

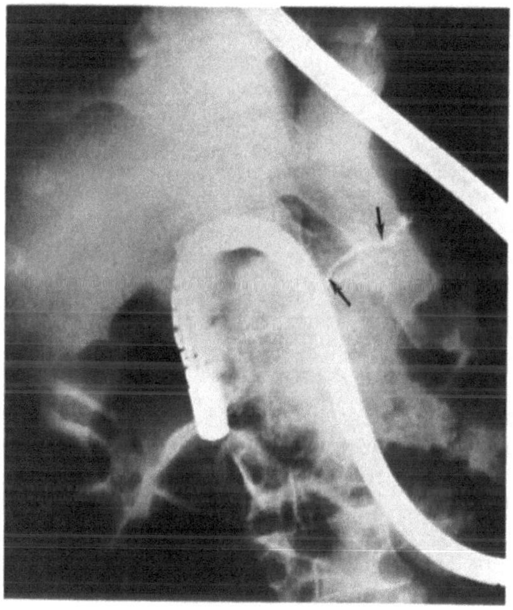

❸ ERCP
Compression and stenosis of the main pancreatic duct is visualized from the body to the tail of the pancreas (→).

④ Angiography

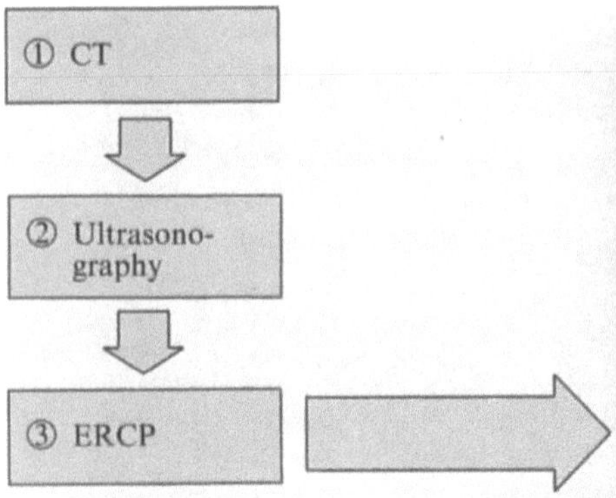

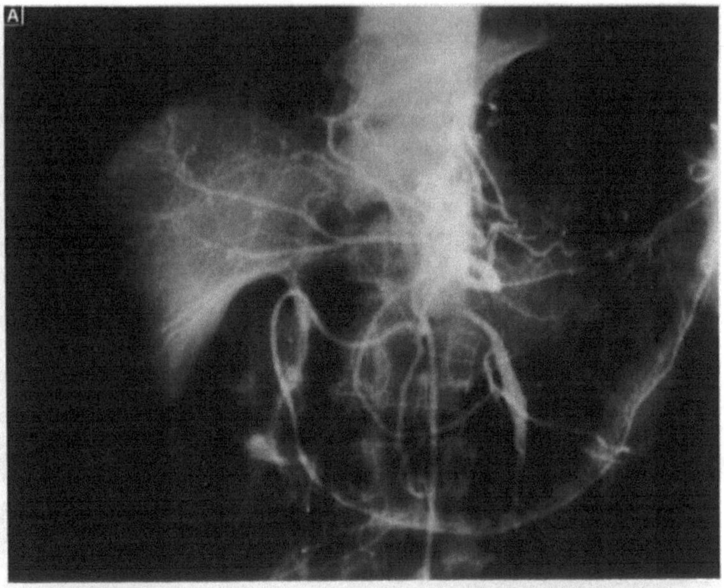

❹ Angiogram
A, A' Stereoscopic celiac arteriogram (arterial phase)
B Celiac arteriogram (venous phase)
C Superior mesenteric arteriogram (venous phase)
D Magnification celiac arteriogram (arterial phase)
The celiac trunk is displaced to the left. The splenic artery (→) shows stenosis and encasement at the origin and intermission. The left gastric artery also shows encasement at the bifurcation, and further encasement is visualized in the dorsal pancreatic artery and the branches feeding the posterior wall of the stomach body (**A, D**). The splenic vein is not opacified and a collateral vein is seen (**B**, →). Compression or occlusion of the splenic vein is suspected. The origin of the superior mesenteric artery is displaced to the left with stenosis about 2 cm long (**A**, ▶). No occlusion is observed in the superior mesenteric vein, but it is displaced to the left.

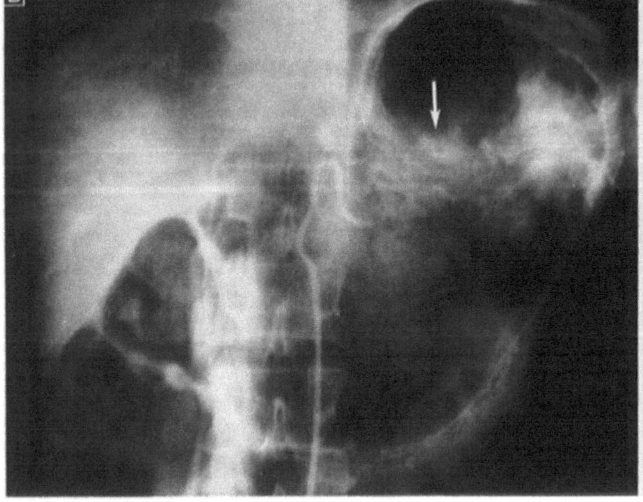

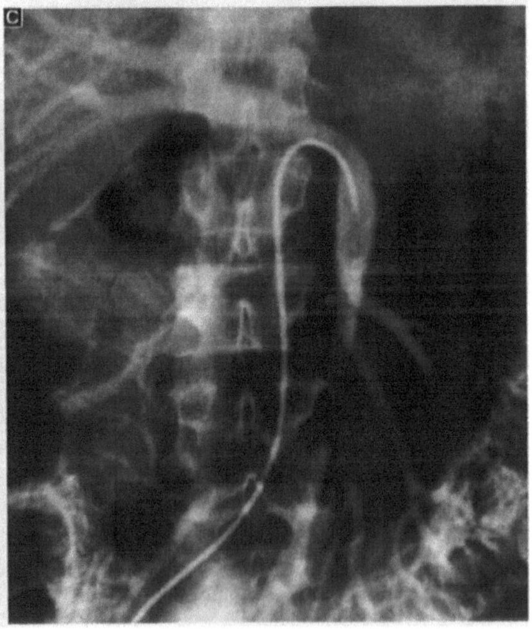

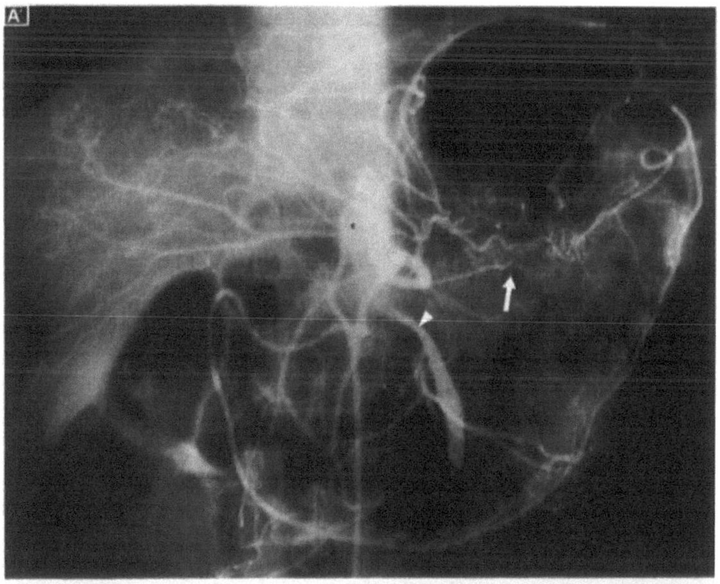
A

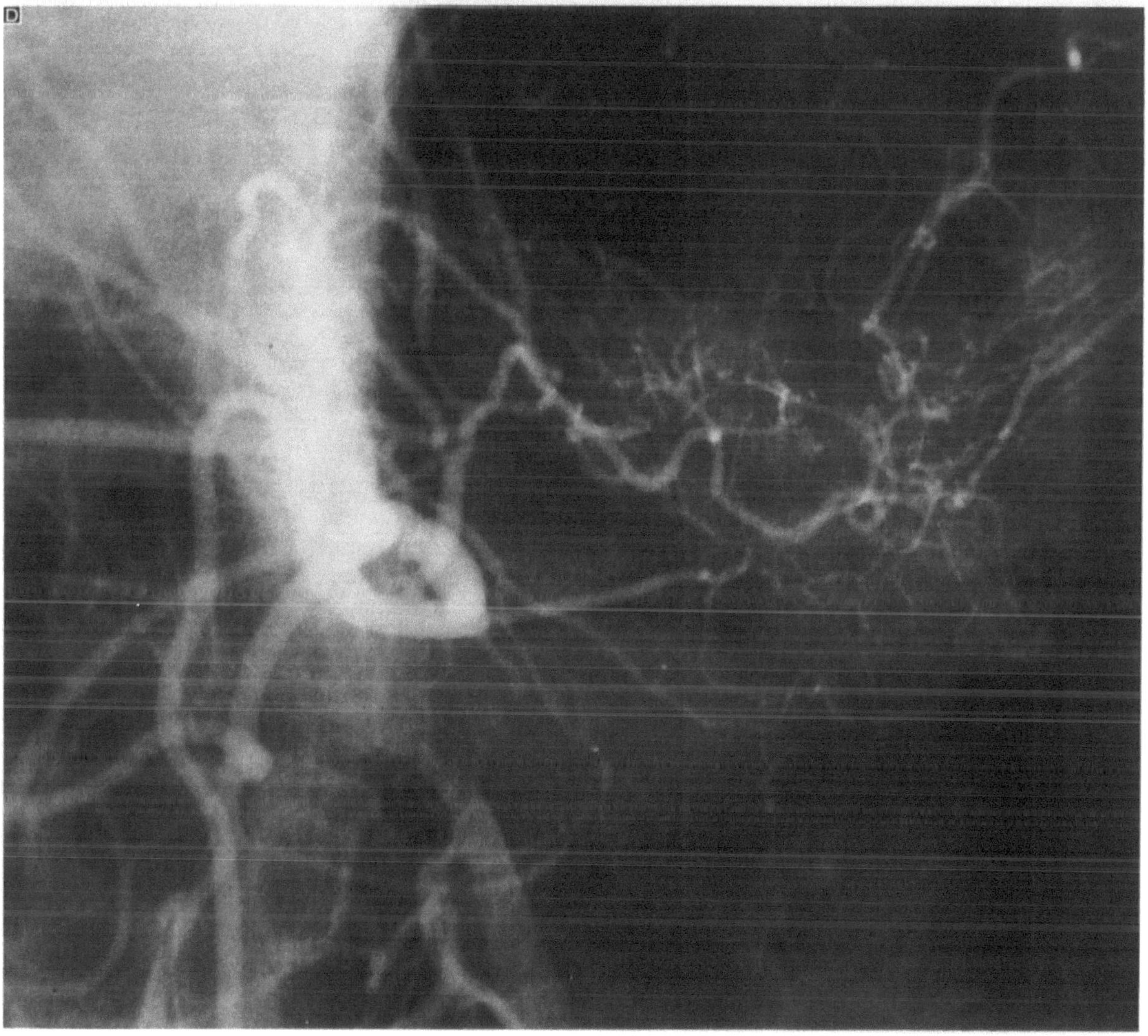
D

Operative Findings. A tumor mass from the body to the tail of the pancreas invading the posterior wall of the stomach at the distal part of the body of the pancreas is observed. Massive lymph node metastasis from the celiac trunk to the origin of the right gastric artery and a pea-sized metastasis at the Douglas' cul-de-sac are also recognized. No metastasis is existent in the porta hepatis and hepatoduodenal ligament.

Significance of Diagnostic Imaging. The localization of a tumor from the body to the tail of the pancreas is easily detected with ultrasonography. Generally, CT is superior to ultrasonography in the study of the extrapancreatic extension of the tumor. CT is also better in cases of lymph node metastasis. However, angiography is required to obtain information about the operability of the cases.

General Matters Concerning Carcinoma of the Pancreas [3, 5, 6, 17, 18]. Tumors in the pancreas are classified into exocrine tumors, endocrine tumors including insuloma, and tumors in supporting tissues. Exocrine tumors are divided into tumors originating in parenchymal (acinar) cells and those in duct cells which consist of solid or cystic tumor. Commonly, carcinoma of the pancreas implies an exocrine tumor.

Recently, the rate of frequency of carcinoma of the pancreas in Japan has been increasing. Comparing the mortality rate in 1978 with that in 1950, it has increased 11.9-fold in males and 14.7-fold in females. The age-adjusted death rate has also risen 5.5-fold in males and 1.2-fold in females, drawing close to the level of Western society.

Histologically, carcinoma of the pancreas principally consists of adenocarcinoma generating from duct cells or acinar cells, but sometimes squamous cell carcinoma, adenosquamous carcinoma, mucoepidermoid carcinoma, or mucinous adenocarcinoma may originate in the pancreatic duct. Of all cases of carcinoma of the pancreas, 60% occur in the head of the pancreas, 30% in the body and tail, and 10% are diffused over the entire pancreas.

Macroscopically, Hayashi classifies the external surface of the carcinoma of the pancreas into the tumor-forming, sclerosing, masked (only detected by cutting or histopathological study), and miscellaneous types and the cutting surface into nodular, infiltrative, and mixed types. Carcinoma originating in the head of the pancreas causes secondary pancreatitis in the tail because of stasis of pancreatic juice due to drainage disturbance in the main pancreatic duct. Therefore, during palpation, a palpable mass does not always indicate carcinoma so that surgical treatment must be carefully performed considering the range of the resection. As carcinoma of the head of the pancreas grows, it infiltrates the intrapancreatic bile duct causing obstructive jaundice. Also, it directly infiltrates the duodenum, stomach, portal vein, transverse mesocolon, root of the small bowel mesentery, and hepatoduodenal ligament. Carcinoma of the body and tail of the pancreas infiltrates the stomach, spleen, adrenal gland, colon, retroperitoneum, and splenic vein. Carcinoma originating from the uncinate process rarely causes obstructive jaundice and infiltrates the wall of the ascending portion of the duodenum. In a carcinoma of the pancreas, continuous or interrupted transductal metastasis in the pancreas takes place. Regional lymph node metastasis includes lymphogenous dissemination within the pancreatic parenchyma and invasion along the perineural lymph vessels in addition to lymph node metastasis anterior or posterior to the pancreas.

Medical treatment is carried out with pancreatoduodenectomy in carcinoma of the head of the pancreas, distal pancreatectomy in carcinoma of the body and tail, and total pancreatectomy is performed in carcinoma expanding entirely over the pancreas. Total pancreatectomy or regional pancreatectomy may be carried out in some cases in which interrupted lesions or continuous extension of the carcinoma through the pancreatic duct are recognizable, but the effects have not yet been clarified. The rate of resectability has been increasing but is still low at 38% in carcinoma of the head of the pancreas, 21% in that of the body and tail, 7% in carcinoma over the entire pancreas, and 31% in general according to Ozaki's statistics in Japan (1976–1979). The 5-year survival rate in resected cases is 10%–20% in carinoma of the head of the pancreas, and in unresected cases treatd merely by laparotomy or anastomosis, half the patients die within 4 months and even the rest almost within 1 year.

2.6 Carcinoma of the Pancreas (Head)

Sequence of Diagnostic Imaging.

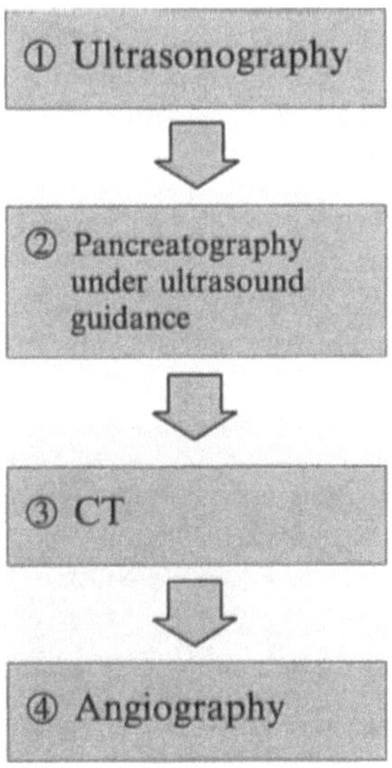

Patient. A 73-year-old male.

Main Complaint. Anorexia.

Present History. The patient was admitted to another hospital complaining of anorexia; hypoproteinemia was diagnosed there, and further examination was performed in our hospital.

Laboratory Data.

SGOT	43 mU/ml	↑	
SGPT	56 mU/ml	↑	
ALP	145 mU/ml	↑	
LDH	247 mU/ml	↑	
γ-GTP	350 mU/ml	↑	
Cho E	192 U/dl	↓	
Total protein	5.1 g/dl	↓	
HBs Ag	(−)		
Serum amylase	286 IU/l	Normal	
Urine amylase	19 IU/l	Normal	
Glucose tolerance test (venous blood)			
Fasting state	1 h	2 h	
101 mg/dl	242 mg/dl	213 mg/dl	Diabetes mellitus type

Purpose of Diagnostic Imaging. To detect disorders of the liver, biliary tract, and pancreas suspected from laboratory data.

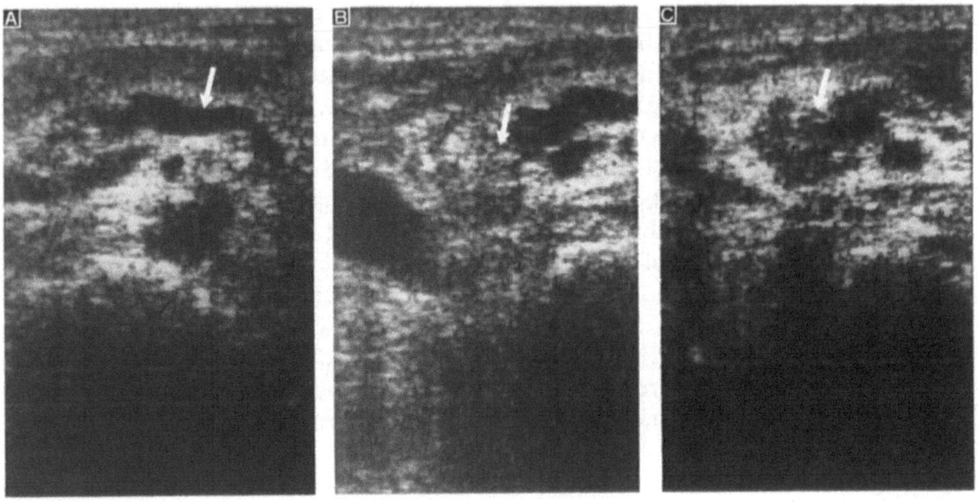

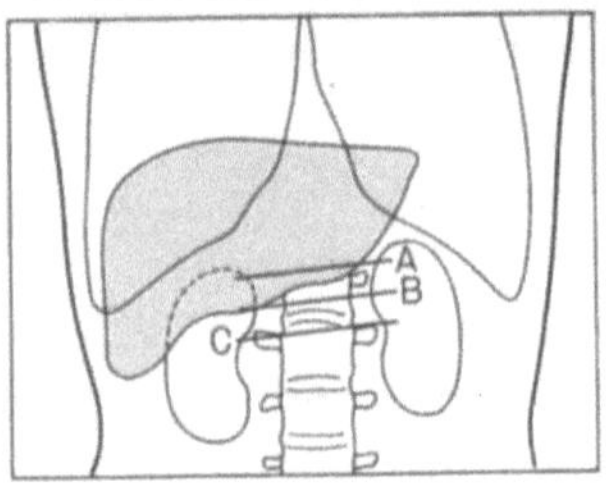

❶ Ultrasonogram
The pancreatic duct is dilated to 7–8 mm from the tail to the head of the pancreas (**A**, →), and an irregular tumor image is seen extending from the head of the pancreas to the uncinate process (**B**, → and **C**, →).

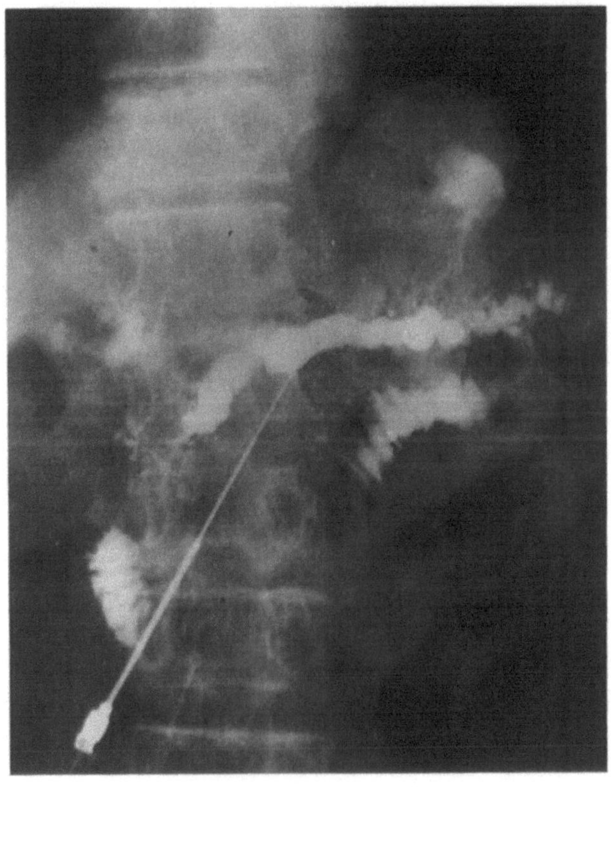

❷ Pancreatogram under ultrasound guidance
Entire dilatation and obstruction near the orifice of the pancreatic duct are observable.

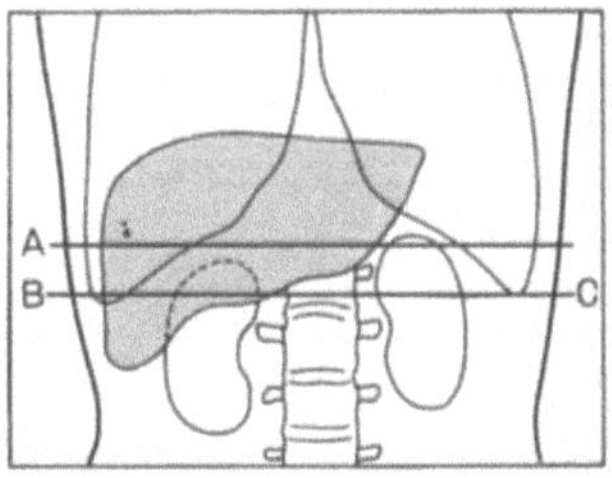

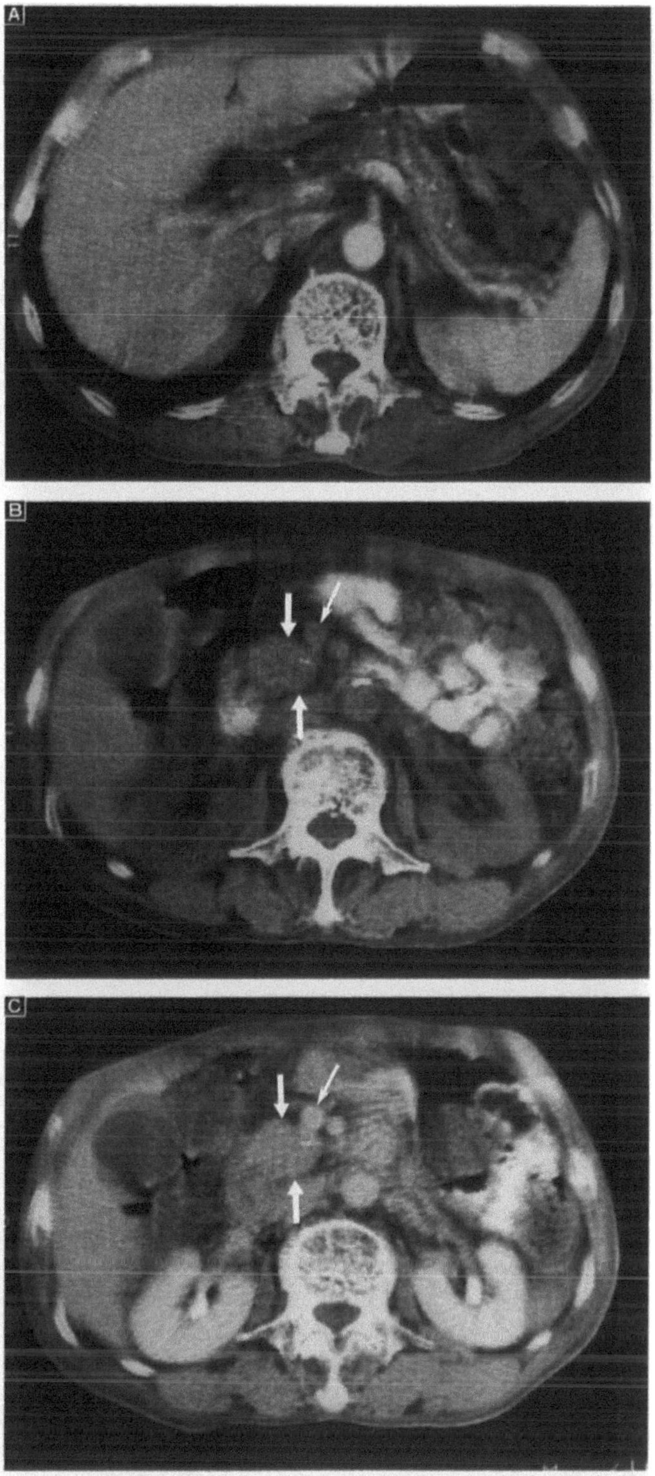

❸ CT image
B Before contrast enhancement
A, **C** After contrast enhancement
In the image (**A**) taken from the body to the tail of the pancreas, the dilated pancreatic duct and pancreatic stones are visualized. The images (**B**, **C**) of the uncinate process level show the pancreatic stones and an entirely swollen uncinate process (→). CT does not demonstrate invasion of the carcinoma into the superior mesenteric vein (→).

④ Angiography

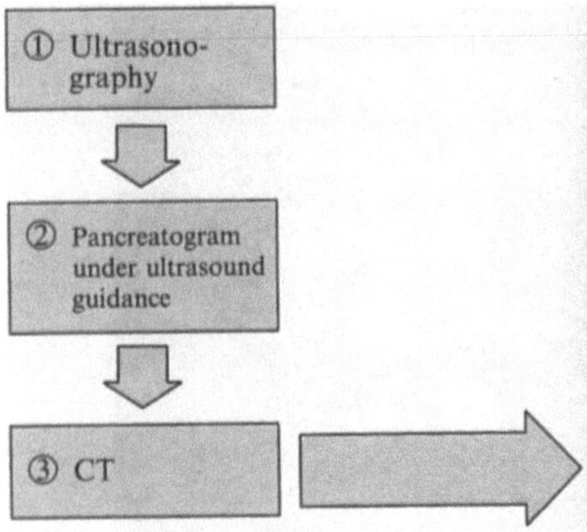

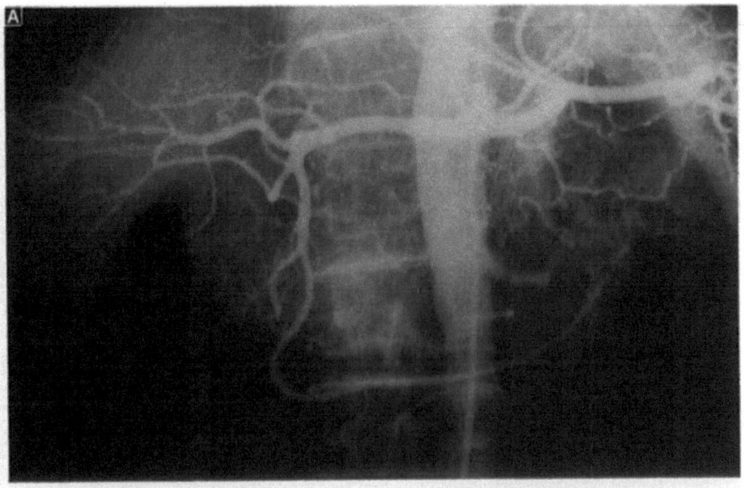

❹ Angiogram
A, A′ Stereoscopic celiac arteriogram (arterial phase)
B Magnification common hepatic arteriogram (arterial phase)
C Magnification common hepatic arteriogram (arterial phase, after intra-arterial noradrenalin injection)
D Superior mesenteric arteriogram (venous phase)
Severe encasement of the posterior superior pancreaticoduodenal artery (branching from the right hepatic artery) and the anterior superior pancreaticoduodenal artery is visible from the head to the uncinate process (**A**, →). Magnification allows clearer observation of this finding (**B**, →) and further, intra-arterial noradrenalin injection makes the region of the tumor distinctly visible (**C**, →). Straightening is shown in a part of the right wall of the superior mesenteric vein (**D**, →) suggesting tumor invasion.

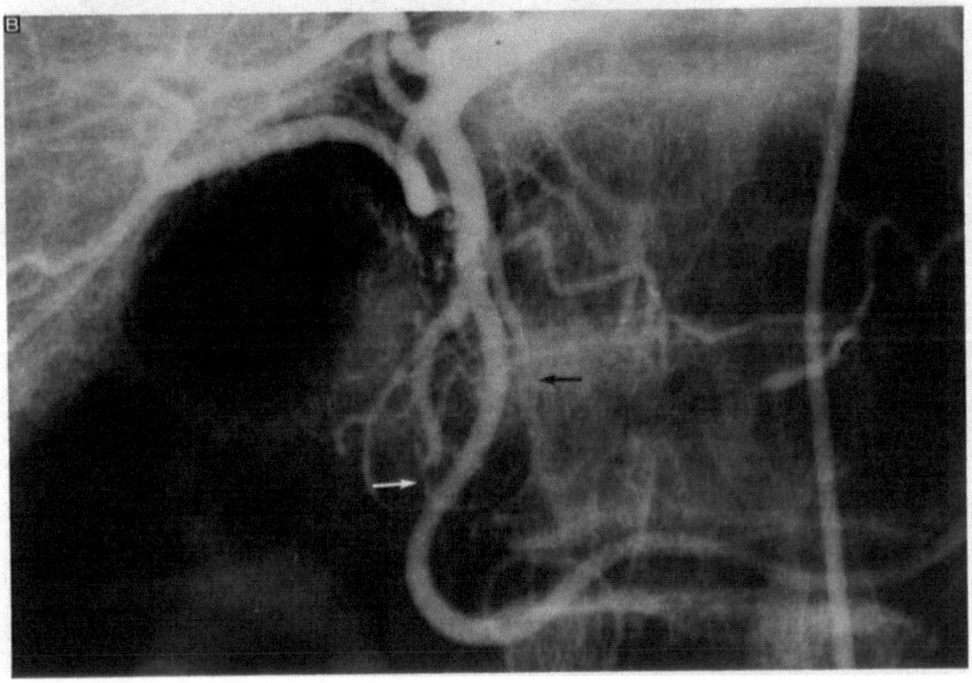

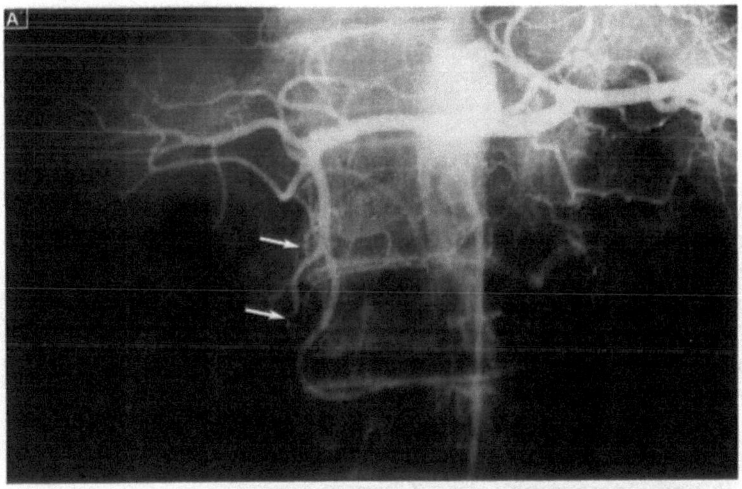
A

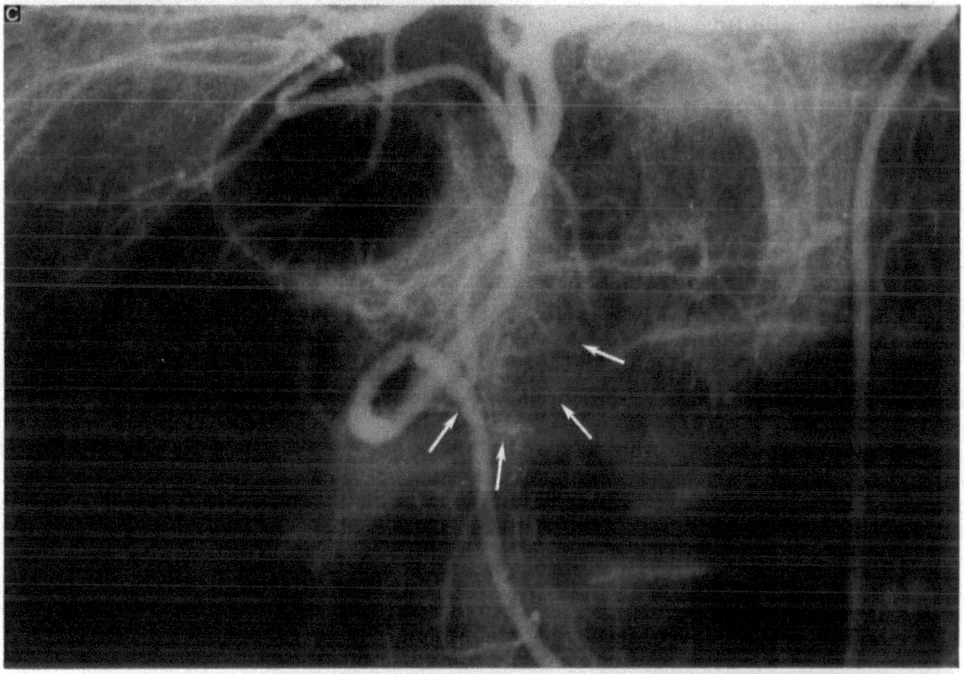
C

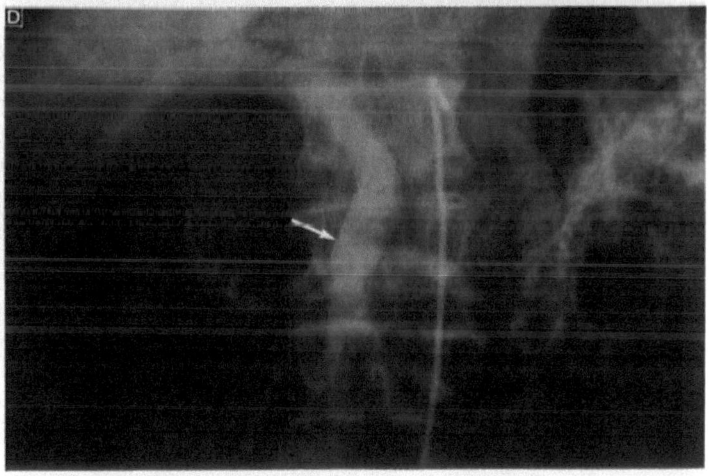
D

Operative Findings. A tumor $5 \times 4 \times 3$ cm in size, ranging from the uncinate process to the head of the pancreas, invaded part of the superior mesenteric artery. Thus, pancreatoduodenectomy with partial resection of the portal vein was performed. The tumor was defined as a well-differentiated adenocarcinoma.

Significance of Diagnostic Imaging. A dilated pancreatic duct and swelling from the head of the pancreas to the uncinate process are detected from ultrasonography, which is performed when diseases of the liver, biliary tract, and pancreas are suspected. The same findings are also obtained with CT, and then carcinoma of the pancreas is determined from angiography. Qualitative diagnosis of carcinoma of the pancreas is not easy, even though the finding of swelling from the head of the pancreas to the uncinate process is obtainable from ultrasonography and CT. The three cases of carcinoma of the pancreas which we had treated, T_2 or T_1 and smaller than this case, could not be detected by ultrasonography or conventional CT. Definite diagnosis was obtained from ERCP and angiography (see Chap. 5, Fig. 5.31). Thus, ultrasonography and conventional CT do not play much role in the qualitative diagnosis of small carcinoma of the pancreas which can be radically operated [1, 21]. Dynamic CT is required to obtain more precise information.

General Matters Concerning Cyst of the Pancreas. See Sect. C 2.5.

2.7 Cystadenocarcinoma of the Pancreas

Sequence of Diagnostic Imaging.

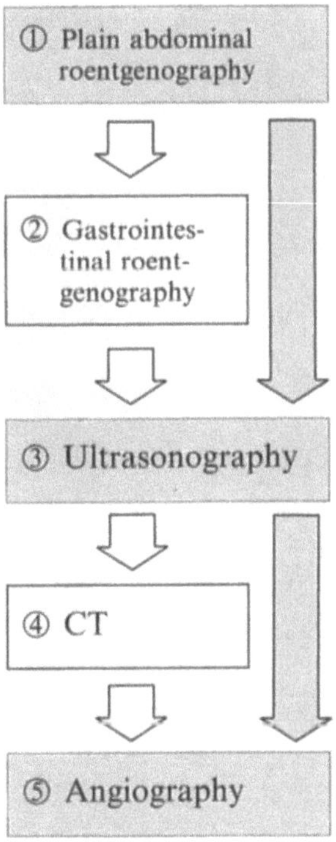

Patient. A 59-year-old woman.

Main Complaint. Epigastralgia and anorexia.

Present History. Epigastralgia and anorexia appeared 2 weeks prior to examination and continued.

Present Status. No jaundice has appeared. A hard, fist-sized mass is palpable at the left hypochondrium with tenderness on pressure.

Laboratory Data.

SGOT	12 mU/ml	Normal
SGPT	9 mU/ml	Normal
ALP	60 mU/ml	Normal
γ-GTP	10 mU/ml	Normal
ZTT	88.7 U	Normal
Serum amylase	65 IU/l	↓
Serum glucose	107 mg/dl	↑
AFP	4.8 mμg/ml	Normal
PS test	Negative	

Purpose of Diagnostic Imaging. To identify the localization of the abdominal mass and obtain a qualitative diagnosis.

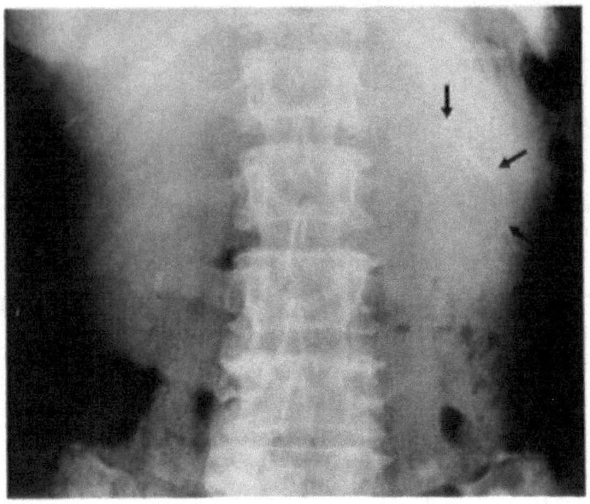

❶ Plain abdominal roentgenogram
An image of soft tissue density with calcification is observable at the left upper abdomen (→).

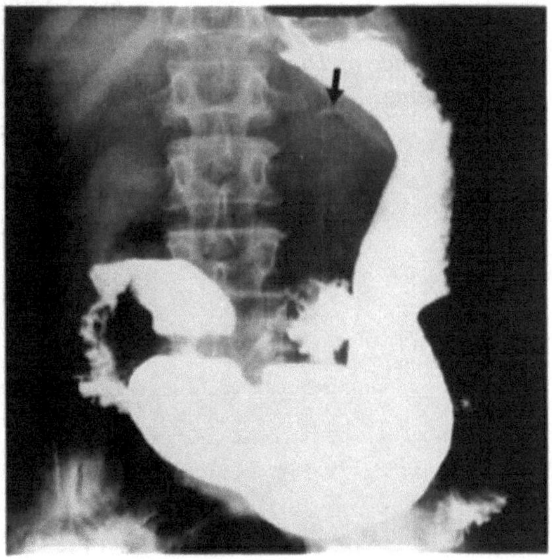

② Gastrointestinal examination with filled stomach in an erect position
The body of the stomach is displaced to the left and anteriorly by the tumor with calcification (→).

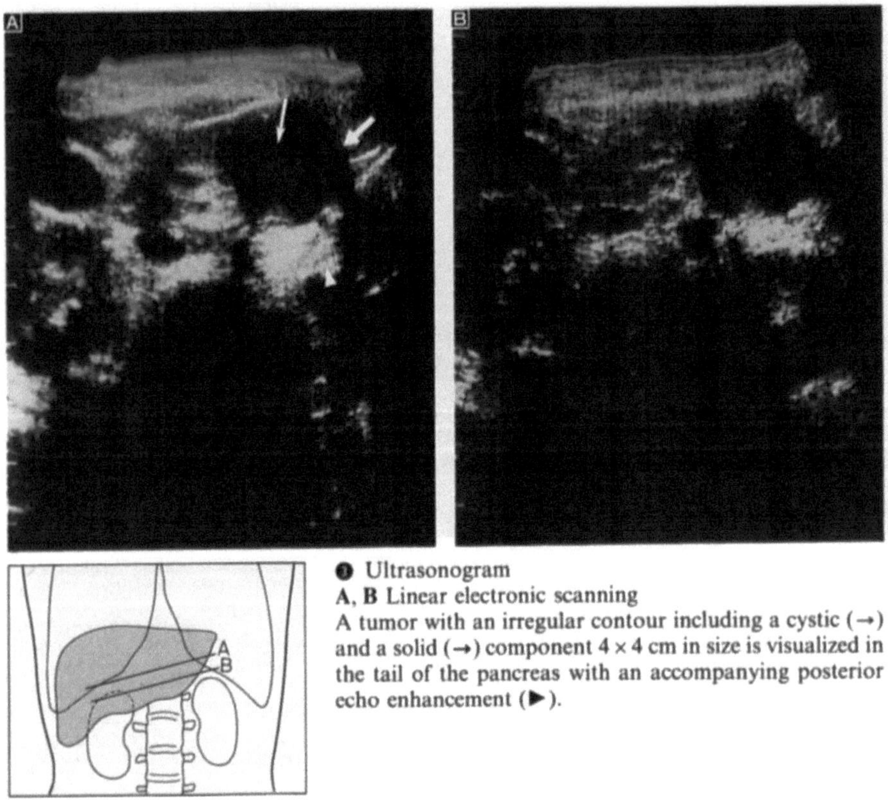

❸ Ultrasonogram
A, B Linear electronic scanning
A tumor with an irregular contour including a cystic (→) and a solid (→) component 4 × 4 cm in size is visualized in the tail of the pancreas with an accompanying posterior echo enhancement (▶).

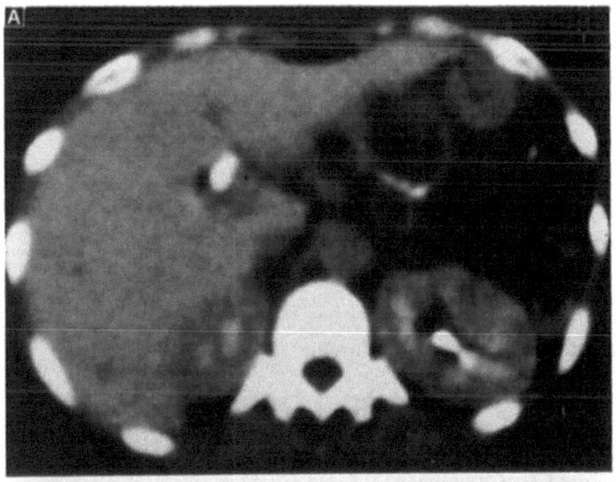

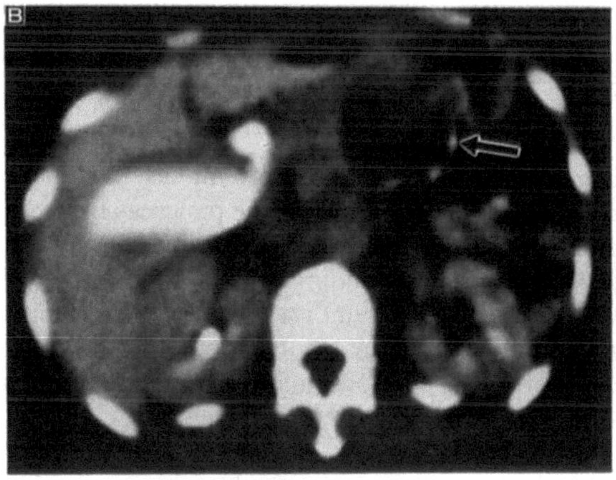

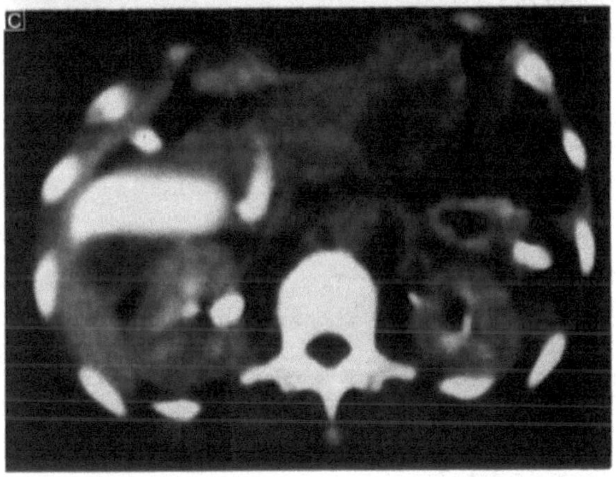

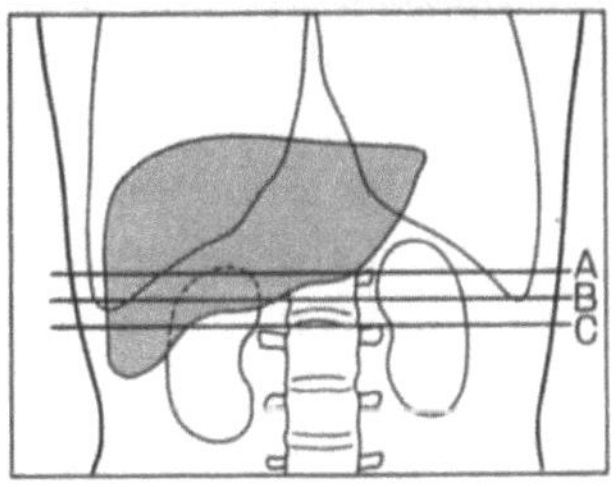

④ CT image
The tumor in the tail of the pancreas is observed with cystic and solid components and calcification of the wall.

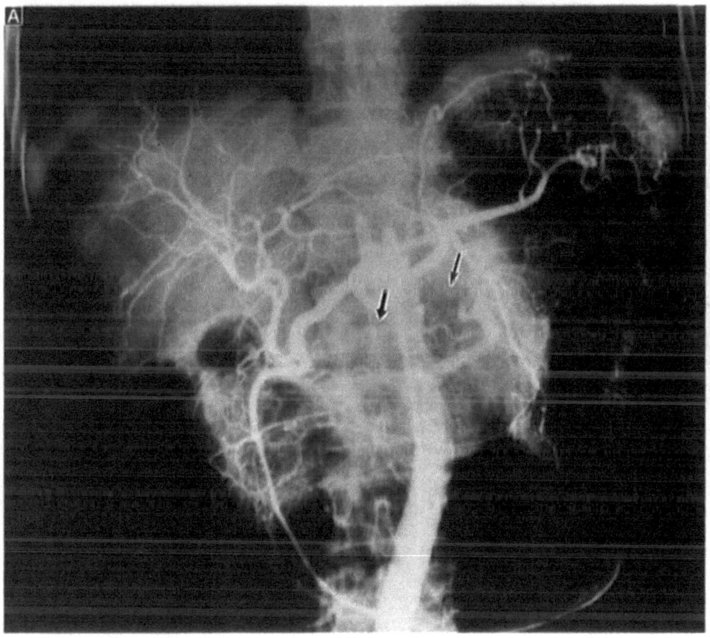

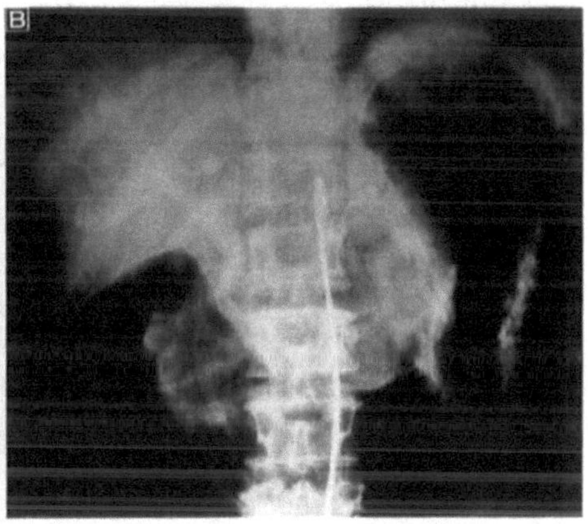

❺ Angiogram
A Celiac arteriogram (arterial phase)
B Celiac arteriogram (venous phase)
The transverse pancreatic artery branching from the dorsal pancreatic artery (→) and a branch from the great pancreatic artery (→) are both irregular. The tumor itself is not particularly hypervascular. In the venous phase, the splenic vein is obstructed by the tumor and drains into the intrahepatic portal vein via the collateral vein.

Clinical Progress. Suddenly after the examinations, the general status became worse, and the patient died 1 month later. Cystadenocarcinoma occupying the body and tail of the pancreas and several metastatic lesions under 1 cm in diameter in the liver were detected from autopsy.

Significance of Diagnostic Imaging. This case was suspected to be a cystadenoma or cystadenocarcinoma of the pancreas from visualization of a mass of soft tissue density with calcification by plain abdominal roentgenography and a solid tumor including cystic components by ultrasonography. CT also visualized the solid tumor with cyst and its calcification. Angiography did not show hypervascularity because of cystic components occupying a large proportion of the solid mass, but malignancy was suggested in some portions.

General Matters Concerning Cystadenocarcinoma of the Pancreas [7]. Cystadenocarcinoma is less frequent than cystadenoma, and only 61 cases have been reported in Japan. The mean age is 51.1 years (9–80 years old), and the male:female ratio is 1:2.17, being more common in females. A tumor often originates in the body or tail of the pancreas (67%) and the major symptom is an abdominal mass without pain (frequent in the upper abdomen).

Histopathologically, it differs from combination cases of carcinoma and cyst in the pancreas, carcinoma originating in a pseudocyst, or cystic formation by central necrosis of carcinoma of the pancreas, but it is a cyst which itself includes a malignant tumor. It is regarded to grow from cystadenoma, which is also frequent in the body and tail of the pancreas and found mostly in the age group of 50-year-old females. Occasionally, benign and malignant components may coexist in the same tumor.

The prognosis of cystadenocarcinoma of the pancreas is considered better compared to adenocarcinoma of the pancreas since the malignancy of cystadenocarcinoma is low. However, according to Kadowaki's statistics, only 3 of the 61 cases survived 5 years.

2.8 Insulinoma of the Pancreas

Sequence of Diagnostic Imaging.

① Ultrasonography
↓
② CT
↓
③ Angiography

Patient. A 42-year-old woman.

Main Complaint. Hypoglycemic symptoms provoked by fasting.

Laboratory Data.

Glucose tolerance test (venous blood)

Fasting state	30 min	60 min	120 min	180 min
24 mg/dl	69 mg/dl	85 mg/dl	67 mg/dl	53 mg/dl

Purpose of Diagnostic Imaging. To identify an insulinoma.

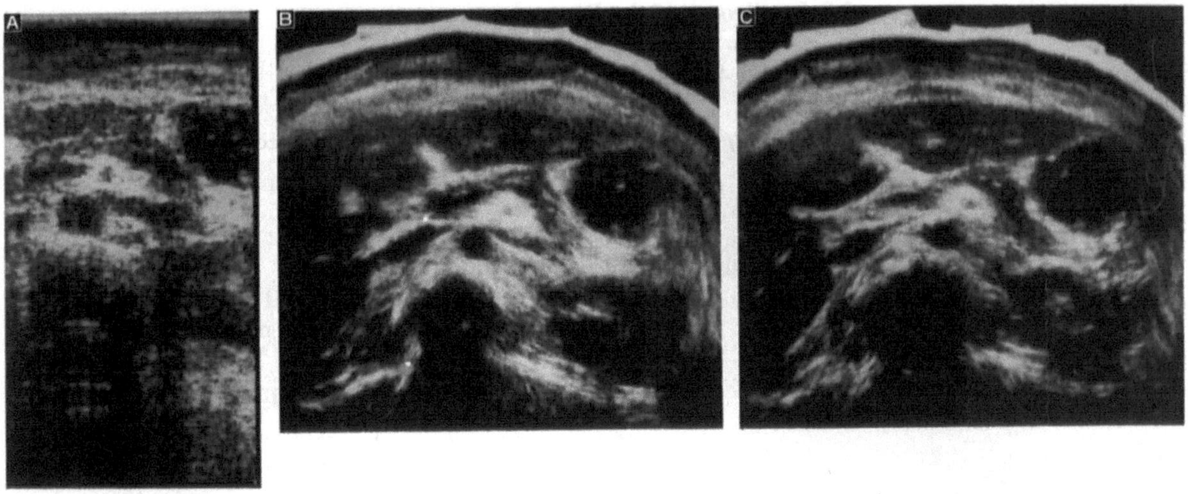

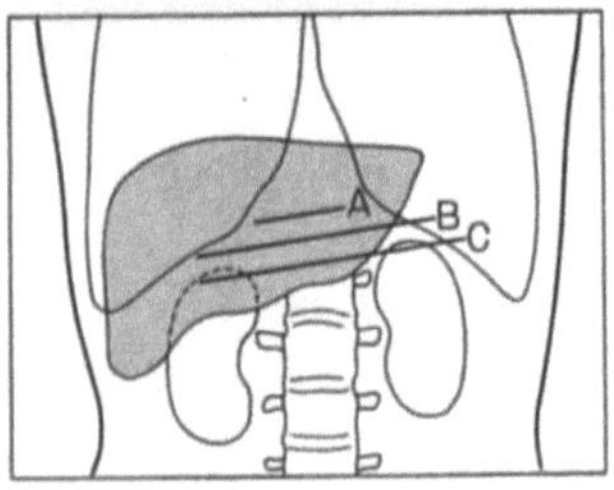

① Ultrasonogram
A Linear electronic scanning
B, C Contact compound scanning
The whole pancreas is visualized. No swelling or abnormality of the internal echo are observed.

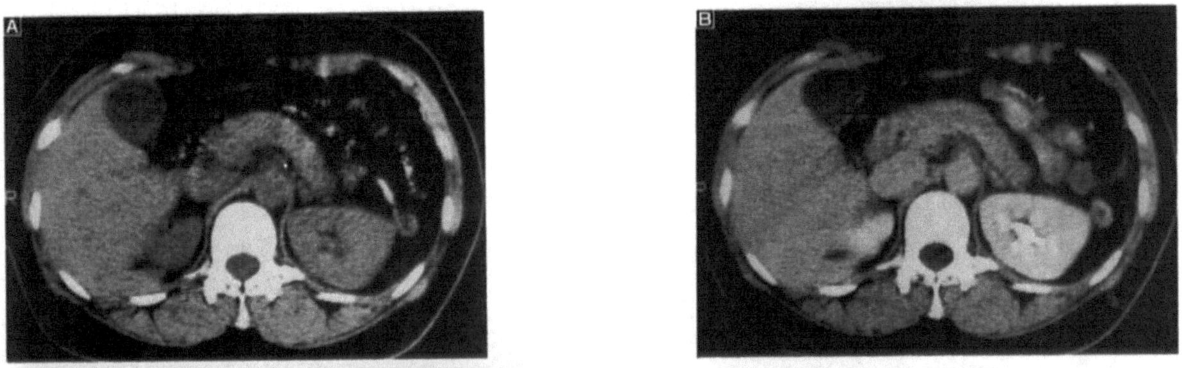

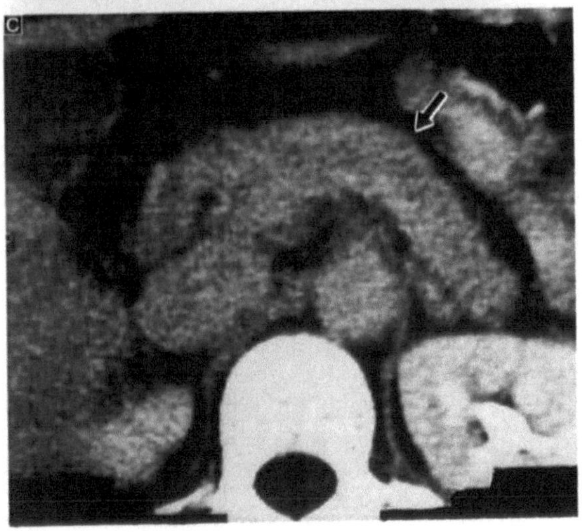

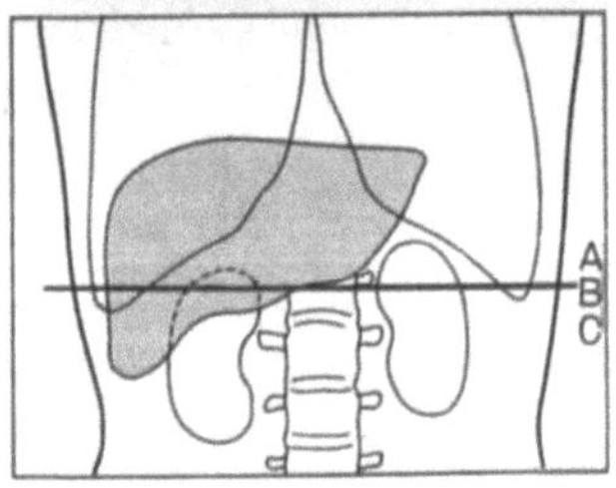

② CT image
A Before contrast enhancement
B After contrast enhancement
C Two fold magnifiction of **B**
The pancreas is clearly visualized, but no abnormality is observable from the CT images before and after the contrast enhancement. The arrow (→) shows the portion of insulinoma at the time of surgery.

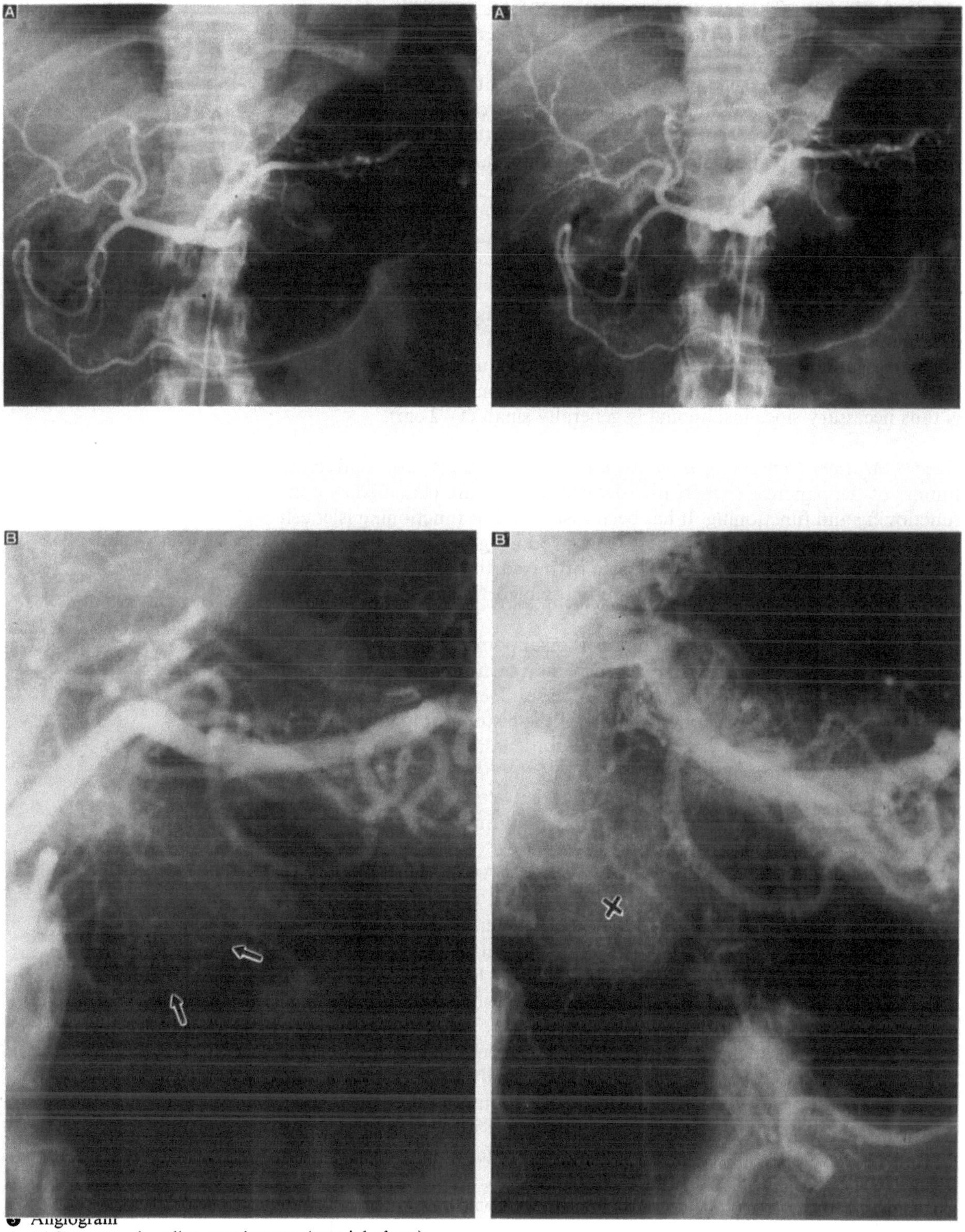

❸ Angiogram
A, A′ Stereoscopic celiac arteriogram (arterial phase)
B, B′ Threefold magnification celiac arteriogram (arterial phase)
A tumor 1 cm in diameter (x) stained in the arterial phase is observed and is fed by the great pancreatic artery. Encasement of the vessel itself is not existent (→). Metastasis to the liver is not suggested.

Operative Findings. The pancreas is normal in color, size, and hardness, and there is no swelling of the regional lymph node. Surgery was performed with enucleation of a tumor at the boundary of the body and tail of the pancreas, which was adjacent to the main pancreatic duct, located slightly anterior in the parenchyma corresponding to the tumor portion on the angiogram. The tumor was $1.7 \times 1.0 \times 0.9$ cm in size, abounding with fine vessels, hemorrhagic, and a histopathologically benign insulinoma.

Clinical Progress. The L-Leucine tolerance test 3 months after surgery was negative, and the glucose tolerance test was normal. Progress is fine at present.

Significance of Diagnostic Imaging. Angiography is highly important in determining the existence of an insulinoma, but CT and ultrasonography are not regarded as valuable. In this case, the insulinoma could not be demonstrated even by CT after contrast enhancement. Dynamic CT study is thus necessary since insulinoma is generally small (1–2 cm).

General Matters Concerning Insulinoma of the Pancreas [8, 16]. Endocrine tumors of the pancreas (pancreatic islet cell tumors) are classified as nonfunctioning and functioning. It has been assumed that functioning islet cell tumors show characteristic symptoms by producing and secreting a hormone. Recently, however, the existence of mixed tumors which produce plural hormones, occasionally including ectopic hormones, has been taken into consideration.

A typical functioning islet cell tumor is insulinoma, which is a beta cell tumor producing insulin. It is mostly a benign adenoma, and malignant adenomas only account for about 10% of cases. Determination of malignant adenoma necessitates not only study of the histopathological findings but also confirming the presence of a metastatic lesion.

It is relatively more frequent in the tail of the pancreas and is usually 1–2 cm in diameter. There is no relationship between the size and clinical symptoms. It occurs at all ages, most frequently in the 30–60 year age group, with no difference between the sexes.

The symptoms are caused by hypoglycemia. At the beginning, with unconsciousness, mental derangement, or coma, it may be misdiagnosed for another disease. The diagnosis is obtained referring to Whipple's triad: (a) spontaneous hypoglycemia accompanied by central nervous and vasomotor system symptoms, (b) repeated blood sugar levels below 50 mg/dl, and (c) relief of symptoms by the oral or intravenous administration of glucose.

Angiography is capable of detecting the insulinoma before operation in 70% of insulinoma cases even when the tumor is only 1–2 cm in diameter.

Radical treatment is performed with enucleation, and the prognosis is fine in benign cases. For nonresectable malignant insulinomas, effective drugs such as inhibitors of insulin release (diazoxide) and antineoplastic drugs (streptozotocin) have been developed.

Functioning endocrine tumors include gastrinoma (gastrin), glucagonoma (glucagon), and WDHA (watery diarrhea, hypokalemia, achlorhydria) syndrome (vasoactive intestinal peptide, VIP) in addition to insulinoma.

2.9 Nonfunctioning Islet Cell Tumor

Sequence of Diagnostic Imaging.

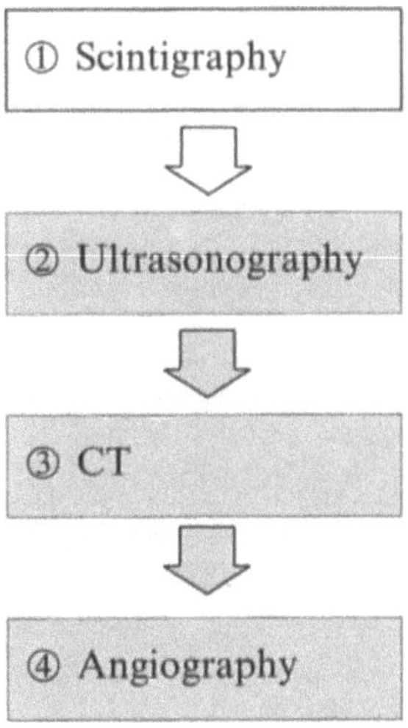

Patient. A 69-year-old woman.

Main Complaint. Abdominal distension and hematemesis.

Present Status. A mass expanding from the right costal margin to the epigastrium and ascites are detected. The esophagogram visualized varices and a tumor 4 × 4 cm in size at the gastric antrum.

Laboratory Data.

SGOT	45 mU/ml	↑
SGPT	49 mU/ml	↑
ALP	193 mU/ml	↑
LDH	159 mU/ml	Normal
γ-GTP	69 mU/ml	↑
Cho E	201 U/dl	Normal
Serum glucose	117 mg/dl	↑
HBs Ag	50 mg/ml	(−)
AFP	50 m g/ml	↑

Purpose of Diagnostic Imaging. To determine the localization and obtain qualitative diagnosis of the abdominal mass.

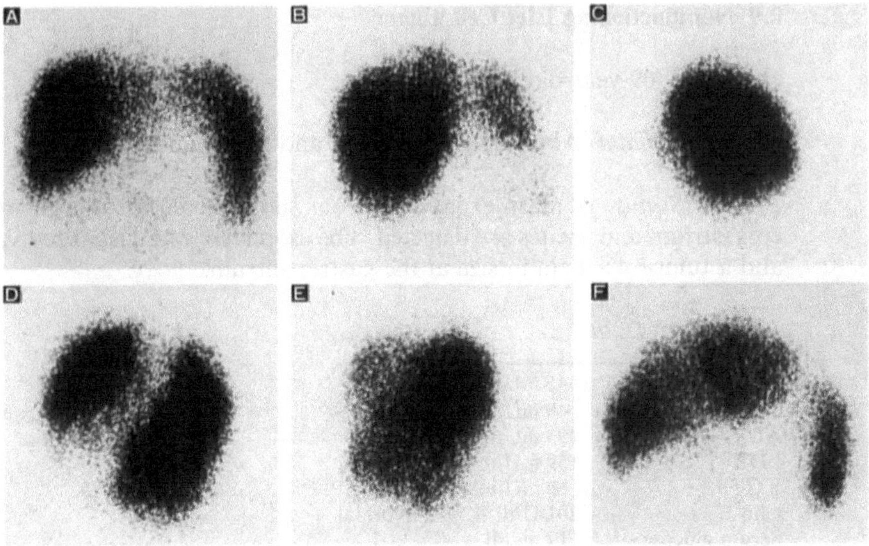

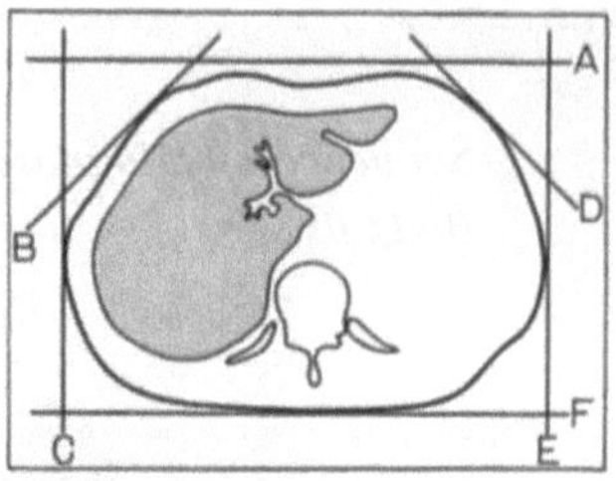

① Liver scintigram
A Frontal view
B Right anterior oblique view
C Right lateral view
D Left anterior oblique view
E Left lateral view
F Posterior view

A pattern of liver cirrhosis with splenomegaly and bone marrow uptake is shown. Space-occupying lesions are suspected in the upper part of the right and left hepatic lobes.

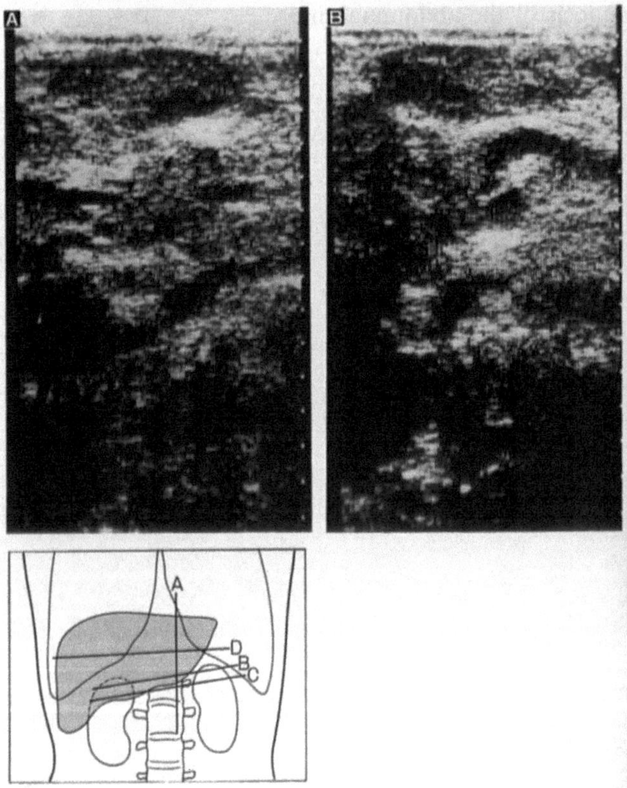

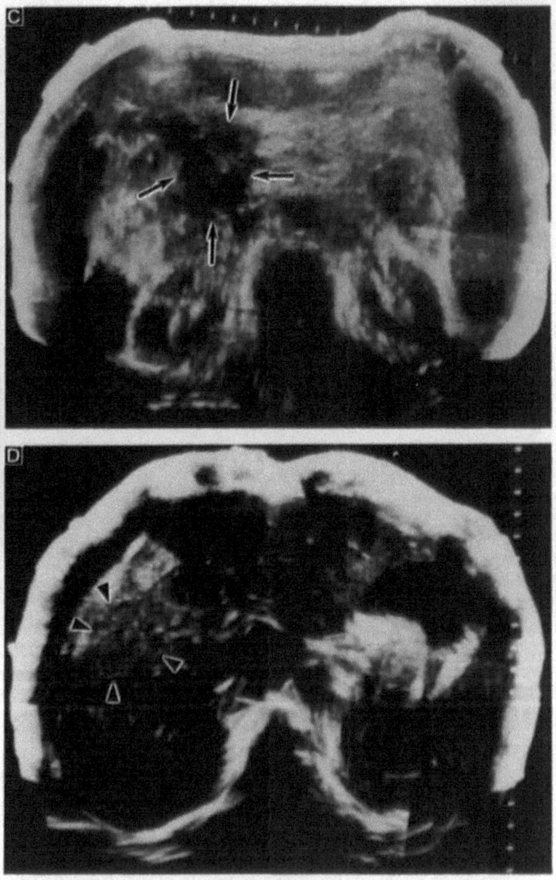

❷ Ultrasonogram
A, B Linear electronic scanning
C, D Contact compound scanning
The head of the pancreas is swollen with an irregular contour and inhomogeneous echogenicity. The echo level of the head of the pancreas is higher than that of the body and tail (→). A tumor in the right hepatic lobe (▶) and a low echo image between the right hepatic lobe and the right abdominal wall suggesting ascites are visualized.

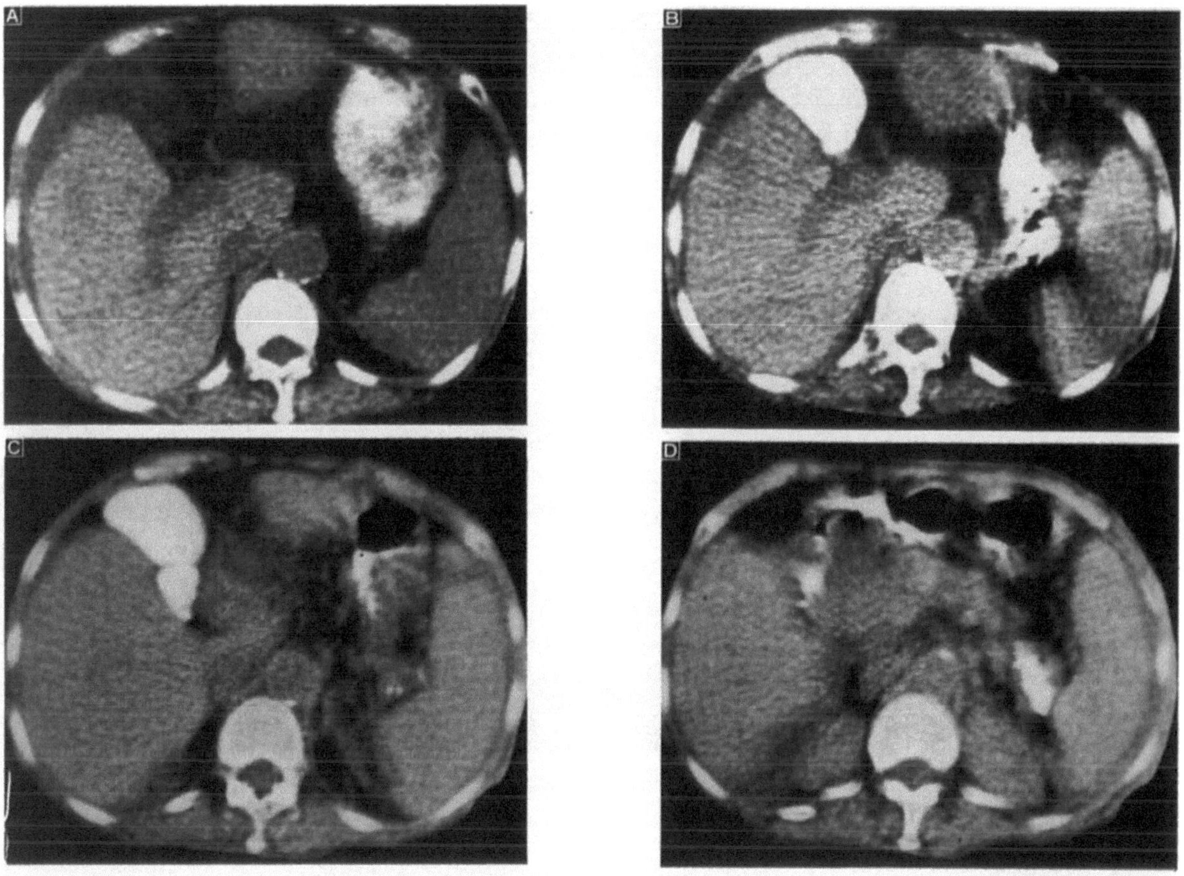

❸ CT image
The swollen head of the pancreas is observable with irregular contours. The disappearence of a posterior fat layer suggests a swelling of the lymph node posterior to the pancreas. The tumor is growing anteriorly; thus, invasion to the antrum of the stomach is suspected. Splenomegaly, ascites, and a low-attenuation area showing space-occupying lesions in both liver lobes are observed.

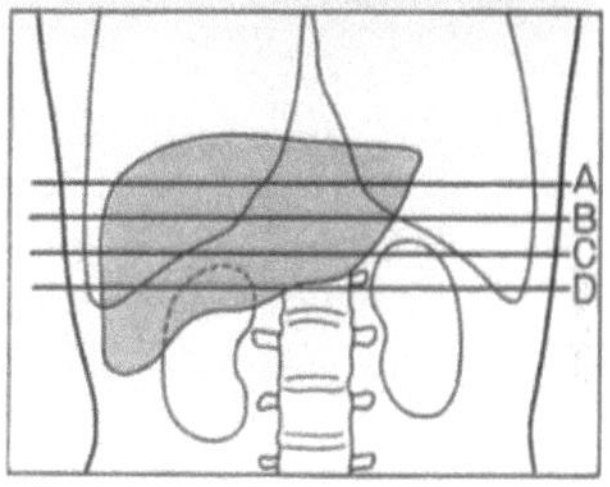

④ Angiography

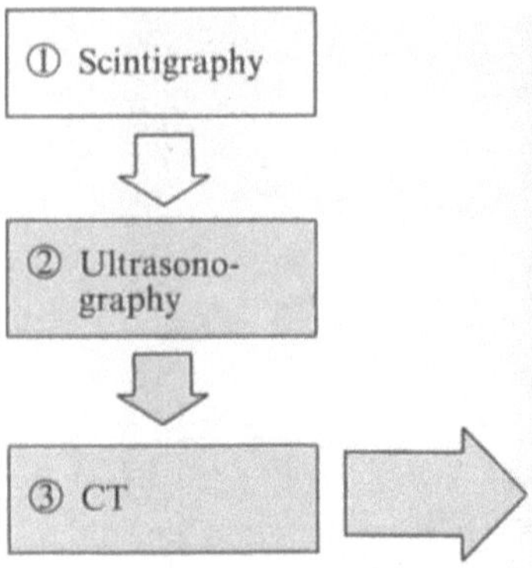

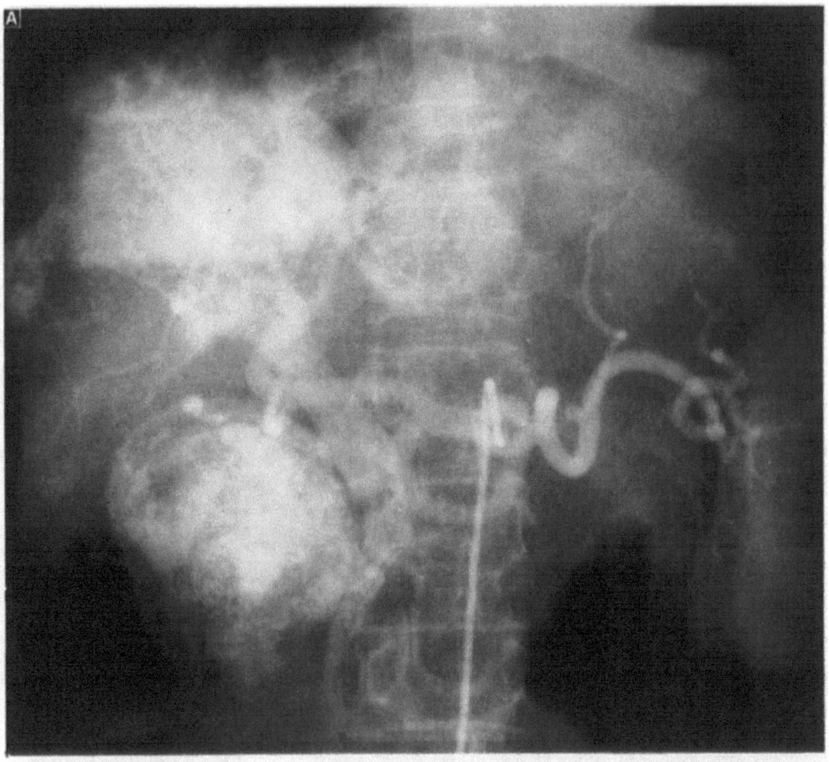

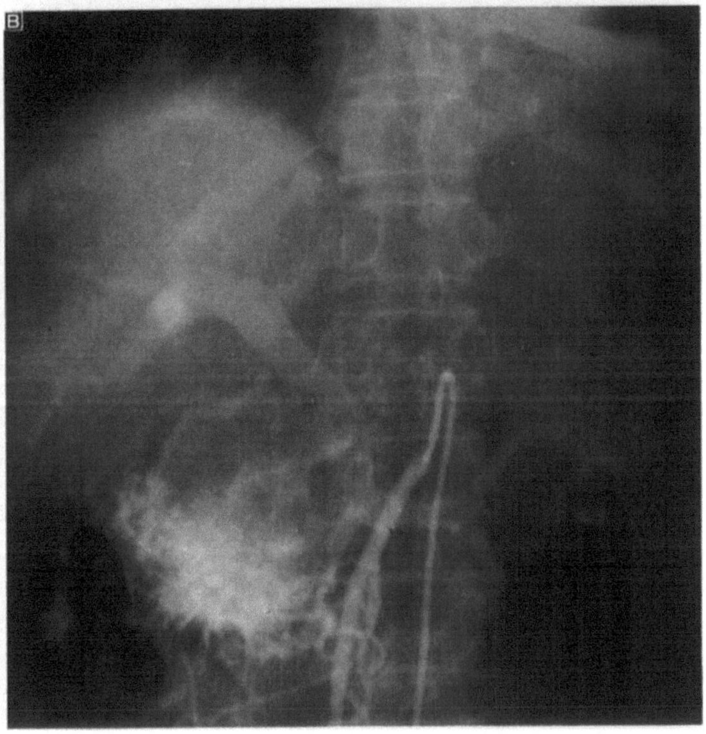

❹ Angiogram
A, A′ Stereoscopic celiac arteriogram (arterial phase)
B, B′ Stereoscopic superior mesenteric arteriogram (venous phase)
A hypervascular tumor is visualized in the right and left lobes of the liver in the early arterial phase. Also, arteriovenous shunt is observed in the early phase. The gastroduodenal artery shows encasement just after the origin, and its branches feed the huge hypervascular tumor. The vessels of the pancreatic arcades which branch from the superior mesenteric artery show hypervascularity and tumor vessels with arterioportal shunt. The right gastric artery and the vessels feeding the transverse colon are also related to the tumor.

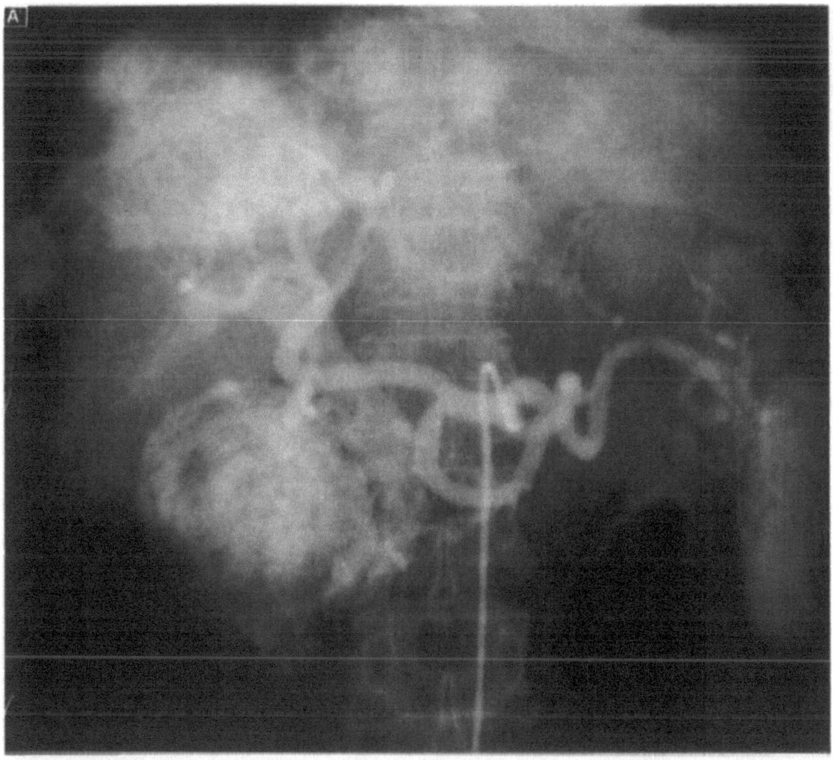
A

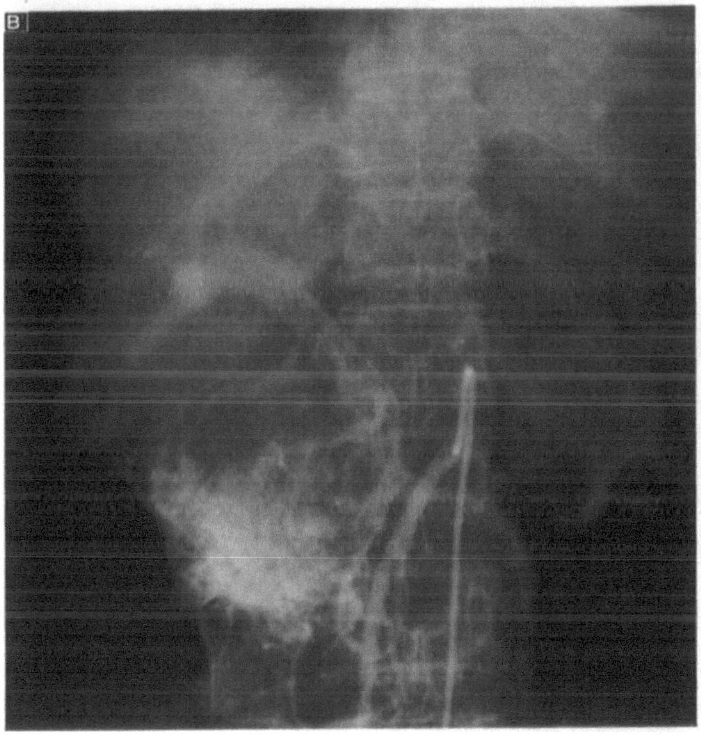
B

Autopsy Findings. An islet cell carcinoma originating in the head of the pancreas was detected with metastasis to the liver and mucosa of the stomach and duodenum. Only degeneration without metastatic lesions was observed in the neighboring lymph nodes of the pancreas. Liver cirrhosis was also found.

Significance of Diagnostic Imaging. The case was suspected to be carcinoma of the pancreas with metastasis to the liver from CT and ultrasonography. Angiography, however, detected a hypervascular tumor. Based on the findings of the gastrointestinal series, leiomyosarcoma or angiosarcoma from the stomach to the duodenum was suspected. Carcinoma of the pancreas was not suspected from the angiogram due to its hypervascularity. In this case, mainly considering the findings of the digestive tract, leiomyosarcoma was strongly suspected but not islet cell carcinoma since its characteristic symptoms were not observed.

General Matters Concerning Insulinoma of the Pancreas. See Sect C. 2.8.

References

C. Disease of Pancreas

1. Ariyama J, Ikenobu H, Sumida M, Shirata I, Shimaguchi S et al (1980) The diagnostic process of the small resectable pancreatic carcinoma (in Japanese): Stomach Intestine 15:611–617
2. Chiba S, Miyashita E, Saito Y, Karino K (1980) A case of pseudocysts penetrating into the spleen (in Japanese). Biliary Tract Pancreas 1:85–93
3. Hayashi K (1979) Pathology of the carcinoma of the pancreas (in Japanese). Intern Med 43:731–736
4. Hayashi K (1979) Pathology of the chronic pancreatitis (in Japanese). Kanehara Shuppan, Tokyo, pp 20–25 (Naika Mook, vol 6)
5. Hirayama T (1980) An epidemiological study of cancer of the pancreas in Japan (in Japanese). Biliary Tract Pancreas 1:533–543
6. Ishikawa K (1981) Current problems in surgery for pancreatic cancer (in Japanese). Biliary Tract Pancreas 2:357–362
7. Kadowaki J, Ueda T, Takeoka H, Kaneko M, Tomita T et al (1981) A resected case of unilocular and multiple cystadenocarcinoma of the pancreas (in Japanese). Biliary Tract Pancreas 2:407–415
8. Kuroda A, Akao S (1979) Functioning tumor of the pancreas (in Japanese). Intern Med 43:738–745
9. Kuroda A, Kubota K (1976) Acute pancreatitis (in Japanese). In: Yamagata S, Kosaka K, Masuda M, Ishii K (eds) Handbook of clinical gastroenterology, vol 4. Kanehara Shuppan, Tokyo, pp 189–209
10. Makino H, Sawabu N, Yoneda M, Nakajima S, Shimazaki K et al (1977) Diagnostic value of various examination methods for pancreatic cancer – in comparison with chronic pancreatitis (in Japanese). Jpn J Gastroenterol 74:1370–1381
11. Maruchi N (1979) Epidemiology of the chronic pancreatitis (in Japanese). Naika Mook vol 6:14–19, Kanehara Shuppan, Tokyo
12. Miyazaki T, Fujita H (1977) Cyst of the pancreas (in Japanese). In: Yoshitoshi Y, Nakao K, Yamagata S, et al (eds) Handbook of internal medicine, vol 25. Nakayama Shoten, Tokyo, pp 347–368
13. Naito S (1977) Cyst of the pancreas (in Japanese). In: Yoshitoshi Y, Nakao K, Yamagata S et al (eds) Handbook of internal medicine, vol 25. Nakayama Shoten, Tokyo, pp 343–246
14. Nakazawa S, Naito H, Kimoto E, Sano H et al (1980) Three cases of calcified pancreatic cyst (in Japanese). Biliary Tract Pancreas 1:103–108

15. Noto N (1980) Pancreatic lithiasis (in Japanese). Biliary Tract Pancreas 1:1129–1139
16. Oda M, Minemura S (1977) Tumor of the pancreas (in Japanese). In: Yoshitoshi Y, Nakao K, Yamagata S et al (eds) Handbook of internal medicine, vol 25. Nakayama Shoten, Tokyo, pp 404–448
17. Ozaki H (1977) Tumor of the pancreas (in Japanese). In: Yoshitoshi Y, Nakao K, Yamagata S, et al (eds) Handbook of internal medicine, vol 25. Nakayama Shoten, Tokyo, pp 371–403
18. Ozaki H, Naito S (1980) Diagnosis of carcinoma of the pancreas in early stage. Review of 1210 cases collected from 63 major clinics in Japan (in Japanese). Jpn J Gastroenterol 77:1979–1983
19. Saito Y, Sekita M, Kita S (1981) Surgical results of chronic pancreatitis in Japan (in Japanese). Biliary Tract Pancreas 2:193–206
20. Sato T, Saito Y (1979) Epidemiology of the chronic pancreatitis (in Japanese). Naika Mook vol 6:5–13 Kanehara Shuppan, Tokyo
21. Takagi, Takahashi T, Hori M, Takekoshi T, Sugiyama N et al (1980) Small carcinoma of head of the pancreas discovered by the clue of transitory elevation of urinary amylase level (in Japanese). Stomach Intestine 15:595–610
22. Toda Y, Hayakawa T (1977) Acute pancreatitis (in Japanese). In: Yoshitoshi Y, Nakao K, Yamagata S et al (eds) Handbook of internal medicine, vol 25. Nakayama Shoten, Tokyo, pp 225–295
23. Yamagata S, Tatebe T (1977) Chronic pancreatitis (in Japanese). In: Yoshitoshi Y, Nakao K, Yamagata S et al (eds) Handbook of internal medicine, vol 25. Nakayama Shoten, Tokyo, pp 299–327

Appendix
Methods of Measurement and Normal Values for Laboratory Data

	Method	Normal values
SGOT	UV	8 ~ 40 mU/ml
SGPT	UV	8 ~ 40 mU/ml
Alkaline phosphatase	Bessey-Lowry	30 ~ 85 mU/ml
Lactate dehydrogenase	Modified Wacker	100 ~ 225 mU/ml
γ-Glutamyl transpeptidase	Modified Rosalki	0 ~ 40 mU/ml
Cholinesterase	Modified Ellman	♂ 193 ~ 551 U/dl ♀ 231 ~ 776 U/dl
Total protein, serum	Biuret	6.5 ~ 8.2 g/dl
Zinc sulfate turbidity test	Method devised by Liver Function Study Group, Japanese Society of Gastroenterology	4.0 ~ 13.0 U
Thymol turbidity test		0 ~ 4.0 U
Total bilirubin, serum	Diazo	under 1.3 mg/dl
Direct bilirubin, serum	Modified Michaellson	under 0.8 mg/dl
Amylase, total blood	Blue Starch/Albumin	105 ~ 440 IU/l
Amylase, urine	Blue Starch/Albumin	265 ~ 2100 IU/l
Cholesterol, total serum	Enzymatic (AA) method	130 ~ 250 mg/dl
Glucose, blood	Glucose oxidase	60 ~ 100 mg/dl
Sodium, serum	Flame photometry	135 ~ 145 mEq/l
Pitassium, serum	Flame photometry	3.5 ~ 4.5 mEq/l
Chlorides, serum	Chloride meter	95 ~ 105 mEq/l
Calcium, serum	OCPC	8.5 ~ 10.5 mg/dl
Urea nitrogen (BUN)	Diacteyl monoxime	10 ~ 20 mg/dl
Albumin, serum	BCP	3.2 ~ 5.0 g/dl
α-Fetoprotein	RIA (Dinabot kit)	0 ~ 20 mμg/ml
HB antigen	RIA (Dinabot kit)	Normal value is within 2.5 times of normal control serum
White blood cell count (WBC)	Electronic particle counter	♂ 4.3 ~ 8.4 ♀ 4.0 ~ 8.8 $\times 10^3/mm^3$
Red blood cell count (RBC)	Electronic particle counter	♂ 4.27 ~ 5.55 ♀ 3.88 ~ 4.83 $\times 10^6/mm^3$
Hemoglobin	Electronic particle counter	♂ 12.5 ~ 16.7 ♀ 11.2 ~ 14.2 g/dl
Hematocrit	Electronic particle counter	♂ 38.4 ~ 49.6 ♀ 33.7 ~ 42.7 %
Platelets	Electronic particle counter	♂ 140 ~ 322 ♀ 132 ~ 386 $\times 10^3/mm^3$

Subject Index

Abscess, pancreas
–, plain abdominal radiography 13
accuracy, CT, gallstone 69
–, –, jaundice 20
–, –, pancreatic carcinoma 73
–, liver scintigraphy 43
–, ultrasonography, gallstone 27
–, –, obstructive jaundice 29
acoustic shadow 27
adenoma, gallbladder, ultrasonography 29
AFP 207
angiography 82
attenuation value, CT, gallbladder 62
– –, –, gallstone 69
– –, –, normal liver parenchyma 61

beaked appearance, liver, CT 68
bile duct, carcinoma 136, 261
– –, common, carcinoma 258
– –, common, ultrasonography 26
– –, congenital dilatation 137, 241, 245
– –, diameter 143
– –, dyskinesia 126
– –, extrahepatic, carcinoma, angiography 97
biliary sludge 28
bolus injections, CT 66
boundary echo 22
bright liver 24, 175
bull's-eye type 23

calcification 10
–, pancreas 13
calculi and calcification, pancreatic, CT 72
Cantlie's line 21, 85, 87
caudate lobe 21, 61
cholangiocarcinoma 215
–, angiography 90
cholecystitis, ultrasonography 29
cholelithiasis 115, 136, 144
–, plain abdominal radiography 11
computed tomography, X-ray, (CT) 58
CT, dynamic 60, 66, 72, 73, 191, 203
cold area, colloid liver scintigraphy 47
colloid liver scintigraphy 43
– – –, normal findings 46
colon-cutoff sign 13
common bile duct, congenital dilatation 125
computed radiography with an imaging plate 7
contact scanning 17
cyst, liver 152, 154
–, –, angiography 93
–, –, colloid liver, scintigraphy 47
–, –, CT 64
–, –, ultrasonography 23
–, pancreas 285, 288
–, pancreatic, angiography 100
cystadenocarcinoma, pancreas 300, 303
–, –, angiography 100
–, –, plain abdominal radiography 13
–, –, ultrasonography 33
cystadenoma, pancreas, angiography 100
–, –, plain abdominal radiography 13
–, –, ultrasonography 33
cystadenoma and cystadenocarcinoma, pancreas, CT 72
cystic artery 96
cystic pattern 23

detection rates of space-occupying lesions with liver scintigraphy, ultrasonography, and X-ray CT examined 149
Doppler effect 18
double-barrel sign, ultrasonography 30
Dubin-Johnson syndrome, hepatobiliary scintigraphy 52

embolization, transcatheter 90, 209
endoscopic retrograde cholangiopancreatography (ERCP) 132
epicholedochal arteries 97
epicholedochal arterial plexus 95
excretory cholecystocholangiography 118
– –, poor opacification 127

falciform ligaments 61
fatty liver 174, 178
– –, CT 67
– –, plain abdominal radiography 9
– –, ultrasonography 24
fissure of the ligamentum teres 22
focal swelling, liver, colloid liver scintigraphy 47

gallbladder, calcified, plain abdominal radiography 12
–, carcinoma 253, 256
gallbladder carcinoma 115
– –, angiography 97
– –, CT 71
– –, percutaneous transhepatic cholangiography 144
– –, plain abdominal radiography 12
– –, ultrasonography 29
gallbladder stones, excretory cholecystocholangiography 126
gallbladder, tumor 29
gallstone, pseudoimage, ultrasonography 28
–, ultrasonography 27
gas in the gallbladder 12
–, in the liver 11
Gilbert's syndromes, hepatobiliary scintigraphy 52
gravel, ultrasonography 28

hemangioma, liver 190, 193
–, –, CT 65
–, –, ultrasonography 24
hemangiomas, liver, angiography 92
hemochromatosis 180
–, CT 68
hemosiderosis and hemochromatosis 183
hemosiderosis, CT 68
hepatic artery 85
– carcinoma, pedunculated 214
– duct, common, carcinoma 263
– –, –, ultrasonography 26
– injury 224, 228
– tumors, benign, angiography 92
– vasculature 85
– vein 87
–, middle 21
–, right 21
hepatitis, acute 25
–, chronic active 160
–, – –, CT 69
–, –, colloid liver scintigraphy 46
–, –, CT 68
–, –, ultrasonography 25
–, lupoid 163
hepatobiliary scintigraphy 49
– –, normal and abnormala findings 51
hepatoblastoma 195, 199
–, angiograhy 91
hepatocellular carcinoma 200, 204, 210
– –, angiography 89

hepatocellular carcinoma
– –, colloid liver scintigraphy 47
– –, CT 65, 66
– –, ultrasonography 24
hepatolithiasis 239
–, and choledocholithiasis 236
hepatomegaly, plain abdominal radiography 9
Hydatid disease, plain abdominal radiograhy 10
hypotonic duodenography 110

intravenous cholangiography 120
islet cell tumors, angiography 100
– – –, nonfunctioning 308
insulinoma of the pancreas 304, 306

jaundice, nonsurgical 51
–, obstructive 29, 69, 70
–, surgical 52

liver abscess 184, 188
–, angiography 94
–, colloid liver, scintigraphy 47
– –, CT 65
– –, plain abdominal radiography 9, 11
– –, ultrasonography 23
limy bile 12
– –, (milk of calcium bile) 11
liver carcinoma 223
liver cirrhosis 164, 167, 169, 173
– –, angiography 94
– –, colloid liver scintigraphy 47
– –, CT 68, 69
– –, ultrasonography 24
–, disease, diffuse, CT 67
ligamentum teres 21
–, venosum 22, 61
lobar fissure, main 21

magnification angiography 82, 86, 90, 96, 98, 100, 101
–, venography 88
metastasis, liver 220
–, –, angiography 91, 92
–, –, colloid liver scintigraphy 47
–, –, CT 66
–, –, ultrasonography 24

necrotizing entiretis 11
nuclear examination 43

pancreas, carcinoma 134, 290, 293, 296,
–, –, angiography 101
–, –, CT 73
–, –, head 116, 144
–, –, ultrasonography 33
–, ultrasonography 31
–, visualization rate, ultrasonography 31
pancreatic duct, dilated 63
– –, main, ultrasonography 31
pancreatitis, acute 13, 32, 71, 271, 274
–, chronic 276, 279, 281
–, chronic, angiography 100
–, –, CT 72
–, –, ultrasonography 32
pancreatolithiasis 281, 283
parallel-channel sign 30
parenchymal hamartoma 156, 159
percutaneous transhepatic cholangiography 140
periportal artery 86
pharmacoangiography 100
plain abdominal radiography 7
polyps, gallbladder, ultrasonography 29
porcelain gallbladder 12
– –, (calcified gallbladder), plain abdominal radiography 11
portal hypertension 95
primary sclerosing cholangitis 247, 252
procedure of diagnostic imaging of the biliary tract 233
– – – –, of the liver 149
– – – –, of the pancreas 269
pseudocyst, pancreas 281, 285
–, –, angiography 100
–, –, CT 72
–, –, ultrasonography 32

radioisotope angiography of the liver 47
real-time scanning 17
Roter's syndorome, hepatobiliary scintigraphy 52

segmental fissure, left 21
– –, right 21
sentinel-loop sign 13
shotgun sign 30
solid mass pattern 23
sonolucent zone, gallbladder 29
– –, liver tumor 23
space-occupying lesions, liver, CT 64
– –, –, nuclear examination 44, 47
– –, –, ultrasonography 24
stereoangiography 82, 96
stones, pancreatic, ultrasonography 32

^{99m}Tc-E-HIDA (^{99m}-Tc-diethyl-IDA) 50
^{99m}Tc-HSA (Human Serum Albumin) 48
^{99m}Tc-sulfur colloid 48
Thorotrast deposits in the liver 9

ultrasonography 17
umbilical portion 21

venography, selective hepatic 88

white liver 172

MIX
Papier aus verantwortungsvollen Quellen
Paper from responsible sources
FSC® C105338

If you have any concerns about our products,
you can contact us on
ProductSafety@springernature.com

In case Publisher is established outside the EU,
the EU authorized representative is:
Springer Nature Customer Service Center GmbH
Europaplatz 3, 69115 Heidelberg, Germany

Printed by Libri Plureos GmbH
in Hamburg, Germany